THE PAPERLESS MEDICAL OFFICE

SECOND EDITION

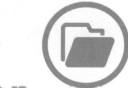

Using Harris CareTracker

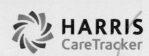

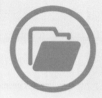

THE PAPERLESS MEDICAL OFFICE

SECOND EDITION

Using Harris CareTracker

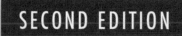

CENGAGE

VIRGINIA FERRARI

Australia • Brazil • Mexico • Singapore • United Kingdom • United States

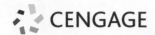

The Paperless Medical Office: Using Harris CareTracker, **2nd Edition**

Virginia Ferrari

SVP, GM Skills & Global Product Management: Jonathan Lau

Product Director: Matthew Seeley

Product Team Manager: Stephen Smith

Senior Director, Development: Marah Bellegarde

Senior Content Development Manager: Juliet Steiner

Content Developer: Kaitlin Schlicht

Product Assistant: Jessica Molesky

Marketing Manager: Jonathan Sheehan

Senior Content Project Manager: Thomas Heffernan

Art Director: Angela Sheehan

Production Service: SPi Global

Cover Images: VAlex/Shutterstock.com, Vectorphoto/Shutterstock.com, smartdesign91/ Shutterstock.com, Bryan Solomon/ Shutterstock.com, Blan-K/Shutterstock.com, Aha-Soft/Shutterstock.com, RedKoala/ Shutterstock.com

For product information and technology assistance, contact us at
Cengage Customer & Sales Support, 1-800-354-9706.

For permission to use material from this text or product,
submit all requests online at **www.cengage.com/permissions**.
Further permissions questions can be emailed to
permissionrequest@cengage.com.

Library of Congress Control Number: 2017957038

ISBN: 978-1-337-61419-1

Cengage
20 Channel Street
Boston, MA 02210
USA

Cengage is a leading provider of customized learning solutions with employees residing in nearly 40 different countries and sales in more than 125 countries around the world. Find your local representative at **www.cengage.com**.

Cengage products are represented in Canada by Nelson Education, Ltd.

For your course and learning solutions, visit **www.cengage.com**.

Purchase any of our products at your local college store or at our preferred online store **www.cengagebrain.com**.

Printed in the United States of America
Print Number: 01   Print Year: 2017

Contents

MODULE 5
Apply Your Skills   571

CHAPTER 11
Applied Learning for the Paperless Medical Office   573

List of Activities

How to Use the Book

CHAPTER OPENERS

Key Terms identify important vocabulary for the chapter. Each term appears in boldface the first time it is used in the chapter and also appears in the glossary with a definition.

Key Terms

abstract
cache
Certification Commission for Health Information Technology (CCHIT®)
classification systems
clearinghouse
clinical templates
clinical vocabularies
Computer Physician Order Entry (CPOE)
covered entity
Current Procedural Terminology (CPT®)
International Classification of Diseases (ICD)
Logical Observation Identifiers Names and Codes (LOINC®)
meaningful use
minimum necessary
modifiers
National Drug Code (NDC)
nomenclature
notice of privacy practices (NPP)
order set

Learning Objectives state chapter goals and outcomes.

Learning Objectives

1. Set up your computer for optimal functionality when using Harris CareTracker PM and EMR.
2. Create a Harris CareTracker training company.
3. Illustrate what occurs in an electronic health network.
4. Explain the process of converting paper health records to electronic health records (EHRs).
5. Summarize administrative workflows in Harris CareTracker.
6. Discuss practice management, front office, billing, and administrative functions.

Real-World Connection

Welcome to Napa Valley Family Health Associates (NVFHA), your Harris CareTracker training company! Our practice is located in the beautiful Napa Valley in California. The practice consists of four providers, six medical assistants, one X-ray technician, and a medical lab scientist who oversees our laboratory. As a medical assisting student, you will rotate among our four providers:

- Amir Raman, DO (Specialty—Internal Medicine)
- Anthony Brockton, MD (Specialty—Family Practice)

The **Real-World Connection** feature at the start of each chapter contains information regarding a day-in-the-life of a medical assistant working in a medical practice using electronic health records. The "real world" scenarios are meant to stimulate thought and critical thinking.

Spotlight boxes highlight important material included throughout the text. It is critical that users of EHR software are familiar with this information. The spotlight boxes include an icon representing the type of information being presented. These types include Administrative, Clinical, and Legal.

 SPOTLIGHT Highlights of the *Patient Registration* module:
- Enter patient demographics
- Enter and record insurance information
- Scan and attach insurance cards and identification cards
- Verify insurance eligibility prior to billing with one click of a button

Alert boxes present critical information to know when completing activities in Harris CareTracker PM and EMR.

ALERT! Due to the evolving nature and continuous upgrades of real-world EMRs such as this one, as you log in and work in your student version of Harris CareTracker there may be a slightly different look to your live screen from the screenshots provided in this text.

When prompted, follow the instructions given in the text to complete the activities.

Step-by-Step Activities, included throughout the text, give instruction on how to complete front and back office functions in Harris CareTracker PM and EMR. They feature detailed information on steps to be performed as well as full color screenshots that illustrate key steps. **Required** icons alert students to activities that are required within a chapter in order for them to proceed with that chapter.

 Activity 2-1
Log in to Harris CareTracker PM and EMR

1. Go to http://www.cengage.com/CareTracker.
2. The domain is set to "Current" by default (Figure 2-1). Leave as is.
3. The product list is set to "Cengage Learning Harris CareTracker Simulation 1.0" by default. Leave as is.

Tip boxes provide helpful hints for using Harris CareTracker PM and EMR.

 TIP Navigate through each field in demographics by pressing the [Tab] key and Harris CareTracker PM and EMR will automatically format the entry, regardless of the way it is entered. For example, by tabbing through the *First Name* and *Last Name* boxes, Harris CareTracker PM and EMR automatically applies title case to the name, meaning the first letter of each name is capitalized. To navigate back to a field, press [SHIFT+TAB].

FYI boxes provide details on functions of Harris CareTracker PM and EMR that are available in real-world settings but are not available in your student version of Harris CareTracker.

 FYI In your student environment, the *Drug Type* list is grayed out and automatically set to "Dispensable." In the real-world version of Harris CareTracker EMR, you can also select "Routed Drug" to record the medication without any dosage information. **Routed** refers to the way that a drug is introduced into the body, such as oral, enteral, mucosal, parenteral, or percutaneous.

SUMMARY

Harris CareTracker PM and EMR provides a robust electronic health record that is fully integrated and interoperable. The *Help* system offers a valuable tool for beginning users and for refresher training as the system continually updates with new features. Medical assistants often advance in their roles in the medical field, and being proficient with electronic health records and health information technology opens many opportunities.

The practice, clinical, and Setup applications you completed in this chapter mimic activities that medical assistants perform in the patient-centered medical environment. Using the *Help* system to seek out additional information enhances proficiency using Harris CareTracker PM and EMR. You now have an understanding of the purpose and location of key features of Harris CareTracker PM and EMR such as the *Main Menu*, *Navigation*, *Home*, and *Dashboard* overview, which makes navigating the EHR seamless.

The **Chapter Summaries** provide an overview and summation of the main learning outcomes within the chapter.

End-of-chapter **Check Your Knowledge** quizzes test the students' retention of information.

CHECK YOUR KNOWLEDGE

Select the best response.

_____ 1. The *Home* module contains three applications. Which of the following is not one of the applications?

    a. Dashboard   c. Messages

    b. Administration   d. News

_____ 2. The *Dashboard* is divided into three tabs. Which of the following is not one of the tabs?

    a. Home   c. Management

    b. Practice   d. Meaningful Use

_____ 3. *Dashboard* represents values that are refreshed overnight. These values are based on the provider and location selected in the batch. Which of the following is not one of the values?

    a. The value indicates all open admissions.   c. The value depicts the total number of patients seen each day.

    b. The value indicates admissions with missing days.   d. None of the above.

CASE STUDIES

Case Study 2-1

Add "Paul T. Endo" to the "Refer Provider To" quick picks list. (Refer to Activity 2-9 for guidance.)

📠 Print a copy of the screen that illustrates your added quick pick. Label the *Paul T. Endo* screenshot as "Case Study 2-1," and place it in your assignment folder.

Case Study 2-2

Create a *ToDo* for patient Kimberly Johnson. (Refer to Activity 2-14 for guidance.) For this case study, enter the following text for the *ToDo*:

"Test ToDo (CS 2-2): Dr. Ayerick, patient Kimberly Johnson called to establish as a New Patient. Your practice is currently restricted to accepting only new pediatric patient. She was referred by Dr. Alfred Peretti who has recently retired. Do you want to accept her as a new patient, or have her schedule with Gabriella?"

📠 Print a copy of the screen that illustrates you created a ToDo for Kimberly Johnson, label it "Case Study 2-2," and place it in your assignment folder.

Case Studies provide additional opportunities for students to test their ability to complete key chapter activities without the benefit of step-by-step instructions. **Note:** Case studies often build on previous case studies from the prior chapters.

Build Your Proficiency activities provide not only additional practice, but also additional activities not previously performed. Completing these activities will elevate the student's level of competency using EHRs.

BUILD YOUR PROFICIENCY

Proficiency Builder 2-1: Add Patient Visit Summary Items

A patient visit summary is printed at the completion of a patient's visit. You can control the items that are included on a patient visit summary print out. To add patient visit summary items, complete the following steps:

1. Click the *Administration* module and then click the *Clinical* tab.

2. Under the *System Administration* column, *Maintenances* header, click the *Visit Summary* link. The application launches the *Patient Visit Summary* application (**Figure 2-55**).

Preface

Electronic technology is the major means through which workers communicate in today's health care environment. *The Paperless Medical Office: Using Harris CareTracker, 2nd edition* is an electronic health record (EHR) solution that integrates instructional theory with a state-of-the-art practice management (PM) and electronic medical record (EMR) software.

Harris CareTracker PM and EMR is one of the most advanced cloud-based PMs and EHRs in the industry. The product is certified through the Certification Commission for Health Information Technology (CCHIT®) and is used by thousands of providers throughout the country. The Harris CareTracker product provides state-of-the-art features and user-friendly software and is compliant with governmental mandates.

The PM side of Harris CareTracker is a sophisticated practice management system that automates time-consuming administrative tasks such as eligibility checks, scheduling, reminders, patient visit documentation, and claims submission. Its features include:

- Interactive dashboards that prioritize work lists automatically
- A rules-based, front-end clinical editing tool that scrubs outgoing claims prior to submission
- An online code lookup software that boosts coding accuracy

The EMR side of Harris CareTracker monitors and measures all clinical data and prioritizes anything that needs attention. Some of the features of Harris CareTracker EMR include:

- Automatic refill requests
- Chart management
- Lab management
- Medication history
- Prescription (Rx) writing
- Report management

PURPOSE OF THE TEXT

The Paperless Medical Office: Using Harris CareTracker, 2nd edition was written to fill a void in today's EHR training market. There are many EHR training solutions available, but this text integrates advanced content on EHR concepts and meaningful use guidelines with 30–40 hours of step-by-step training activities that simulate typical workflows in ambulatory health organizations. This text takes students through critical information on integrating EHR software into the medical practice, and then offers step-by-step guidance on how those principles can be applied using the Harris CareTracker PM and EMR software.

Chapter 1 serves as an introduction to the EHR, including its benefits and core functions. Activities in Chapter 1 guide students through how to set up their computers for optimal performance, register their credentials, and create their personal Harris CareTracker training companies. Chapters 2 through 10 contain step-by-step front and back office activities for the students to complete. At the end of each activity, students are asked to print a screenshot or report that captures the work they have completed. Students are encouraged to keep this documentation in an "assignments" folder to be turned in to their instructor. Chapter 11 provides comprehensive case studies without the benefit of step-by-step instructions. Completing the Chapter 11 Case Studies affirms proficiency using Harris CareTracker PM and EMR.

ORGANIZATION OF THE TEXT

The Paperless Medical Office is organized to match the daily flow of an office. Chapters 1 and 2 address theoretical EHR concepts that are essential to foundational learning. Beginning with Chapter 3, Patient Demographics and Registration, and continuing throughout the text, students follow the logical sequence of what occurs from the time the patient registers and schedules an appointment through to processing the insurance claim form generated from the patient's visit.

The following breakdown summarizes what is included in each chapter:

Chapter 1: Introduction to the Paperless Medical Office
- This chapter discusses the process of converting paper health records to electronic health records and illustrates what occurs in an electronic health network. Students are provided with a list of common acronyms and terms associated with EHR and PM technology. A variety of common coding and classifications systems are presented in this chapter. Students will learn how set up their computer for optimal performance, register their credentials, and create their Harris CareTracker training company.

Chapter 2: Introduction to Harris CareTracker PM and EMR
- Students will learn how to log in to Harris CareTracker in this chapter and use the *Help* system. Basic navigation functions of the *Main Menu*, *Home*, and *Dashboard* are presented here as well as the discussion of administrative features available within Harris CareTracker PM. Students will gain a firm understanding of using an electronic messaging system and will demonstrate their knowledge by performing messaging activities.

Chapter 3: Patient Demographics and Registration
- In this chapter, students will learn the fundamentals of entering patient demographics, registering new patients, and viewing and performing eligibility checks.

Chapter 4: Appointment Scheduling
- Scheduling is the central theme of this chapter. Students will learn how to book, reschedule, and cancel appointments; add patients to the wait list; and perform activities managing the daily schedule. Users will also learn how to check in patients, create a batch, accept payments, print patient receipts, run a journal, and post the batch.

Chapter 5: Preliminary Duties in the EMR
- This chapter is where the EMR side of Harris CareTracker is introduced. Students will learn the significance of meaningful use and receive training in how to activate the care management registries. In this chapter, users will perform basic maintenance functions such as adding a room, adding a custom resource, and managing immunizations. Learning how to navigate through the medical record is a large focus of the chapter.

Chapter 6: Patient Work-Up
- In this chapter, students will learn the major applications of the *Clinical Today* module—the clinical or EMR side of Harris CareTracker. Students will perform basic check-in duties, and track patients throughout the visit. Learning how to read the tasks menu and complete those tasks is a central focus in this chapter. Tasks may include items such as prescription renewals, electronic *ToDos*, outstanding lab reports or lab reports waiting for a response, and managing open encounters. This chapter emphasizes the importance of time management. In addition to these items, students will learn how to record vital signs

and chief complaints, view and create flow sheets, create and print growth charts, update the patient on preventive testing and health maintenance items, and create progress notes.

Chapter 7: Completing the Visit

- This chapter focuses on what occurs following the patient's examination. Students will learn how to input medication, laboratory, and radiology orders. Users will also learn how to access the correspondence application, create outgoing and incoming referrals, and complete the visit by capturing ICD and CPT® codes required for billing services.

Chapter 8: Other Clinical Documentation

- In this chapter, users will learn how to edit progress notes, add addendums, sign progress notes, and enter results into the patient's medical record. Students will learn how to view, customize, graph, and print patient results and record messages. Additionally, users will create and update patient recall letters, and use the clinical export feature to run an immunization report.

Chapter 9: Billing

- Students switch back to administrative tasks in this chapter. Once the visit is completed the financial activities begin. Creating a batch for financial activities, manually entering charges, and editing an unposted charge are just a few of the activities in this chapter. Users will also learn how to generate electronic and paper claims and perform activities related to electronic remittance.

Chapter 10: ClaimsManager and Collections

- In this chapter, users will learn how to use the *ClaimsManager* feature in Harris CareTracker and will check the status of unpaid or inactive claims. Generating patient statements and collection letters are also introduced in this chapter.

Chapter 11: Applied Learning for the Paperless Medical Office

- This chapter is the finale of the text. It includes several case studies that test the users' comprehension of the material presented throughout the text without providing step-by-step instructions. Students will build both competence and confidence from performing activities in this chapter.

NEW TO THIS EDITION

The second edition of this text has been revised to improve student support. Updates include:

- A **Best Practices** guide at the beginning of the book outlines key tips for working in Harris CareTracker PM and EMR.
- A **Student Companion Website** includes a blank Patient Registration Form for additional practice, some video tutorials, and a mapping grid showing chapter activities you can reference for help when completing the Applied Learning Case Studies (Chapter 11).
- To show greater distinction between the different tasks performed in a PM/EMR, the text has been divided into five **modules**: Get Started, Administrative Skills, Clinical Skills, Billing Skills, and Apply Your Skills.
- A **Quick Start Guide** begins each module. This Quick Start Guide identifies the prerequisite activities required to advance with the module. Students can review this Quick Start Guide prior to starting a module to ensure that they have not missed any key steps. Students on a wheel curriculum will be able to start the text at four different points (Get Started, Administrative Skills, Clinical Skills, or Billing Skills) by starting with a Quick Start Guide.
- A **Real-World Connection** feature begins each chapter which helps the student make the connection between what they are learning to how they will apply what they've learned on the job.
- **Required icons** appear next to chapter activities that are required in order to proceed. This helps prevent students from skipping over necessary activities.

- **Build Your Proficiency** content and activities provide students with optional supplemental practice for skills they've learned and teach new skills that aren't required for completion of the book, but that will help prepare students for the workforce. These activities help build the student into an advanced EMR user.

As a result of these changes, activities in each chapter have been reorganized and some activities have also been rewritten for greater clarification. In addition to reorganizing the text and updating activities, some content updates have been made. Major content updates include:

- Focus on ICD-10 coding with reference to ICD-9 only for historical information
- Enhanced demographics update
- Blank registration templates for use in creating additional patients
- Notation of required activities

FEATURES

The *Help* system within the Harris CareTracker software includes a plethora of educational materials and training tutorials that provide tips for using Harris CareTracker PM and EMR. In addition to text materials, the Harris CareTracker *Help* system provides training videos that walk users through each function within the system. Because this product is a live program, updated training materials containing the most recent information for meaningful use, ICD-10, and HIPAA are available.

The 30–40 hours of hands-on, step-by-step training activities include critical thinking components. The students not only learn how to use the different functions of the Harris CareTracker software but also how to change settings in the software to meet meaningful use goals and to satisfy individual preferences. The *Clinical Today* module within Harris CareTracker PM and EMR assists students in learning how to manage daily, weekly, and monthly tasks, promoting organization and time management.

Unique features of the text also include:

- Full color screenshots throughout the text illustrate the step-by-step activities and allow students to check their work.
- **Key Terms** identify important vocabulary for the chapter. Each term appears in boldface the first time it is used in the chapter and also appears in the glossary with a definition.
- **Learning Objectives** state chapter goals and outcomes.
- The **Real-World Connection** feature at the start of each chapter contains information regarding a day-in-the-life of a medical assistant working in a medical practice using electronic health records. The "real world" scenarios are meant to stimulate thought and critical thinking.
- **Spotlight** boxes highlight important material included throughout the text. It is critical that users of EHR software are familiar with this information. The spotlight boxes include an icon representing the type of information being presented. These types include Administrative, Clinical, and Legal.
- **Alert** boxes present critical information to know when completing activities in Harris CareTracker PM and EMR.
- **Required** icons alert students to activities that are required within a chapter in order for them to proceed with that chapter.
- **Tip** boxes provide helpful hints for using Harris CareTracker PM and EMR.
- **FYI** boxes provide details on functions of Harris CareTracker PM and EMR that are available in real-world settings but are not available in your student version of Harris CareTracker.
- The **Chapter Summaries** provide an overview and summation of the main learning outcomes within the chapter.

- End-of-chapter **Check Your Knowledge** quizzes test the students' retention of information.
- **Case Studies** provide additional opportunities for students to test their ability to complete key chapter activities without the benefit of step-by-step instructions. **Note:** Case studies often build on previous case studies from the prior chapters.
- **Build Your Proficiency** activities provide not only additional practice, but also additional activities not previously performed. Completing these activities will elevate the student's level of competency using EHRs.

DISCLAIMER

Due to the evolving nature and continuous upgrades of real-world EMRs such as this one, as you log in and work in your student version of Harris CareTracker, there may be a slightly different look to your live screen from the screenshots provided in the text.

Keep in mind that you will be asked to work in "current dates" when completing activities, so your appointment and encounter dates will not match those used in the textbook screenshots.

When prompted, follow the instructions given in the text to complete the activities.

LEARNING PACKAGE FOR THE STUDENT

Student Companion Website

Cengage's Student Companion Website to accompany *The Paperless Medical Office: Using Harris CareTracker, 2nd Edition* is a complementary resource that includes additional support such as a blank Patient Registration Form for additional practice, some video tutorials, and a mapping grid showing which chapter activities you can reference for help when completing the Applied Learning Case Studies (Chapter 11). To access the Student Companion Website from CengageBrain, go to http://www.cengagebrain.com, and key the author, title, or ISBN in the **Search** window. Locate the desired product and click on the title. Scroll to the bottom of the page and click on the **Free Materials** tab, then **Save to MyHome**. Once you have added it to "My Home," click on the product under "My Products" to access the Student Companion Website.

The Paperless Medical Office Workbook, 2nd Edition

(ISBN 978-1-337-61421-4)

The Paperless Medical Office Workbook, 2nd edition is a modified and shortened version of *The Paperless Medical Office, 2nd edition*. This workbook focuses on the step-by-step activities presented in *The Paperless Medical Office,* but reduces the amount of general content presented in the chapter and does not include Build Your Proficiency activities.

Billers and Coders Workbook, 2nd Edition

(ISBN 978-1-337-61420-7)

The Paperless Medical Office for Billers and Coders, 2nd edition workbook provides hands-on practice that is focused on billing and coding activities within Harris CareTracker PM and EMR. This workbook contains 8–10 hours of activities with screenshots and step-by-step instructions.

TEACHING PACKAGE FOR THE INSTRUCTOR

Instructor Companion Website

(ISBN 978-1-337-61422-1)

Spend less time planning and more time teaching with Cengage's Instructor Companion Website to accompany *The Paperless Medical Office: Using Harris CareTracker, 2nd Edition.* As an instructor, you will have access to all of your resources online, anywhere and at any time. All instructor resources can be accessed by going to www.cengage.com/login to create a unique user log-in. The password-protected instructor resources include the following:

- An electronic *Instructor's Manual* that includes information about how to use this textbook and answer keys for all chapter activities, Case Studies, Proficiency Builders, and Check Your Knowledge quizzes. Customizable PowerPoints® for each chapter outline key concepts to assist with lectures.
- *Cengage Testing Powered by Cognero*, which is a flexible, online system that allows you to author, edit, and manage test bank content from multiple Cengage solutions; create multiple test versions in an instant; and deliver tests from your learning management system (LMS), classroom, or elsewhere.
- Mapping of the Applied Learning Case Studies (Chapter 11) to the in-text Activity number for reference.
- Spreadsheet showing which patients appear in which activities as well as what activities are required.
- Blank Patient Registration Forms to use for additional assignment/practice.

ABOUT THE AUTHORS

Virginia Ferrari is a former adjunct faculty member at Solano Community College in the Career Technical Education/Business division, where she taught medical front office, medical coding, and small business courses. In addition, she has been a contributing author for other Cengage Learning textbooks, including the Seventh and Eighth Editions of *Medical Assisting: Administrative and Clinical Competencies* and the Second Edition of *Clinical Medical Assisting: A Professional, Field Smart Approach to the Workplace.* Prior to joining Solano Community College, Virginia served as the manager of extended services for one of the fastest-growing physician networks in the San Francisco Bay area. In addition to overseeing the conversion and implementation of electronic medical records, she served on the Best Practice Committee, Customer Satisfaction Committee, Pilot Project for Risk Adjust Coding, and Team Up for Health, a national collaborative for Diabetes Self-Management Education. Virginia holds dual bachelor degrees in sociology and family and consumer studies from Central Washington University and a master's degree in health administration from the University of Phoenix. Virginia also holds certification from the National Healthcareer Association as a Certified Electronic Health Record Specialist (CEHRS), is a previous member of the AAMA Editorial Advisory Committee, and current member of the AAMA Leadership Committee.

ACKNOWLEDGMENTS

To Guy, my husband and best friend, who has believed in me from the day we met more than 40 years ago. Thank you for your inspiration and unwavering support. Thank you for sharing me with all my personal and professional commitments, for keeping me focused, and offering encouragement when I needed it most.

To the entire team at Cengage Learning, and especially Stephen Smith and Kaitlin Schlicht, thank you for the opportunity to write and share my passion for learning, leadership, and excellence. Your continued support, guidance, attention to detail, and utmost professionalism (always going above and beyond) to see this project through has been invaluable. To Mark Turner, thank you for all the assistance to the entire team working on this project and countless reviews to ensure accuracy for the best possible learning experience for students. To Lauren Whalen, thank you for all your guidance and support while we worked as a team to bring the vision of this book and product to its first edition.

A very special thanks to my colleague and coauthor, Michelle Heller. Your inspiration and creativity shine throughout the book. To Dr. Blake Busey, thank you for sharing your knowledge and passion for the medical field and expertise as a practicing physician.

—Virginia Ferrari

System Requirements for Harris CareTracker

MINIMUM REQUIREMENTS

- Intel core or Xeon processor
- Operating System: Windows 7, Windows 8, Windows 10, iPad IOS6
- Windows 7: 8 GB
- Microsoft Internet Explorer 11
- Acrobat Reader
- Adobe Flash
- Java
- 1024 × 768 resolution

THIRD-PARTY SOFTWARE

Third-party software (such as Yahoo! and Google toolbars, or Norton and McAfee) does not follow the rules setup in Internet options; therefore, it tends to block Harris CareTracker functionality with respect to pop-ups. If this does happen, then you need to add training.caretracker.com and rapidrelease.caretracker.com to the allowed or safe sites lists of those programs. Follow the instructions in the next section, Internet Settings (Add as Trusted Site).

INTERNET SETTINGS

Add as Trusted Site

1. Open Internet Explorer browser window.
2. On the menu bar, click Tools and then select Internet Options from the menu. Internet Explorer displays the Internet Options dialog box.
3. Click the Security tab and then click Trusted Sites.
4. Click Sites. Internet Explorer displays the Trusted Sites dialog box.
5. In the Add this website to the zone box, type: training.caretracker.com
6. Click Add. Internet Explorer adds the address to trusted sites.
7. Repeat steps 5 and 6 for rapidrelease.caretracker.com.
8. Deselect the Require server verification (https:) for all sites in this zone checkbox.
9. Click Close to close the Trusted Sites box.
10. Click OK on the Internet Options box to save your changes.

Compatibility View Settings

1. In Internet Explorer 11, launch the website for which you want to disable Compatibility View (www.cengage.com/caretracker).
2. If the menu bar is not visible, press the **Alt** key to display the browser menu.
3. On the browser menu, click the Tools > Compatibility View Settings. The browser opens the Compatibility View Settings window.
4. In the "Websites you've added to Compatibility View" section, remove caretracker.com if it appears there.

BANDWIDTH RECOMMENDATIONS

If there are multiple workstations utilizing Harris CareTracker, then each will require a minimum of 300 kb of bandwidth per active workstation with a DSL or Cable connection. For a T1 or Dedicated connection, a minimum of 60 kb per workstation is required.

RECOMMENDED SCREEN RESOLUTION

The recommended screen resolution is 1024 × 768.

SUPPORTED BROWSER

Harris CareTracker supports only Internet Explorer 11 for desktop devices. Safari for iPad may also be used. Mozilla Firefox and Google Chrome are not yet supported.

Best Practices for Harris CareTracker

Certain best practices should be followed whenever you are working in Harris CareTracker. A list of these best practices is provided below. Continue reading for more information on these best practices.

- Before beginning work each day, check the News application in CareTracker for updates from Harris CareTracker and Cengage. To do so, click on the Home Module and then click on the News tab.
- When you are instructed to complete an activity, read all of the activity directions first, before completing any steps. This is a proven method for reducing data entry errors.
- Check your browser. Use only Internet Explorer 11 (IE 11) or Safari for iPad.
- Check Compatibility View settings. "Display intranet sites in Compatibility View" and "Use Microsoft compatibility lists" should be unchecked.
- Clear your cache each time you start working in Harris CareTracker.
- If you receive a "Duplicate Session" error message, close your browser window. Then open a new Internet Explorer browser window. In the new window, select File>New Session.
- When directed to "print," if a print button is not available in Harris CareTracker, take a screenshot of your work.
- Properly log out when you are finished working.
- For technical support questions, check your student companion website for solutions. If you can't find a solution to your issue, contact Cengage.

Check Your Browser

Harris CareTracker supports only Internet Explorer 11 and Safari for iPad.

To Determine Your Browser

You can determine the basic type of browser you are using by looking at the icon at the bottom of your computer screen, in the Start Menu, on the Desktop, or on your Task Bar. Internet Explorer or Safari for iPad are required for using Harris CareTracker. **Figure 1** shows the Internet Explorer icon. **Figure 2** shows the Safari icon

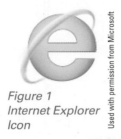

Figure 1
Internet Explorer
Icon

Used with permission from Microsoft

Figure 2
Safari Icon

Used with permission of Apple Inc.

(which is compatible with Harris CareTracker for iPads only). **Figure 3** shows other icons that are *not* compatible with Harris CareTracker (Google Chrome, Microsoft Edge, and Mozilla Firefox).

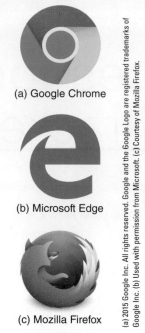

(a) Google Chrome

(b) Microsoft Edge

(c) Mozilla Firefox

Figure 3 Unsupported Browsers

To Determine Your Browser Version

There are multiple versions of Internet Explorer. You must be working in Internet Explorer 11 to use Harris Care-Tracker. To determine which version you have, click on the Internet Explorer icon on your device. In the browser window, click on "Help" to bring up the Help menu (**Figure 4**). Click "About Internet Explorer" and you will see the pop up showing what version of IE you are using (**Figure 5**).

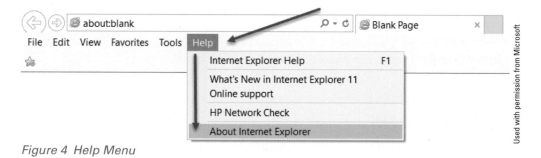

Figure 4 Help Menu

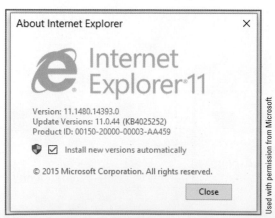

Figure 5 About Internet Explorer

To Locate Internet Explorer in Windows 10

Newer Windows computers may not have Internet Explorer installed and you will need to install prior to working in Harris CareTracker. To locate IE 11 in Windows 10, select the Start button and search for "Internet Explorer." If IE 11 is installed, you will see it pop up at the top of the search results. Search Microsoft's Support page for more help if needed, or to install IE 11 on your Windows computer.

Check Compatibility View Settings

You will need to change your Compatibility View Settings as follows.

1. Open up Internet Explorer 11 (IE 11).
2. Click on the Tools menu tab.
3. Select the Compatibility View settings option (**Figure 6**).

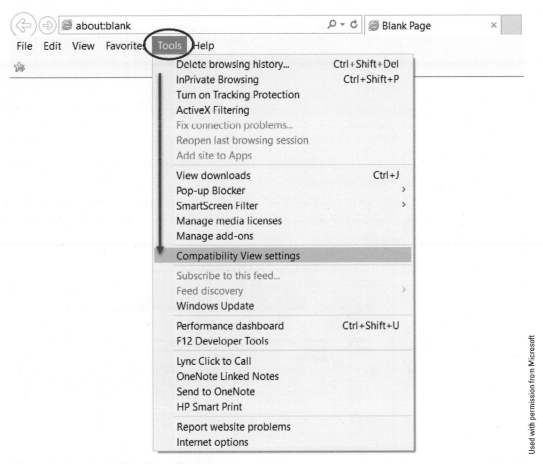

Figure 6 Compatibility View Settings

Used with permission from Microsoft

4. In the resulting popup, uncheck the "Display intranet sites in Compatibility View" option (Figure 7).
5. Uncheck "Use Microsoft compatibility lists" (**Figure 7**).
6. Click Close.

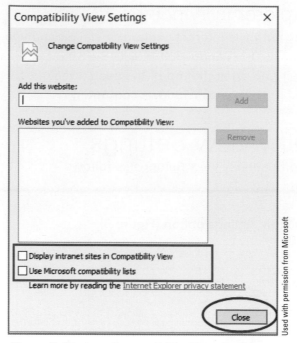

Figure 7 Change Compatibility View Settings

Clear Your Cache

You should clear your cache each time you begin working in CareTracker. To clear your cache in Internet Explorer 11:

1. Open an Internet Explorer® browser window.
2. From the *Tools* menu, select *Internet Options*. Windows® displays the *Internet Options* dialog box.
3. On the *General* tab, in the *Browsing history* section, click *Delete...* (**Figure 8**). Windows® displays the *Delete Browsing History* dialog box.

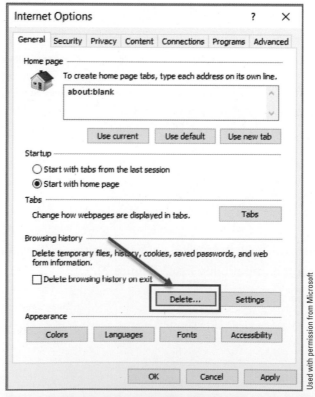

Figure 8 Delete Browsing History

4. Deselect the *Preserve Favorites website data* checkbox (**Figure 9**).

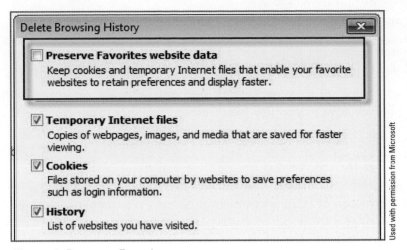

Figure 9 Preserve Favorites

5. Select the *Temporary Internet files and website files, Cookies and website data,* and *History* checkboxes only.
6. Click *Delete.*
7. Click *OK* when finished.

To clear your cache in Safari for iPad:

1. Tap *Settings* from your iPad® home screen.
2. Tap *Safari®* from the *Settings* pane on the left. The *Safari®* pane displays *Clear History, Clear Cache,* and *Clear Cookies* at the bottom (**Figure 10**).

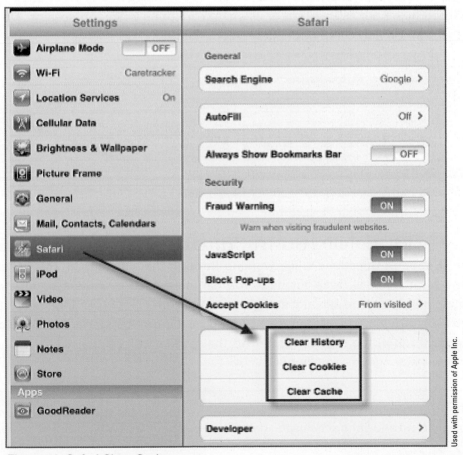

Figure 10 Safari Clear Cache

3. Tap *Clear History*. iPad® displays a confirmation window.
4. Tap *Clear* in the confirmation window.
5. Repeat steps 3 and 4 to clear your cache and cookies (refer to Figure 10).

Resolve a "Duplicate Session" Error Message

If you receive a "Duplicate Session" error message, close your browser window. Open a new Internet Explorer browser window. In the new window, select File > New Session. You should now be able to access Harris CareTracker.

Take a Screenshot

Throughout the text you will be instructed to "print" or in some cases, take a screen shot, of your work to submit to your instructor as confirmation of activity completion. To take a screenshot with your PC:

1. Find the screen you need to print out (this will usually be noted in your "end of activity print instruction").
2. Press the Print Screen [PrtSc] key on your computer keypad to capture your entire screen. Alternatively, press the key [Alt] and [PrtSc] to capture only the active window.
3. Open a Word document.
4. Using the Paste command, paste the image from the screen onto your Word document. This can also be accomplished by either right clicking your mouse and choosing one of the Paste options, or by left clicking anywhere in the Word document and pressing the keys [Ctrl] and [V] to paste the image onto the Word document.
5. Save the Word document and submit the document to your instructor as advised (electronically or paper).

Log Out of Harris CareTracker

It is important to properly log out of CareTracker when you are done with your session. Do not simply close the window, but instead, click on *Log Off* in Harris CareTracker (**Figure 11**).

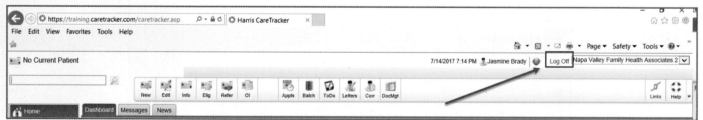

Figure 11 *Properly Log Off Harris CareTracker PM and Physician EMR*   Courtesy of Harris CareTracker PM and Physician EMR

Contact Cengage for Technical Support When Needed

If you have technical support questions while working through the activities in *The Paperless Medical Office,* check your student companion website for help. You can access your student companion website through logging in or creating a free student account at login.cengage.com, clicking on Find Free Study Tools, searching for and adding the ISBN 9781337614191 and then clicking on the product under My Products. If you are unable to resolve your issue through the support posted to the student companion website, then contact Cengage technical support at www.cengage.com/support.

 ALERT! WARNING!! Do not purchase a "used textbook," as the credentials would have already been registered and cannot be used again. You must have a new textbook with your own credentials in order to be able to create your training company for work in Harris CareTracker.

MODULE 1
Get Started

This module includes:

- Chapter 1: Introduction to the Paperless Medical Office
- Chapter 2: Introduction to Harris CareTracker PM and EMR

In order to complete activities in Harris CareTracker, you must first set up your computer for optimal functionality. You will then register your credentials and create your Harris CareTracker training company.

If you are beginning your work starting with this module, follow along from the beginning and complete all the Required ⚑ activities as you move sequentially through the text.

Introduction to the Paperless Medical Office

Key Terms

abstract
cache
Certification Commission for Health Information Technology (CCHIT®)
classification systems
clearinghouse
clinical templates
clinical vocabularies
Computer Physician Order Entry (CPOE)
covered entity
Current Procedural Terminology (CPT®)
credentials
designated record sets (DRS)
electronic health record (EHR)
electronic medical record (EMR)
electronic protected health information (ePHI)
EncoderPro®
Health Insurance Portability and Accountability Act (HIPAA)
Health Level 7 (HL7)
hybrid conversion
International Classification of Diseases (ICD)
Logical Observation Identifiers Names and Codes (LOINC®)
meaningful use
minimum necessary
modifiers
National Drug Code (NDC)
nomenclature
notice of privacy practices (NPP)
order set
protected health information (PHI)
providers
scope of practice
scrub
sequelae
sustainability
Systemized Nomenclature of Medicine, Clinical Terms (SNOMED-CT®)
total conversion
treatment, payment, and operations (TPO)
Unified Medical Language System (UMLS®)
workflow

Learning Objectives

1. Set up your computer for optimal functionality when using Harris CareTracker PM and EMR.
2. Create a Harris CareTracker training company.
3. Illustrate what occurs in an electronic health network.
4. Explain the process of converting paper health records to electronic health records (EHRs).
5. Summarize administrative workflows in Harris CareTracker.
6. Discuss practice management, front office, billing, and administrative functions.
7. Define classification systems.
8. Distinguish between coding systems such as the International Classification of Diseases (ICD), Healthcare Common Procedural Coding System (HCPCS), and Current Procedural Terminology (CPT®).
9. Identify clinical components of the EHR and clinical workflows in Harris CareTracker.
10. List common acronyms and terminology associated with EHRs.

Real-World Connection

Welcome to Napa Valley Family Health Associates (NVFHA), your Harris CareTracker training company! Our practice is located in the beautiful Napa Valley in California. The practice consists of four providers, six medical assistants, one X-ray technician, and a medical lab scientist who oversees our laboratory. As a medical assisting student, you will rotate among our four providers:

- Amir Raman, DO (Specialty—Internal Medicine)
- Anthony Brockton, MD (Specialty—Family Practice)

(*continues*)

Real-World Connection (*continued*)

- Rebecca Ayerick, MD (Specialty—Family Practice/Pediatrics)
- Gabrielle Torres, NP (Specialty—Family Practice)

We are a busy family health center and take care of patients across the lifespan. To be considered for a job in our practice, you must have a caring attitude, have strong administrative and clinical skills, and get along well with people of all ages and all socioeconomic backgrounds.

We are a practice that believes in a proactive approach to health care. We look for ways to improve patient outcomes while driving down health care costs. As a matter of fact, we recently applied for and received NCQA Patient-Centered Medical Home (PCMH) Recognition. The PCMH is a care delivery model whereby patient treatment is coordinated through their primary care provider to ensure the patient receives the necessary care when and where they need it, in a manner they can understand. Becoming a PCMH is a way of organizing primary care that emphasizes care coordination and communication to transform primary care into "what patients want it to be." Medical homes are intended to lead to higher quality care, lower costs, and improved outcomes. We chose Harris CareTracker PM and Physician EMR as our electronic health record system because of its robust functions and reporting capabilities, which are essential to a PCMH model.

This textbook focuses on technical skills, but do not be surprised if you learn a few other skills along the way! Throughout the text, you will be challenged to think critically and perform to the best of your ability. Your first challenge is to carefully read the instructions and implement all of the settings for the activities/features outlined in this first chapter. Failure to implement the recommended settings may result in an inability to perform some activities. Let's get started!

INTRODUCTION

Harris CareTracker PM and EMR is a fully integrated **Certification Commission for Health Information Technology (CCHIT®)** and ONC-ATCB–certified complete practice management (PM) and electronic health record (EHR). You often hear the terms *EMR* and *EHR* used interchangeably, but there is a distinction between the two. **Electronic medical records (EMRs)** are patient records in a digital format. **Electronic health records (EHRs)** refer to the interoperability of electronic medical records, or the ability to share medical records with other health care facilities.

Harris CareTracker PM and EMR is an ONC-Certified HIT (**Figure 1-1**), meaning that, among other things, it supports meaningful use, which is discussed later in the chapter. ONC is an acronym for "The Office of the National Coordinator", the entity that is the main certification authority for EHR technology.

Harris CareTracker PM is a powerful cloud-based application that gives medical practices new levels of efficiency, integration, and accountability. Harris CareTracker PM features a sophisticated infrastructure within a simple user experience that:

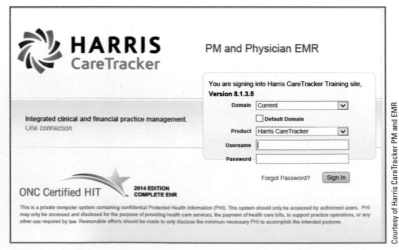

Figure 1-1 Harris CareTracker PM and EMR Login Page

- Automates patient scheduling and registration
- Verifies eligibility at every step
- Scrubs outgoing claims prior to submission (to **scrub** a claim means to verify its technical and coding accuracy before it is filed by identifying potential problems that will cause claim rejection or reduction in payment. The claim scrubber provides a comprehensive set of coding and technical edits.)
- Maximizes "pay at first pass"
- Returns to payers daily to check claim status
- Monitors contracts for underpayment
- Routes issues to billing staff and managers
- Ensures accountability at all levels

Harris CareTracker PM and EMR is fully integrated with all the operational functions of a medical practice. Harris CareTracker EMR gives providers a new way to manage tasks, streamline their workflow, and improve the quality of patient care. With Harris CareTracker EMR you can:

- Capture patient visits electronically using *QuickText*, dictation, and structured templates
- Manage and document patient communications quickly and efficiently
- Generate and process prescription refills
- Complete office workflow tasks with detail or summarize patient information that includes medications, allergies, and more
- Attach patient documents, images, X-rays, or other files in electronic format
- Evaluate patient information using graphs and flow sheets
- Manage medication and allergy interactions
- Generate patient education information

This chapter introduces you to concepts and terminology relating to health information technology (HIT), medical practice workflows, coding systems, and rules implemented by the HHS and the Centers for Medicare and Medicaid Services (CMS). As with all aspects of medical care, the field of EHRs is constantly evolving and improving. As such, medical practices find it desirable to hire employees who are proficient using EHRs.

SET UP COMPUTER FOR OPTIMAL FUNCTIONALITY

Learning Objective 1: Set up your computer for optimal functionality when using Harris CareTracker PM and EMR.

In order to complete activities in Harris CareTracker, you must first set up your computer for optimal functionality. You will then register your credentials and create your Harris CareTracker training company. Because it may take up to 24 hours for your student company to be created, you will complete the activities in Learning Objectives 1 and 2 now.

Readiness Requirements

In order to use Harris CareTracker you must meet the minimum system requirements and update your browser settings. You'll walk through these requirements in the activities in this chapter. In addition, the most current System Requirements can be found on your Student Companion site.

 TIP You will find up-to-date *System Requirements and Recommendations* in the *Help* system of Harris CareTracker at *Help > Contents* tab > *System Requirements and Recommendations folder*. Chapter 2 will introduce you to *Help* and the various content and training available.

To use Harris CareTracker PM and EMR, your computer must have Internet Explorer® version 11. Other browsing software (outside of Safari® for iPad®) may work differently with the application. See the System Requirements section for further technology requirements. Chrome and Firefox are not currently supported. While iPads® are compatible with Harris CareTracker, Macs cannot be used to register an access code, also known as your credentials. In an EHR, **credentials** are the login information required to access the software, which is the assigned username and password.

Disable Third-Party Toolbars

Remove all third-party toolbars (Google, Yahoo!, Bing, AOL, etc.) from Internet Explorer®. Third-party toolbars cause random performance and functionality issues within Harris CareTracker PM and EMR. Complete Activity 1-1 to disable toolbars.

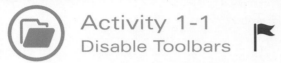

Activity 1-1
Disable Toolbars

1. Open an Internet Explorer® browser window.

2. Right-click on the menu bar (at the top of your browser window). The browser displays a list of toolbars. Active toolbars appear with a check mark to the left of the name (**Figure 1-2**).

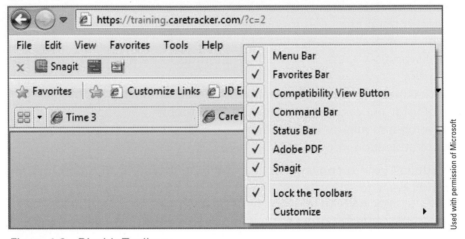

Figure 1-2   Disable Toolbars

3. Uncheck the toolbars you want to disable (Google, Yahoo!, Bing, AOL, etc. if displaying). Internet Explorer® disables the toolbar if that toolbar does not have a check mark next to it. Leave a check-mark next to "Menu Bar."

Setting Up Tabbed Browsing

Tabbed browsing allows you to open multiple websites in a single browser window. It is very important to set this up to access several patient charts at one time in a single browser. This will make switching between patients much easier and enables you to have multiple items open on the task bar. Complete Activity 1-2 to set up tabbed browsing.

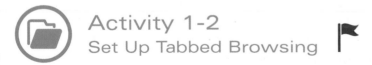

Activity 1-2
Set Up Tabbed Browsing

1. Open an Internet Explorer® browser window.

2. Select *Tools > Internet Options* from the browser menu. The *Internet Options* dialog box displays.

3. In the *Tabs* section, click *Tabs*. The *Tabbed Browsing Settings* dialog box displays.

4. Select the following options noted below and in **Figure 1-3**:

   • Warn me when closing multiple tabs

   • Always switch to new tabs when they are created

   • Show previews for individual tabs in the taskbar*

   • Enable Tab Groups*

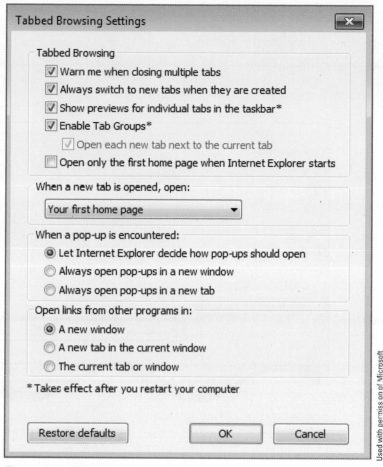

Figure 1-3   Tabbed Browser Settings

- When a new tab is opened, open: Your first home page
- When a pop-up is encountered: Let Internet Explorer® decide on how pop-ups should open
- Open links from other programs in: A new window

  *Takes effect after you restart your computer

5. Click *OK* to close the *Tabbed Browsing Settings* box.

6. Click *OK* on the *Internet Options* box to save your changes.

Disable Pop-Up Blocker

A pop-up window is a small web browser window that appears on top of the website you are viewing. This allows you to avoid having to navigate away from the current window you are viewing. Harris CareTracker PM and EMR uses the pop-up mechanism, enabling an efficient workflow. Many computers have firewall protectors that alleviate nonsense pop-up ads from displaying as you work on a website. However, you must enable pop-ups to use the functionality within Harris CareTracker PM and EMR. Complete Activity 1-3 to turn off pop-up blocker in Internet Explorer® and Safari®.

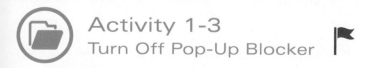

Activity 1-3
Turn Off Pop-Up Blocker

1. To disable pop-up blocker in Internet Explorer®, open an Internet Explorer® browser window.

2. Select *Tools > Pop-up Blocker > Turn Off Pop-up Blocker* from the browser menu.

To disable pop-up blocker in Safari® for iPad®:

1. Tap *Settings* from your iPad® home screen.

2. Tap *Safari®* from the *Settings* panes on the left. The *Safari®* pane displays the browser options.

3. Tap *Block Pop-ups* to turn off pop-up blocker (**Figure 1-4**).

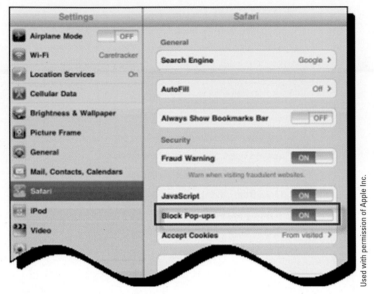

Figure 1-4   Safari Pop-up Blocker

Change the Page Setup

It is important to change the default margin, header, and footer settings to print letters, forms, and claims in Harris CareTracker PM and EMR. Complete Activity 1-4 to change page setup.

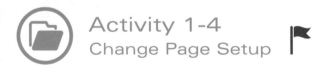

Activity 1-4
Change Page Setup

1. Open an Internet Explorer® browser window (one such as your Harris CareTracker training company). *Note:* You must have an actual website up, not just a blank/new tab.

2. On the browser menu bar, click *File*. Then choose *Page setup* from the menu. Internet Explorer® launches the *Page Setup* dialog box.

3. Delete the values in the *Margins* (*inches*) fields. Leaving these fields blank will automatically set their value to zero.

4. Select *Empty* in each of the *Header* and *Footer* fields. Click *OK*.

Downloading Plug-ins

A plug-in is a program that works with Harris CareTracker PM and EMR to give added functionality. Follow each link to download the required plug-in for free, if you don't have the plug-in already.

- Adobe Reader (*www.adobe.com, search for "Reader"*)
  - *To view, navigate, and print PDF files.*

- Adobe Flash (*www.adobe.com, search for "Flash Player"*)
  - *To view animation and interactive content.*
- Java (*www.java.com*)
  - *To run applications and applets that use Java technology. Java is required to view prerecorded sessions.*

Adding Trusted Sites

Add *training.caretracker.com* and *rapidrelease.caretracker.com* to the trusted site list. Otherwise some functionality may be blocked, such as running ActiveX controls and installing browser plug-ins. Adding trusted sites also allows your computer to distinguish between secured sites and harmful sites. Complete Activity 1-5 to add trusted sites.

Activity 1-5
Add Harris CareTracker to Trusted Sites

1. Open an Internet Explorer® browser window.

2. On the menu bar, click *Tools* and then select *Internet Options* from the menu. Internet Explorer® displays the *Internet Options* dialog box.

3. Click the *Security* tab and then click *Trusted Sites*.

4. Click *Sites*. Internet Explorer® displays the *Trusted sites* dialog box.

5. Deselect the *Require server verification (https:) for all sites in this zone* checkbox.

6. In the *Add this website to the zone* box, type: *training.caretracker.com*.

7. Click *Add*. Internet Explorer® adds the address to trusted sites.

8. In the *Add this website to the zone* box, type: *rapidrelease.caretracker.com*.

9. Click *Add*. Internet Explorer® adds the address to trusted sites (**Figure 1-5**).

10. Click *Close* to close the *Trusted Sites* box.

11. Click *OK* on the *Internet Options* box to save your changes.

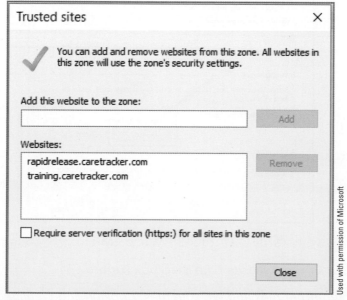

Figure 1-5   Trusted Sites

Clearing the Cache

The **cache** is a space in your computer's hard drive and random access memory (RAM) where your browser saves copies of recently visited web pages. Typically these items are stored in the *Temporary Internet Files* folder. It is important to clear your cache on a regular basis and at every release for Harris CareTracker PM and EMR to function more efficiently.

 IMPORTANT!! You must clear your cache prior to logging in to Harris CareTracker PM and EMR. If you are already logged in, log out of Harris CareTracker before clearing your cache.

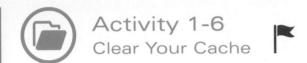

Activity 1-6
Clear Your Cache

To clear your cache in Microsoft Internet Explorer® 11:

1. Open an Internet Explorer® browser window.

2. From the Internet Explorer® 11 *Tools* menu, select *Internet Options*. Windows® displays the *Internet Options* dialog box.

3. On the *General* tab, in the *Browsing history* section, click *Delete...* (**Figure 1-6**). Windows® displays the *Delete Browsing History* dialog box.

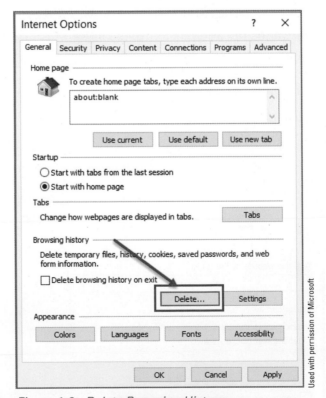

Figure 1-6   Delete Browsing History

4. Deselect the *Preserve Favorites website data* checkbox (**Figure 1-7**).

5. Select the *Temporary Internet files and website files*, *Cookies and website data*, and *History* checkboxes only.

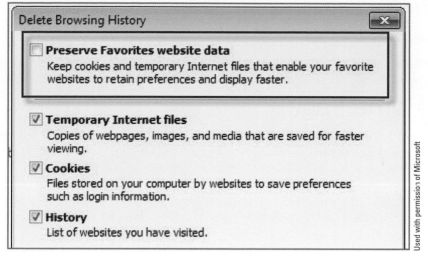

Figure 1-7   Preserve Favorites

6. Click *Delete.*

7. Click *OK* when finished.

To clear your cache in Safari® for iPad®:

1. Tap *Settings* from your iPad® home screen.

2. Tap *Safari®* from the *Settings* pane on the left. The *Safari®* pane displays *Clear History, Clear Cache,* and *Clear Cookies* at the bottom (**Figure 1-8**).

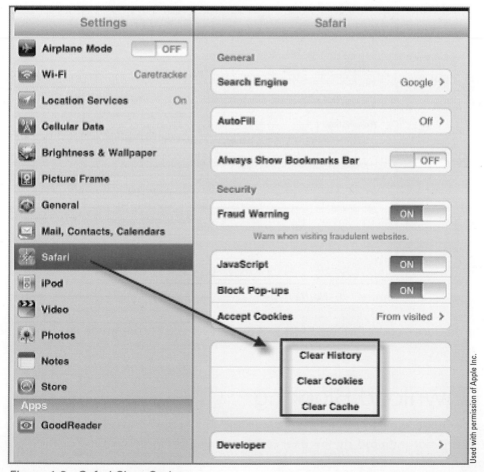

Figure 1-8   Safari Clear Cache

3. Tap *Clear History*. iPad® displays a confirmation window.

4. Tap *Clear* in the confirmation window.

5. Repeat steps 3 and 4 to clear your cache and cookies (refer to **Figure 1-8**).

Setting Your Home Page

Your home page is displayed when Internet Explorer® first opens. You can choose to set Harris CareTracker PM and EMR as your home page if necessary.

Activity 1-7
Setting Harris CareTracker as Home Page

1. Open an Internet Explorer® browser window.

2. Select *Tools > Internet Options* from the browser menu. The *Internet Options* dialog box displays.

3. In the *Address* box of the *Home page* section, type: *http://www.cengage.com/CareTracker* (**Figure 1-9**).

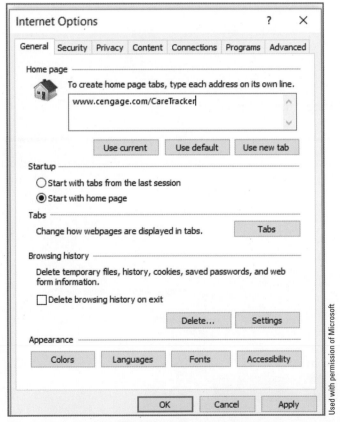

Figure 1-9   Home Page

4. Click *OK*. Harris CareTracker PM and EMR will display as your home page the next time you open Internet Explorer®.

Disable Download Blocking

The automatic download blocking in Internet Explorer® is a security feature that blocks all file download dialog boxes that are not initiated by the user (such as by clicking the mouse or hitting a key). Complete Activity 1-8 to disable download blocking.

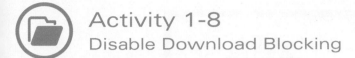

Activity 1-8
Disable Download Blocking

1. Open an Internet Explorer® browser window.

2. Select *Tools* > *Internet Options* from the browser menu. The browser displays the *Internet Options* dialog box.

3. Click the *Security* tab.

4. Click the *Internet* (globe) link.

5. Click the *Custom level...* button.

6. Scroll down to the *Downloads* section.

7. In the *File Download* section, click *Enable*. Click *OK*.

8. Click *OK* in the *Internet Options* window to close it.

Now that you have set your computer to the required settings to work in Harris CareTracker PM and EMR, you will register your credentials and log in to begin your training.

REGISTER YOUR CREDENTIALS AND CREATE YOUR HARRIS CARETRACKER TRAINING COMPANY

Learning Objective 2: Create a Harris CareTracker training company.

You will be assigned a user name and password (your credentials) to log in to Harris CareTracker PM and EMR. Your preassigned user name and password can be found on the inside front cover of your textbook. Your password must be changed the first time you log in to Harris CareTracker PM and EMR. You will also be prompted to change your password every 00 days for security reasons. The password must consist of at least eight characters with one capital and one numeric character. As best practice, write your new password and the date created on the inside cover of your textbook each time you change it.

Before beginning any activities, clear your cache as instructed in Activity 1-6. If you are using a personal computer (PC), only work in Internet Explorer®. Use Safari® for iPad®. Once the cache has been cleared, you may continue by registering your credentials and creating your Harris CareTracker training company (Activity 1-9).

Activity 1-9
Register Your Credentials and Create Your Harris CareTracker PM and EMR Training Company

1. Go to *http://www.cengage.com/CareTracker* (**Figure 1-10**).

2. The "Domain" is set to *Current*. Do not change this setting—leave as is.

3. The *Product* list is set to "Cengage Learning Harris CareTracker Simulation 1.0" by default. Leave as is.

4. In the *Username* box, enter the username preassigned to you on the inside front cover of your textbook.

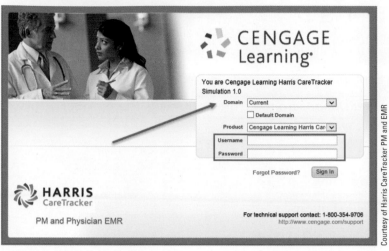

Figure 1-10 Login Screen

5. In the *Password* box, enter your password. If this is your first time logging in to Harris CareTracker PM and EMR, use the preassigned password located on the inside front cover of your textbook. Then click *Sign In*. On your first login, you will be prompted to change your temporary password and complete the *Security Information* and *General Information* fields in the *Operators Settings* dialog box.

TIP Both the username and password are case sensitive.
Your new password:
- Must differ from your old password by at least one character
- Must consist of at least eight characters
- Must contain at least one capital letter and one number; for example: Password5
- Must be reentered in the *Verify Password* field

6. Complete the *Security Information* fields by selecting a security question and providing the answer.

7. In the *General Information* fields, enter your *Phone* number (best contact), your *Email* (best contact), and skip the *Direct Email Address* field.

8. Record your new password on the inside cover of your text book and the date the password was created. This allows for easy reference in case of a lost or an expired password.

9. After changing your password and completing the *Security* and *General Information* fields, click *Save*. A message will display indicating that your operator settings have been updated.

10. Close out of the *Success* box. Harris CareTracker will now create your training account and you will receive a notification email when the process is complete. **Figure 1-11** is an example of the notification email you will receive. **Note:** You will not be able to log in to Harris CareTracker until you have received the notification email. It may take up to 24 hours for your Harris CareTracker training company to be created and to receive the notification.

Hello cengage238032,

Your training company has been successfully created. Log in and begin using CareTracker's training environment

Harris CareTracker has worked with tens of thousands of physicians to create healthier practices and healthier patients. The training environment is a lite version of the complete practice management and EMR solutions we offer to our customers. We look forward to working with you in the future.

Sincerely,
The Harris CareTracker Practice Management and EMR Team

Figure 1-11 Welcome Login Email

Note: On subsequent logins, you will receive a *Message from webpage* that says "There is no Operator Batch Control for this Group". Click "OK" and a dialog box called *Operator Encounter Batch Control* will display when you first sign in. Close out of this box by clicking the *Save* button and then clicking the "X" at the top right of the box (**Figure 1-12**).

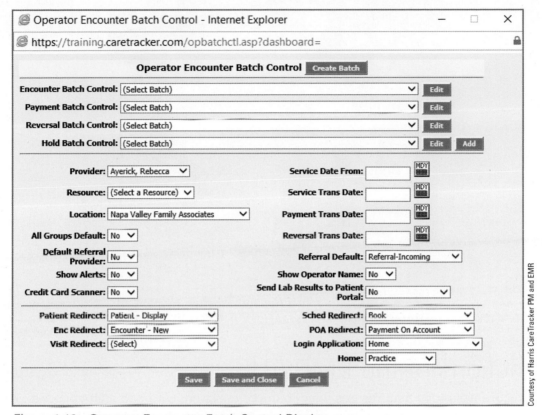

Figure 1-12   *Operator Encounter Batch Control Display*

ELECTRONIC MEDICAL RECORDS

Learning Objective 3: Illustrate what occurs in an electronic health network.

Electronic medical records (EMRs) are patient records in digital format. EMRs can refer to a hospital's electronic patient records, a physician's office electronic patient records, or the EHRs of any other health care establishment. EHR refers to the interoperability of EMRs or the ability to share medical records with other health care entities. **Figure 1-13** illustrates what occurs within an electronic health network.

- The connection is initiated when the primary care provider (PCP) requests the medical assistant to order diagnostic tests for the patient (a).

- The medical assistant sends electronic orders to the facility where the tests are to be performed (b).

- The testing facility receives the orders, performs the tests, and electronically sends the results back to the PCP (c).

- The PCP reviews the results and electronically signs (commits) the results into the patient's medical record (d).

- The patient enters the emergency department with chest pain. The patient alerts the ED physician that he or she just had a physical and diagnostic testing performed at his or her physician's office. A representative from the ED looks up the patient's records in the EHR which contains the PCP records and tests (e).

- In a matter of minutes, the ED physician has vital information that is needed for determining necessary testing, making a diagnosis, and treating the patient (f).

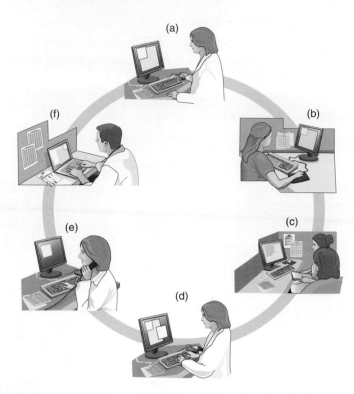

Figure 1-13 A Computer Network Provides Health Care Workers with the Necessary Information with Just a Click of a Button

Core Functions of the EMR/EHR

The electronic record has many features designed to improve patient care and staff efficiency. The type of software that a medical practice selects will depend on many factors including the type of practice, the goals of the practice, the cost of the software, and individual preferences of the clinicians and staff. Following is an overview of the various functions within Harris CareTracker EMR, a widely used, real-world EHR.

- Allows multiple users to access different parts of the chart at the same time

- Creates a chart summary, which identifies key components of the patient's medical history on one screen, including open activities or orders, active problems, active medications, allergy status, immunization status, a listing of the patient's last vital sign measurements, a listing of the patient's progress note history, documents downloaded into the chart, lab results, and correspondence information. This summary can be shared electronically with other providers who see the patient

- Creates customized progress notes through standardized templates

- Creates customized clinical letters

- Enables the provider and staff members to print, send electronically, or fax progress notes, prescriptions, and other orders directly from the point of care

- Automatically files and displays lab results in a variety of different formats

- Graphs lab values, pediatric growth chart patterns, and vital signs

- Provides electronic tasking features to improve efficiency and communication between staff members

- Provides reporting and benchmarking capabilities that allow users to compare patient outcomes or to track other statistical data

- Interfaces with the practice management side of Harris CareTracker, making billing more efficient

- Provides full remote access of patient records for those authorized to use them

Through a public and private collaborative effort to advance the adoption of EHR systems, the Institute of Medicine (IOM) and the HHS formed a committee that identified a set of eight core care delivery functions that EHR systems should be capable of performing to promote greater safety, quality, and efficiency in health care delivery. As discussed earlier in the chapter, the 2003 report, titled "Key Capabilities of an Electronic Health Record System," enumerated the eight core functions of an EHR system (**Table 1-1**).

Advantages of Electronic Medical/Health Records

An EMR system is an electronic platform that facilitates the needs of a medical practice. An advantage of using a fully integrated practice management and EMR such as Harris CareTracker is that it automates the overall workflow to the greatest extent possible to achieve the maximum amount of practice efficiency. Patient care coordination is improved, and there is a demonstrated reduction in errors, which previously resulted from illegible notes or prescriptions. According to information published by the National Healthcareer Association (NHA) (n.d.), errors in prescribing medicine harm almost one million Americans per year. These errors range from prescribing a drug that interacts with a drug that the patient is already taking to dispensing the wrong medication

Table 1-1	Key Capabilities of an Electronic Health Record System
Health Information and Data	Designed to have immediate access to essential patient information (e.g., diagnoses, allergies, lab results, and medications). The system holds the information that would be expected in a paper chart—problem lists, medication lists, test results, etc.
Results Management	Has the ability for all health care providers participating in the patient's care to quickly access new and past test results from multiple settings. An EHR enables the importation of lab results, radiology reports, and X-ray images electronically.
Order Management	Contains the ability to enter and store orders in a computer-based system for tests, prescriptions, and other services. Medication order entry and e-prescribing, laboratory, microbiology, pathology, radiology, nursing, and supply orders, as well as ancillary services and consults. In Harris CareTracker PM and EMR, the *Patient Care Management* module provides important tracking to indicate overdue orders and consults.
Clinical Decision Support	Uses technology to improve best clinical practice with reminders, prompts, and computerized decision-support systems to improve compliance, ensure regular screenings and other preventative care practices, identify possible drug interactions, and facilitate diagnoses and treatment. An EHR should warn clinicians about drug–drug and drug–allergy interactions and make available evidence-based guidelines to help providers consider treatment options.
Electronic Communication and Connectivity	Provides access to communications among providers and patients that is efficient, secure, and readily accessible. Providers should be able to efficiently communicate with their staff as well as other care partners (other clinicians, lab, radiology, and pharmacy staff, etc.). EHR systems may also provide options for communicating directly with patients.
Patient Support	Allows patients to access their health records, interactive patient education, and to improve chronic conditions through home-monitoring and self-testing. Patients can access educational materials and enter data themselves through online questionnaires and home-monitoring devices.
Administrative Processes	Improves hospital and clinic efficiency and provides more timely services to patients using electronic administrative tools, such as scheduling systems. The system enhances the overall efficiency of standard practice management functions, aiding with billing and claims management, authorizations, referrals, etc.
Reporting and Population Management	Using electronic data storage with uniform data standards to enable health care organizations to respond quickly to federal, state, and private reporting requirements. An EHR will help organizations adhere to multiple public and private sector reporting requirements at the federal, state, and local levels for patient safety and quality, as well as for public health.

Adapted from the Institute of Medicine.

due to poor handwriting. Although functions vary widely in EHR programs, the ability to e-prescribe is a feature most EHR programs provide. One of the main advantages of e-prescribing is the ability to quickly perform safety checks. EHR programs will send alerts for potential prescription problems.

In 2011, the National Center for Biotechnology Information published an article titled "Benefits and Drawbacks of Electronic Health Record Systems." It was reported that researchers examined the benefits of EHRs by considering clinical, organizational, and societal outcomes. Clinical outcomes include improvements in the quality of care, a reduction in medical errors, and other improvements in patient-level measures that describe the appropriateness of care. Organizational outcomes, on the other hand, have included such items as improvement in financial and operational performance as well as satisfaction among patients and clinicians who use EHRs. Lastly, societal outcomes include being better able to conduct research and achieving improved population health (Menachemi & Collum, 2011). Other unintended results include increased success of litigation.

Duties of an EHR Specialist

The EHR specialist will perform duties that assist health care facilities and federal government agencies in the proper handling of electronic patient data, including document management, privacy and security, electronic procedures, and compliancy.

According to the U.S. Department of Labor, Bureau of Labor Statistics, medical records and health information technicians organize and manage health information data by ensuring their quality, accuracy, accessibility, and security in both paper and electronic systems by using various classification systems to code and categorize patient information for insurance reimbursement purposes, for databases and registries, and to maintain patients' medical and treatment histories.

EHR specialists are responsible for documenting patients' health information, including the medical history, symptoms, examination and test results, treatments, and other information about health care provider services. Duties will vary according to the size of the facility in which the specialist works, but typical duties include the following:

- Review patient records for timeliness, completeness, accuracy, and appropriateness of health data
- Organize and maintain data for clinical databases and registries
- Track patient outcomes for quality assessment
- Use classification software to assign clinical codes for reimbursement and data analysis
- Electronically record data for collection, storage, analysis, retrieval, and reporting
- Protect patients' health information for confidentiality, authorized access for treatment, and data security
- Although EHR specialists do not provide direct patient care, they work regularly with physicians and other health care professionals. They meet with these workers to clarify diagnoses or to obtain additional information to make sure that records are complete and accurate.

With the predominant use of EHRs, job responsibilities of medical records and health information technicians will continue to change and evolve. Specialists will need to be familiar with, or be able to learn, EHR software, follow EHR security and privacy practices, and analyze electronic data to improve health care information as more health care providers adopt EHR systems. Medical records and health information technicians can specialize in many aspects of health information. Even if a specific role such as biller and coder does not require actual documenting in the patient chart, having knowledge of the EHR software functionality is vital, such as the knowledge of how to access, record, and update information in order to ensure payment for services rendered.

Facilities in Which an EHR Specialist May Work

An EHR specialist may obtain positions in a variety of health care facilities. Most medical records and health information technicians work in hospitals or physician offices. Some work for the government. **Table 1-2** lists the industries that employed the most medical records and health information technicians in 2014, as reported by the Department of Labor.

Table 1-2 EHR Specialist—Employment by Industry	
Hospitals: state, local, and private	38%
Physician Offices	21%
Nursing Care Facilities (skilled nursing facilities)	7%
Administrative and Support Services	6%
Professional, Scientific, and Technical Services	5%

Source: U.S. Department of Labor (2014).

Use of EHRs in Ambulatory Care vs. a Hospital

There are distinct differences between the hospital-based EHR and the ambulatory EHR. Dr. Robert Rowley, in his article titled "Ambulatory vs. Hospital EHRs" (2011), identified key elements of each. Ambulatory EHRs address the workflows in the physician's office. These workflows vary (sometimes significantly) from one specialty to another. The Stage 1 criteria for Meaningful Use describe some fundamental elements needed for such systems.

Dr. Rowley describes ambulatory practices as "service nodes" in a larger ecosystem, with much of the work done in concert with other pieces of the delivery system—referring physicians, consultants, pharmacies, outside laboratories, outside X-ray and imaging centers, and so on, focusing on connectivity.

The hospital environment is quite different and tends to be more self-contained as far as the services provided, and the workflows involved are about communication between different hospital departments, generally under the same roof. The EHR in a hospital is extremely important in patient care. The EHR compiles data from multiple clinical systems and provides a single source of information about a particular patient. In addition, the EHR will capture and store information about the patient's care and will assist in managing transactions such as medicine prescribed, tests ordered/test results, and improving the quality of patient care.

Hospital information systems are quite complex. In addition to providing quality care for patients, there are other contributing factors that affect the care the patient receives, such as the financial aspect of a patient's stay, lab tests ordered, pharmacy information, picture archiving, radiology information, and clinical information.

The primary benefits of a hospital EHR are the unlimited access to patients' information, decreased waiting time for medication delivery as well as test results, and increased efficiency and accuracy in overall patient care.

Pitfalls of the Electronic Health Record

EHRs have many benefits as described earlier, but there are also a few pitfalls. In the same article by the National Center for Biotechnology Information (Menachemi & Collum, 2011), it was noted that despite the growing consensus on benefits of EHR functionalities, there are some potential disadvantages associated with this technology. These include financial issues, changes in workflow, temporary loss of productivity associated with EHR adoption, privacy and security concerns, problems that occur when the system goes down, and other unintended consequences.

The financial issues related to the EHR, including adoption and implementation costs, ongoing maintenance costs, loss of revenue associated with temporary loss of productivity, and declines in revenue, present a disincentive for hospitals and physicians. These disincentives have been partially offset with the monetary incentives provided by the federal government for providers and health care facilities to adopt EHRs.

Implementation costs for an EHR adoption include purchasing and installing hardware and software, converting paper charts to electronic ones, and training end-users. EHR maintenance can also be costly. Hardware must be replaced and software must be upgraded on a regular basis as technology improves and changes in regulations occur. In addition, ongoing training and support must be available to providers and for all users of an EHR.

Patients and providers express concern over privacy issues related to EHRs and the personal information collected by the federal government. The Affordable Care Act (ACA) mandates the IRS as the collection and enforcement arm for the federal government, which troubles many Americans. In addition, the Department of Health and Human Services (HHS) of the Obama administration issued additional rules pertaining to the ACA, that resulted in more intrusion into a patient's medical files, with the patient's privacy being sacrificed. The possible repeal and replacement of the ACA is an ongoing debate in Congress, and may result in slight or significant changes to the law. Absent any changes in the law, it is expected that some of the rules and regulations will be changed to fix some of the ACA's obvious shortcomings and deficiencies. Examples include mental health questions (e.g., "Do you, or have you ever, felt depressed?") and questions regarding relationship status, including number of sexual partners. Data-mining patients' personal health information is made easily accessible through EHRs. Many private citizens and those in the medical field question how these data will be used and by whom. For example, will the required question regarding "felt depressed" (mental health screening) then create an automatic link to the government (federal, state, and/or local) regarding the Second Amendment rights of gun ownership? Have you given thought to or do you find yourself hesitating to answer personal questions that your physician asks you during a medical exam?

PAPER RECORDS vs. PAPERLESS RECORDS

Learning Objective 4: Explain the process of converting paper health records to electronic health records (EHRs).

It is important that you have knowledge and understanding of the concepts of both paper and electronic medical records. The medical record is an important business and legal document used to support treatment decisions and to document services provided. The medical record can also be subpoenaed and used as a legal document in a court of law.

SPOTLIGHT The release of records requires a written authorization from the patient or a subpoena. Always follow office policy regarding the release of **protected health information (PHI)**. PHI is all individually identifiable health information held or maintained by a **covered entity** or its business associates acting for the covered entity that is transmitted or maintained in any form or medium. Covered entities can include health plans, health care clearinghouses, and health care providers. A **clearinghouse** is any company that processes health information and executes electronic transactions.

Important factors enter into the decision for a medical practice to convert from paper records to electronic records. Primary considerations are improved accuracy and outcomes and coordination of patient care. In addition, the federal government implemented regulations concerning the adoption and use of EHRs that provided the medical profession financial incentives for using a qualified EHR and penalties if it does not. For example, if Medicare eligible professionals (EPs) have not adopted EHR technology by 2015, the EPs fee schedule amount for covered services will be adjusted down by 1% each year. The adjustment schedule is as follows:

- 2015—99 % of Medicare physician fee schedule covered amount
- 2016—98 % of Medicare physician fee schedule covered amount
- 2017 and each subsequent year—97% of Medicare physician fee schedule covered amount
- If less than 75% of EPs have become meaningful users of EHRs by 2018, the adjustment will change by 1% point each year to a maximum of 5% (95% of Medicare covered amount).

The American Recovery and Reinvestment Act (ARRA) allows for hardship exception from the payment adjustment in certain instances. The exemption must be renewed each year and will not be given for more than five years (HealthIT.gov).

Sustainability

There has been a broad consensus among professionals in the medical field and the federal government that changes and developments in technology would better meet the needs of providers and patients than traditional patient charts. Rising health care costs and persistent errors in patient documentation have led many to advocate for the use of EHRs as an opportunity to improve upon the patient's coordination of care.

EMRs contribute to greater **sustainability** (the responsible use of resources) and coordination of patient care and also cut down on the use of printed resources. Most practices will find the process of electronic charting vs. paper charting to be time-neutral; however, safety, quality, stewardship of resources, and efficiency will be improved.

TIP   Consider this . . . Is there a greener way of doing things?

Throughout the text you will be completing Activities in Harris CareTracker PM and EMR. When you are instructed to "Print" the completed activity and place it in your assignment folder, consider saving the page to an electronic file on a thumb drive if this format is preapproved by your instructor. Always follow your instructor's direction for printing activities and for creation/submission of your assignment folder.

Government Health Initiatives

Government laws and initiatives outline the roles and responsibilities of the medical assistant. The practice of medicine is governed by the Medical Practice Act and the Board of Medical Examiners. These boards have ruled that physicians are accountable for the actions of medical assistants in their employ. Medical assistants, regardless of their amount of education, training, and experience, must act within their **scope of practice** and within certain laws and limitations. Laws and scope of practice vary from state to state, and it is the responsibility of medical assistants to research the specific requirements and restrictions that apply within their state because there is no single definition of a medical assistant and his or her scope of practice.

SPOTLIGHT   All medical assistants must work under the direction of a physician or licensed health care professional. The employer is ultimately responsible and accountable for the actions of the medical assistant, known by the Latin term *Respondeat Superior*. A medical assistant is not allowed to independently assess or triage patients, make medical evaluations, independently refill prescriptions, or give out drug samples without the approval of the physician.

CRITICAL THINKING   As a medical assistant at Napa Valley Family Health Associates (NVFHA), log on to the Medical Board of California website *http://www.mbc.ca.gov*, and search for "FAQ – Medical Assistants." Navigate to the FAQ and pick a topic. Write a one-page analysis on the subject explaining how you would apply the information learned to your position as a medical assistant. Present the paper to your instructor for class discussion.

There are a number of government initiatives that affect health care professionals and it is important to understand what these laws mean to you as a medical assistant.

HIPAA

The **Health Insurance Portability and Accountability Act (HIPAA)** law was passed in 1996, providing new directives for protecting patient information and providing security measures as well as specific requirements for electronically transmitting patient data. HIPAA privacy rules apply to all PHI regardless of the method in which the information is acquired, stored, or distributed. Covered entities are required to protect and guard against the misuse of individually identifiable health information. The amount of PHI used or disclosed should be the minimum necessary to do the job.

There are instances that a patient's PHI may be shared. For example, the HIPAA privacy regulations do not require that you obtain a patients' consent to use their PHI for routine disclosures, such as those related to treatment, payment, or health care operations (TPO). The regulations do, however, mandate that you obtain written patient consent before releasing their information for any reason other than TPO (e.g., disclosure of psychotherapy notes) (AAPP 2003).

Title I of HIPAA was intended to protect health insurance coverage for workers and their families when they change or lose their jobs. Title II of HIPAA requires the HHS to establish national standards for electronic health care transactions and national identifiers for providers, health plans, and employers. It also addresses the security and privacy of health data.

SPOTLIGHT HIPAA's minimum necessary rule:

- Must provide only PHI in the **minimum necessary** amount to accomplish the purpose for which use or disclosure is sought

- Does not apply when patients provide a valid, signed authorization for release of PHI

- De-identify information: PHI with all HIPAA identifiers removed

---

Incentives for EHR Implementation

In his 2004 State of the Union address, President Bush noted: "By computerizing health records, we can avoid dangerous medical mistakes, reduce costs, and improve care" and set a 10-year goal for all Americans to be using EHRs. Many applauded this statement, recognizing that EHRs represent an enormous opportunity to improve patient care and health system operations. However, efforts to develop the EHR represent a long journey from early visions to today's reality. The EHR is not a simple computer application; rather, it represents a carefully constructed set of systems that are highly integrated and require a significant investment of time, money, process change, and human factor reengineering.

The economic stimulus package of 2009 (the ARRA) dedicated $19 billion to the cause of accelerating the adoption of progressive health information technologies such as EHRs. Payment incentive funds were distributed in the form of incentives under Medicare and Medicaid. Medicare incentives were provided to physicians in ambulatory medical facilities that use EHRs. The total amount of Medicare incentive was $44,000 per physician, paid out over a period of five years, and paid directly to the health care professional or employer. Incentive bonus payments were also paid to physicians demonstrating they are meaningful users of a certified EHR system.

Medicaid eligible physicians received cash incentives of up to $63,750 for purchasing and using qualified EHRs. Under the Medicaid program, $21,250 was offered to every physician to assist in the procurement and implementation of a qualified EHR system. The deadline for purchasing the EHR system was 2016 to be eligible for these incentives. After the adoption of an EHR system, the Medicaid incentive program further provided $8,500 to every physician for persisting with a meaningful use of the EHR configuration.

As the government continues its attempts to lower health care costs and improve patient care, new regulations are implemented. One of those programs is the Quality Payment Program (QPP), which took effect in 2017. The Medicare Access and CHIP Reauthorization Act of 2015 (MACRA) ended the Sustainable Growth Rate formula. The QPP provides new tools and resources to help providers give patients the best possible care, such as the Merit-based Incentive Payment System (MIPS). For providers that registered, participated, and recorded data for the year 2017, Medicare will analyze the data in 2018, and providers may earn a 5% incentive payment in 2019.

Meaningful Use

Meaningful use is the set of standards defined by CMS incentive programs that governs the use of EHRs and allows eligible providers and hospitals to earn incentive payments by meeting specific criteria. For EMR software to be certified, it must meet meaningful use. These standards ensure that providers are using their EMR software to its fullest potential, promoting accuracy, access, patient empowerment, and better coordination of care. Chapter 5 expands on meaningful use and its specific stages.

Affordable Care Act

The Affordable Care Act (ACA) was passed by Congress and then signed into law by President Obama on March 23, 2010. On June 28, 2012, the Supreme Court rendered a final decision to uphold a key provision of the health care law, citing the authority of Congress to impose a tax. The Internal Revenue Service (IRS) is responsible for the collection and taxation provisions of the ACA. Many crucial elements of the ACA law were written after the passage of the law in 2010. The debate over the ACA, including the benefits of the law and also its negative aspects continues. While more people are covered with the Medicaid expansion, the mandates and costs of health insurance have shifted to the middle class, which makes their coverage even more unaffordable.

There are also the unintended consequences from such extensive legislation to overhaul the health care industry. Contrary to the promises that passage of the ACA would lower health care costs and health care insurance costs, insurance premiums have skyrocketed and the law still does not cover all uninsured or underinsured Americans. At the passage of the ACA in 2010 it was claimed there were approximately 30 million uninsured, yet the *Fiscal Times* and the Kaiser Family Foundation reported there were still as many as 29 million Americans uninsured in 2016, a negligible change, especially considering all the costs associated with the law. The mandate that every American must purchase health insurance, and insurance that meets government requirements, has taken away the freedom of choice of an individual to purchase insurance or not, or to purchase a policy that meets his or her individual needs. There is a shift in sentiment with less people favoring the law as they become familiar with more of the regulations involved, including significant increases in premiums, increases in out-of-pocket expenses, and significantly higher deductibles. During the health care debate of 2009, President Obama promised "First of all, if you've got health insurance, you like your doctors, you like your plan, you can keep your doctor, you can keep your plan" (ABCNews.com, 2009). However, many employers dropped coverage for employees due to the skyrocketing costs, or in the alternative, were forced to find ways to be exempt from the legislation (e.g., reduce hours for employees to less than 30 hours per week). Insurance companies are issuing policy cancellations and increases in premiums at an alarming rate, citing ACA mandates in coverage that rendered many of the pre-ACA existing policies noncompliant. Many insurers have pulled out of the government health exchanges, offering few or no options in some states. There are states and counties with only one health insurer in the exchange, if any at all. This has severely restricted choice and caused premiums to spike. In addition, some providers are retiring or no longer accepting Medicare or Medicaid patients due to the burdensome regulations, reductions in fees paid to them, and restrictions on how providers are able to care for their patients. This is creating a growing shortage of doctors, especially primary care physicians.

There is significant debate ongoing whether to "repeal", "replace", or "repeal and replace" the ACA. The overwhelming volume of regulations makes changes to the law difficult at best. Congress and the Trump administration have focused on changes to the law and reaching solutions to address the failures of the current law but have yet to reach consensus.

Converting the Practice

Although most medical practices have converted to electronic health records, there are still some that have not, mostly solo practitioners. The cost to convert a medical practice from paper records to electronic records can be expensive and time-consuming. Costs include the EHR program (software), the technical components (hardware, e.g., computer, scanner, and wireless connectivity), the time to **abstract** data from the paper charts, and to train and provide support to employees and physicians. To abstract data means to condense a record. In the context of medical records, entering data from the patients' paper chart into an EHR is abstracting. For example, the patient's problem list, current medications, allergies, and personal and family history are entered into the electronic chart as a baseline of medical history.

A **total conversion** is when all paper records are converted to electronic records at once. This method can be costly and often would need to be outsourced so as not to interrupt services to patients. Many practices convert their paper records to electronic in a gradual or an incremental process, adding components as the staff becomes familiar with the application. A gradual or an incremental conversion tends to lower the initial cash outlay and provides a smooth transition. Some practices will use a combination of paper and electronic data, often referred to as **hybrid conversion**. Regardless of the format used, the provider is the one that must complete the patient examination and progress note.

An analysis of workflow changes and a prearranged schedule can be quite helpful in determining the stages of implementation. For example, once the EHR product has been selected (e.g., Harris CareTracker), the practice will determine a "go-live" date that accounts for acquisition and installation of hardware, training for the staff, and reducing the patient schedule during the initial transition. (Learning Objective 5 more fully addresses workflow in the medical office.)

 CRITICAL THINKING Drawing from your personal experience as a medical assistant and as a patient, describe your present medical office. Has the practice converted from paper to electronic records? If so, when? What advantages/disadvantages have you observed? If not, how would you advocate for the transition? Support your position with facts and personal experience.

The EHR Specialist—Administrative and Practice Management

To promote greater safety, quality, and efficiency in health care delivery, a committee of the Institute of Medicine of the National Academies identified a set of eight core care delivery functions that EHR systems should be capable of performing. The committee's report was sponsored by the U.S. Department of Health and Human Services and is one part of a public and private collaborative effort to advance the adoption of EHR systems. The list of key capabilities will be used by **Health Level 7 (HL7)**, one of the world's leading developers of health care standards for exchanging information between medical applications, to devise a common industry standard for EHR functionality that will guide the efforts of software developers. HL7 is known as a messaging standard used to transfer data between applications. The eight core functions are listed next and described further in **Table 1-1**:

1. Health information and data
2. Result management
3. Order management
4. Decision support

5. Electronic communication and connectivity

6. Patient support

7. Administrative processes and reporting

8. Reporting and population health management

The EHR specialist is expected to know how to input information into an EHR and will commonly find work in physician offices, laboratories, urgent care centers, nursing home facilities, wellness clinics, and hospitals. In addition to traditional occupations, new technology will open many opportunities. The HIT field will provide new, often high-paying, positions such as clinical analyst, health information technician, and records and information coordinator.

A key element of your position as a medical assistant and EHR specialist is to be an active listener and demonstrate respect in your communications, both verbal and nonverbal, with coworkers, patients, providers, and visitors. Always be patient, courteous, and respectful. Refrain from using a negative tone, remark, or expression.

ADMINISTRATIVE WORKFLOWS IN HARRIS CARETRACKER

Learning Objective 5: Summarize administrative workflows in Harris CareTracker.

Workflow is defined as how tasks are performed throughout the office (usually in a specific order), for example, the patient is checked in, insurance cards are scanned, copay is collected, and then the patient is taken to the exam room where vital signs are taken/recorded, and so on. Conducting a comprehensive workflow analysis is a critical step in EHR implementation. Workflow analysis allows health care organizations to critically look at how work is currently being done in the practice. In general, workflow analysis should be conducted prior to EHR implementation. This will provide a benchmark of current workflows, which can then be refined during the implementation process. **Figure 1-14** is an example of patient flow.

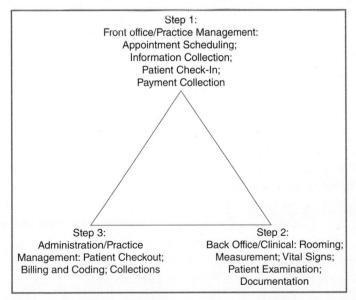

Figure 1-14   Patient Flow

PRACTICE MANAGEMENT

Learning Objective 6: Discuss practice management, front office, billing, and administrative functions.

Practice management (PM) software runs the business side of health care, from registering a new patient and scheduling patient visits to coding and billing the patient encounter and generating monthly reports. Harris CareTracker PM software can be customized to user preferences. PM software maximizes provider productivity and meets rigorous scheduling demands. Alert messages, a master index, and insurance profiles help reduce error and administrative expenses during registration and charge entry.

Front Office

Front office duties begin with patient demographics (searching for an existing patient, registering a new patient, and editing patient information). Once patient demographics and insurance information are recorded, appointments are scheduled. Much of the patient contact in the front office takes place on the telephone, such as when a patient will call in to the office to make an appointment. Not only must you carefully record the patient's demographic information, you must screen the call to determine the most appropriate appointment type and availability. Your knowledge and skills as a medical assistant will be invaluable in determining the urgency of the patient's condition. While operating within your scope of practice, you can take a message for your provider or schedule a routine appointment. If the call is urgent, you must follow office policy and either refer the patient to emergency services or contact the provider for additional instructions.

Accurate documentation in the electronic record is crucial. You must be certain that you are documenting in the correct patient's chart, recording messages for the provider with utmost accuracy, as well as documenting the chief complaint and prescription details. When there is to be a call back to the patient, confirm the telephone number(s) and best time to call. Repeat information you have recorded back to the caller to verify accuracy. Be polite, courteous, and professional at all times.

Your front office duties will also include patient interactions in the office. You will greet the patient upon arrival, accept insurance cards for copying, collect copays, and check the patient in for his or her visit. Each activity or transaction is recorded in Harris CareTracker PM. Once a patient has completed his or her visit, he or she may be asked to schedule a follow-up appointment. Taking instruction from the provider, schedule future appointments and provide any patient education (health information) materials as advised.

The Harris CareTracker PM task sheet (**Figure 1-15**) provides a quick reference guide to the daily, weekly, and monthly tasks for front office, billing, and administrative duties of the medical assistant.

Billing

Entering a patient's insurance information accurately in the *Insurance* section of the *Demographics* application ensures that insurance companies will pay claims in a timely manner. Accurate and complete information begins with the required fields entered into a patient's demographic screen. Any required information that is missing will prevent a claim from being submitted and/or paid and will affect the revenue cycle of the practice.

Although appointments may be booked for the patient with only the name fields populated, insurance claims cannot be processed until the remainder of the *Demographics* information is complete. If a patient lives outside of the United States, his or her address must be entered differently than a patient who lives in the country. Statements will *not* be sent to foreign addresses, but setting up the patient's *Demographics* correctly will prevent the claim from becoming an unbilled claim due to the patient's address. If a patient's sex is not entered, claims for the patient will *not* be electronically transmitted to the insurance company. Any claim lacking a specified sex will become an unbilled claim and will remain as such until an operator specifies a sex and re-bills the claim. The billing functions of Harris CareTracker PM are featured in Chapter 9.

Harris CareTracker Practice Management PM Task Sheet   HARRIS CareTracker

DAILY TASKS

FRONT OFFICE			BILLING		ADMINISTRATIVE
Before Appointment	*Day of*	*End of Day*	[ ] Review NEWS	[ ] Review/work open	[ ] Review/work open
[ ] Clear cache	[ ] Create batch	[ ] Review visits and		To Dos, Faxes and Mail	To Dos, Faxes and Mail
[ ] Review NEWS	[ ] Review/work open	charges on hold	[ ] Clear cache	[ ] Work credit balances by batch	[ ] Clear cache
[ ] Review missing	To Dos, Faxes and Mail	[ ] Run journal and	[ ] Create batch	[ ] Work denials	[ ] Review NEWS
information	[ ] Enter demographics	balance deposit	[ ] Work the claims worklist	[ ] Print journal and	
[ ] Work eligibility work list	[ ] Enter ref/auth/cases	[ ] Post batch	[ ] Review electronic	balance payments	
[ ] Print encounter forms and	[ ] Book appointments	[ ] Cancel no shows	reports received	[ ] Run verify payments	
appointment list		[ ] Review appointment	[ ] Correct errors and rebill	[ ] Review/reconcile unapplied cash	
[ ] Confirm appointments		conflicts	[ ] Close open electronic	[ ] Save admission visits	
[ ] Review/Reschedule	*Patient Contact*		claim batches	[ ] Post batch	
wait list appointments	[ ] Check-in		[ ] Print paper claims	[ ] Check on new insurances	
[ ] Print unprinted	[ ] Verify insurance and		/flag as printed	[ ] Send To Do(s) to others	
correspondence	other patient info		[ ] Enter charges or	where help is req	
	[ ] Check eligibility (walk-ins,		save bulk charges	[ ] Work unpaid/inactive	
Harris CareTracker	new patients, changes)		[ ] Review and save	claims	
Patient Portal	[ ] Post co-payment		admissions entered	[ ] Generate claims	
[ ] Accept/deny patient	[ ] Print receipt		[ ] Post payments (manually		
demographic updates	[ ] Print encounter form		and electronically)		
[ ] Work appointment	[ ] Enter visit (MD or staff)		[ ] Close electronic remit		
requests			files/or make inactive		

WEEKLY TASKS

FRONT OFFICE	BILLING	ADMINISTRATIVE	
[ ] Weekly call w/Account Manager*	[ ] Verify claims are on file for major payors	[ ] Verify users have the	[ ] Review Rx refill requests
[ ] Print unprinted correspondence	[ ] Electronic claim verification	correct permissions	[ ] Review lab results
[ ] Review missing encounters	[ ] Review unbilled procedure balances	[ ] Review and close	[ ] Review charts
[ ] Open To Do(s) -- open and	[ ] Work collection accounts	To Do(s) out to	[ ] Review notes entered
closed client review		terminated employees	[ ] Review new Rx's
[ ] Recalls -- past due follow up		[ ] Remove terminated	[ ] Check on Rx's
[ ] Review undeliverable/forwarded		employees from list	that may have failed
statements/ letters		of operators	transmission
		[ ] Reset employee passwords	[ ] Review orders
		as needed	[ ] Review visits

MONTHLY TASKS

FRONT OFFICE	BILLING	
[ ] Send recalls	[ ] Run bulk apply unapplieds	[ ] Print month end reports
	[ ] Month end close period	[ ] Review credit balances
	[ ] Open new fiscal period	

QUARTERLY TASKS

FRONT OFFICE	BILLING	ADMINISTRATIVE
[ ] Read release notes	[ ] Read release notes	[ ] Ensure employees read release notes
[ ] Attend live or view recorded release training	[ ] Attend live or view recorded release training	[ ] Ensure employees attend live or view recorded release training

Harris CareTracker Practice Management TASKS

[ ] Transmit claims
[ ] Software support
[ ] Software updates
* Only for Full Service Clients

Courtesy of Harris CareTracker PM and EMR

Figure 1-15   *Harris CareTracker PM Task Sheet*

Administrative

The *Administration* module contains the *Administration* application, which is divided into three tabs: *Practice, Clinical,* and *Setup*. Functions of the *Practice* tab (**Figure 1-16**) include *Daily Administration, System Administration, Import/Export,* and *Knowledgebase*. These functions contain financial, forms and letters, security logs, messages, and patient security. The *Clinical* tab (**Figure 1-17**) includes *Daily Administration, System Administration,* and *Import/Export* functions, which contain forms and letters, security logs, clinical setup, and maintenance. The *Setup* tab (**Figure 1-18**) is where you set up PM features. Each tab is organized into sections containing links to other applications in Harris CareTracker PM. Chapter 2 introduces *Administration* features and activities associated with Harris CareTracker.

Every operator must have a user name and a password to log into Harris CareTracker PM and EMR. You are required to change your password every 90 days. Harris CareTracker PM and EMR reminds users seven days before their password expires and gives them the option to change their password at any time after they begin using Harris CareTracker PM and EMR, even prior to the system requirement.

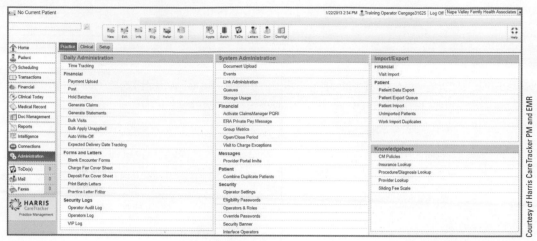

Figure 1-16   Administration/Practice Tab

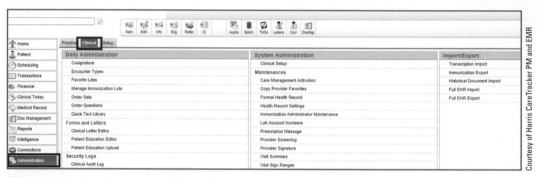

Figure 1-17   Administration/Clinical Tab

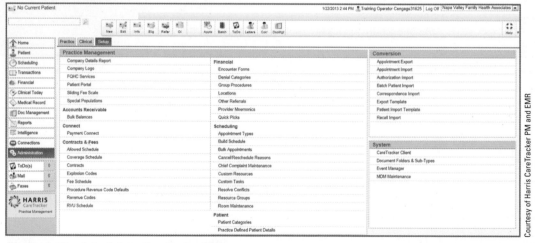

Figure 1-18   Administration/Setup Tab

CLASSIFICATION SYSTEMS

Learning Objective 7: Define classification systems.

Classification systems organize related terms into categories for easy retrieval. These classification systems are used for billing and reimbursement, statistical reporting, and administrative functions. There is the expectation with EHRs that the terminology and classification systems work in concert together and support both efficient and effective clinical information and administrative needs for health care organizations. Classifications and terminologies meet diverse user data requirements and are designed for distinctly different purposes. Clinical terminologies are considered the input format, whereas classification systems are the output format.

HIPAA required the HHS to establish national standards, some of which include specific code sets and electronic transactions. The following code set standards were named by HIPAA:

- CPT® (outpatient procedure codes)

- HCPCS (items and supplies and nonphysician services not covered by CPT®-IV)

- ICD-10-CM and ICD-10-PCS (the current diagnosis coding system [implemented October 1, 2015])

- **National Drug Code (NDC)**—a code that identifies all medications recognized by the Food and Drug Administration (FDA) by vendor (manufacturer), product, and package size.

Examples of output systems would be ICD-10-CM and ICD-10-PCS. These are typically used for external reporting requirements and are not intended or designed for the primary documentation of clinical care. The input systems, such as SNOMED-CT®, are designed for the primary documentation of clinical care. Together, clinical terminologies and classification systems represent a common medical language that allows data to be shared.

The **Systemized Nomenclature of Medicine, Clinical Terms (SNOMED-CT®)** is the most comprehensive clinical health care terminology in the world, contributing to the advancement of patient care by improving the recording of EHR information, allowing health care facilities to better communicate. **Nomenclature** is a system of terms used in a particular science. SNOMED-CT® is defined as a comprehensive clinical terminology covering diseases, clinical findings, and procedures that allows for a consistent way of indexing, storing, retrieving, and aggregating clinical data across specialties and sites of care. SNOMED-CT® terminology helps structure the electronic medical record.

The universal terms and code system for the identification and electronic exchange of laboratory and clinical observations is known as **Logical Observation Identifiers Names and Codes (LOINC®)**. LOINC® enables the exchange and aggregation of electronic health data from many independent systems and includes standardized terms for all kinds of observations and measurements. The **Unified Medical Language System (UMLS®)** is another clinical standard. It is a set of files and software that brings together many health and biomedical vocabularies and standards to enable interoperability between EHRs, that is, a thesaurus database of medical terminology.

CODING SYSTEMS

Learning Objective 8: Distinguish between coding systems such as the International Classification of Diseases (ICD), Healthcare Common Procedural Coding System (HCPCS), and Current Procedural Terminology (CPT®).

Harris CareTracker features an automatic coding process that checks procedure and diagnosis codes for accuracy. For a provider to receive reimbursement for services, every procedure and diagnosis must be documented in the patient's medical record. Integrating automated coding with billing facilitates claims processing. Computer-assisted coding in EHRs works in a variety of ways, with some systems using keywords or analysis of words, phrases, and sentences. Harris CareTracker features *ClaimsManager* and *EncoderPro*®. When all the appropriate CPT® and ICD codes are entered, *EncoderPro*®, Harris CareTracker's partner for online code verification, can be run to verify all the procedures, diagnoses, and modifiers entered for a patient. Clicking on the *EncoderPro.com*® button (**Figure 1-19**) helps to ensure that correct coding information is entered and that claims are processed and paid quickly (**Figure 1-20**).

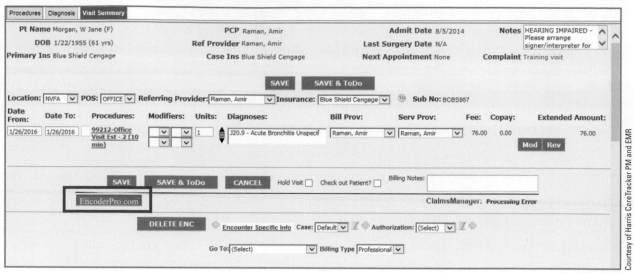

Figure 1-19   EncoderPro Button

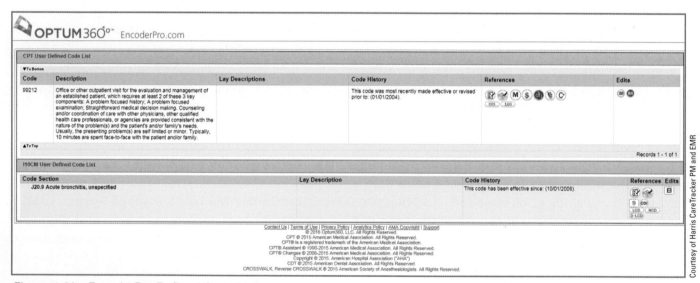

Figure 1-20   EncoderPro Defined Code List

Coding Fundamentals

Most EHRs have features that automate the coding process. Although the features of each EHR may vary, the codes are checked for accuracy by a coding specialist or program. Harris CareTracker's automated coding process is the *ClaimsManager* feature, and it utilizes *EncoderPro.com*® to provide further coding detail.

Every service submitted for payment must be documented in the patient's medical record. To receive reimbursement, providers must document each service provided to the patient. The integration of automated coding with the billing system facilitates claims processing.

International Classification of Diseases (ICD)

As of October 1, 2015, the **International Classification of Diseases** code set of ICD-10 is the internationally recognizable code set representing medical conditions or signs and symptoms (standardized categorization of diseases/diagnosis codes) in a health care setting, developed by the World Health Organization (WHO).

SPOTLIGHT Characteristics of the ICD-10-CM Coding book format used in the outpatient setting:

- Single codebook, with two parts.
- The Index to Diseases and Injuries is an alphabetic listing of terms and corresponding codes.
- The two sections of the alphabetic index are the Index to Diseases and Injuries and the Index to External Causes of Injury. A Neoplasm Table and Table of Drugs and Chemicals are also included in the Index.
- The Tabular List of Diseases and Injuries is an alphanumeric list of codes. The Tabular List is divided into chapters based on body systems (anatomical site) or condition (etiology).

ICD-10 is the international classification that contains the most significant changes in the history of ICD. The alphanumeric format provides a better structure than did ICD-9. ICD-10 allows considerable space for future revision without disrupting the numbering system.

ICD-10 codes consist of up to seven alphanumeric digits, with the seventh digit extension representing the visit encounter or **sequelae** (an aftereffect of disease, condition, or injury; a secondary result) for injuries and external causes. **Table 1-3** outlines the features of ICD-10-CM codes. The change was transformational to the health care industry.

Table 1-3 Features of ICD-10-CM Codes

FEATURE	DETAILS
Number of codes	Approximately 68,000
Code length	Three to seven characters
Code structure	Three-character category Fourth, fifth, sixth characters for etiology, anatomic site, severity Seventh character extension for additional information
First character	First character is always alphabetic
Subsequent characters	Second character is always numeric; all other characters may be alphabetic or numeric
Decimal point	Mandatory after the third character on all codes
Extensions	Some codes use a seventh character as an extension to provide additional information
Placeholders	Character "X" is used as a placeholder in certain six- and seven-character codes

Healthcare Common Procedural Coding System (HCPCS)

In 1983, Medicare developed a new coding system to supplement CPT® Level I, which is currently known as the Healthcare Common Procedural Coding System (HCPCS). HCPCS is divided into two principal subsystems, referred to as Level I and Level II of the HCPCS. Level I is used to represent a service provided by health care providers in an outpatient setting. Level II of the HCPCS is a standardized coding system that is used primarily to identify products, supplies, and services not included in the CPT® codes (such as ambulance services and durable medical equipment [DME]). HCPCS Level II codes are maintained and distributed by the CMS. **Modifiers**, which append the HCPCS codes, are two-digit (alphanumeric or numeric) characters and different from those listed in CPT®. A modifier is a two-character code added to a CPT® or HCPCS code that is used to help in the reimbursement process. For example, a modifier is used to explain that a procedure not normally covered when billed on the same day as another is actually a separate and significant process, or that it is a rural health procedure that gets higher reimbursement. Up to four modifiers can be attached to each CPT® code, although in most cases only one or two are used. Modifiers should be appended to Medicare claims whenever applicable.

Current Procedural Terminology (CPT®) (HCPCS Level I)

Current Procedural Terminology (CPT®) is a nationally recognized numeric or alphanumeric coding system maintained by the American Medical Association (AMA) and represents a service provided by health care providers in an outpatient setting. CPT® is Level I of the Healthcare Common Procedural Coding System (HCPCS). Level I does not include codes needed to separately report medical items or services that are regularly billed by suppliers other than physicians. The CPT® codebook is divided into sections and code ranges as noted in **Table 1-4**.

Table 1-4   HCPCS Level I Codes and Descriptions Section/Code Range of CPT®

SECTION	CODE RANGE
Evaluation and Management	99201-99499
Anesthesia	00100-01999, 99100-99140
Surgery	10021-69990
Radiology (Including Nuclear Medicine and Diagnostic Ultrasound)	70010-79999
Pathology and Laboratory	80047-89398
Medicine (except Anesthesiology)	90281-99199, 99500-99607

Source: Current Procedural Terminology © 2017 American Medical Association.

HCPCS Level II

Table 1-5 provides a section/code range for HCPCS Level II codes.

Table 1-5   HCPCS Level II Codes and Descriptions

SECTION	CODE RANGE
Transportation Services Including Ambulance	A0021-A9999
Enteral and Parenteral Therapy	B4034-B9999
Outpatient PPS	C1713-C9899
Durable Medical Equipment (DME)	E0100-E8002

SECTION	CODE RANGE
Procedures/Professional Services (Temporary)	G0008-G9862
Alcohol and Drug Abuse Treatment	H0001-H2037
Drugs Administered Other than Oral Method	J0120-J7685
Chemotherapy Drugs	J7686-J9999
Temporary Codes	K0001-K0900
Orthotic Devices and Procedures	L0112-L4631
Prosthetic Procedures	K5000-L8695
Medical Services	M0075-M0301
Pathology and Laboratory Services	P2028-P9615
Q Codes (Temporary Codes)	Q0035-Q9983
Diagnostic Radiology Services	R0070-R0076
Temporary National Codes (Non-Medicare)	S0012-S9999
National T Codes Established for State Medicaid Agencies (State Medicaid)	T1000-T5999
Vision Services	V2020-V2799
Hearing Services	V5008-V5364
Appendix 1—Table of Drugs and Biologicals	
Appendix 2—Modifiers	
Appendix 3—Abbreviations and Acronyms	
Appendix 4—Internet-only Manuals (IOMs)	
Appendix 5 New, Changed, Deleted, and Reinstated HCPCS Codes	
Appendix 6—Place of Service and Type of Service	

CLINICAL COMPONENTS AND CLINICAL WORKFLOWS IN HARRIS CARETRACKER

Learning Objective 9: Identify clinical components of the EHR and clinical workflows in Harris CareTracker.

In addition to the administrative and practice management functions, it is vital to have an understanding of clinical duties and definitions. **Table 1-6** provides an explanation of clinical components of the EHR.

Table 1-6 Clinical Components of the EHR

Allergies	A list of the patient's allergies as well as his or her reactions to each one
Chief Complaint	A verbal account made by the patient describing his or her problems
Diagnosis and Assessment	The physician's conclusion regarding the cause of the patient's problem
Family History	Information regarding the medical problems of the patient's family
HPI (History of Present Illness)	A compilation of information regarding all aspects of the patient's present illness
Medication List	Information regarding the dosage and frequency of the patient's medications
Past Medical History	Information regarding the patient's past medical problems, conditions, or surgeries
Plan and Treatment	The physician's recommended plan of action to cure or manage the patient's condition
Progress Notes	Documentation of the care delivered to a patient along with necessary information regarding diagnosis and treatment
ROS (Review of Systems)	An inventory of body systems in which the patient reports signs or symptoms he or she is currently having or has had in the past
Social History	Information regarding the patient's lifestyle such as smoking and drinking habits, relationship status, and sexual history
Vital Signs	Measurements of the patient's temperature, respirations, pulse, and blood pressure

Computer Physician Order Entry

The EHR improves clinical documentation and orders by use of **Computer Physician Order Entry (CPOE)**. CPOE is an application used by physicians and other health care providers to enter patient care information. EHRs with the CPOE feature also provide support tools that result in improved care and patient outcomes. eMars work with the CPOE system to increase patient safety by electronically tracking medication administration. eMars is Electronic [Customized] Medication Administration Records.

An **order set** is a grouping of treatment options for a specific diagnosis or condition. Using an order set, rather than individual orders, helps standardize patient care, expedite order entry, and minimize possible delays due to inconsistent or incomplete orders. Order sets are predefined groupings of standard orders for a condition, disease, or procedure. These order sets make it easier to deliver patient care by eliminating errors and providing easy access to clinical content. You must have the appropriate security setting on your user profile to access the *Administration* module in Harris CareTracker to modify order sets.

As addressed in the administrative workflow (Learning Objective 5) discussion, it is helpful to follow a workflow assessment guide and checklist. Harris CareTracker *Help* provides an EHR Task Sheet (**Figure 1-21**) outlining clinical workflows.

 CRITICAL THINKING Familiarize yourself with the task sheet of Clinical Workflows (refer to Figure 1-21) and then complete **Table 1-7** by identifying the action and describing how the workflow of electronic vs. paper records would differ, and which role would perform visit workflow responsibilities. The first answer has been stated for you as an example.

HARRIS CareTracker

Harris Caretracker EMR Task Sheet

CLINICAL

Visit	Daily	Weekly and Quarterly
Patient Visit (or Encounter) Activities [ ] Review/Update Patient's Clinical Information [ ] Enter Chief Complaint & Vital Signs [ ] Review/Update History & Immunization Panes [ ] Lab/Imaging Results Committed to Chart & Orders are Linked/Completed [ ] Document Progress Note [ ] Review/Resolve Open Activities [ ] Review/Resolve Pt Care Management Items [ ] Medications (New/Refills) Completed [ ] Lab/Imaging Orders Created [ ] Patient Education, Referrals, Clinical Letters, Recalls, & ToDo's Created [ ] Progress Note Signed [ ] Communication to Referring Provider & Patient as needed (HT&RPP) [ ] Visit Capture Complete [ ] Patient Provided Copy of Chart Summary	*Daily Activities* [ ] Read Harris CareTracker Mail [ ] ToDo(s) Completed(inc.messages from Provider Portal) [ ] Rx Refills Completed Within 48 Hours* [ ] Review/Submit Saved or Failed Rx(s) New & Renewals [ ] Link Lab/Radiology Results to Open Orders [ ] Lab/Radiology Results Committed [ ] Open Encounter [ ] Visits Captured [ ] Progress Notes Signed [ ] Incoming Documents [ ] Scanned or Paper Results Manually Entered [ ] Matched [ ] Signed [ ] Voice Attachments [ ] Untranscribed Notes [ ] Print Scheduled Charts (for next day) [ ] Enter Admissions (if applicable)	*Weekly Activities*** [ ] Print Scheduled Charts (every Friday) [ ] Administrative Review of Quick Tasks (for all providers) [ ] Order Tracking/Run Overdue Orders Report [ ] Repopulate Registries [ ] Read Harris CareTracker News [ ] Clear Your Cache *Quarterly Activities*** [ ] Ensure employees read release notes [ ] Ensure employees attend live or view recorded release training
*Surescript requirement		**Also see Administrative Tasks related to Clinical Oversight on the PM Task Sheet

Visit Workflow Responsibilities	Which Role?
Check In	
Take Back	
Vital Signs & Chief Complaint (if done prior to PN)	
Problem List	
Med List	
Allergy	
Update History Pane & Immunizations	
Open Activity/Patient Care Mgmt Review	
Complete Orders/Link/Manual Enter Results	
Progress Note/ Data Entered & Signed	
ePrescriptions/printed scripts	
Clinical Orders (Labs/Referrals/Immunizations)	
Clinical Letters	
Recall Creation or ToDo for Next Appt	
Patient Education Handouts	
Visit Capture	
Check Out Including ToDos	

Figure 1-21 Clinical Workflows—Task Sheet

Table 1-7 Clinical Workflows and Actions

WORKFLOW	ACTIONS	PAPER VS. ELECTRONIC RECORDS
Visit	List patient visit (or encounter) activities: *Review/Update Patient's Clinical Information*	Describe how the workflow of electronic vs. paper records would differ: *MA would enter data using a computer into an EMR vs. writing on paper*
Daily Activities	List daily clinical activities ____________	Describe how the workflow of electronic vs. paper records would differ ____________
Weekly Activities	List weekly clinical activities ____________	Describe how the workflow of electronic vs. paper records would differ ____________
Quarterly Activities	List quarterly clinical activities ____________	Describe how the workflow of electronic vs. paper records would differ ____________
Visit Workflow Responsibilities	List visit workflow responsibilities ____________	Which role would perform each of these duties? ____________

COMMON ACRONYMS AND TERMINOLOGY

Learning Objective 10: List common acronyms and terminology associated with EHRs.

Throughout this text and during your career as a medical assistant, you must be familiar with common acronyms and terminology associated with the medical field and often used in EHRs. In addition to the key terms identified throughout the text, **Table 1-8** provides a comprehensive list of acronyms and terminology that are aligned with EHRs. Additional key terms and medical terminology are available on your Student Companion site.

Table 1-8 Common Acronyms and Terminology Associated with Electronic Health Records

TERMS/ACRONYMS	DEFINITIONS
AC (prescription abbreviation)	Take before meals
acute care	Treat patient with urgent problem
ambulatory care	Treatment without admission
clinical standards	Ensure consistency, reliability, safety
clinical templates	Progress notes made within the EHR; allows documentation into the EHR; *must be interoperable*
clinical vocabularies	A standardized system of medical terminology; set of common definitions for medical terms
computer-based, stand alone	Personal health records that patients can access using a software program that has been downloaded onto a patient's personal computer, or by accessing through a secure website
CVX	Vaccine Administered *Immunizations*
designated record sets (DRS)	Any item, collection, or grouping of information that includes PHI and is maintained by a covered entity
DICOM (Digital Imaging and Communication in Medicine)	A standardized system used in the outpatient setting; imaging information to workstations
eMars (electronic medication administration records)	The rights of medication administration: right patient, right medication, right dose, right time, right route, right documentation, right reason, right response
ePHI (electronic protected health information)	Protected health information that is created, received, maintained, or transmitted in electronic format
general authorization	Required for uses other than TPO
health plan	Insurance plan; provides or pays for medical care
HIT (health information technology)	The use of technology as a resource to manage patient health care information
HPI	History of Present Illness

TERMS/ACRONYMS	DEFINITIONS
h.s. (prescription abbreviation)	Take at bedtime
ICD (International Classification of Disease)	Standards developed by WHO Diagnosis codes used in health care setting to include diseases, signs, symptoms, conditions, and preventive care
• ICD-10 Diagnosis Usage	Inpatient and outpatient Three to seven alphanumeric characters Of the approximately 155,000 ICD-10 codes total, there are roughly 68,000 diagnosis codes (CM)
• ICD-10-PCS Procedure Usage	Inpatient Seven alphanumeric characters Approximately 87,000 codes of the total ICD-10 codes are procedure usage (PCS)
IEEE (Institute of Electric and Electronics Engineering)	Device/device connectivity; used to provide communication between medical devices
incremental conversion	Gradual change; smoother; less impact on office; lower cost. Disadvantages: paper still used; not all data available
Internet-based network and interoperable	A networked PHR that allows the transfer of patient information, providers, and health care organizations such as insurance carriers and pharmacies. A networked PHR is continually updated. Potential disadvantage is that networked PHRs do not ensure complete privacy and security
Internet-based, tethered	Patients gain access to their PHR through an outside organization (e.g., insurance company or patient's provider). May have limited editing capabilities. Ownership is maintained by the organization that provides access to the patient (user)
Internet-based, untethered	Patients granted access to their PHR through a web-based application. After creating a user name and password, patient is able to create and update information as needed
medication reconciliation	Obtain and update list of patients meds
MVX	Manufacturers of Vaccines *Immunizations*
National Health Information Network	Links medical records across the country
NCPDP (National Council for Prescription Drug Program)	Retail pharmacy transactions, Standardized system used to transfer prescription information
NIP	National Immunization Program
Notice of privacy practices (NPP)	Document that describes practices regarding the use and disclosure of protected health information; a requirement of HIPAA
ONC-HIT (Office of the National Coordinator-HIT)	Group that identified standards for electronic exchange
PHR (personal health record)	Patient's life history in electronic format; does not replace legal record; patient owns
p.o. (prescription abbreviation)	Per oral (take by mouth)

(*continues*)

Table 1-8 Common Acronyms and Terminology Associated with Electronic Health Records *(continued)*

TERMS/ACRONYMS	DEFINITIONS
Providers	People or organizations that furnish, bill, or are paid for health care services in the normal course of business
Rights of Individuals	Notice of privacy act given to patient; *right to access and inspect a copy of PHI; request amendment of record; request restrictions on uses and disclosure;file complaint with Office of Civil Rights*
specific authorization	Required for HIV, STD, drug and alcohol abuse
standards	Commonly agreed-upon specification
total conversion	All data converted at once; office still operates; can be outsourced; costly
TPO (treatment, plan, and operations)	Conditions under which PHI can be released without consent of the patient

Medical Terminology

In addition to the many common acronyms and EHR terminology contained in Table 1-8, to further understand health care terminology you must perform word analysis. Words are broken down into word roots, prefixes, suffixes, and combining vowels and forms.

- Word roots, or base words, are the foundation of the health care term.
- A suffix is a word ending.
- A prefix is a word beginning.
- A combining vowel (usually "o") links the root to the suffix or to another root.
- The combining form is the word root plus the appropriate combining vowel.

Word analysis example: osteoarthritis (oste/o/arthr/itis)

- oste (bone)
- o (combining vowel)
- arthr (joint)
- itis (inflammation)

Additional medical terminology resources are available on your Student Companion site. Included are examples of some prefixes and their meanings, examples of some suffixes and their meanings, additional suffixes used to describe therapeutic interventions, combining forms and their meanings, positional and directional terms, and action terms.

CRITICAL THINKING Now that you have completed your Chapter 1 activities, how did the challenge put forth in the Real-World Connection apply? Did you carefully read and implement all of the directions when setting up your computer for the first time? Were you able to successfully create your Harris CareTracker training company? Elaborate on your successes and any challenges you encountered.

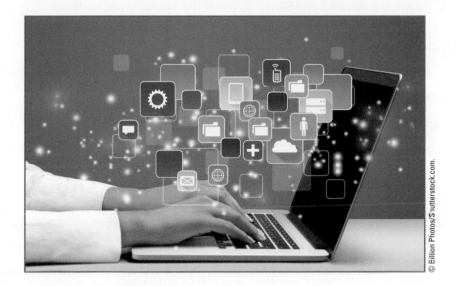

© Billion Photos/Shutterstock.com.

SUMMARY

Chapter 1 has introduced you to the paperless medical office and provided you with the background and steps to set up your computer for optimum functionality and to complete the registration of your Harris CareTracker training company credentials.

Remember that electronic medical records (EMRs) refer to patient records in a digital format, whereas the electronic health record (EHR) refers to the interoperability of EMRs or the ability to share medical records with other health care facilities. Workflows of the paper vs. electronic record medical practice were reviewed and you can use your critical thinking skills to determine how you would best adapt to and improve workflows in your current workplace.

You are now familiar with some of the many government health initiatives, rules, and laws surrounding the creation of, implementation of, and current and ongoing regulatory reforms regarding EHRs in the medical practice. The Affordable Care Act (ACA) was signed into law in 2010 but the debate continues. Burdensome rules and mandates have made the ACA unaffordable to many. The Congress and administration are likely to amend, repealed, or modify the law. The debate over access to health care and health insurance costs will likely continue as attempts to control costs and provide access are formulated.

Health information technology (HIT) is in a constant state of evolution, improving functionalities and compliance with new and changing laws. Harris CareTracker PM and EMR is a fully integrated CCHIT® and ONC-ATCB–certified complete practice management (PM) and electronic medical record (EMR). You will be introduced to the specific features and functionalities of the Harris CareTracker PM and EMR program in Chapter 2.

CHECK YOUR KNOWLEDGE

_____ 1. Which law provides incentive payments to providers for converting from paper records to electronic health records?

        a. Affordable Care Act (ACA)

        b. Health Insurance Portability and Accountability Act (HIPAA)

        c. American Recovery and Reinvestment Act (ARRA)

        d. None of the above

_____ 2. An unbilled claim can result from:

        a. sex missing in demographic field

        b. a patient with a foreign address

        c. only the patient name fields being populated

        d. a and c

_____ 3. Which is known as Level I of HCPCS?

        a. HIPAA

        b. HCPCS/DME

        c. CPT®

        d. ICD

_____ 4. Which is not a function of practice management (PM)?

        a. Recording a patient's vital signs

        b. Recording patient demographics

        c. Billing

        d. Scheduling appointments

_____ 5. In addition to front and back office medical assisting positions, an electronic health records specialist would find employment opportunities in:

        a. coding

        b. HIPAA compliance

        c. abstracting

        d. All of the above

_____ 6. A universal code system for identifying laboratory and clinical observations is known as:

        a. SNOMED-CT®

        b. LOINC®

        c. HIPAA

        d. NDC

_____ 7. Which of the following is NOT an advantage of an EMR?

        a. Patient coordination

        b. Reduction in errors

        c. Patient privacy

        d. Medical research

_____ 8. Information regarding the patient's lifestyle such as smoking and drinking habits, relationship status, and sexual history are considered:

        a. past medical history

        b. social history

        c. review of symptoms

        d. diagnosis and assessment

_____ 9. Word analysis breaks words down into:

        a. word roots

        b. prefixes and suffixes

        c. combining vowels and forms

        d. All of the above

_____ 10. Conditions under which protected health information can be released without consent from the patient are known as:

        a. ePHI (Electronic Protected Health Information)

        b. DRS (Designated Record Sets)

        c. TPO (Treatment, Payment, and Operations)

        d. None of the above

Introduction to Harris CareTracker PM and EMR

2

Key Terms

accounts receivable (A/R)
clearinghouse
fee schedule
Knowledge Base
open order
override
recall
resource
revenue code
role
task class

Learning Objectives

1. Log in to Harris CareTracker to complete activities.
2. Use the *Help* system to become familiar with key features of Harris CareTracker PM and EMR and to access step-by-step instructions on using each aspect of the system to quickly and successfully complete required tasks.
3. Explain the purpose and location of the *Main Menu*, *Navigation*, *Home*, and *Dashboard*.
4. Identify *Administration* features and functions for *Practice Management* and Electronic Medical Records.
5. Use the *Message Center* components for appropriate EHR tasks.

Real-World Connection

Prior to using the EHR software in our practice, medical assistants at NVFHA are required to become certified as "Super Users" of Harris CareTracker PM and EMR, a widely recognized and utilized EHR program. The training that employees receive to obtain this status is similar to the training you will receive throughout this textbook. This chapter introduces you to the *Help* system, which features a variety of video links and written training materials that elaborate on the training outlined in each chapter. Employees who utilize these materials typically perform at a higher level than those who do not. Your challenge is to use the *Help* content to enhance the training process and expand your knowledge.

INTRODUCTION

Welcome to Harris CareTracker PM and EMR, a fully integrated CCHIT® and ONC-ATCB–certified complete Practice Management (PM) and Electronic Health Record (EHR). Harris CareTracker Practice Management (PM) is a cloud-based application that enables physician practices to achieve greater efficiency by streamlining their administrative workflows. Harris CareTracker EMR is fully integrated with all the operational functions of the practice.

This chapter introduces the features and function of *Practice Management*, *Clinical*, and *Billing* activities in a live Electronic Medical Record (EMR) program and the related workflows. Throughout this text book you will perform real-world activities, including *Patient Demographics* and *Registration*, *Appointment Scheduling*, *EHR Clinical Duties* (patient work-up, completing the visit, and clinical documentation), *Billing*, and *Collections*. At the end of each chapter, there are *Case Studies* to complete as a "day in the life" of the medical assistant. These case studies will test your ability to apply what you have learned throughout the chapter. You will also find *Build Your Proficiency* activities at the end of each chapter. These activities offer the opportunity to not only practice what you've learned in the chapter, but also to gain new skills and embrace new challenges, to build yourself into an expert EHR user.

Throughout this book you will review the subject matter of the text, follow detailed step-by-step instructions, and refer to associated screenshot(s) to complete activities in your personal Harris CareTracker PM and EMR environment.

 ALERT! Due to the evolving nature and continuous upgrades of real-world EMRs such as this one, as you log in and work in your student version of Harris CareTracker there may be a slightly different look to your live screen from the screenshots provided in this text.

When prompted, follow the instructions given in the text to complete the activities.

Before you begin the activities in this chapter, review the Best Practices list on page xxiii of this textbook. These Best Practices are provided to help you complete work quickly and accurately in Harris CareTracker PM and EMR. Review these Best Practices periodically so that they become second nature. For your convenience, this list is also posted to the student companion website.

LOG IN TO HARRIS CARETRACKER

Learning Objective 1: Log in to Harris CareTracker to complete activities.

There are system readiness requirements that must be met before logging in to Harris CareTracker. These instructions are found in Chapter 1, Activities 1-1 through 1-8 and must be completed prior to working in Harris CareTracker. You must "clear your cache" (Activity 1-6) before logging in for each session.

In Chapter 1, Activity 1-9, you registered your credentials and created your Harris CareTracker PM and EMR training company using your preassigned user name located on the inside front cover of your book and the password you created when setting up your training company. Before beginning the activities, clear your cache. If you are using a personal computer (PC), only work in Internet Explorer 11®. Use Safari® for iPad®. Once the cache has been cleared, you may continue by logging in to your student version of Harris CareTracker (Activity 2-1).

 ## Activity 2-1
Log in to Harris CareTracker PM and EMR

1. Go to http://www.cengage.com/CareTracker.

2. The domain is set to "Current" by default (**Figure 2-1**). Leave as is.

3. The product list is set to "Cengage Learning Harris CareTracker Simulation 1.0" by default. Leave as is.

4. In the *Username* box, enter the username preassigned to you. **Note:** Both the username and password are case sensitive.

5. In the *Password* box, enter your password you created in Chapter 1, Activity 1-9. Then click *Sign In.* **Note:** As noted in Chapter 1, on each subsequent login, a dialog box called *Operator Encounter Batch Control* will display when you first sign in. Close out of this box by clicking the *Save* button and then clicking the "X" at the top right of the box (refer to Figure 1-12).

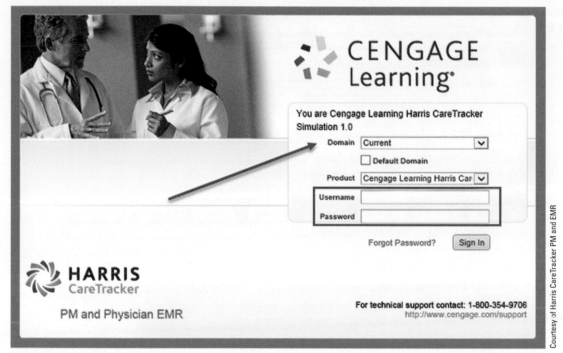

Figure 2-1   Login Screen

Courtesy of Harris CareTracker PM and EMR

HELP SYSTEM

Learning Objective 2: Use the *Help* system to become familiar with key features of Harris CareTracker PM and EMR and to access step-by-step instructions on using each aspect of the system to quickly and successfully complete required tasks.

Harris CareTracker PM and EMR *Online Help* ⊙ integrates product help, recorded training sessions, live webinars, support documentation, and quick reference tools to help you learn about and use Harris CareTracker PM and EMR effectively. The Harris CareTracker PM and EMR *Help* system offers an invaluable one-stop resource for both novice and advanced users. It is designed to familiarize the user with key features of Harris CareTracker PM and EMR, and it provides step-by-step instructions on using each aspect of the system to quickly and successfully complete required tasks.

As with all live programs, there are continual updates. The same is true for Harris CareTracker. While Harris CareTracker strives to have the most current information available in *Help*, there are instances where you may notice an update in the program that has not been updated in *Help*. This may include a reference to "Optum" PM & Physician EMR and "Ingenix." The content is the same, regardless of the title reference.

Harris CareTracker PM and EMR's *Help* system is intended for all staff in the practice with different levels of expertise and job functions. The user can range from front office staff handling appointment scheduling to a physician providing patient care.

Using the Harris CareTracker PM and EMR Help Window

The *Help* system includes left- and right-hand panes (**Figure 2-2**) and a toolbar (**Figure 2-3**). Each tool button contains various methods of navigating. The *Help* system is designed to open in the user's default web browser. To become familiar with the *Help* feature, log in to Harris CareTracker, click on *Help* ⊙, and explore the various *Help* topics and materials. This section goes into more detail about the resources available in the *Help* feature. **Figure 2-4** offers a description of conventions used in the *Help* system.

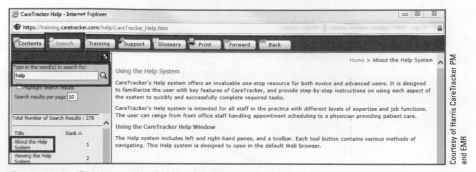

Figure 2-2 Right- and Left-Hand Panes

Courtesy of Harris CareTracker PM and EMR

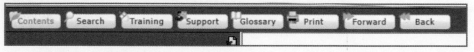

Figure 2-3 Help Toolbar

Courtesy of Harris CareTracker PM and EMR

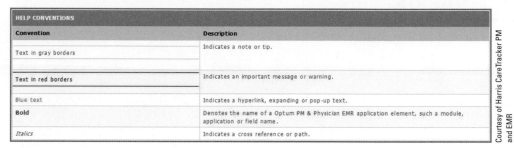

HELP CONVENTIONS	
Convention	**Description**
Text in gray borders	Indicates a note or tip.
Text in red borders	Indicates an important message or warning.
Blue text	Indicates a hyperlink, expanding or pop-up text.
Bold	Denotes the name of a Optum PM & Physician EMR application element, such as a module, application or field name.
Italics	Indicates a cross reference or path.

Figure 2-4 Help Conventions

Courtesy of Harris CareTracker PM and EMR

Contents

The *Contents* tab displays the table of contents that includes folders and pages in the left-hand pane. Each folder or page represents categories of information in the *Help* system. When a closed folder 📁 is clicked, it displays subfolders and pages. When an open folder 📂 is clicked, it closes. When pages 📄 are clicked, the selected topic displays in the right-hand pane.

Search

The *Search* tab provides a way to explore the content of topics and find matches to user-defined queries. Clicking any topic from the search results list displays the page in the right-hand pane (**Figure 2-5**). Ways to use the *Search* tab include using a phrase, singular words, a substring, or customizing your search.

- Phrase search—To search for a phrase, the best practice is to enter the phrase in quotation marks in the search box, although this is not required.

- Search singular words—Search using singular instead of plural words to return better results. For example, search for "prescription" instead of "prescriptions."

- Substring search—If you search for "log" the system returns topics containing the words "catalog" and "logarithm" among others. Substring search takes longer than whole-string search.

- Customize search results list—By default, 10 search results appear at a time. In these two outputs, the *Search* pane contains an option for the maximum number of search results to show in a list.

Training

In addition to the folders in the *Contents* tab, there are also *Live Webinars, Recorded Training,* and *Snipit Training* available in *Help* found in the *Training* tab. *Live Webinars* lists the instructor-led training schedule for the calendar year, registration information, and related webinar material.

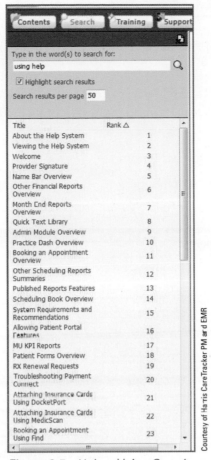

Figure 2-5   Help—Using Search

Recorded Training

Recorded training sessions are a series of self-paced online trainings that focus on different features in Harris CareTracker PM and EMR. Because these sessions are recorded, you can replay them as often as you need. *Recorded Training* displays a list of recorded web tutorials that give users more information about the features in Harris CareTracker PM and EMR (**Figure 2-6**). *Recorded Training* provides the flexibility of following each video at your own pace. To become familiar with *Recorded Training* features, click on *Help* ⚙, *Training* tab, *Recorded Training,* and scroll down through the available topics where you will find the title and topic of the recorded training. Titles with an (S) following the name refer to Snipits (abbreviated, short recorded trainings).

To learn more about Harris CareTracker and the *Help* features provided, click on the *General Navigation and Help System* training under *Getting Started* in the *Practice Management Recorded Training* header and view the video (Activity 2-2). The most current versions of documents are always available in *Help* for easy reference. Refer back to the recorded trainings throughout your studies as needed.

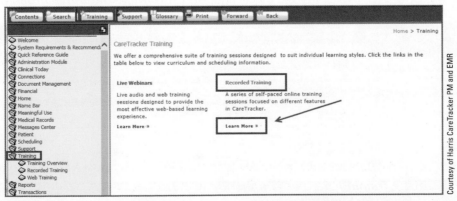

Figure 2-6   Recorded Training

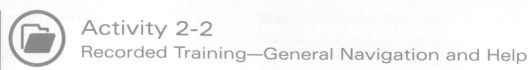

Activity 2-2
Recorded Training—General Navigation and Help

1. Click on *Help* ✪.

2. At the top of the screen, click on the *Training* button. (**Note:** The *Training* button is to the left of the *Support* button.)

3. Click on "Learn More" under *Recorded Training*.

4. Scroll down to *Practice Management*.

5. Click on the *General Navigation and Help System* topic (**Figure 2-7**) under the *Getting Started* header.

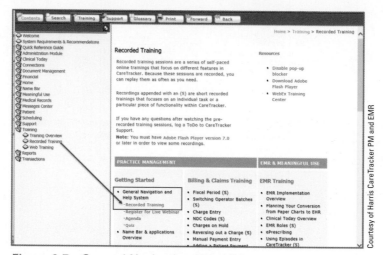

Figure 2-7   General Navigation Help Video

6. Click on the *Recorded Training* link to watch the video.

🖨 **Print a screenshot taken during your viewing of the Recorded Training, label it "Activity 2-2," and place it in your assignment folder.**

7. After you finish viewing the *Recorded Training*, click on the "X" in the upper-right corner of the *Recorded Training* box. Do not close out of Harris CareTracker.

Snipit Training

A "Snipit" is a short recorded training that focuses on an individual task or a particular piece of functionality within Harris CareTracker PM and EMR. Snipits are identified with an (S) following the topic header. If you have any questions after watching a Snipit (S) video, you can watch one of the longer recorded training sessions that include the topic. You will view a Snipit (S) in Activity 2-3 by clicking on *Learn More* under *Recorded Training* (**Figure 2-8**).

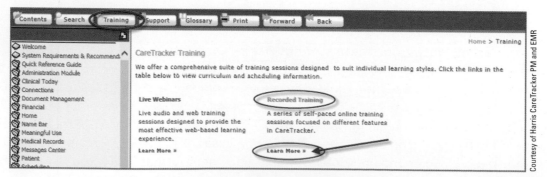

Figure 2-8   Help Snipit Learn More

To become familiar with *Snipit (S)* recordings, complete Activity 2-3 to review the *Snipit (S)* on *Fiscal Period*. Refer back to Snipits (S) as needed throughout your training for additional reference.

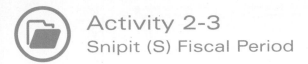

Activity 2-3
Snipit (S) Fiscal Period

1. Click on *Help* ⊕.

2. Click on the *Training* button on the toolbar.

3. Click on "Learn More" under *Recorded Training.*

4. Scroll down to the *Practice Management* section. The recorded trainings are grouped by topic area. Any training with an "(S)" at the end of the title is a Snipit training.

5. Click on the *Fiscal Period (S)* topic under "Billing & Claims Training" (**Figure 2-9**).

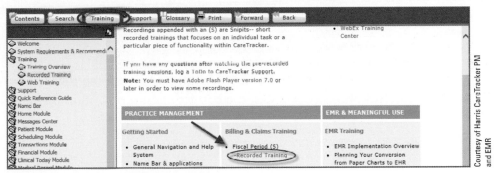

Figure 2-9   Help–Snipit Fiscal Period

6. Click on the *Recorded Training* link to watch the video.

    *   You must have Adobe Flash Player version 7.0 or later to view a *Snipit (S)* recording. The first time you view a recorded training you may be prompted to download and install the Adobe Flash Player if you do not already have it installed.

    *   If you find that the *Recording Training* or *Snipits (S)* are running slow or freezing, you may need to log out, clear your cache, and log back in to begin your activities.

🖫 **Print the Snipit Fiscal Period screen, label it "Activity 2-3," and place it in your assignment folder.**

Support

Support displays a list of innovative and comprehensive resources to assist in performing Harris CareTracker PM and EMR tasks. *Support Knowledge Base* displays a list of documents and articles that include tips and tricks, procedures, trends in the industry, and much more helpful information. The *Knowledge Base* is a repository of constantly updated product troubleshooting tips and procedures. The list of support resources available can make all the difference in terms of support, guidance, and inspiration. The support resources are a combination of an online knowledge base and the knowledge and expertise of *CareTracker Customer Service* (**Figure 2-10**).

PDF Documents can be found online in *Help* on topics for many of the Harris CareTracker applications and modules and are found by clicking on the *Support Knowledge Base* link in the *Support* tab/folder. *PDF Documents* displays a list of available documents in Adobe portable document format (PDF). You have the flexibility and option of viewing, printing, or saving the documents.

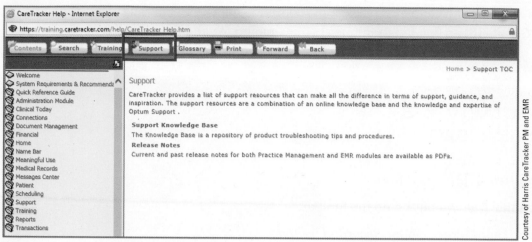

Figure 2-10 Support Tab in Help

Release Notes display the current and last release notes that include information on new and enhanced features. Current and past release notes for both Practice Management and EMR modules are available as PDFs.

Glossary

The *Glossary* tab displays a *Glossary* in the left-hand pane of the window (**Figure 2-11**). The *Glossary* is similar to one found in a printed publication and provides a list of words with the associated definition. When a term is selected from the top pane ("Term") of the *Glossary* tab, the corresponding definition displays in the lower pane ("Definition").

Print

Print enables printing of the current page that displays in the right-hand pane of the *Help* system (**Figure 2-12**). An alternate method of printing is to right-click your mouse, then click *Print* on the shortcut menu.

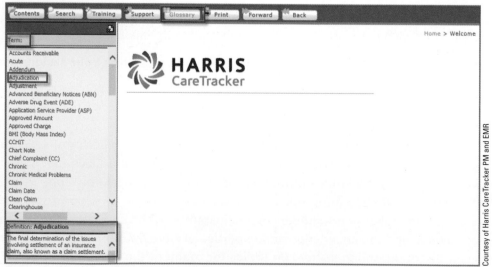

Figure 2-11 Help–Glossary

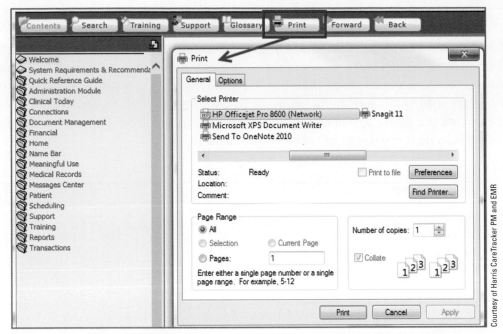

Figure 2-12   Help—Print

Forward and Back

The *Forward* and *Back* tabs guide you through topics based on the history of visited topics. By clicking on the *Forward* or *Back* tabs, your screen will go to the previous topic visited in *Help* (**Figure 2-13**).

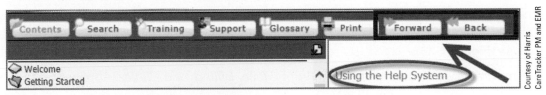

Figure 2-13   Forward and Back Tabs in Help

MAIN MENU AND NAVIGATION

Learning Objective 3: Explain the purpose and location of the Main Menu, Navigation, Home, and Dashboard.

There are three applications contained in the *Home* module: *Dashboard*, *Messages*, and *News* (**Figure 2-14** and **Table 2-1**). There are also three tabs: *Practice*, *Management*, and *Meaningful Use*. Your Harris CareTracker PM and EMR role determines which applications you can access. Your *Home* screen is set to default to the *Home > Dashboard > Practice* screen.

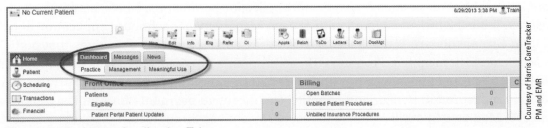

Figure 2-14   Home Application Tabs

Home Overview

In Harris CareTracker PM and EMR, the *Dashboard* is where you find your quick links to front office, billing, and clinical functions and features. The *Messages* application is a communication tool used to manage *ToDos*, mail messages, and faxes. The *News* application provides the ability to post messages to patients and employees, ensuring that important information is made available in a timely manner. In your student version of Harris CareTracker, you can visit the *News* application for important messages from Cengage and Harris CareTracker, but you will not be able to post messages yourself (**Figure 2-15**).

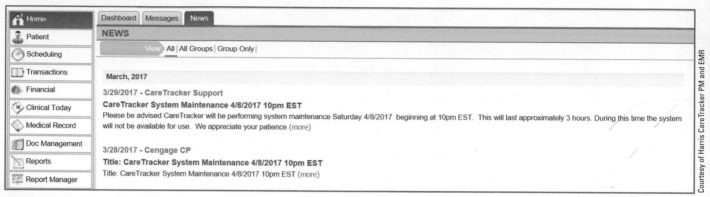

Figure 2-15   News Dashboard

Dashboard Overview

In Harris CareTracker PM and EMR, the *Dashboard* is considered "information central." At a quick glance, you can see a summary of what activity has taken place in your practice, and you can also see what key indicators need to be addressed, such as inactive claims. The *Dashboard* is divided into three tabs: *Practice*, *Management*, and *Meaningful Use* (**Figure 2-16**).

- *Practice.* The *Practice* dashboard contains *Front Office, Billing,* and *Clinical* application summaries.

- *Management.* The *Management* dashboard includes the practice's financial and management functions.

- *Meaningful Use.* The *Meaningful Use* dashboard measures and tracks a provider's progress toward meeting each of the Meaningful Use requirements and to qualify for the Medicaid and Medicare EHR incentive programs.

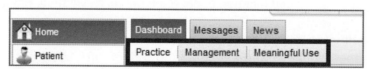

Figure 2-16   Dashboard Tabs
Courtesy of Harris CareTracker PM and EMR

Table 2-1 provides a summary of each *Practice* application and description.

The *Management* dashboard contains *Management* application summaries, *Financials* application summaries, and *Staff Measures*. **Table 2-2** provides a summary of each *Management* dashboard application and description.

The *Meaningful Use* dashboard is designed to assist providers in meeting objectives that participate in the Medicare and Medicaid EHR Incentive Programs. These programs provided incentive payments to eligible providers that have demonstrated they are using certified EHR technology, such as Harris CareTracker PM and EMR, in ways that can be measured in quality and quantity. The incentive payments for Medicare eligible providers (EPs) ended in 2016. Medicaid EPs will continue to receive incentives through 2021. Beginning in 2015, Medicare EPs who do not successfully demonstrate meaningful use will be subject to a payment adjustment (incentive reduction).

Table 2-1   Practice Dashboard Application Summaries

FRONT OFFICE APPLICATION SUMMARIES

APPLICATION	DESCRIPTION
Show Figures for All Groups	The *Show Figures for All Groups* checkbox is included on both the *Practice* and *Management* dashboards. Select this checkbox to refresh the dashboard and display totals for all of your company's groups. Note: This feature works only in a live practice, not in your educational training company.
Links	The *Links* application is included on both the *Practice* and *Management* dashboards. *Links* displays sites that are saved as favorites via the *Link Administration* application in the *Administration* module. This link enables you to quickly access the frequently used sites.
Eligibility	Every evening Harris CareTracker PM and EMR will automatically batch check patient eligibility for the primary insurance saved on each patient's *Demographic* record. This automated eligibility check will be performed for all patients with an appointment scheduled in Harris CareTracker PM and EMR within the next five days. Electronic insurance eligibility checks return a status of *Eligible, Ineligible,* or *Unknown*. The list of *Ineligible* or *Unknown* patients is accessible by clicking on the *Eligibility* link. The application is updated overnight.
Patient Portal Patient Updates	This application allows an operator to approve demographic data changes a patient makes via the *Patient Portal* website.
Missing Patient Information	Any patient with a scheduled appointment whose record is missing or contains inaccurate demographic information essential for billing and submitting insurance claims will be listed in this application. From the *Missing Info* list, you can determine the necessary information to be added to or edited in the patient's record. This application is updated overnight.
New Insurance	Patients who were originally registered in Harris CareTracker PM and EMR without insurance information but have since had insurance information entered onto their account are flagged by this application to ensure that all previously entered charges are billed to the new insurance. The application is updated overnight.
Unprinted Correspondence	By clicking this link, you access the *Unprinted Correspondence* application, a queue for form letters generated and saved for patients in Harris CareTracker PM and EMR that need to be printed. These letters can be printed from this application for either all patients or just the patient in context. This application can also be accessed in a window by clicking on the *Corr* button in the *Name Bar*. This application is updated overnight.
Appointments	This link shows the total number of appointments scheduled for the current day for either the entire group or for the specific resource you selected as the resource default when you created your batch. From this screen, you can check in patients, transfer patients, check out patients, print encounter forms, capture visits, cancel an appointment, view appointment details, and enter copayments. This application is updated in real time.
Wait List	An appointment wait list of patients who would like an appointment with a provider prior to their currently scheduled appointment can be generated by clicking on the *Wait List* link under the *My Lists* section of the *Dashboard*. The *Wait List* link will identify all patients who are currently on the *Wait List* for which an open appointment slot in Harris CareTracker PM and EMR may be available based on a patient's appointment criteria. It will also flag for you the available appointment slot that matches the patient's *Wait List* appointment criteria. The application is updated in real time.
Appointment Conflicts	This link alerts you to any upcoming appointments that are in conflict. From this link, you can cancel and reschedule conflicted appointments. This application is updated overnight.

(continues)

Table 2-1 Practice Dashboard Application Summaries (*continued*)

FRONT OFFICE APPLICATION SUMMARIES

APPLICATION	DESCRIPTION
Patient Portal Appointment Requests	This link lists all appointment requests submitted by patients via the *Patient Portal* application.
Expired Reoccurring Appointments	Physical therapy and occupational therapy practices often schedule reoccurring appointments for their patients. The *Expired Reoccurring Appointments* application in the *Front Office* section of the Dashboard identifies patients whose reoccurring appointments will soon expire because additional authorizations or referrals may be required before future appointments.
Appointment Outreach	The *Appointment Outreach* application tracks the confirmation status of upcoming appointments. The default view for the *Appointment Outreach* work list displays unconfirmed appointments for the current day plus the next two days. The outreach result column displays either the result returned by *Patient Notifications* or a message manually entered by an operator in the *Appt Outreach Result field* in the *Appointment* window.
Missing Encounters	This link ensures that all appointments scheduled in Harris CareTracker PM and EMR have a visit saved for them and that all visits saved have been turned into charges. From the *Missing Encounters* link, appointments can be canceled, bulk visits can be saved, and bulk charges can be saved. This application is updated overnight.
Open Admissions/Missing Admissions	The *Admissions* application is not only a fast and convenient way to keep track of all patients a provider sees during hospital rounds, but will also help boost revenue by ensuring that all your valuable services in a hospital are ultimately billed for. The *Dashboard* represents two values that are refreshed overnight. These values are based on the provider and location selected in the batch. The first value indicates all open admissions. The second value indicates admissions with missing days. It is important to review and work both values daily. This application is updated overnight.
Visits on Hold	The *Visits On Hold* application displays all visits in the "Hold" status. This enables you to work and save the held visits. Held visits do not display in the *Bulk Charges* application and therefore are not billable until the *Claims Manager* screening is passed. This application is updated in real time.
Charges on Hold	The *Charges On Hold* application displays all charges in the "Hold" status, making it easy to work the list to send out the claims. Held charges do not move to *Accounts Receivable* and therefore are not billable to send out as a claim. The held charges are assigned to a *Hold Batch* that is set up when creating a batch for the day. The application is updated in real time.

BILLING APPLICATION SUMMARIES

Open Batches	You must create a batch to enter any financial information into Harris CareTracker PM and EMR (e.g., charges, payments, and adjustments). After running a journal to verify your batch information, click this link to view all open batches and to post your batch into the system. Posting a batch permanently stores all financial transactions linked to it in Harris CareTracker PM and EMR. This application is updated in real time.
Unbilled Patient Procedures and Unbilled Insurance Procedures	*Unbilled Procedures* identifies any procedure that has not been billed. For example, procedures that are paid by Medicare (primary) and then "piggybacked" (crossover claims) to Medex are considered "unbilled procedure balances" (e.g., Medicare paid its portion of the procedure; the remaining balance is transferred to Medex, but the procedure will not be billed because Medicare will notify Medex of its responsibility). This application is updated in real time.
Unapplied Payments	The *Unapplied Payments* link identifies any patient payments entered into Harris CareTracker PM and EMR that have not been applied to a specific date of service. This application is updated in real time.

BILLING APPLICATION SUMMARIES (*continued*)

APPLICATION	DESCRIPTION
Electronic Remittances	The total number and sum of remittances received electronically into Harris CareTracker PM displays on the *Dashboard,* and a list of the received remittances that need to be posted into the system is accessed by clicking on the *Electronic Remittances* link. They should only be posted after the check is received from the insurance company. This application is updated overnight.
Denials	Denials are claims that an insurance company has determined they will not pay due to a specific reason. The number of denials and the total monetary value of the denials for a specific period, batch, or group, is identified by the *Denials* link and from this link, denials can be worked accordingly. The application is updated overnight.
Credit Balances	A credit balance is created when either a patient or an insurance company pays more money for a specific procedure for a specific date of service than what was billed. The credit balances that are displayed are for both patients and insurance companies and can be identified for a specific batch, for a specific group, or for all groups. The application is updated in real time.
Verify Payments	*Verify Payments* compares the money an insurance company has paid for a procedure to the allowed amount an insurance company will pay for the same procedure. This feature can only be used for primary payments and is designed to make you aware of instances when you are paid less than the actual allowed amount.
Statements	Harris CareTracker PM and EMR generates and prints patient statements on a weekly basis; however, patients will only receive one statement every 28 days regardless of the number of services they have had. This link identifies the batch of patients who qualify to receive a statement from *ExpressBill* as well as patients who did not receive a statement because of a bad or forwarded address. Once the statements are printed, the status of the batch will be changed to "printed" so they will no longer be identified on the *Dashboard*. This application is updated overnight.
Collections	This link identifies patients eligible to receive different types of collection letters including "Collection Letter 1," "Past Due," "Delinquent," "Final Notice," and "75 Collections." Collection letters are generated from this link as well. Generated collection letters must be printed from the *Print Batch Letters* link under the *Daily Administration* section of the *Administration* module. This application is updated in real time.
Claims Worklist	This link contains all claims identified by Harris CareTracker PM and EMR as those with missing or incorrect information and will not be forwarded to the respective insurance companies until they are corrected accordingly and rebilled, which can be accomplished by clicking on the *Claims Worklist* link. This application is updated overnight.
Open Claims	Open claims are claims that have been submitted to an insurance company but have not been paid yet. An inactive claim would be a claim that not only is unpaid, but has not had any follow-up activity on that claim for the last 30 days. The application is updated overnight.
Unprinted Paper Claim Batches	Harris CareTracker PM and EMR automatically sends all electronic claim batches to the appropriate insurance company or **clearinghouse** and will capture all claims that cannot be transmitted electronically in *Unprinted Paper Claim Batches*. This link identifies the paper claim batches that are ready to be printed. This application is updated overnight. In the medical field, a clearinghouse is a private or public company that provides connectivity and often serves as a "middleman" between physicians and billing entities, payers, and other health care partners (e.g., American Medical Association) for transmission and translation of claims information (primarily electronic) into the specific format required by payers.

(*continues*)

Table 2-1   Practice Dashboard Application Summaries (*continued*)

BILLING APPLICATION SUMMARIES

APPLICATION	DESCRIPTION
Open Electronic Claim Batches	Harris CareTracker PM and EMR sends claims electronically to insurance companies and to clearinghouses. The insurance companies and clearinghouses send an electronic response to Harris CareTracker PM and EMR indicating whether or not they have accepted the claims. All responses must be reviewed and if there are any errors indicated, you must fix and rebill those claims. If the claims have been accepted, the open electronic claim batch may be closed. The application is updated overnight.
Batch Level Rejections	The *Batch Level Rejections* application allows you to view batch level claim rejections received from the Clearinghouse/EDI Services®.

CLINICAL APPLICATION SUMMARIES

Open Encounters	This link identifies patient encounters with missing/unsigned notes and missing/unbilled procedures. *Missing/Unsigned Notes* identifies patients who have an encounter but no encounter note, and *Missing/Unbilled Procedures* identifies patients who have an encounter note but no visit information. **Note:** Operators must have either the "VIP Patient Access" or the "VIP Patient Access Break Glass" override included in their operator profile to access this application for a VIP patient.
Overdue Recalls and Letters	This link identifies patients who have upcoming or overdue recalls. A **recall** is a reminder to the patient to schedule a specific appointment. An overdue recall is a patient who has not yet scheduled a specific appointment and needs to be contacted. From this link, you can generate and print appointment recall letters or labels to send to patients as a reminder that they need to schedule an appointment. This application is updated overnight.
Open Orders	An **open order** is a test that the provider has ordered for a patient, but the practice has not received the results of that test. This link totals all of the open orders for all patients in the group. You can enter and save the test results for all patients by clicking on the *Open Orders* link. *Test Results* for an individual patient can be entered in the *Open Orders* application of the *Clinical* module. The application is updated in real time. **Note:** Operators must have either the "VIP Patient Access" or the "VIP Patient Access Break Glass" override included in their operator profile to access this application for a VIP patient.
Results	Patient lab results transmitted from a laboratory are received into and stored in the *Lab Results* link until the results are reviewed and analyzed by a provider. When a provider has reviewed them, the lab results are saved in the corresponding patient's record. The application is updated in real time. **Note:** Operators must have either the "VIP Patient Access" or the "VIP Patient Access Break Glass" override included in their operator profile to access this application for a VIP patient.
Prescriptions	This link flags all patient prescription refill requests electronically transmitted from pharmacies, and from this link each request should be approved or denied. Approvals and denials of each refill request are in turn transmitted back to the pharmacy. The application is updated in real time. Additionally, this application lists all prescription renewal requests submitted by patients through the *Patient Portal* website. **Note:** Operators must have either the "VIP Patient Access" or the "VIP Patient Access Break Glass" override included in their operator profile to access this application for a VIP patient.
Untranscribed Voice Attachments	This link identifies all audio files, such as dictations, patient interviews, voice mail messages, and more, that require transcription. These audio files are created using the *Attachment* application in the *Medical Record* module. The *Untranscribed Voice Attachment* application supports in-house and third-party transcription by enabling you to directly transcribe through the application or download the file to the computer. The application is updated in real time. **Note:** Operators must have either the "VIP Patient Access" or the "VIP Patient Access Break Glass" override included in their operator profile to access this application for a VIP patient.

Table 2-2 Management Dashboard Application Summaries

MANAGEMENT APPLICATION SUMMARIES	
APPLICATION	**DESCRIPTION**
Show Figures for All Groups	The *Show Figures for All Groups* checkbox is included on both the *Practice* and *Management* dashboards. Select this checkbox to refresh the dashboard and to display totals for all of your company's groups.
Links	The *Links* application is included on both the *Practice* and *Management* dashboards. *Links* displays sites that are saved as favorites via the *Link Administration* application in the *Administration* module. This link enables you to quickly access the frequently used sites.
Appointments Scheduled	The number that displays here is the total number of appointments scheduled for the month for the entire practice. This is a display-only field. This application is updated overnight.
Accounts Receivable	This link displays the group's total **accounts receivable (A/R)**, which is money that is owed to your group broken out by financial class (e.g., Private Pay, Medicare, Blue Shield, Commercial), and also by age (e.g., current to 30 days old, 31–60 days old). You can see the list of patients that comprise a specific financial class A/R by clicking on the *Total* column of the desired financial class. This application is updated overnight.
Visits by Day	Harris CareTracker PM displays the total number of visits that have been entered into the system for the current period. By clicking on this link, you can see a breakdown of the number of visits entered per day for a particular period. This application is updated overnight.
Batch Deposits	The total number of bank deposits made for the current month thus far displays next to this link. By clicking this link, you can view the date and amount of each deposit as well as the source of the money deposited. This application is updated overnight.
FINANCIALS APPLICATION SUMMARIES	
Charges	Harris CareTracker PM displays the total amount of charges generated thus far for the entire group and for the current month. Clicking this link will give you charges breakdown by day. This application is updated overnight.
Payments	Harris CareTracker PM displays the total amount of payments received thus far for the entire group and for the current month. Clicking on this link will give a payment breakdown by day. This application is updated overnight.
Adjustments	Harris CareTracker PM displays the total amount of adjustments made thus far for the entire group and for the current month. This link displays adjustments by day. This application is updated overnight.
STAFF MEASURES APPLICATION SUMMARY	
User Access Audit	In this link, you can see the total number of operators who worked in Harris CareTracker PM and EMR for a particular date and can drill down to see which operators did what on a specific date. This application is updated overnight.
Dual Coding Review	Companies configured for dual coding (coding claims for both ICD-9 and ICD-10 diagnosis codes) can review dual-coded charges and a history of ClaimsManager edits from this application. When launched, this application displays a list of all dual-coded charges entered for the group in context for the last seven days. This application is not available in your student version.

Providers must demonstrate meaningful use and then submit report data or self-attest (legally state) to the Centers for Medicare and Medicaid Services (CMS) that they have met the requirements. HealthIT.gov provides the following meaningful use definition and objectives:

Meaningful use is using certified electronic health record (EHR) technology to:

- Improve quality, safety, efficiency, and reduce health disparities
- Engage patients and family
- Improve care coordination, and population and public health
- Maintain privacy and security of patient health information

Ultimately, it is hoped that the meaningful use compliance will result in:

- Better clinical outcomes
- Improved population health outcomes
- Increased transparency and efficiency
- Empowered individuals
- More robust research data on health systems

Meaningful use sets specific objectives that eligible professionals (EPs) and hospitals must achieve to qualify for Centers for Medicare & Medicaid Services (CMS) Incentive Programs.

The *Meaningful Use* dashboard (**Figure 2-17**) measures and tracks a provider's progress toward meeting each of the meaningful use requirements. From the dashboard, you can:

- Customize the requirements displayed on the dashboard for each participating provider
- View a status of a provider's progress (percentages are updated nightly) (**Figure 2-18**)

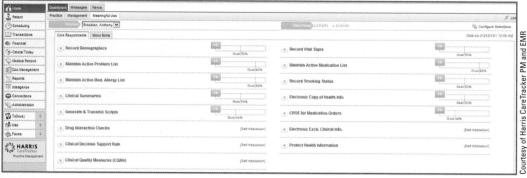

Figure 2-17   Meaningful Use Dashboard

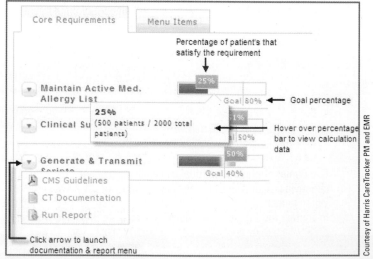

Figure 2-18   Meaningful Use Core Requirements

- Hover over the percentage bar to review the data used to calculate the provider's percentage
- Click the *Menu Items* tab to download reference documents or run Key Performance Indicator (KPI) reports

ADMINISTRATION FEATURES AND FUNCTIONS

Learning Objective 4: Identify Administration features and functions for Practice Management and Electronic Medical Records.

The *Administration* module contains the *Administration* application, which is divided into three tabs: *Practice, Clinical,* and *Setup*. Each tab is organized into sections containing links to other applications in Harris CareTracker PM.

Practice—Daily Administration

Although there are numerous features in the *Administration* module, we will focus on the applications you will use during the course of your training relative to practice management. In the *Practice* tab, you will find the *Daily Administration, System Administration, Import/Export* (**Figure 2-19**), and *Knowledgebase* (**Figure 2-20**) applications. Under each application tab, you can perform various functions by clicking on the associated tab. We will explore *Administration > Practice > Daily Administration* features that provide tools for operators to follow that help maintain compliance with HIPAA privacy rules: the *Operator Audit Log, Operator Log,* and *VIP Log*. The *Knowledgebase* tab (**Figure 2-20**) summarizes features that are useful in your daily Practice Management activities.

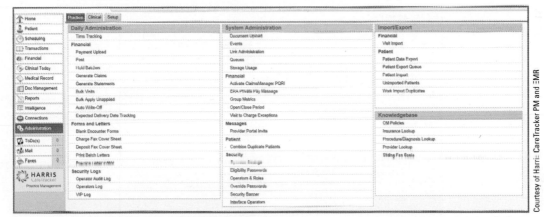

Figure 2-19   Administration Module–Practice Tab

PRACTICE TAB: KNOWLEDGBASE	
Application	**Description**
CM Policies	The CM Policies application enables you to view and/or search the list of all active, attached policies and/or URLs saved into Harris CareTracker PM and EMR. This will enable the user to click on a mnemonic and view the linked policy if a ClaimsManager edit is triggered during the claim generation process.
Insurance Lookup	A search of all insurance plans compiled in Harris CareTrackers PM and EMR's Insurance database can be performed by clicking on this link.
Procedure/Diagnosis Lookup	From this link you can search Harris CareTracker PM and EMR's database for a procedure or diagnosis code.
Provider Lookup	A search of all providers compiled in Harris CareTracker PM and EMR's Provider database can be performed by clicking on this link.
Sliding Fee Scale	Discounts used to equitably charge patients for services rendered. Fees are set based on the federal poverty guidelines and patient eligibility is determined by annual income and family size.

Figure 2-20   Knowledgebase

Operator Audit Log

The *Operator Audit Log* maintains an audit trail of all actions performed in Harris CareTracker PM and EMR by each operator. This log is helpful to monitor each operator's usage. You can customize the log by operator, activity type, and date range. Regardless of the filters you set, the operator log always includes the date, time, operator's log-in identification (ID), operator's name, the name of the patient whose record was accessed, the group in which the action was taken, and a comment (the action performed). After you have completed activities in later chapters, you will again be asked to generate an *Operator Audit Log* (part of your Applied Learning Case Studies in Chapter 11).

The *Operator Audit Log* and *Operators Log* are typically part of the manager's role and responsibilities, but it is helpful for your knowledge and understanding regarding privacy issues and the "digital footprint" recorded for each and every action you take in the EHR.

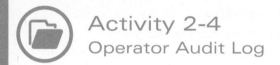

Activity 2-4
Operator Audit Log

1. Click the *Administration* module. The application opens the *Practice* tab.

2. Click the *Operator Audit Log* link under *Security Logs* (**Figure 2-21**). The application launches the *Operator Audit Log.* **Note:** This may take a few moments to populate.

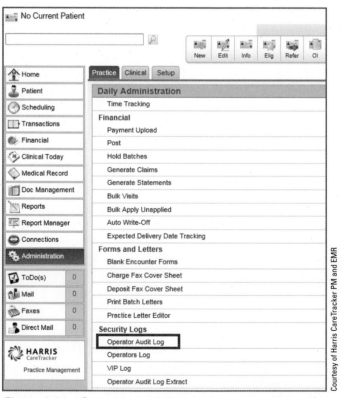

Figure 2-21   Operator Audit Log Link

3. From the *Type* list, select the type of activity for which you want to view a log. Leave as "-Select-" to view a log of all activities. (**Note:** View the drop-down to see the various "Type(s)" of logs available to create.)

4. From the *Operator* list, select the operator for whom you want to generate an audit log (Current Operator). To see a log of all operator activities, you would leave the field as "-Select-."

5. In the *Date* boxes, enter the dates to include in the audit log. (Leave the dates as they are set to run a report for the past seven days.)

6. Click *Show Log*. Harris CareTracker PM displays the log in the bottom half of the screen (**Figure 2-22**). **Note:** This may take a few moments to populate.

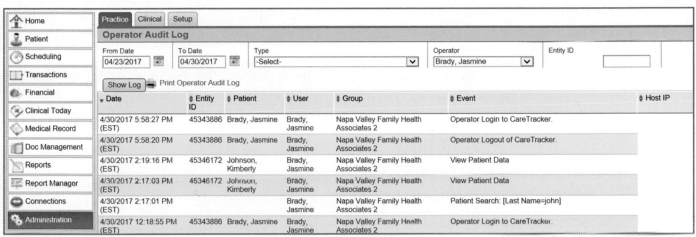

Figure 2-22   *Operator Audit Log*

Courtesy of Harris CareTracker PM and EMR

🖫 **To print the log, right-click your mouse on the log and then select Print from the shortcut menu. Label the Operators Audit Log "Activity 2-4" and place it in your assignment folder.**

Operators Log

The *Operators Log* tracks the number of operators who log in to Harris CareTracker PM and EMR each day. You can view the log for the current month or for a specific time period. Instructions to create and view the *Operators Log* are found in Proficiency Builder 2-4 at the end of the chapter.

VIP Log

There are many reasons to flag a patient as a VIP. Doing so allows you to restrict operator access to the patient's demographic information. Any operator may flag a high-profile patient as a VIP, but only operators assigned either the "VIP Patient Access" or the "VIP Patient Access Break Glass" override in their profile can access a VIP demographic.

"Break the glass" privileges allow an operator limited access to a VIP patient's information. The access is only available during the operator's current Harris CareTracker PM and EMR session and the operator must provide a reason why the record is being accessed.

Each time an operator accesses a VIP patient demographic, Harris CareTracker PM and EMR creates an entry in the *VIP Patient Log*. The log lists the patient name, the operator who accessed the record, and the date and time the record was accessed. This too is referred to as a "digital footprint." Because you have not yet flagged any patients as "VIP," there will currently be no information displayed in the log. However, in Chapter 3, Activity 3-2 and Case Study 3-1, you will be instructed to register patient(s) and flag them as VIP. You will then be able to view the *VIP Log* using the instructions in Chapter 3, Proficiency Builder 3-4.

SPOTLIGHT

IMPORTANT!! Your operator role must include a VIP Patient Log security override to view the *VIP Patient Log*. By default, only the practice administrator ("Fin-Practice Admin" role) is assigned access to view VIP patients and the VIP log. The practice administrator can approve a request for an override. Operator access to both VIP patient demographics and the *VIP Patient Log* is set by the practice administrator in the *Operators & Roles* application in the *Administration* module.

Practice—System Administration

In the *Administration > Practice > System Administration* setting, you will find features including *Financial, Messages* (provider portal), *Patient* (combining duplicate patient accounts), and *Security* sections. Vital *System Administration* functions to be reviewed are the *Open/Close Period, Operator Settings,* and *Operators & Roles.*

Open/Close Period

Working in the correct fiscal period is crucial to the electronic health record. Transactions and entries are permanently linked to a fiscal period and must be accurate. You must define the fiscal periods for your practice before any charges or payments are entered into Harris CareTracker PM and EMR. You can manage the practice's financials by opening each fiscal period. You can post financials to multiple open periods, but you cannot post financials or create a batch for a closed period. The fiscal period and year you are working in displays in all financial transaction applications, such as *Charge, Bulk Charges,* and *Payments on Account.* All reports are linked to the established fiscal periods, not the periods of the calendar year.

Depending on when you begin using this textbook, you may be required to change the fiscal year in addition to opening and closing fiscal periods. Activity 2-5 instructs you how to open a new fiscal year.

Activity 2-5
Open a New Fiscal Year

1. Click the *Administration* module. Harris CareTracker PM displays the *Practice* tab.

2. Under the *System Administration* column, in the *Financial* section, click the *Open/Close Period* link (**Figure 2-23**). Harris CareTracker PM displays all of your fiscal periods for the current fiscal year.

3. Enter the year in the *Fiscal Year* field. **Note:** If the *Fiscal Year* already displays for the current year you are working, move on to the next step. If you need to change the fiscal year, enter the current year and click *Go.*

4. To open a fiscal year for all groups within your company, select *Y* from the *All Groups* list and then click *Go* (**Figure 2-24**).

5. By default, the beginning and end date of each period is set to the first and last day of the month. Leave as is.

6. Click *Save.*

7. Continue with Activity 2-6 to open a new fiscal period.

📄 **Print the Open Fiscal Period screen, label it "Activity 2-5," and place it in your assignment folder.**

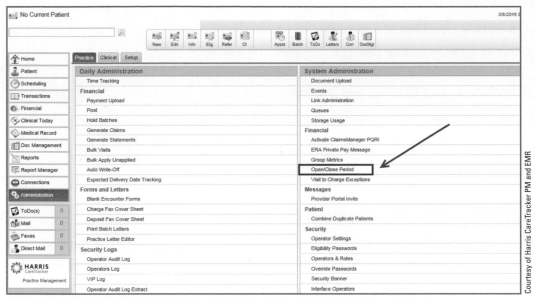

Figure 2-23   Open/Close Period

Figure 2-24   Open/Close Fiscal Year

On the first day of a new period, the practice administrator must change the status of the period to *Open* to begin posting financials to that period. You can also open a period prior to the first day of the period. It is typical for a practice to have multiple periods open.

You will have to open periods while working throughout the text to reflect the current date(s) of the activities you are working in.

ALERT! Do *not* close a fiscal period unless instructed to do so.

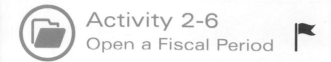

Activity 2-6
Open a Fiscal Period

1. Continue from Activity 2-5. If you had already logged out:

   a. Click the *Administration* module. Harris CareTracker PM displays the *Practice* tab.

   b. Under *System Administration/Financial*, click the *Open/Close Period* link. Harris CareTracker PM displays all of your fiscal periods for the current fiscal year.

   c. For multigroup companies, select *Y* from the *All Groups* list and then click *Go* to open a fiscal period for all groups in the company.

2. From the list in the *Status* column, use the drop down and select "OPEN" for the period you want to open. Open the period (month/year) you are currently working in (for example, if the day you complete this activity is January 20, 2018, you would open fiscal period January 2018). **Note:** As you continue your work/activities in Harris CareTracker, you may need to open additional fiscal periods as well. Refer to this activity throughout the text when you need to open additional fiscal periods.

3. Click *Save.* You can now create batches and post financials for this period (**Figure 2-25**).

Fiscal Year: 2017   **All Groups:** Y   GO

	PERIOD	FISCAL YEAR MONTH	BEGIN DATE	END DATE	STATUS	CLOSED DATE OPERATOR
	1	2017 January	1/1/2017	1/31/2017	(Select)	
	2	2017 February	2/1/2017	2/28/2017	(Select)	
	3	2017 March	3/1/2017	3/31/2017	(Select)	
EXISTS	4	2017 April	4/1/2017	4/30/2017	OPEN	Jasmine Brady
	5	2017 May	5/1/2017	5/31/2017	(Select)	
	6	2017 June	6/1/2017	6/30/2017	(Select)	
	7	2017 July	7/1/2017	7/31/2017	(Select)	
	8	2017 August	8/1/2017	8/31/2017	(Select)	
	9	2017 September	9/1/2017	9/30/2017	(Select)	
	10	2017 October	10/1/2017	10/31/2017	(Select)	
	11	2017 November	11/1/2017	11/30/2017	(Select)	
	12	2017 December	12/1/2017	12/31/2017	(Select)	
	13	2017 CONTROL			(Select)	

Save

Courtesy of Harris CareTracker PM and EMR

Figure 2-25   Fiscal Period Open

Print the Open Fiscal Period screen, label it "Activity 2-6," and place it in your assignment folder.

When all financials have been posted into a period, only the practice administrator will change the status of the period to "Closed." Once a period is closed, financials cannot be posted into it. <u>Never</u> close a period until all financials for that period have been posted, and <u>never</u> close a period unless specifically instructed to do so. A closed period cannot be reopened and financials cannot be posted into a closed period.

Operator Settings

Every operator must have a user name and a password to log into Harris CareTracker PM and EMR. You are required to change your password every 90 days. Harris CareTracker PM and EMR reminds users seven days before their password expires and gives you the option of changing the password at that time. If your password expires, you can reset it without having to log a *ToDo* to *Support*. You can also use *Operator Settings* to change your password at any time after you begin using Harris CareTracker PM and EMR, even prior to being required to by the system.

The *Operator Settings* application is also used to store the operator's contact information. This information is used by *CareTracker Customer Service* to contact operators for support issues or in response to *ToDos*. For security reasons, passwords expire every 90 days. You will be prompted by Harris CareTracker PM and EMR when the 90-day period is approaching. In Activity 2-7, you will change your password for practice with this feature.

 TIP It is important that you keep the *General Information* section of the operator settings updated with your current phone number and email address. The application will prompt the operator for an email address if a valid address is not already saved for the operator.

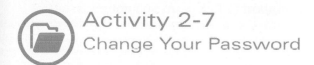

Activity 2-7
Change Your Password

1. Click the *Administration* module. The application displays the *Practice* tab.

2. Under the *System Administration* column, in the *Security* section, click the *Operator Settings* link (**Figure 2-26**). Harris CareTracker PM and EMR launches the *Operator Settings* application.

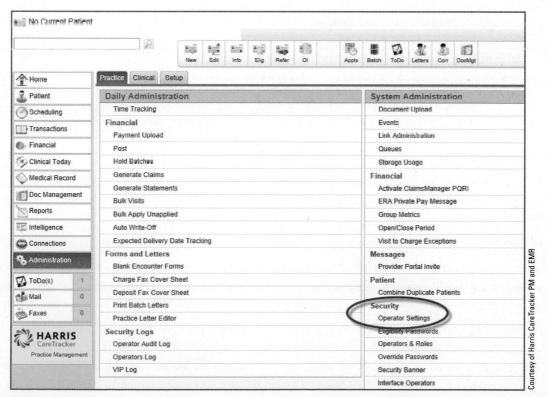

Figure 2-26   Operator Settings

3. In the *Old Password* box, enter your current password (the one you created in Activity 1-9).

4. In the *New Password* field, enter your new password (enter a personal password you will remember). Record your user ID and new password for future reference:

   a. User Name: _____

   b. New Password: _____

   The new password must meet the following criteria:
   - The new password must differ from your old password by at least one character.
   - The new password must consist of at least eight characters.
   - At least one of the eight characters must be a capital letter and at least one must be a number. For example: "Password5."

5. In the *Verify Password* box, reenter your new password.

6. From the *Question* list, select a security question.

7. In the *Answer* box, enter the answer to the security question.

8. In the *Phone* and *Email* fields, enter your phone number and email address. It is important to keep this contact information up to date because it is used by *Support* to follow up on support issues or *ToDos*. (See **Figure 2-27**.)

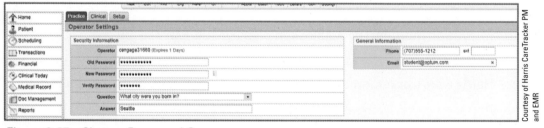

Figure 2-27   *Change Password Screen*

9. Click *Save*, and you will receive a *Success* pop-up box. Click *Close* on the pop-up box.

💾 **Print the Change Your Password screen, label it "Activity 2-7," and place it in your assignment folder.**

Operators and Roles

All Harris CareTracker PM and EMR operators are set up with a user profile based on their responsibilities and duties in a practice. An operator's privileges in Harris CareTracker PM and EMR are determined by the *Role(s)* and *Override(s)* assigned to his or her profile:

- **Roles** determine which Harris CareTracker PM and EMR modules and applications an operator can access.

- **Overrides** are used either to restrict an operator's access to a certain application and functionality or to grant an operator additional privileges that may not be included in his or her role. For example, if an operator needs access to only one application within the *Financial* module, you could add an override to the operator's profile to allow him or her to access just a particular financial application.

From the *Operator & Roles* application you can add an operator, edit an existing operator's roles/override, remove an operator from your practice, and monitor operator activities. When viewing the *Operator's*

Activity Log located in the *Operators & Roles* link, at the far right of the operator's name are four buttons as noted below:

- A: generates a list of operator activity for the last seven days
- L: generates a list of operator activity for the last 30 days including the date and time each operator logged in and from what IP address
- O: Creates an Operator Account Log for every login by the operator.
- R: lists each operator's access rights for all Harris CareTracker applications or for all applications of a particular module in a pop-up window

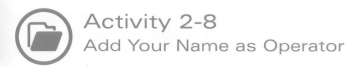

Activity 2-8
Add Your Name as Operator

In order to provide a customized user experience, you will now add your name as operator. This also helps easily identify your "training company" operator name as user.

1. Click the *Administration* module. The application displays the *Practice* tab.

2. Under the Security header, click the *Operators & Roles* link. The application displays the *Group Operators* list.

3. Click on your operator name. The information will display below your operator name.

4. In the *Name* section:

   a. Skip the *Title* box (not used for operators).

   b. In the *First Name* box, enter your first name.

   c. Skip the *Middle* name box (not used for operators).

   d. In the *Last Name* box, enter your last name.

5. Click *Save*. The application updates your operator name.

6. Log out of Harris CareTracker, and then log back in. Your name will now be listed as the operator (**Figure 2-28**).

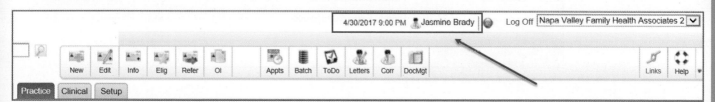

Figure 2-28   Add Your Name as Operator

Courtesy of Harris CareTracker PM and EMR

Print the Updated Operator Name screen, label it "Activity 2-8," and place it in your assignment folder.

In the end-of-chapter Build Your Proficiency activities you will complete steps to add key information to operator settings, such as the "idle time" (wait time) period (Proficiency Builder 2-7). You can also add, edit, override, and remove operator settings. Instructions are provided in *Help*.

In addition to the *Security Logs* link, the *Operator Activity Log* can be accessed from the *Operators & Roles* application. This allows you to monitor each operator's activity. This is an important feature and one more reason never to share your login and password with anyone.

CRITICAL THINKING Identify the buttons in the *Action* column of the *Operator Activity Log* as noted in the *Operators & Roles* link and provide a description of their use. In your judgment, rank them in order of importance, explaining your reasons why. Assess the value of the *Operator Activity Log* in maintaining compliance with HIPAA privacy laws. How would you use the *Log* in your duties as a practice manager?

Clinical–Daily Administration

In a live practice, the average employee may not have access to this module as this is more of managerial rights and features. The functions that every employee would do can also be accessed in other modules of the program.

The *Administration > Clinical* module is where you will find EMR features that include *Daily Administration, System Administration,* and *Import/Export*. For example, if you click *Favorite Labs* on the *Administration > Clinical > Daily Administration* column (**Figure 2-29**), you can view the providers available, the lab name (by using the drop-down feature), add a new lab (**Figure 2-30**), or change the order in which the labs appear on the screen.

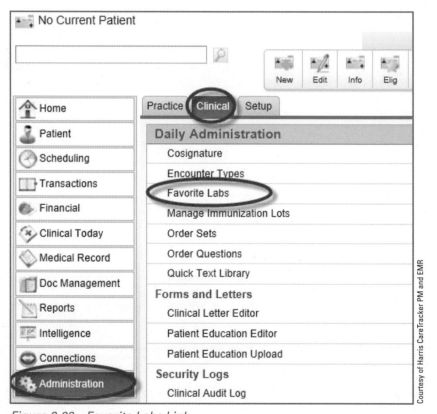

Figure 2-29   *Favorite Labs Link*

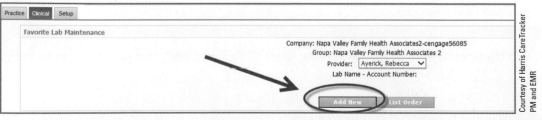

Figure 2-30   *Add a New Lab*

In the *Favorite Labs* application, you can create a list of commonly used labs. This expedites the ordering process by avoiding the need to go through a long list of facilities supported by Harris CareTracker PM and EMR each time you create an order.

Adding labs is only one example of the many features and functions in the *Daily Administration > Clinical* module. To view additional topics, log in to *Help* and open the *Administration Module > Clinical Administration > Daily Administration* folder in the *Contents* section.

Clinical–System Administration

The *Clinical > System Administration* module is where you will find EMR features that include *Clinical Setup* and *Maintenance* links. For example, if you click on the *Visit Summary* link in the *Administration > Clinical > System Administration* column (**Figure 2-31**), you can view the checklist for items to include on the *Patient Visit Summary Print Out* (see **Figure 2-32**). To make changes, you can select *All* or *None*. By selecting *None*, you can choose only the items you want to include on the *Patient Visit Summary Print Out*, or, alternatively, you can deselect items (by clicking on the check mark) to remove them from the list. Complete Proficiency Builder 2-1 at the end of the chapter to learn how to set up your *Patient Visit Summary* items.

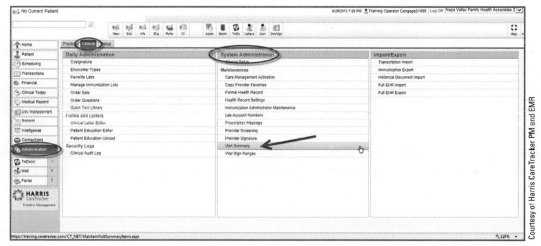

Figure 2-31   *Visit Summary Link*

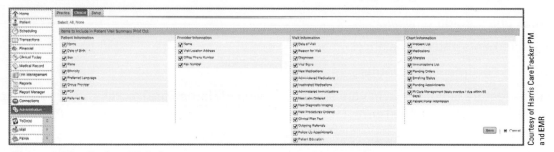

Figure 2-32   *Patient Visit Summary*

Updating patient visit summaries is only one example of the many features and functions in the *Administration* Module > *Clinical* tab *System Administration* column. To view additional topics, log in to *Help* and open the *Administration Module > Clinical Administration > System Administration* folder in the *Contents* section.

Clinical Import/Export

Although your student version of Harris CareTracker does not allow access to the *Clinical–Import/Export* tabs, in a live environment the following activities would be performed:

- *Transcription Import*
  - In the *Transcription Import* application, you can build transcription templates and upload transcription files. Harris CareTracker PM and EMR automatically saves the transcription to the corresponding

patient's record. After upload, you can access transcription files in the *Progress Notes* application of the *Medical Records* module.

- *Immunization Export*
  - o The *Immunization Export* application allows a practice to generate a record of all vaccinations given during a specified period. The application pulls the Harris CareTracker PM and EMR data into a state-specific format that can be downloaded and then sent to the state's department of health.
- *Historical Document Import*
- *Full EHR Import*
- *Full EHR Export (PDF) and Full EHR Export (CDA)*
  - o The *Full EHR Export* tool provides you the ability to export a batch of patient clinical data in PDF format. You can select the period to cover and the level of patient information to include.

Log in to *Help* and click on the *Home > Administration Module > Clinical > Import/Export* link to view more information.

Setup

The *Administration > Setup* module is where you will find *Practice Management* features that include the *Patient Portal, Contracts & Fees, Financial, Scheduling* functions and more.

Patient Portal

The *Patient Portal* is a secure web-based portal that allows patients to track and manage their personal health information online (**Figure 2-33**). In the *Patient Portal*, patients can:

- Communicate with the provider's office via secure messaging
- Request and confirm appointments
- Update personal information
- View portions of their health record
- Request prescription renewals
- View statements and pay balances
- Download documents and forms

Although this feature is not active in your student version of Harris CareTracker, most medical practices offer a patient portal feature. In the live Harris CareTracker program, you must enable the *Patient Portal* and then

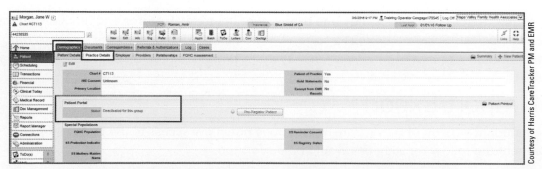

Figure 2-33   Patient Portal Feature in Practice Details of Patient Demographics

CRITICAL THINKING Describe the activities that a patient can perform in the *Patient Portal* feature. Provide an analysis of each of the activities and how might they affect the relationship between patients and providers.

configure the site's appearance and features. You can then customize the content, functionality, and colors; upload a logo; and add locations and taglines. Refer to *Help* features of the *Patient Portal*.

Contracts & Fees

Fee schedules determine the amount charged for each CPT® code entered into Harris CareTracker PM and EMR. Although the fee schedule is initially set up when the practice enrolls with Harris CareTracker PM and EMR, you can edit existing schedules or create new fee schedules for your practice at any time using the *Fee Schedule* application in the *Administration* module.

Revenue Codes. **Revenue codes** are practice-specific codes that give you an alternative way of reporting financial data in Harris CareTracker PM and EMR. Revenue codes can either be linked to specific CPT® codes on your fee schedule (e.g., "New Patient Office Visits") or be selected during visit or charge entry to represent a specific servicing provider, billing provider, and location combination (e.g., "Evening Clinic").

For reporting purposes, you can group *Month End* reports by revenue codes. When you create a revenue code to use during visit or charge entry, you can link a billing provider, servicing provider, or location you choose to code. However, a revenue code does not have to be linked to a billing provider, servicing provider, or a location.

Financial

In the *Financial* application of *Setup,* there are commonly used features such as *Encounter Form Maintenance, Locations*, and *Quick Picks,* (which will be reviewed later in the textbook).

Encounter Form Maintenance. The Harris CareTracker PM and EMR Enrollment Department builds encounter forms for clients when they decide to use Harris CareTracker PM and EMR as their practice management system; however, you can use the *Encounter Form Maintenance* application to build a custom encounter form for your practice. In a live practice, you can print the encounter forms based on appointments scheduled in the *Book* application either individually or in a batch.

When a provider uses paper encounter forms to capture CPT® and ICD-10 codes for a patient's visit, you must manually enter the procedure and diagnosis codes into Harris CareTracker PM and EMR via the *Visit* window or the *Charge* application of the *Transactions* module.

Locations. The *Locations* application allows you to add locations where services are rendered and to search all locations saved in the Harris CareTracker PM and EMR's global database. Global locations are created by Harris CareTracker PM and EMR Support, but operators can create new locations specific to their company and group. In a live practice, you must have the *Location Maintenance* override included in your operator profile to add and edit locations. To learn how to search and add new locations, complete Proficiency Builder 2-2 at the end of the chapter.

Quick Picks. Throughout Harris CareTracker PM and EMR, drop-down lists are available from which you can select field-specific data to help create a more efficient work flow, known as *Quick Picks.* Options available in a drop-down list are built for each practice and are group specific. Your practice can build drop-down options for locations, employers, insurance companies, and financial transactions.

In order for certain data fields to be available as you work in Harris CareTracker PM and EMR, they need to be added to your "quick picks" list. You can add or remove options from a drop-down list in the *Quick Picks* application in the *Setup* tab.

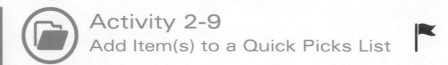

Activity 2-9
Add Item(s) to a Quick Picks List

1. Click the *Administration* module and then click the *Setup* tab.

2. Under the *Financial* header, click the *Quick Picks* link (**Figure 2-34**). Harris CareTracker PM and EMR launches the *Quick Picks* application.

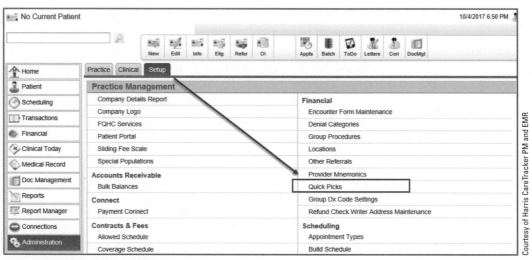

Figure 2-34   Quick Picks Link

Courtesy of Harris CareTracker PM and EMR

3. From the *Screen Type* drop-down list, select the quick picks list to which you want to add an item (select "Form Letters"). The application displays the "quick picks list."

4. Verify that the item you want to add (New Referral) is not already included in the current "quick picks" list.

5. Enter the item you want to add in the *Search* box (enter "New") and then click the *Search* icon. The application displays a search window containing a list of possible matches (**Figure 2-35**). Click on the desired result to select it (select "New Referral"). The application closes the search window and adds the data as an option in the list (**Figure 2-36**).

6. Click on "X" or "Close" to close out of the "Success" dialog box.

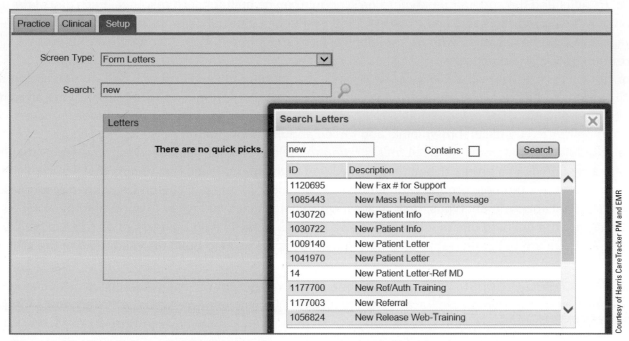

Figure 2-35   New Referral Form Letter

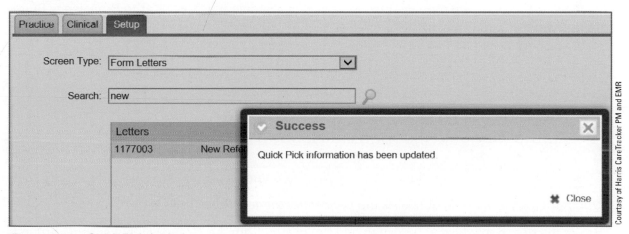

Figure 2-36   Quick Pick Added

💾 **Print the Quick Picks screen, label it "Activity 2-9," and place it in your assignment folder.**

Scheduling

In the *Scheduling* application of the *Administration* module you will use features such as *Build Schedules, Appointment Types, Cancel and Reschedule Reasons, Chief Complaint Maintenance, Room Maintenance, Custom Resources* and more.

You can create appointment types that allow you to customize your schedule for each resource or group in your practice. You can also set up your schedule so that only certain appointment types can be booked at certain times.

For example, an appointment could be "Established Patient Physical" that has a duration of 30 minutes. This appointment type could then be linked to an "Established Patient" task. Now, when someone is booking an "Established Patient Physical," he or she will only be able to book that appointment type during an "Established Patient" available task time.

After establishing the appointment types, the schedule can be built for each resource. Each day of the week is set up with the appropriate tasks and corresponding availability. Special days, such as holidays, personal days, and vacations, can be set aside with no availability. Also, appointment types can be linked to a specific group or all of the groups in a practice.

You can customize your schedule by color coding appointment types. For example, you can assign a color to help quickly identify new patient visits on the schedule. The color is applied to the border of the appointment in the *Book* application. The color assigned to an appointment type overrides the default border colors used to identify appointment conflicts (brown/pink) and forced appointments (blue).

The schedule template built in the *Administration* module is the interface used to generate availability for each of the resources in a group. Scheduling is executed at the group level. This means that a parent company, or practice, can have multiple groups with different schedules. A group can customize its own resources, availability, tasks, and appointment types. **Task classes**, which determine what types of appointments can be seen at what times, are the building blocks for a resource's schedule. A day is then built based on the availability of the task classes. Days are built into weeks and then those weeks are used to build the resource's entire schedule.

Cancel/Reschedule Reasons. The schedule for Napa Valley Family Health Associates has been built into your student version of Harris CareTracker. The practice is responsible for maintaining the schedule template, making changes, and opening future availability, which may be an activity you perform. Refer to *Help* (*Administration Module > Setup > Scheduling*) for steps to make changes in scheduling.

The *Cancel/Reschedule Reasons* application enables you to create company- or group-specific cancellation and reschedule reasons. Once a reason is added and made active, it is available when cancelling or rescheduling appointments via the *Scheduling* module. To view cancel/reschedule reasons, refer to Proficiency Builder 2-6 at the end of the chapter.

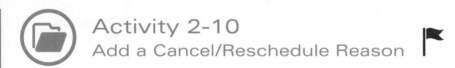

Activity 2-10
Add a Cancel/Reschedule Reason

1. Click the *Administration* module and then click the *Setup* tab.

2. Under the *Scheduling* section, click the *Cancel/Reschedule Reasons* link.

3. Select the group to which you want to add the reason from the *Group* list. If a specific group is not selected, the reason will be added to all groups in the company (select "Napa Valley Family Health Associates 2").

4. Select the type of reason to add from the *Reason Type* list. There are three options (listed next). For this activity, select "Cancel".
    *   (All): Includes both Cancel and Reschedule.
    *   Cancel: Makes the reason available when cancelling an appointment via the *Scheduling* module.
    *   Reschedule: Makes the reason available when rescheduling an appointment via the *Scheduling* module.

5. Click *Add Reason*.

6. Enter a description of the reason in the *Reason Name* box (enter "Pt went to emergency room").

7. Enter an abbreviated name for the reason in the *Short Name* box (enter "ER").

8. From the *Active* list, select *Yes* to make the reason available for use (**Figure 2-37**).

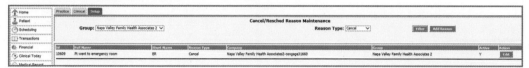

Figure 2-37   Add Cancel Reason   Courtesy of Harris CareTracker PM and EMR

9. Click *Save*.

10. Click on *Filter* and view your cancel reason added (**Figure 2-38**).

Figure 2-38   Cancel Reason Added   Courtesy of Harris CareTracker PM and EMR

🖫 **Print the Cancel Reason screen, label it "Activity 2-10," and place it in your assignment folder.**

Chief Complaint Maintenance. The *Chief Complaint Maintenance* application allows you to create a favorite list of MEDCIN-based chief complaints that are available to select from when booking appointments. You can create a chief complaint that is specific to a group or available to all groups in the company. If the chief complaint is not assigned to a specific group, it is automatically available to all groups in the company.

You can link chief complaints to a progress note template. If the chief complaint is linked to a progress note template, Harris CareTracker PM and EMR will automatically apply the linked template to the *Chief Complaint* section of the progress note for that visit. Harris CareTracker PM and EMR uses the following hierarchy to determine which template is applied to the progress note:

- By default, Harris CareTracker PM and EMR will apply the progress note template linked to the chief complaint selected in the *Book Appointment* window.

- If the chief complaint for the appointment is not linked to a progress note template, then Harris CareTracker PM and EMR will apply the template linked to the appointment type.

- If there is no template linked to either the chief complaint or the appointment type, Harris CareTracker PM and EMR will apply the operator's default template.

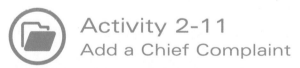

Activity 2-11
Add a Chief Complaint

1. Click the *Administration* module and then click the *Setup* tab.

2. Under the *Scheduling* section, click the *Chief Complaint Maintenance* link. The application launches the *Chief Complaint Maintenance* feature.

3. Click the + *New Complaint* link. The application displays the *Add New Complaint* dialog box.

4. From the *Group* list, select the group for which you want to add a chief complaint (select "Napa Valley Family Health Associates 2").

5. In the *Chief Complaint* field, click the *Search* icon. The application displays the *Complaint* search window. Note: If the name of the complaint is known enter the full or partial name of the complaint in the *Search* box. For this step just click on the *Search* icon. The application returns the available results.

6. Scroll down and click on the complaint you want to add (select "New Patient (1000248)," **Figure 2-39**). The application populates the *Chief Complaint* box with the selected complaint. **Note:** This may take a few moments to populate. Wait until *New Patient* is added to the *Chief Complaint* box before moving on.

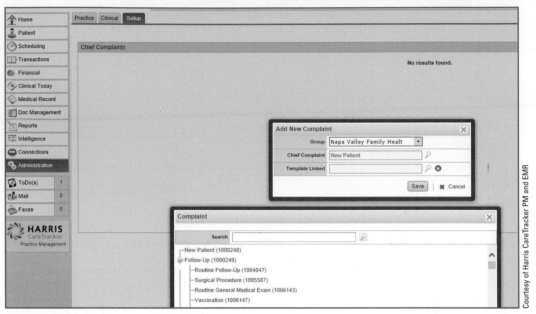

Figure 2-39   Chief Complaint Maintenance

7. In the *Template Linked* field, click the *Search* icon. The application displays the *Template* search window. Scroll down and click the "+" sign next to "Internal Medicine." Scroll down and select "IM OV Option 4 (v4) w/A&P."

8. Click *Save*. The new complaint is now added to the *Chief Complaint Maintenance* screen (**Figure 2-40**). Note again, this may take a few moments to populate. Do not click on Save more than once or you may receive an error message.

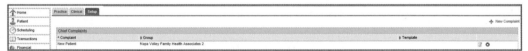

Figure 2-40   New Complaint Saved
Courtesy of Harris CareTracker PM and EMR

🖶 **Print the New Patient *Chief Complaint* screen, label it "Activity 2-11," and place it in your assignment folder.**

You can also edit and delete a *Chief Complaint* in this application. To remove the selected template, click the delete icon (the red "x"). Refer to the instructions in *Help* (*Administration Module > Setup > Scheduling > Chief Complaint Maintenance*).

Custom Resources. The *Custom Resources* application of the *Administration* module is where you can add, define options, and assign classes for resources. **Resources** can be people, places, or things. Providers are always considered a resource, but an exam room or a piece of equipment can also be considered a resource. Something that requires a schedule is considered a resource because it has specific availability with the days and times it can provide certain services. If the resource does not need a set schedule, then it is not considered a "resource" in Harris CareTracker PM and EMR.

After a resource is entered in the system, you can customize the resource, assign it to resource classes, and assign it to a resource group for scheduling purposes. Then, an operator can book that resource when scheduling an appointment that requires the resource.

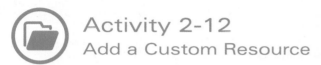

Activity 2-12
Add a Custom Resource

1. Click the *Administration* module and then click the *Setup* tab.

2. In the *Scheduling* section, click the *Custom Resources* link. Harris CareTracker PM displays the *Resource* page. All providers in the practice are listed as *Available Resources*.

3. (FYI only) If you are adding the custom resource for a particular provider in your group, select the provider from the *Provider* list and then click the left arrow button.

4. Click *New* next to the *Available Resources* list. Harris CareTracker PM displays a dialog box, prompting you to enter a name for the resource.

5. In the dialog box, enter a name for the resource you are creating. Enter "Obstetric 2-D Ultrasound Machine" (**Figure 2-41**).

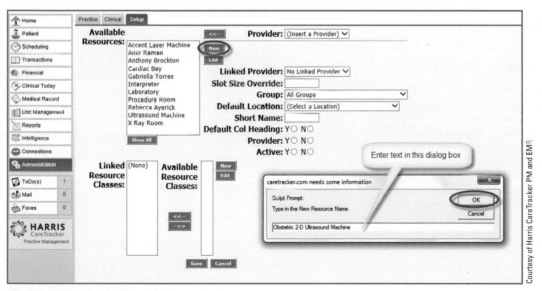

Figure 2-41   Add a Resource

6. Click *OK*. The application adds the resource to the *Available Resources* list (**Figure 2-42**).

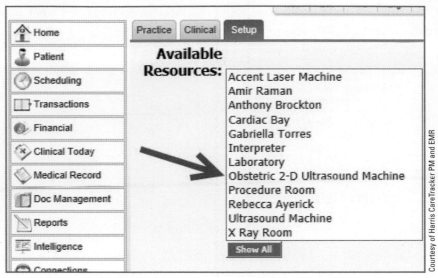

Figure 2-42   Added Resource

💾 **Print the Added Resource screen, label it "Activity 2-12," and place it in your assignment folder.**

Room Maintenance. It is important to have an efficient appointment workflow to better serve patients. The *Room Maintenance* feature helps you set up rooms to keep track of where the patients are during their visit by updating their location throughout their appointment (e.g., exam room one, nursing station).

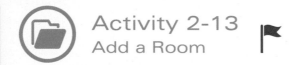

Activity 2-13
Add a Room ⚑

1. Click the *Administration* module and then click the *Setup* tab.

2. In the *Scheduling* section, click the *Room Maintenance* link.

3. Click *Add*.

4. Enter the name you want to assign to the room in the *Room Name* box (enter "Exam Room # 2").

5. Enter an abbreviated name for the room in the *Room Short Name* box (enter "Ex 2").

6. Select the group you want to assign to the new room from the *Group* list. This determines whether the room is shared among all groups in your practice or if it is only used by one group (select "All Groups").

7. Select where the room is located from the *Location* list. This is useful if you are a multilocation practice or if you want to set up floors for specific hospitals when using the *Admissions* application (select "All Locations").

8. By default, the *Active* field is set to *Y*. This means the room is active (**Figure 2-43**).

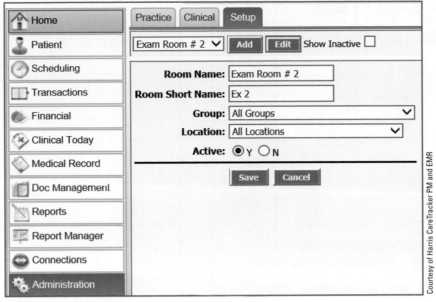

Figure 2-43   Add a Room

9. Click *Save.* The application adds the room.

10. Click back on the *Administration > Setup > Room Maintenance* link to view the newly added "Exam Room # 2" in the drop-down list (**Figure 2-44**).

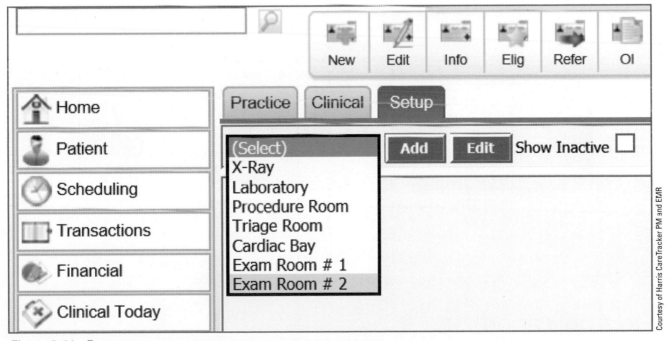

Figure 2-44   Rooms

▣ **Print the Add a Room screen, label it "Activity 2-13," and place it in your assignment folder.**

MESSAGE CENTER

Learning Objective 5: Use the Message Center components for appropriate EHR tasks.

The *Message* application is a communication tool that allows you to manage customer, staff, and patient communications. The *Message* application is a combination of the following features:

- *ToDos.* *ToDos* are Harris CareTracker PM and EMR's internal messaging system that serve two primary functions: assigning a coworker a task and communicating with the Harris CareTracker PM and EMR Support team.

- *Mail.* The *Mail* application is similar to any standard email application and allows you to send, receive, organize, and reply to internal email messages.

- *Queues.* *Queues* allow you to send *ToDos* to a group of people instead of an individual person.

- *Fax.* The *Fax* feature provides the ability to send and receive electronic faxes through Harris CareTracker PM and EMR.

Accessing the Messages Application

There are several ways to access the *Message Center*:

- Click on the *ToDo* 📝 icon on the name bar.

- Click the *Home* module and then click the *Messages* tab. The *Messages* application displays. By default, the application displays all open *ToDos* that pertain to you. You can access and manage other communication methods such as mail, fax, and queues by clicking on the panes on the right-hand side of the window. Each category is further subdivided based on the status. Once you have been entering data in Harris CareTracker, when you click on the *Home-Messages* tab, your messages screen will include information as shown in **Figure 2-45** and more.

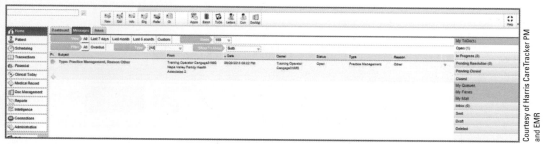

Figure 2-45 Home Messages

- Click the *ToDos* or *Mail* links in the left navigation pane.

- Click the *Clinical Today* module and then click *ToDos* in the *Quick Tasks* menu.

ToDo Application

The *ToDo* application is Harris CareTracker PM and EMR's internal messaging system that allows you to assign administrative and patient-related tasks within your practice as well as communicate with the Harris CareTracker PM and EMR support team. You will know you have an open *ToDo* if a number appears next to the *ToDo* link in the left navigation pane. In the *ToDo* application, you can review each *ToDo* that has been sent to you, reply to a *ToDo*, transfer a *ToDo*, take ownership of a *ToDo*, or close a *ToDo*. The application is updated in real time.

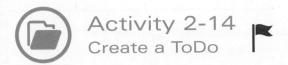

Activity 2-14
Create a ToDo

1. Click the *Home* module and then click the *Messages* tab. The *Messages* application displays all of your open *ToDo*(s).

2. Click on the *ToDo* ✅ icon on the *Name Bar*. The application displays the *New ToDo* window (**Figure 2-46**).

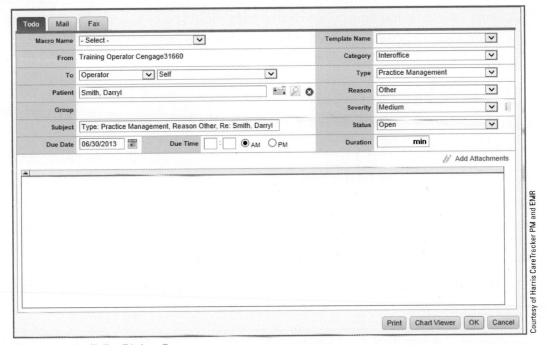

Figure 2-46   *ToDo Dialog Box*

3. Leave the *Macro Name* blank.

4. By default, the *From* list displays your name.

5. In the *To* list, click the required options. The *To* list includes the categories described in **Figure 2-47**. Select "Operator" in the first field and "Self" in the second field.

TO LIST OPTIONS	
Field	**Description**
Operator	Enables you to select a Optum PM and Physician EMR user from your company.
Queue	Enables you to select a work queue set up for the practice. This will redirect the ToDo to the queue. For example, you can send a ToDo to the Support queue and an operator in the queue will respond to the ToDo.
Participant	Enables you to select a participant in the ToDo. This can be a person or a queue that participated in the ToDo.

Figure 2-47   *List Options for ToDo*

6. If you are sending a *ToDo* to a patient, enter his or her full or partial last name in the *Patient* box (enter "Smith") and then click the *Search* icon. When the search window opens, click on the name of the patient in the search results (select "Smith, Darryl").

> **TIP** If the *ToDo* is not patient related, you would click the *Delete* icon ⊗ to remove the name from the *Patient* field. You can click the *Info* icon to view the patient's contact information in the "At a Glance" patient information window.

7. By default, the *Subject* box displays information based on the selection in the *Type* and *Reason* lists in the right-hand column. However, you can change the subject if necessary. Leave as "Practice Management, Reason Other."

8. The *Due Date* automatically defaults to today's date and *Due Time* box defaults blank. Depending on the ToDo, enter the date and time by which the *ToDo* should be completed. This is important to track overdue items. For this activity, leave *Due Date* as today's date and leave the *Due Time* blank.

9. Leave the *Template Name* field blank.

10. From the *Category* list, select the *ToDo* category (leave as "Interoffice").

11. In the *Type* list, click/confirm the type of the *ToDo* (leave as "Practice Management").

12. In the *Reason* list, click/confirm the reason for the *ToDo* (leave as "Other").

13. In the *Severity* list, select the priority level of the *ToDo* (leave as "Medium").

14. The *Status* list is set to "Open" by default. Leave as is.

15. In the *Duration* box, enter the total time spent working on the *ToDo* (enter "5").

16. In the content box, type in "Test ToDo."

17. Click *OK*. The *ToDo* will disappear and show in your *Messages Dashboard* (**Figure 2-48**).

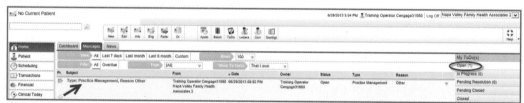

Figure 2-48 Student-Created ToDo

Courtesy of Harris CareTracker PM and EMR

💾 **Print the *Messages* dashboard with the completed *ToDo*, label it "Activity 2-14," and place it in your assignment folder.**

To view additional information regarding the *ToDo* features of Harris CareTracker, use the *Help* system by going to *Messages Center > ToDos* folder (**Figure 2-49**).

Mail

The *Mail* application allows you to communicate electronically with staff members, providers in your *Provider Portal*, and patients activated in the *Patient Portal*. The mail feature works the same as other email applications, enabling you to open, view, create, send and receive, and delete messages. In addition, you can link attachments such as patient encounter notes, documents, results, referrals and authorization forms, set priorities, and more.

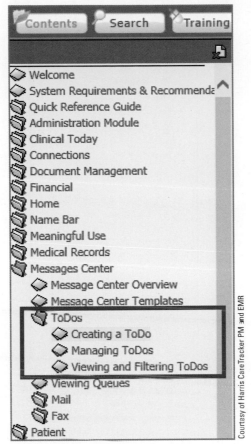

Figure 2-49   Help ToDo Pane

You can use templates to create preformatted content for mail messages. For example, you can create a standard mail message used for outgoing referrals. Any time that template is selected the mail message is automatically populated with the text in the template. Templates are created in the *Event Manager* application in the *Administration* module.

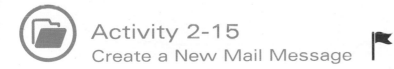

Activity 2-15
Create a New Mail Message

1. Click the *Home* module and then click the *Messages* tab. The *Messages Center* opens and displays all of your open *ToDos*.

2. Click *Send Mail*, located on the bottom right of the page (**Figure 2-50**). The application displays the *Message* dialog box.

3. Leave the *Macro Name* as is: (-Select-).

4. The *From* list defaults to the operator creating the mail message and cannot be edited.

5. In the *To* field, click the *Search* icon. Harris CareTracker PM and EMR opens the *Select Operators* dialog box.

6. Place a check mark in the box by <u>your</u> login name (see example in **Figure 2-51**). **Note:** The last name field will either include your last name or your CareTracker username.

7. Click *Select.* The application closes the *Select Operators* dialog box.

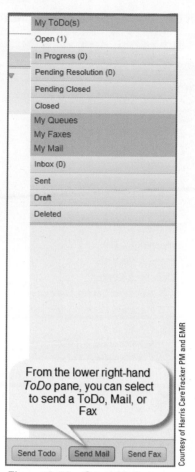

Figure 2-50   Send Mail

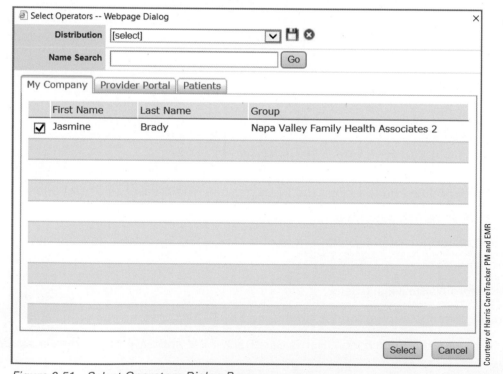

Figure 2-51   Select Operators Dialog Box

8. If a patient is in context, the patient name displays in the *Patient* box. However, you can also send a mail message about a different patient by clicking the *Search* icon. For this activity, you will leave the

patient field blank. If a patient is in context, click the red "x" at the end of the patient name field to remove the patient from context.

9. In the *Subject* box, enter the subject of the mail message (enter "Test Mail Message").

10. Leave the *Template Name* field blank.

11. By default, the *Severity* list displays "Medium." However, you can change the priority of the mail message if necessary. Leave as is.

12. (FYI only) To link patient data or to add attachments, refer to the instructions in *Help*. Do not link or add any data.

13. In the message dialog box, enter the message and format the information if necessary. Enter "Test Mail Message" (**Figure 2-52**).

14. Click *Send*. If you did not want to send the message immediately you would click *Save Draft* to save the message and send later. For this activity, click *Send*.

15. To view your sent message, click the *Sent* link on the *My ToDo(s)* pane on the right side of the screen (**Figure 2-53**) or the *Mail* link on the left-hand side of your screen.

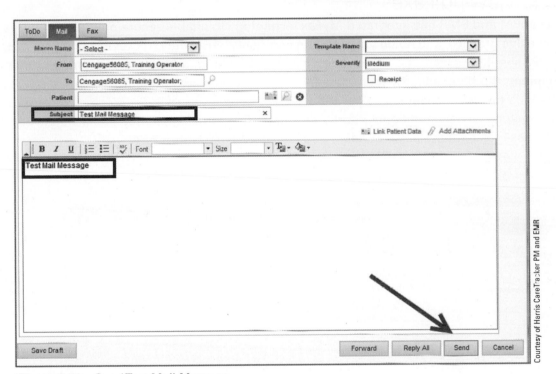

Figure 2-52   Send Test Mail Message

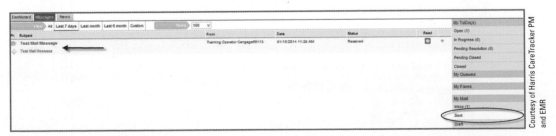

Figure 2-53   Sent Mail Message

💾 **Print the Sent Message screen, label it "Activity 2-15," and place it in your assignment folder.**

Queue

Queues are used to organize and group *ToDos*, mail, and faxes in the *Messages Center*. Queues help manage tasks more efficiently by allowing you to route *ToDos* to a group rather than to one individual. At the top of each queue is a set of filters you can use to sort *ToDos*, mail messages, and faxes.

Harris CareTracker PM and EMR provides several global queues, such as the *Support* and *Mail* queues. You can also create custom queues for your company for routing *ToDos* or sending and receiving faxes. Queues are created in the *Queues* application in the *Administration* module.

Fax Capabilities of Harris CareTracker

In order to utilize the *Fax* feature of Harris CareTracker, you must receive a confirmation email from *Protus* that your *MyFax* number has been linked to your Harris CareTracker PM and EMR account before you can begin faxing. This function is not active in your student version of Harris CareTracker. To check faxing activity, you would log in to your *MyFax* account to view the faxing activity on your account, including the total number of incoming and outgoing faxes.

Sending and Viewing Faxes

Harris CareTracker PM and EMR has integrated *MyFax* technology to enable secure online faxing. This feature is only available in a live practice, and not in your training company. Harris CareTracker PM and EMR automatically generates a cover sheet for faxes. The cover sheet displays the name, address, and phone number of the fax sender and recipient, the date, and any text entered in the *Notes* box when the fax was created. You have the option not to include the cover sheet.

Use the *Help* system to view additional information regarding the *Fax* features of Harris CareTracker at the *Contents tab > Messages Center > Fax > Sending and Viewing Faxes* (**Figure 2-54**).

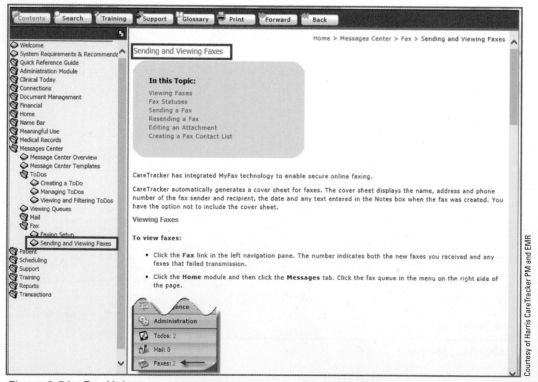

Figure 2-54   Fax Help

There you will find instructions on:

- Viewing Faxes
- Fax statuses
- Sending a Fax
- Resending a Fax
- Editing an attachment
- Creating a Fax contact list

 CRITICAL THINKING In the beginning of this chapter, your challenge was to utilize the *Help* materials to enhance the training process and expand your knowledge. Which features in *Help* did you access? What topics did you find most helpful? If you experienced any challenges completing the activities, did you log in to *Help* to look for support? If not, why not?

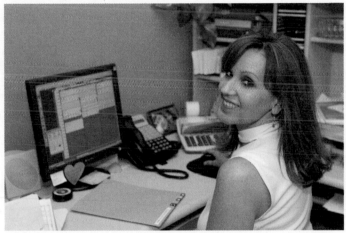

© B. Franklin/Shutterstock.com.

SUMMARY

Harris CareTracker PM and EMR provides a robust electronic health record that is fully integrated and interoperable. The *Help* system offers a valuable tool for beginning users and for refresher training as the system continually updates with new features. Medical assistants often advance in their roles in the medical field, and being proficient with electronic health records and health information technology opens many opportunities.

The practice, clinical, and Setup applications you completed in this chapter mimic activities that medical assistants perform in the patient-centered medical environment. Using the *Help* system to seek out additional information enhances proficiency using Harris CareTracker PM and EMR. You now have an understanding of the purpose and location of key features of Harris CareTracker PM and EMR such as the *Main Menu*, *Navigation*, *Home*, and *Dashboard* overview, which makes navigating the EHR seamless.

CHECK YOUR KNOWLEDGE

Select the best response.

_____ 1. The *Home* module contains three applications. Which of the following is not one of the applications?

    a. Dashboard   c. Messages

    b. Administration   d. News

_____ 2. The *Dashboard* is divided into three tabs. Which of the following is not one of the tabs?

    a. Home   c. Management

    b. Practice   d. Meaningful Use

_____ 3. *Dashboard* represents values that are refreshed overnight. These values are based on the provider and location selected in the batch. Which of the following is not one of the values?

    a. The value indicates all open admissions.   c. The value depicts the total number of patients seen each day.

    b. The value indicates admissions with missing days.   d. None of the above.

_____ 4. An appointment wait list of patients who would like an appointment with a provider prior to their currently scheduled appointment can be generated by clicking on the:

    a. *Wait List* link under the *Appointments* section of the *Dashboard.*   c. *Wait List* link under the *Setup* tab in the *Administration* module.

    b. *Wait List* link under the *Administration* module of the *Home* page.   d. *My Lists* section of the *Dashboard* under *Practice* tab.

_____ 5. An inactive claim would be a claim that not only is unpaid, but has not had any follow-up activity for the last _____ days.

    a. 7   c. 30

    b. 14   d. 60

_____ 6. What feature can only be used for primary payments and is designed to make you aware of instances when you are paid less than the actual allowed amount?

    a. Inactive claims   c. Open encounters

    b. Verify payments   d. Unbilled claims

_____ 7. In the _____ link, you can see the total number of operators who worked in Harris CareTracker PM and EMR for a particular date and can drill down to see which operators did what on a specific date.

    a. Batch deposits   c. Adjustments

    b. Notes   d. User access audits

_____ 8. Which of the following is not on the operator log, regardless of the filters you set?

    a. Date and time   c. Name of the patient whose record was accessed, the group in which the action was taken, and a comment

    b. Operator's login ID and operator's name

                                   d. Provider and account receivable

_____ 9. What application is a communication tool that allows you to manage customer, staff, and patient communications?

    a. Maintenance   c. Resources

    b. Messages   d. Setup

_____ 10. Where would you find the *Provider Lookup* link?

    a. *Administration > Daily Administration*   c. *Home > Dashboard > Staff Measures*

    b. *Home > Dashboard > Management*   d. *Administration > Knowledgebase*

CASE STUDIES

Case Study 2-1

Add "Paul T. Endo" to the "Refer Provider To" quick picks list. (Refer to Activity 2-9 for guidance.)

Print a copy of the screen that illustrates your added quick pick. Label the *Paul T. Endo* screenshot as "Case Study 2-1," and place it in your assignment folder.

Case Study 2-2

Create a *ToDo* for patient Kimberly Johnson. (Refer to Activity 2-14 for guidance.) For this case study, enter the following text for the *ToDo*:

> "Test ToDo (CS 2-2): Dr. Ayerick, patient Kimberly Johnson called to establish as a New Patient. Your practice is currently restricted to accepting only new pediatric patient. She was referred by Dr. Alfred Peretti who has recently retired. Do you want to accept her as a new patient, or have her schedule with Gabriella?"

Print a copy of the screen that illustrates you created a ToDo for Kimberly Johnson, label it "Case Study 2-2," and place it in your assignment folder.

BUILD YOUR PROFICIENCY

Proficiency Builder 2-1: Add Patient Visit Summary Items

A patient visit summary is printed at the completion of a patient's visit. You can control the items that are included on a patient visit summary print out. To add patient visit summary items, complete the following steps:

1. Click the *Administration* module and then click the *Clinical* tab.

2. Under the *System Administration* column, *Maintenances* header, click the *Visit Summary* link. The application launches the *Patient Visit Summary* application (**Figure 2-55**).

(continues)

BUILD YOUR PROFICIENCY *(continued)*

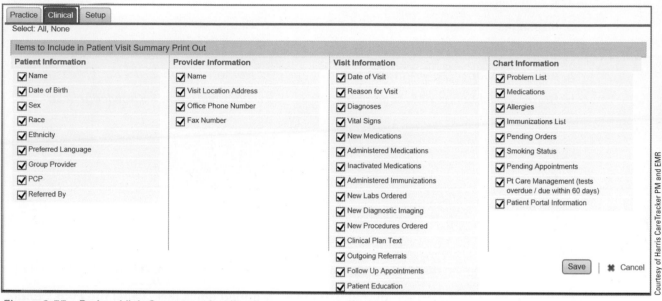

Figure 2-55   *Patient Visit Summary Application*

3. Deselect *Inactivated Medications* by clicking on the checkbox (removes the check mark).

4. Deselect *Patient Portal Information* by clicking on the checkbox (removes the check mark) (**Figure 2-56**).

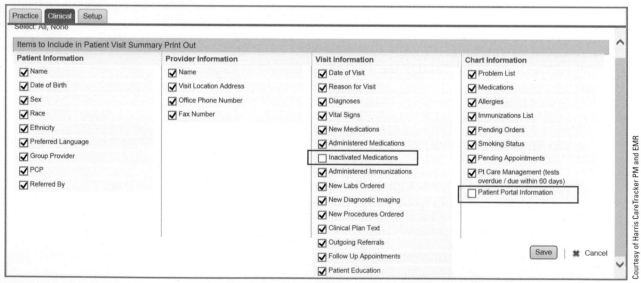

Figure 2-56   *Deselect Patient Visit Summary Items*

5. Click *Save. Patient Visit Summary Print Out* has been successfully updated.

6. Return to the *Administration > Clinical* tab, click on the *Visit Summary* link, and see that the changes have been saved.

🖶 **Print the Patient Visit Summary Items List screen, label it "BYP 2-1," and place it in your assignment folder.**

Proficiency Builder 2-2: Search for, then Add a New Location

You can search for other locations to add to your database. You would do this because it is a time-saving feature to enter frequently used locations.

1. Click the *Administration* module and then click the *Setup* tab.

2. Under the *Financial* header, click the *Locations* link (**Figure 2-57**). Harris CareTracker PM and EMR launches the *Locations* application.

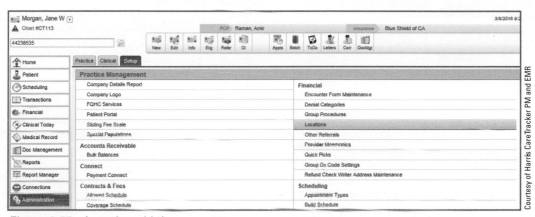

Figure 2-57   Locations Link

3. Enter the search criteria in one or more of the *Name, Modified,* or *Location* fields and then click *Search.* The application displays a list of search results in the bottom half of the screen (enter "Queen of" in the *Location Full Name* box and "CA" in the *State* box, then click *Search*). The application search will display "Queen of the Valley Medical Center" in Napa, California (**Figure 2-58**).

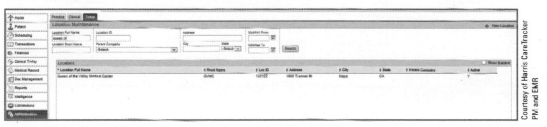

Figure 2-58   Search Location Queen of the Valley Medical Center

📠 **Print the Search Location screen, label it "BYP 2-2A," and place it in your assignment folder.**

4. Click on the location you want to review (Queen of the Valley Medical Center). The application displays the location details.

   You can also add or edit locations from this application.

(continues)

BUILD YOUR PROFICIENCY (continued)

5. To add a new location, click on the plus sign next to *New Location* (**Figure 2-59**).

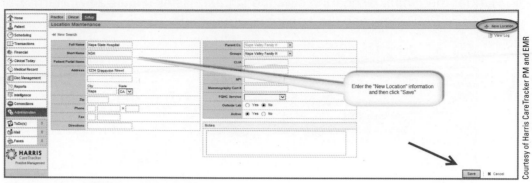

Figure 2-59 Add New Location–NSH

6. Enter the new location information:

   a. In the *Full Name* field, enter "Napa State Hospital"

   b. In the *Short Name* field, enter "NSH"

   c. In the *Address* fields, enter, 1234 Grapevine Street, Napa, CA, 94558

   d. Leave the other fields blank or leave as defaulted.

   e. Click *Save.*

7. Your new location is now saved. Click back on the *Administration* module > *Setup* tab > *Locations* link, enter short name of "NSH," and enter "CA" in the *State* field, and hit *Search*.

8. Your new location is now displayed (**Figure 2-60**).

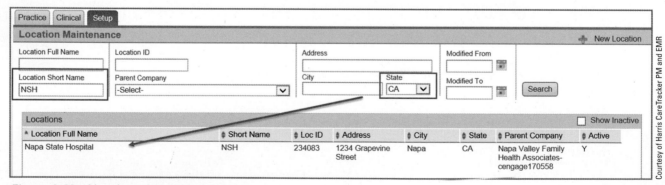

Figure 2-60 New Location Added–NSH

💾 Print the Search Location screen, label it "BYP 2-2B," and place it in your assignment folder.

Proficiency Builder 2-3: Additional Practice with Recorded Training

Look for "Operators & Roles" under *Administration Training* in the *Recorded Training* section of the *Help* feature. (Refer to Activity 2-2 for guidance in using this feature.) Review the "Operator & Roles" training session. Once you have completed the review, click on "Quiz." Take the *Quiz* and submit to your instructor for grading.

🖷 **Print the Quiz, label it "BYP 2-3," and place it in your assignment folder.**

You may repeat this activity to search for additional topics and quizzes, such as "Front Office Dashboard Overview" and more.

Proficiency Builder 2-4: Steps to View the Operators Log

The *Operators Log* tracks the activity of operators that log in to CareTracker. Operators can search the audit log by a date range (within the last 30 days).

1. Click the *Administration* module. Harris CareTracker PM displays the *Practice* tab.

2. Click the *Operators Log* link in the *Security Logs* section of the *Daily Administration* menu. Harris CareTracker PM displays the operators log for the current month.

3. To view the *Operators Log* for a particular date range (current month):

    a. Enter the beginning and ending dates for the range in the *Date From* (enter the first day of the month/year you are currently working in, and in the *Date To* box enter today's date). Use the calendars to look up the dates if necessary.

    b. Click *Go*. Harris CareTracker PM displays the operators log with the date and number of operators for the specified date range (**Figure 2-61**).

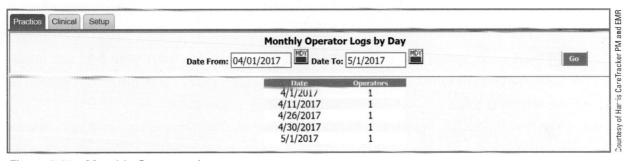

Figure 2-61   Monthly Operators Log

🖷 **Print the Operator's Log screen, label it "BYP 2-4," and place it in your assignment folder.**

Proficiency Builder 2-5: Additional Practice with Quick Picks Lists (Add and then Remove a Form Letter)

1. Add "Light Duty" to the "Form Letters" Quick Picks list. (Refer to Activity 2-9 if you need guidance to complete this activity.)

🖷 **Print the Quick Picks screen, label it "BYP 2-5a," and place it in your assignment folder.**

2. Now delete "Light Duty" from the "Form Letters" Quick Picks list by clicking the *Delete* icon next to the item you want to remove.

3. Click *Yes* to remove the item from the list.

🖷 **Print the Quick Picks screen, label it "BYP 2-5b," and place it in your assignment folder.**

(continues)

BUILD YOUR PROFICIENCY *(continued)*

Proficiency Builder 2-6: View Cancel/Reschedule Reasons; Add Reason

1. Click the *Administration* module and then click the *Setup* tab.

2. Click the *Cancel/Reschedule Reasons* link under the *Scheduling* header.

3. Select the "Napa Valley Family Health Associates2" from the *Group* list.

4. Select the type of reason to view from the *Reason Type* list. Select "(All)" then click *Filter*. Harris CareTracker PM displays a list of reasons if any have been created. If necessary, you can edit the reason details by clicking the *Edit* button.

5. Click back on the *Administration* module, *Setup* tab.

6. Click the *Cancel/Reschedule Reasons* link under the *Scheduling* header.

7. Select the "Napa Valley Family Health Associates2" from the *Group* list.

8. From the Reason Type, select "Cancel" and then click *Filter*.

9. From the Reason Type, select "Reschedule," then click *Filter*.

10. If no "Reasons" display, click on *Add Reason*.

11. Leave the *Group* as "Napa Valley Family Health Associates2."

12. Select *Reason Type*: "Reschedule."

13. In the *Reason Name* field, enter "Provider Unavailable."

14. In the *Short Name* field, enter "ProviderCx."

15. In the *Active Y/N* field, select "Yes."

🖼 **Print a screenshot of the Cancel/Reschedule Reason(S), label it "BYP 2-6," and place it in your assignment folder.**

16. Click on *Save*.

You may repeat this Proficiency Builder and enter additional cancel or reschedule reasons.

Proficiency Builder 2-7: Key Information to Add to Operator Settings

The maximum idle time in Harris CareTracker PM is 180 minutes. For security reasons, in a live practice it is best practice to keep the idle time short, such as 5–10 minutes. The time zone defaults to Eastern Standard Time (EST) if no time zone is set for the operator. Because this is an educational environment, a longer idle time is suggested as you work on your activities. This proficiency builder provides instructions to change the idle time that best suits your needs.

1. Click the *Administration* module. The application displays the *Practice* tab.

2. Click the *Operators & Roles* link in the *Security* section. The application displays the *Group Operators* list.

3. Click on your Operator Name. The details of your settings will then display in the lower portion of the screen.

4. In the *Timeout* box, enter the amount of time (in minutes) that the Harris CareTracker PM system can be idle before the operator is automatically logged out (enter "30").

5. From the *Time Zone* list, select the time zone in which you are located (for example, select "US/Pacific" if you are in Napa, California). The application calculates the check-in, take-back, and check-out time based on the operator's time zone setting. Additionally, the time stamp in the clinical log, progress note, and appointment list are also based on the time zone set for the operator.

6. From the *Position* list, select a position for the operator (select "Site Admin").

7. Click *Save*. The application adds the operator setting (**Figure 2-62**).

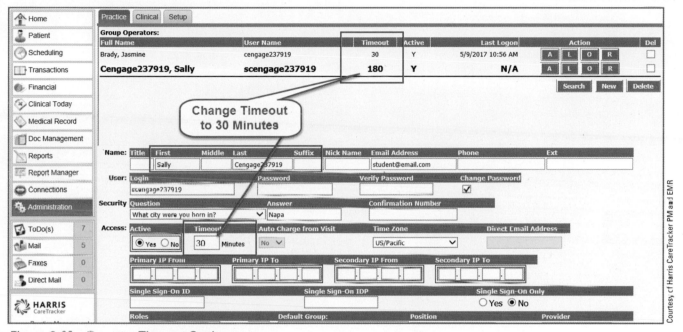

Figure 2-62   *Operator Timeout Setting*

Print the New Operator Added screen, label it "BYP 2-7," and place it in your assignment folder.

MODULE 2
Administrative Skills

This module includes:

- Chapter 3: Patient Demographics and Registration
- Chapter 4: Appointment Scheduling

As a health care professional, you may use Harris CareTracker PM and EMR to search for patients in the database, edit a patient's demographics, register a new patient, perform eligibility checks, and schedule appointments. These tasks are performed first in the practice workflow, before the patient sees the provider. A patient must be registered in the database in order to perform any administrative, clinical, or financial tasks. All the activities you complete in this module mimic a real-world setting using the administrative features of electronic health records.

QUICK START

Because Harris CareTracker is a live EMR, you will need to complete several tasks to optimize your computer for using the EMR software. **If you have been following along in this book from the beginning and have completed all Required ▐ activities as you've moved sequentially through the text, then you have already completed the activities below and can move forward. If you are beginning with this module, then you will need to complete the activities below *before* you can complete any other activities in this module.**

Be sure you are working in a supported browser (Internet Explorer 11 or Safari for iPad) before you begin. Other browsers (such as Chrome and Firefox) are not supported. Review Best Practices, included on page xxiii of this textbook.

- ❑ Activity 1-1: Disable Toolbars
- ❑ Activity 1-2: Set Up Tabbed Browsing
- ❑ Activity 1-3: Turn Off Pop-Up Blocker
- ❑ Activity 1-4: Change Page Setup
- ❑ Activity 1-5: Add Harris CareTracker to Trusted Sites
- ❑ Activity 1-6: Clear Your Cache
  - *Note: Remember that you should clear your cache each time before you begin working in CareTracker.*
- ❑ Activity 1-8: Disable Download Blocking
  - *Note: Once you have completed the system set-up requirements (Activities 1-1, 1-2, 1-3, 1-4, 1-5, 1-6, and 1-8), you will not need to repeat these activities unless you change the device you are using or the settings automatically default back to prior settings.*

❏ Activity 1-9: Register Your Credentials and Create Your Harris CareTracker PM and EMR Training Company
  • *Note: It will take up to 24 hours for your CareTracker ``Student Company'' to be created. Plan accordingly.*

❏ Activity 2-1: Log in to Harris CareTracker PM and EMR
  • *Note: Be sure to write down your new password inside the front cover of your book for easy reference.*

❏ Activity 2-5: Open a New Fiscal Year
  • *Note: Every January 1, you will need to open a new fiscal year.*

❏ Activity 2-6: Open a Fiscal Period
  • *Note: Every first of the month, you will need to open a new fiscal period.*

Patient Demographics and Registration

Key Terms

batch
carve-out
context
demographic
edit
eligibility
encryption
group number
guarantor
member number
non-participating
notice of privacy
   practices (NPP)

Practice Management
primary
protected health
   information (PHI)
responsible party
secondary
subscriber
subscriber number
tertiary
unknown status
workflow

Learning Objectives

1. Identify components of the Name Bar.
2. Describe the Patient Module and Demographics features in Harris CareTracker.
3. Search for a patient within Harris CareTracker PM.
4. Register a new patient in Harris CareTracker.
5. Edit patient information in Harris CareTracker.
6. View and perform eligibility checks.

Real-World Connection

Here at NVFHA, we conduct reference checks on all job applicants who make it to a second interview. Our goal is to hire applicants who have a high capacity for "attention to detail." When entering patient demographic information in the electronic health record, it is critical to pay attention to detail because this information impacts so many departments within our practice. If you misspell a patient's name, or put in incorrect address information, it creates havoc for the clinical team searching for the patient's chart, the billing team that has to send out a second billing statement due to incorrect address information, and even the insurance company that reviews a claim for the second time due to demographic discrepancies with the first claim. These types of errors are costly to the practice because they increase employee hours needed to correct the errors and delay reimbursement for service that affect the revenue cycle.

As you go through the activities in this chapter, pay particular attention to your ability to enter information correctly. If you struggle in this area, you may want to slow down a bit and make certain that you're reading the instructions carefully and thoroughly, and are entering the correct information the first time around. Keep this information in mind as you begin your activities. At the end of the chapter, you will be asked to summarize your experience. Are you up for the challenge? Let's get started!

INTRODUCTION

Harris CareTracker Practice Management and Physician EMR is a cloud-based application that enables physician practices to achieve greater efficiency by streamlining their administrative workflows. **Practice Management** (PM) refers to the "front office" of a medical practice: functions that include the patient's financial, demographic, and nonmedical information. **Workflow** refers to how tasks are performed throughout the office (usually in a specific order); for instance, the patient is checked in and his or her insurance cards are scanned, and then taken to the exam room where vital signs are taken/recorded, and so on.

The *Patient* module in Harris CareTracker PM and EMR is where you register patients into the system. The information stored in this module includes the patient's basic and detailed demographics, health insurance information, and referrals and authorizations. **Demographics** comprise the basic patient-identifying information, for example, full name, address, phone number, sex, Social Security number, date of birth, and health insurance information; and is defined as relating to the dynamic balance of a population, especially with regard to density and capacity for expansion or decline. Some practices may refer to the Demographics form as a "Face Sheet." Entering accurate patient information is essential because Harris CareTracker PM and EMR pulls the information from the *Patient* module to print and send insurance claims for billing purposes. The PM module makes registration simple and improves service by centralizing billing and demographics details at the first stage of the patient encounter.

SPOTLIGHT   Highlights of the *Patient Registration* module:

- Enter patient demographics
- Enter and record insurance information
- Scan and attach insurance cards and identification cards
- Verify insurance eligibility prior to billing with one click of a button

In this chapter, you will learn the role of patient demographics and registration in the paperless medical office. You will complete activities in the PM system such as searching for a patient, registering a new patient, and then **edit** (modifying the content of the input by inserting, deleting, or moving characters, numbers, or data) patient information, and perform **eligibility** checks (determining whether a person is entitled to receive insurance benefits for health care services). These tasks mimic actual duties you will be performing as a medical assistant. You will learn and discover the many attributes of working in a paperless medical office, along with gaining an understanding of the responsibilities associated with your position.

> Before you begin the activities in this chapter, refresh your memory on working with Harris CareTracker by referring back to the Best Practices list on page xxiii of this textbook. This list is also posted to the student companion website. Following best practices will help you complete work quickly and accurately.

NAME BAR

Learning Objective 1: Identify components of the Name Bar.

The *Name Bar*, located across the top of the Harris CareTracker window, provides quick access to the most frequently used Harris CareTracker applications (**Figure 3-1**). A quick reference guide to the various applications launched from the *Name Bar* illustrates each button and a description of the function (**Figure 3-2**). The *Name Bar* allows you to pull a patient into **context** to perform specific tasks. A patient is "in context" when his or her information appears in the *Name* list and *ID* box, as illustrated on the *Name Bar* picture. To pull a patient into context, you will type in either the patient account number or the first letters of the patient's last name and click *Enter*.

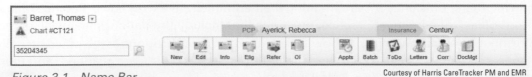

Figure 3-1   Name Bar   Courtesy of Harris CareTracker PM and EMR

Alternatively, you can click on the search patient icon (**Figure 3-3**) 🔍. When the pop-up screen appears, you will enter the first three letters of the last name and first one to three letters of the first name and click on the *Search* button (see **Figure 3-4**) to search. Always verify at least two patient identifiers (such as name, date of birth, last four of the Social Security number, etc.) to confirm you have selected the correct patient. Click on the patient, and he or she will be pulled into context. If no patient is found in the search, you will proceed to creating a new account by registering the new patient.

NAME BAR	
Button	**Description**
🔍 **Search**	Pulls patients into context by Harris CareTracker PM and EMR ID number, chart number, claim ID, or last name. Enter the patient's first name, last name, or at least three letters of each name to display the Advanced Search dialog box that enables you to select a patient.
⚠ **Alert**	Displays the Patient Alerts window. The Patient Alerts window notifies the operator when key information is missing from a patient's demographics or if any problems exist with the patient's account.
Edit	Launches the Demographics application in edit mode for the patient in context.
New	Launches the Demographics application, enabling you to register a new patient in Harris CareTracker PM and EMR.
Info	Displays a read only summary of the patient's information, including address, contact information, family members, balance information, insurance, etc.
Elig	Displays a history of eligibility checks and enables you to perform an individual electronic eligibility check to ensure that the patient is covered by the insurance company listed as the primary insurance.
Refer	Launches the Referral/Authorization application.
Appts	Displays a list of upcoming patient appointments. In addition, you can view and confirm an appointment, check in/check out a patient, print the encounter form, and perform various other tasks pertaining to the appointment.
OI	Displays information pertaining to dates of service. For example, you can obtain information such as associated procedures, financial transactions and claim activity, and make financial transactions such as payments, adjustments, refunds, and more.
Batch	Launches the Batch application, allowing you to create a new batch to enter charges and post payments and adjustments. In addition, you can also set up personal settings when using Harris CareTracker PM and EMR. For example, the main application to launch when logged on to Harris CareTracker PM and EMR.
ToDo	Launches the Harris CareTracker PM and EMR messaging tool, allowing you to communicate with other staff and the Harris CareTracker PM and EMR Support Department.
Letters	Generated and prints letters to send a patient.
Corr	Displays a queue of letters generated and enables you to print the letters to send to patients.

Figure 3-2   Description of Name Bar Applications

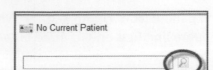

Figure 3-3   Search Patient
Courtesy of Harris CareTracker PM and EMR

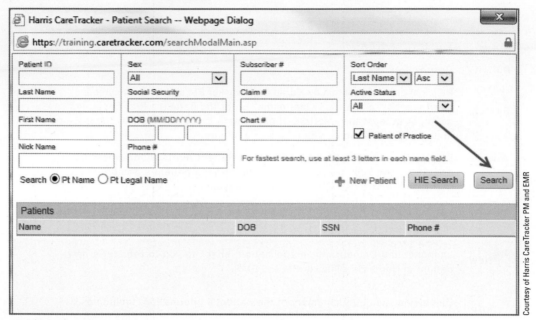

Figure 3-4   Patient Search Window

To access a patient previously in context, click the arrow next to the patient's name (**Figure 3-5**). To remove the patient from context, select *None*.

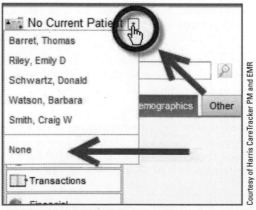

Figure 3-5   Patients Previously in Context

Click the *Info* icon (also known as the "At a Glance" patient info icon) on the left-hand side next to the patient's name to view patient demographic information, *Patient Portal* status, primary/secondary insurance information, primary/secondary copayment amounts, previous and pending appointment details, and provider information (**Figure 3-6**). To launch the *Patient Information* window, click the *View Complete Patient Information* link at the bottom-right side of the window.

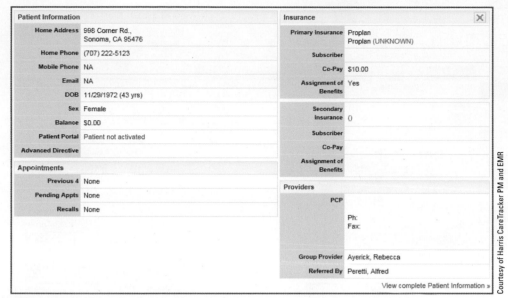

Figure 3-6   Patient Information

Your student version of Harris CareTracker will not have access to *Patient Portal* (the Personal Health Record feature of Harris CareTracker). For medical offices that have the fully integrated Harris CareTracker PM and EMR, medical assistants would click the *Patient Portal* tab to launch the *Patient Portal* in the *Patient* module, which allows patients to communicate electronically and securely with their provider.

DEMOGRAPHICS

Learning Objective 2: Describe the Patient Module and Demographics features in Harris CareTracker.

The *Demographics* application in the *Patient* module is where new patients are registered and added into the Harris CareTracker PM and EMR system. A patient's record will contain basic identifying information and is where pertinent health insurance information is captured. You will record a patient's personal information such as his or her name, address, phone number, date of birth (DOB), Social Security number, marital status, sex, insurance, and employment information necessary to create a patient registration and electronic chart. Demographics in the medical field can be described as defining or descriptive information on the patient (e.g., name, address, phone number[s], sex, insurance information, DOB [age], ethnicity) (**Figure 3-7**).

The minimum required information to create a patient record in Harris CareTracker PM and EMR is a patient's first and last names. Harris CareTracker PM and EMR will allow you to save this information and navigate away from the *Demographics* application. However, whenever this patient is pulled into context in the *Name Bar*, an alert will pop up, indicating the patient's record is missing necessary information. Although appointments may be booked for the patient with only the name fields populated, insurance claims cannot be processed until the remainder of the *Demographics* information is complete. In addition, the pop-up alert will notify you if information such as preferred *Language, Race,* and *Ethnicity* are missing when you check the box "Trigger Patient Flash Note" (in the lower right-hand corner on the left side of the *Save* button). Information is entered by clicking the *Patient Details* tab, clicking *Edit*, then populating the fields, and then clicking on *Save* (**Figure 3-8**).

CRITICAL THINKING Describe what would happen to the revenue cycle (billing/income to the practice) if a full registration is not completed prior to a patient's visit. Explain how you reached your conclusions.

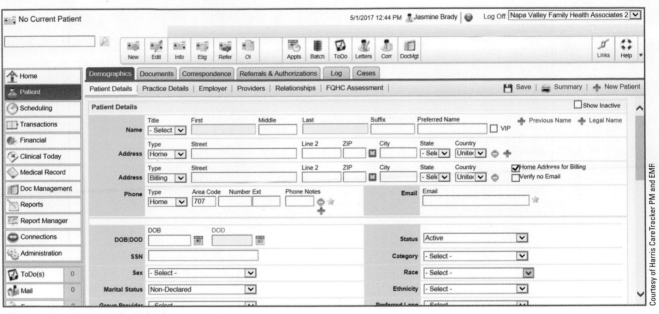

Figure 3-7   Demographics Screen

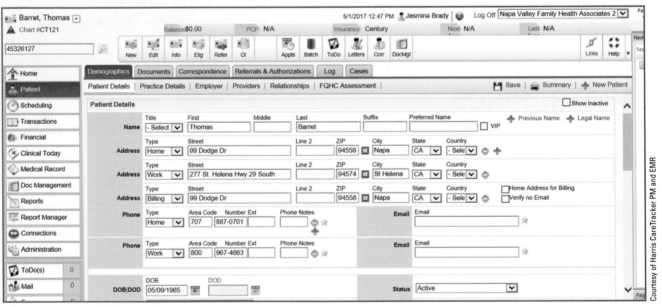

Figure 3-8   Patient Details Window

Patient Search

You must take care not to create duplicate patient accounts because it requires significant administrative research and work to confirm patient information and consolidate into one account, to maintain chart integrity, and patient care coordination. Only use the patient's legal name (e.g., William vs. Bill) and verify with the patient's ID and insurance card. Before creating a new patient account, always search for the patient in the database for previous registration by using at least two patient identifiers (e.g., last name [first three letters], first name [first one to three letters], DOB, or Social Security number) (**Figure 3-9**).

Harris CareTracker PM and EMR will alert you if it appears that a duplicate patient record is being created. If duplicate patient records are mistakenly created, those records must be combined into one account using the *Combine Duplicate Patients* application in the *Administration* module.

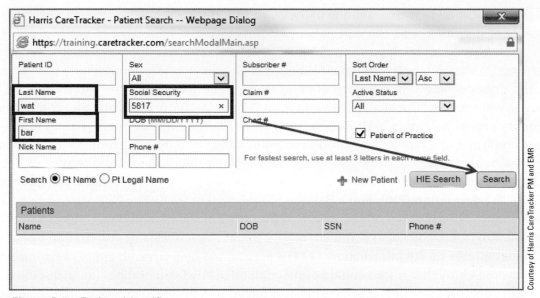

Figure 3-9   Patient Identifiers

Patient Alerts

The *Patient Alerts* window notifies the operator when key information is missing from a patient's demographics, or if any problems exist with the patient's account. With a patient in context, you can access *Patient Alerts* by clicking the *Alert* ⚠ icon next to the patient's chart number on the *Name Bar*. Certain conditions trigger Harris CareTracker PM and EMR to display the *Patient Alerts* window. When setting up your batch, you can set alerts to automatically display. A new **batch** must be created to enter financial transactions. A batch establishes defaults and assigns a name to a batch (group) of financial transactions you will be entering into Harris CareTracker PM and EMR. The *Patient Alerts* window is divided into four sections (see **Figure 3-10**):

1. Patient Demographics

2. Eligibility

3. Other Alerts

4. Notes for this Patient

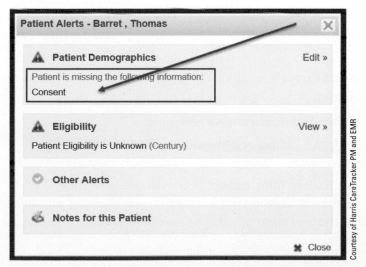

Figure 3-10   View Patient Alerts

To launch the application that corresponds to the alert, click the *View* link.

From the *Patient Alert* box, you can edit patient information. It is important to verify accuracy and update information when a patient schedules an appointment or checks in for an appointment. This makes the treatment process faster and avoids unnecessary complications in billing resulting from outdated information. The pop-up alert will let the operator know what information is missing. In the case of the *View Patient Alerts* example (Figure 3-10), you will see that "Consent" is missing from *Patient Demographics*, and that eligibility is "unknown" from the example provided (**Figure 3-11**). The *Patient Alert* acts as a form of internal audit of the demographic record. Always confirm in the patient's electronic record that the written registration forms contain the required documentation with a valid signature. These documents include the consent form; **notice of privacy practices (NPP)**, a document that describes medical practices policies and procedures regarding the use and disclosure of **protected health information (PHI)**; and a Release of Information (ROI). The NPP should also list the name of the HIPAA Compliance Officer at the office/clinic, and the name of the person/department, determined by state, if they feel a violation has occurred, to complain to. The Department of Health and Human Services defines PHI as individually identifiable health information, held or maintained by a covered entity or its business associates acting for the covered entity that is transmitted or maintained in any form or medium (including the individually identifiable health information of non-U.S. citizens). This includes identifiable demographic and other information relating to the past, present, or future; physical or mental health; or condition of an individual; or the provision or payment of health care to an individual that is created or received by a health care provider, health plan, employer, or health care clearinghouse. For purposes of the Privacy Rule, genetic information is considered to be health information (HHS/NIH).

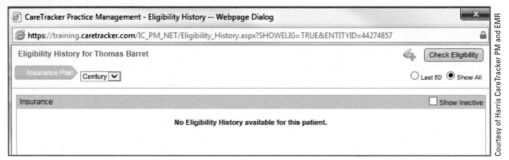

Figure 3-11   View Eligibility

An individuals' right under HIPAA to access their health information empowers them to be more in control of decision-making regarding his or her health choices. The Privacy Rule gives the individual the right to:

1. inspect, review, and obtain a copy of their PHI,

2. request a change or amendment to their medical or billing record if they think the information is incorrect,

3. access the PHI for as long as the information is maintained by a covered entity, regardless of the date the information was created,

4. request restrictions on uses and disclosures of PHI, and

5. file a complaint about a HIPAA violation with the Office of Civil Rights.
    (*Source:* U.S Department of Health and Human Services)

In addition to documenting patient information, you must de-identify PHI when directed. Methods include **encryption** in the electronic record, shredding paper records, and blacking out information that would identify a patient. Encryption refers to the conversion of letter or numbers to code or symbols so that its contents cannot be viewed or understood.

CRITICAL THINKING Describe identifiable demographic and other information relating to the past, present, or future; physical or mental health; or condition of an individual that would be considered PHI. How would you assess the information? Provide a comparison of what you would consider PHI and non-PHI.

Name

Registering a new patient begins with entering the patient's name in the *Name* section of the *Demographics* application. If you are doing a mini-registration, you can save just the patient's name to create a patient record. Some practices save only a new patient's name to book an appointment and then complete the remainder of the demographic information when the patient comes into the office. Always follow the established office protocol. It is important to review and compare the patient registration form to the demographics as entered into Harris CareTracker to identify any discrepancies.

Photos

Many practices now require photo identification of their patients to protect against medical identify theft, ensure the integrity of the patient's chart, and maintain privacy (HIPAA compliance). Harris CareTracker PM provides a means of adding a photo or a copy of a driver's license to the patient's demographic record (**Figure 3-12**). You will not be able to insert or scan documents in your student version of Harris CareTracker PM.

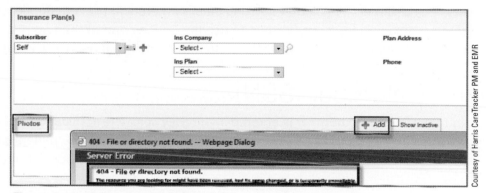

Figure 3-12   Add a Picture in Patient Demographics

Addresses

If the home and the billing addresses are the same, you do not have to enter a billing address. However, if a patient's statements are going to be sent to a different address, add a separate billing address; otherwise the home address becomes the billing address by default (you can also place a check mark in the "Home Address for Billing" box). If only a billing address is entered for the patient, the home address defaults to the same address when patient information is saved.

When a patient lives outside of the United States, his or her address must be entered differently than a patient who lives in the country. Please keep in mind, statements will not be sent to foreign addresses, but setting up the patient's *Demographics* correctly will prevent the claim from being unbilled due to the patient's address. Refer to Harris CareTracker's *Help* feature for more information on entering a foreign address.

Phones

Entering a patient's phone number into Harris CareTracker PM and EMR is similar to entering a patient's address. A phone number can be deactivated at any time and you can add as many phone numbers as needed. Harris CareTracker PM and EMR prints the patient's *Home* and *Work* phone numbers on the appointment list.

Chart Number

When registering a patient, it is not necessary to enter or assign a chart number to the patient in the *Chart Number* field unless the practice prefers that a specific chart number be manually entered for internal purposes. If a practice has converted from another medical management system to Harris CareTracker PM and EMR and chart numbers were previously used, they will cross over and appear in the *Chart Number* field. This makes it possible to search the database for established patients from the previous system (**Figure 3-13**).

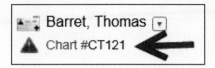

Figure 3-13   Chart Number

When new patients are registered in Harris CareTracker PM and EMR, the chart number becomes the same as the *ID* number that is automatically assigned by Harris CareTracker PM and EMR.

Date of Birth

Date of Birth (DOB) displays the patient's date of birth. You can enter the date of birth manually in MM/DD/YYYY format, or click the *Calendar* icon ⊞ to select the date. If by error you enter a future date in the *Date of Birth* box, an error message prompts to notify you that a wrong date is entered. To prevent duplicate patient accounts and to speed the patient search option, it is advisable to use the DOB as one of the two patient identifiers. The *Date of Death* (DOD) field is only enabled when the *Status* field has been changed to "Deceased."

Social Security Number (SSN)

The patient's nine-digit Social Security number is entered in the *SSN* field. The application will automatically add the hyphen when you [Tab] to the next field. For security purposes, after saving the patient's demographic, the *SSN* is encrypted and only the last four digits are displayed (**Figure 3-14**). Encryption is a method of de-identifying PHI.

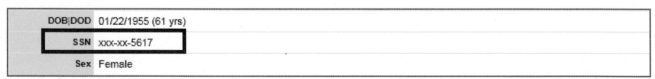

Figure 3-14   Last Four Digits of Patient's SSN

With the passage of the Affordable Care Act (ACA), commonly referred to as "Obamacare," the Internal Revenue Service (IRS) requires health insurance companies to provide Form 1095-B regarding health coverage on the insured. The law requires SSNs to be reported on Form 1095-B.

Sex

The *Sex* list in the *Demographics* application contains two options: *Male* and *Female*. If a patient's sex is not entered, claims for the patient will not be electronically transmitted to the insurance company. Any claim lacking a specified sex will become an unbilled claim and will remain as such until an operator specifies a sex and re-bills the claim (**Figure 3-15**).

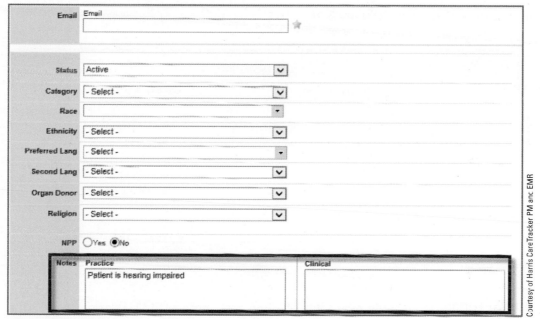

Figure 3-15   Sex Field in Demographics Screen
Courtesy of Harris CareTracker PM and EMR

Notes

In the *Notes* field, you can free-type any important patient information to which users may need to be alerted. For example, if a patient is hearing-impaired or does not speak English, you could type that information in the *Notes* field, and the note would be saved in the patient's demographic (**Figure 3-16**). There is a 249-character limit for the *Notes* field. There are two fields, *Practice* and *Clinical*. Notes entered in the *Clinical Notes* field are displayed in the *Clinical Alert* window when an operator launches a patient's health record.

Figure 3-16   Notes Field in Patient Demographics Screen

CRITICAL THINKING   Flash Notes: When you select the *Trigger Patient Flash Note* checkbox, it creates a flash note for the patient. When this checkbox is selected, Harris CareTracker PM and EMR will display the note in an alert each time the patient is pulled into context. The note will also be displayed in the *Notes* field in the *Patient Details* application of the *Patient* module *Demographics* tab.
    Provide examples of what type of information and when it would be appropriate to enter information for use *Patient Flash Notes*.

VIP Flag

Flagging a patient as a *VIP* allows the practice to restrict operator access to the patient's demographic. Any operator may flag a high-profile patient as a *VIP*, but only operators assigned either the *VIP Patient Access* or the *VIP Patient Access Break Glass* override in their profile can access a *VIP* demographic (**Figure 3-17**). *Important*—By default, only the practice administrator ("Fin-Practice Admin" role) is assigned access to view *VIP* demographics and the *VIP Log*. The practice administrator is responsible for assigning access to other operators in the group by adding a security override to their user profile.

Demographics	Documents	Correspondence	Referrals & Authorizations	Log	Cases

Patient Details	Practice Details	Employer	Providers	Relationships	FQHC Assessment

Patient Details

	Title	First	Middle	Last	Suffix	Preferred Name	☑ VIP	+ Previous Name + Legal Name
Name	- Select - ▾	Thomas		Barret				

	Type	Street		Line 2	ZIP	City	State	Country	
Address	Home ▾	99 Dodge Dr			94558 ⊠	Napa	CA ▾	United States ▾ ⊖ ✛	

Figure 3-17 VIP Flag

Courtesy of Harris CareTracker PM and EMR

SPOTLIGHT Break the glass privileges allow an operator limited access to a VIP patient's information. The access is only available during the operator's current Harris CareTracker PM and EMR session, and the operator must provide a reason why the record is being accessed. An operator must have either the *VIP Patient Access* or the *VIP Patient Access Break Glass* override included in his or her operator profile to access a VIP patient. Each time an operator accesses a VIP patient demographic, Harris CareTracker PM and EMR creates an entry in the VIP Patient Log. The log lists the patient's name, the operator who accessed the record, and the date and time the record was accessed (**Figure 3-18**).

VIP Patient Log

Date From	Date To	Log Type	
4/8/2010 📅	5/8/2010 📅	VIP Access ▾	**Search**

	VIP	Username	Last Access Date
✚	1. Adams, Brian	Rajan, G	4/16/2010 9:55:12 AM EST
✚	2. Babcock, M	Robinson, D	5/7/2010 11:39:35 AM EST
✚	3. Bolte, H	Reis, D	5/7/2010 4:57:04 PM EST

Figure 3-18 VIP Patient Log

Courtesy of Harris CareTracker PM and EMR

CRITICAL THINKING Provide examples of when a patient should be flagged as a VIP, and why.

CRITICAL THINKING What law prohibits the unauthorized access of patient charts? What provisions apply? Identify consequences of accessing a patient chart without reason.

Responsible Party

The patient's **responsible party** (also referred to as **guarantor**) is the individual who is responsible for any private pay balances; the remaining amount, if any, after insurance has paid its portion. Patient statements are addressed to the person indicated in the *Responsible* field, and *Self* is the default option for the *Responsible* field in the *Demographics* application. Patients over the age of 18 are considered responsible parties. For patients under the age of 18, parents or guardians are usually the responsible parties.

If the responsible party does not appear in the list, search the database:

1. Click the *Add* icon next to the *Responsible Party* field. The application displays the *Add Responsible Party* window.

2. From the *Type* list, select the type of responsible party.

3. In the *Responsible Party* field, either select the name from the list, or click the *Search* icon to search the database.

4. From the *Relationship* list, select the relationship of the responsible party to the patient. **Note:** This field is only enabled when the responsible party type is "Patient."

5. Click *Save*.

6. Click *Save* on the *Patient Details* tab.

Note: If the responsible party is a patient, but is not found in the search, you can add the patient to the CareTracker database. Click the *Add* icon next to the *Responsible Party* field or the *New Patient* link in the search window and register the responsible party.

Insurance Plan(s)

Entering a patient's insurance information accurately in the *Insurance* section of the *Demographics* application ensures that insurance companies will pay claims in a timely manner. A list of the practice's most frequently accepted insurance companies and plans can be created in the *Quick Picks* application or you can search the Harris CareTracker PM and EMR database (this is not a student task/function). When an insurance company or plan is not listed in Harris CareTracker PM and EMR's database, it can be added using *Pending Insurance* as a placeholder.

Employers

The *Employer* tab of the *Demographics* application is where a practice can track patient employment information. Often, the patient's employment history and insurance history go hand-in-hand. Having a patient's employment information is essential for any work-related injuries covered by workers' compensation. This ensures the practice has the necessary information on hand for a workers' compensation claim to be paid.

SEARCH FOR A PATIENT

Learning Objective 3: Search for a patient within Harris CareTracker PM.

Now that you have reviewed the patient registration and demographics segment, you will complete activities to demonstrate your knowledge and ability to perform tasks within Harris CareTracker PM. The first activity is to *Search* for a patient (one that is already in the database). Follow the step-by-step instructions to complete the activities for this chapter. Log into Harris CareTracker PM with your user ID and password provided with your materials. Remain logged in as long as you are completing activities. Properly log out when finished.

It is important to have a patient in context for every patient-specific function such as editing demographics, booking an appointment, entering referral/authorization information, and more. The basic methods to pull a patient into context are by the last name, ID number, chart number, claim number, and Social Security number. It is recommended that you always use two identifiers to verify that you are viewing the correct chart and do not create a duplicate account.

Activity 3-1
Search for a Patient by Name *(currently in the database)*

PATIENT: Frank Powell

1. In the *ID* search box on the *Name Bar* located under the patient name (or No Current Patient), enter the first three letters of the patient's last name ("Pow"), and hit [Enter] (see Figures 3-1 and 3-2 for help). The pop-up will list any patient matching your search criteria (**Figure 3-19**). Click on patient Frank Powell and the patient will be pulled into context. Note: If you receive a pop-up asking if you want to navigate away from this page (**Figure 3-20**), select "OK" and Harris CareTracker PM will launch the *Patient Demographics* application, displaying the patient's demographics screen.

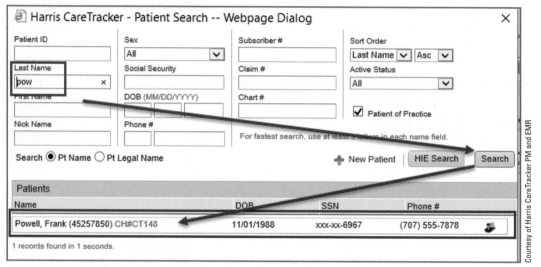

Figure 3-19 Search by First Three Letters of patient's Last Name

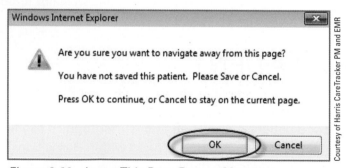

Figure 3-20 Leave This Page Pop-up Message

 TIP An alternate method to search for existing patients is:

1. Remove a patient in context by clicking on the drop-down list at the end of the patient's name (**Figure 3-21**) and select "None." The name in the patient field will be removed and "No current patient" will display.

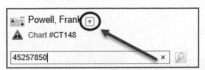

Figure 3-21   Remove Patient from Context Drop-Down
Courtesy of Harris CareTracker PM and EMR

2. With "no current patient" in the ID search box, click on the *Search* icon 🔍, which will bring up the *Patient Search* box.

3. In the *Patient Search* box, enter at least three letters of the patient's last ("Pow") and first name ("Fra"). A previous name such as a maiden name or an alias cannot be used to search for a patient.

4. Click the *Search* button. The *Patient Search* box displays a list of patients that match the information entered (see Figure 3-19), along with the patient ID and chart number.

5. Click the *Family* icon 👥 to view the patient's family members registered in Harris CareTracker PM and EMR (if applicable).

6. Verify the "second identifier" such as DOB or last four numbers of the Social Security number, and then click the specific name to launch the patient into context (see Figure 3-19).

2. Record the patient's ID number, chart number, and Social Security number for additional activities related to searching for a patient. _____

📧 **Print the Patient Demographic screen displayed, label it "Activity 3-1A," and place it in your assignment folder.**

3. Repeat Activity 3-1 by searching for four additional established patients by name. Record their ID number, chart number, and Social Security number for future searches.

a. Kevin Johnson _____

b. Jane Morgan _____

c. Kirk Johnson _____

d. Abby Zuffante _____

📧 **Print the Search Results screen for each patient, label it "Activity 3-1B," and place it in your assignment folder.**

REGISTER NEW PATIENTS

Learning Objective 4: Register a new patient in Harris CareTracker.

Your next activity is to register a new patient, one who is not in the current database (**Figures 3-22** and **3-23**). It is important to register all patients in the Harris CareTracker PM and EMR system with their demographics information such as name, contact information, date of birth, insurance and employer information, and more. This information is required to ensure proper treatment as well as to facilitate billing. Prior to registering a new patient, always search the database to be certain that the patient has never been registered. Use two patient identifiers when searching to avoid creating a duplicate account.

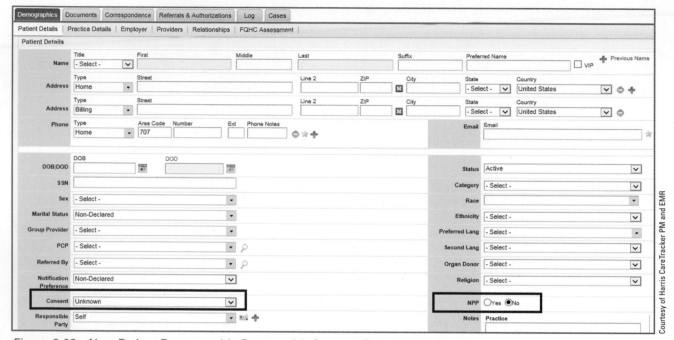

Figure 3-22 New Patient Link

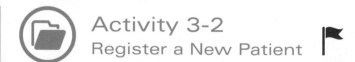

Figure 3-23 New Patient Demographic Screen with Consent Fields Highlighted

> **TIP** Navigate through each field in demographics by pressing the [Tab] key and Harris CareTracker PM and EMR will automatically format the entry, regardless of the way it is entered. For example, by tabbing through the *First Name* and *Last Name* boxes, Harris CareTracker PM and EMR automatically applies title case to the name, meaning the first letter of each name is capitalized. To navigate back to a field, press [SHIFT+TAB].

Activity 3-2
Register a New Patient

To register new patient Jordyn Lyndsey, refer to Source Document 3-1 (Patient Registration Form) and Source Document 3-2 (NPP) found at the end of this activity (pages 120–121). First, search the existing database to confirm the patient (Jordyn Lyndsey) has never been registered. After confirming she is not in the system, click *New* on the *Name Bar*. Harris CareTracker PM displays the *Patient Details* window. Register "New Patient" Jordyn Lyndsey's demographic information, responsible party, insurance, and employer information from her patient registration form. When finished, click *Save*.

1. *Name*: Enter the patient's full legal name. Include a nickname if used, for example, Jordy for Jordyn in the *Preferred Name* box/field.

2. Ms. Lyndsey is considered a "VIP." Place a check mark next to the *VIP* box at the end of the *Name* line.

3. *Address*:

    a. In the *Line 1* box, enter the patient's street address (house number + street name).

    b. In the *Line 2* box, enter the patient's apartment or condominium number, if applicable.

    c. In the *Zip* box, enter the patient's zip code (**Figure 3-24**).

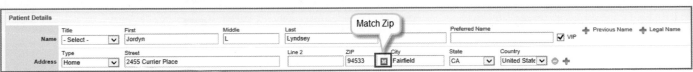

Figure 3-24   Patient Address Fields

Courtesy of Harris CareTracker PM and EMR

    d. Press the [Enter] key. Harris CareTracker PM automatically populates the *City, State,* and *Country* fields based on the zip code. Note: Unless a separate billing address is entered, the patient's home address becomes the billing address by default.

    e. Confirm that a check mark is in the "Home Address for Billing" box. If not, click on the box.

    f. If needed, click the + icon to add additional address fields.

4. *Phone*:

    a. The phone number field will default to the patient's home phone number. You can also use the drop-down feature from the *Type* list to select the type of phone number you are entering (**Figure 3-25**).

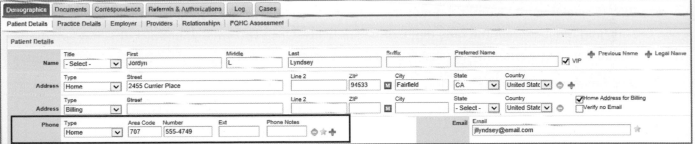

Figure 3-25   Patient Phone Number Fields

Courtesy of Harris CareTracker PM and EMR

    b. In the *Area Code* field, enter the area code if not already populated.

    c. In the *Number* field, enter the phone number. You do not need to enter a hyphen (it will automatically be added as you enter the phone number).

    d. (FYI) If the phone number entered requires an extension, enter the extension in the *Ext* field.

    e. In the *Phone Notes* field, enter any notes related to the patient's contact information, for example, "OK to leave message, do not call after 8 P.M." and so on. (Enter whether okay to leave detailed message as noted in Source Document 3-1 here.)

f. Click on the *Set as Preferred Contact* ⭐ icon at the end of the line.

TIP   Steps to deactivate or activate a phone number:

*   If a patient's phone number is no longer active, click the *Deactivate* icon at the end of the phone number line to make it inactive (**Figure 3-26**). By clicking on the *Deactivate* icon, the phone number will be deactivated but will remain in the patient's record. Harris CareTracker PM and EMR grays out deactivated phone numbers as a visual reminder.
*   Click the *Activate* icon to reactivate a phone number.

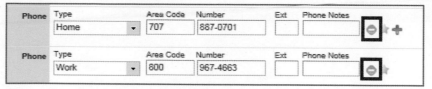

Figure 3-26   *Deactivate a Patient Phone Number*
Courtesy of Harris CareTracker PM and EMR

---

g. In the *Email* field, enter the patient's email address on the same line as the patient's home phone number. Enter the email address exactly as you would if you were sending an email. Harris Care-Tracker PM will validate the email address format when the record is saved. Note: If a patient does not have an email address, place a check mark in the "Verify no Email" box. When checked, the *Email* field will be grayed out.

CRITICAL THINKING   Although email is listed as an optional field, most practices are required to collect of the patient's email address. Identify reasons why the practice would want to have a patient's email address.

---

5. *Date of Birth* (DOB) (Age): Enter the date of birth in MM/DD/YYYY (or mm/dd/yy—six-digit) format, or click on the *Calendar* icon ▦ to select a DOB.

6. *SSN* (Social Security Number): Enter the patient's Social Security number. Do not include dashes. This field must contain the nine digits or be left blank. Once you save your edits, the first five digits will be encrypted and only the last four digits display.

7. *Sex*: Enter the patient's sex. If no sex is entered, a claim cannot be sent.

8. *Marital Status*: Enter the patient's marital status, if known or declared. Choose the status from the drop-down list.

9. *Group Provider*: Select from the drop-down list the provider listed on the patient registration form.

10. *PCP* (Primary Care Provider): Select the PCP for the patient noted on the registration form from the drop-down list. (**Note:** If you were searching for a provider who is not on the list, you would click the Search icon 🔍 to the right of the field, type in as much information as you have [minimally last name and state], and search for providers. [**Figure 3-27**]). You would normally select the provider listed on the patient registration form.

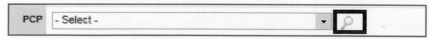

Figure 3-27   *PCP Search Icon*
Courtesy of Harris CareTracker PM and EMR

11. *Referred By*: This field is referring to what physician, if any, referred the patient to the practice. From the drop-down list, select the most appropriate. If you do not find the referring physician in the drop-down list, you can search the National Provider Identifier (NPI) database. For this activity, the referring providers are in your quick-pick drop-down list.

12. *Notification Preference*: From the drop-down list, select the preferred method of communication noted in Source Document 3-1.

13. *Consent*: From the drop-down box, select from the options: Unknown, Yes, No, or Revoked. Review Source Documents 3-1 and 3-2 and determine if *Consent* and *NPP* have been given. Enter the appropriate response in each field.

14. *Advance Directive*: The *Yes* and *No* fields are grayed out and cannot be changed in your student environment. Using the drop-down in the -Select- field, select "Patient Refusal" for this activity. **Note:** In a live environment, you would have to add the Advance Directive Document to the system before the *Yes* can be checked by clicking the plus sign to the right and add the document. Then *No* will change to *Yes* once the document is saved.

15. *Responsible Party*: Enter the responsible party information from the patient registration form and insurance card. The only option available from the drop-down list is "Self." Leave as "Self" for new patient Jordyn Lyndsey. **Note:** If you click on the + icon to the right of the field, the *Add Responsible Party* dialog box will pop up (**Figure 3-28**), and you can add a responsible party if it is other than "Self." Using the *Search* icon 🔍 in the *Add Responsible Party* box allows you to search the practice's database. There is also a *Relationship* field, and from the *Relationship* list you can select the patient whose demographic information is being completed. When a relationship is selected, the patient's name is displayed in the *Responsible Party* field.

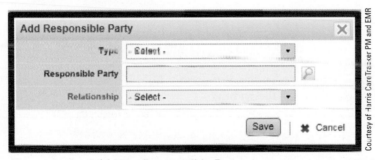

Figure 3-28   Add New Responsible Party

16. *Status*: This field is used to note the patient's status. Choose "Active" for new patients. (Other choices from the drop-down list would be used as appropriate, for example, Deceased, Discharged, Followed by Another M.D., Inactive, Moved Out of Area, or Not a Patient of Practice.)

17. *Category*: From the drop-down list, select the most appropriate category (if any). Leave Category as "-Select-" when registering a new patient. Categories available are Bad address, Collections, and High deductible. (**Note:** Additional categories can be added through the *Administration* module if the practice chooses to do so.)

18. *Race*: In the drop-down menu, select from the following options: American Indian or Alaskan Native, Asian, Black or African American, Native Hawaiian or other Pacific Islander, Patient Refusal, or White.

19. *Ethnicity*: In the drop-down menu, select from the following options: Hispanic or Latino, Not Hispanic or Latino, or Patient Refusal.

20. *Preferred Lang*: Select the preferred language of the patient from the drop-down menu.

21. *Second Lang*: Select the patient's second language from the drop-down menu, if applicable.

22. *Organ Donor*: Identify whether the patient is an organ donor (if noted on the patient registration form).

23. *Religion*: Select the patient's religion from the drop-down menu (if noted on the patient registration form).

24. *NPP* (Notice of Privacy Practices): Referring to the Patient Registration packet, select the radio dial button "Yes" or "No" indicating whether the NPP has been signed/recorded. Always confirm if the *Consent* and *NPP* were signed by the patient, and check "Yes" on the demographics screen. Harris CareTracker will automatically "date stamp" when the *NPP* and *Consent* information were entered.

25. *Notes* (*Practice* or *Clinical*): Enter any notes that you want to include for this patient. In the lower right-hand corner of the demographics screen, check the box *Trigger Patient Flash Note*. That will activate the notes to flash when you pull the patient into context. For example, "requires electric exam table."

26. *Insurance Plan(s)*: Complete the fields with information from the patient registration form (Source Document 3-1).

    a. A **subscriber** (policy holder) is an individual who is a member of a benefits plan. For example, in the case of family coverage, one adult is ordinarily the subscriber. A spouse and children would ordinarily be dependents. The *Subscriber* field defaults to "Self." Leave this selection if the patient is the subscriber. (Jordyn Lyndsey is the subscriber, so leave as "Self.") If an individual other than the patient or the responsible party is the subscriber, click on the + icon at the end of the *Subscriber* field.

TIP To Add a New Subscriber

In this activity, you do <u>not</u> need to add a new subscriber, but you may need to add a new subscriber in future activities and certainly in the real-world setting. To add a new subscriber:

1. Click the + icon next to the *Subscriber* field (**Figure 3-29**). Harris CareTracker PM displays the *Add Subscriber* dialog box.

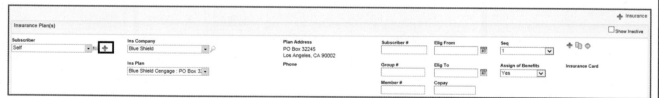

Figure 3-29 *Search Icon in the Subscriber Field*   Courtesy of Harris CareTracker PM and EMR

2. In the *Add Subscriber* dialog box, you will select the appropriate *Type, Subscriber,* and *Relationship.*

3. To search for the *Subscriber,* click on the *Search* 🔍 icon. (Note: Only search the database if the subscriber was ever a patient of the practice.) If the subscriber is not found in the database, close the *Search Patients* window and click the *Copy* icon in the *Add Subscriber* dialog box. Harris CareTracker PM displays demographic fields for the new subscriber information.

4. Complete the demographic information for the subscriber in the fields provided. You must enter the subscriber's *Name, SSN, DOB, Sex,* and *Insurance* information at a minimum.

b. In the *Ins Company* field, select the subscriber's insurance company from the drop-down list (**Figure 3-30**). Verify that you have the correct insurance plan by double-checking the address displayed next to the insurance plan name. The insurance plan will populate with the name and address if you select a plan from the drop-down list. If the plan name is not in the list, search the Harris CareTracker PM database.

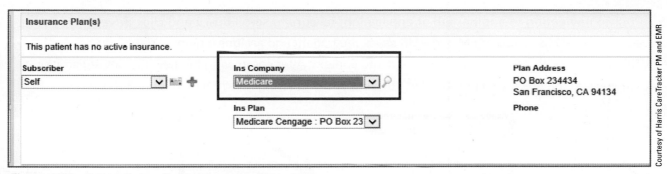

Figure 3-30   *Select Subscriber's Insurance Plan*

c. In the *Subscriber #* field, enter the subscriber number listed. The **subscriber number** refers to the insurance policy number.

d. (If applicable) Enter the group number in the *Group #* field. The **group number** typically identifies the employer. The use of group numbers varies among insurance carriers, so be sure to enter the numbers in accordance with each carrier's numbering policy.

e. (If applicable) Enter the member number in the *Member #* field. (There is no member number for this patient.) The **member number** is typically assigned to individual family members on the policy.

f. In the *Elig From* and *Elig To* fields, enter the subscriber's effective dates of coverage with a particular insurance carrier. Often the date entered in the *Elig From* field will match the patient's employment start date if the patient is covered through that employer. The *Elig To* field remains blank until the patient changes insurance plans. To complete the eligibility fields, you can either enter the dates manually in MM/DD/YYYY format, or you can click the *Calendar* 🗓 icon and select a date. In the case of Jordyn Lyndsey, the *Elig From* date would have been her 65th birthday, since she is a Medicare patient.

g. If the subscriber is required to pay a copayment, enter the copayment amount in the *Copay* field. Do not use dollar signs. When charges are entered for the patient, Harris CareTracker PM will automatically calculate and **carve-out** the copayment amount for private pay (the amount for which the patient is responsible). The carve-out occurs only if the copay amount is entered in the *Copay* field.

h. The *Sequence* field indicates whether the insurance plan entered for the patient is the **primary** (first in order), **secondary** (second in order), or **tertiary** (third in order) insurance. The number of insurance plans entered on a patient's demographic determines the numbers that display on the *Sequence* list. Select "1" for the primary insurance, select "2" for the secondary insurance, and so on. For example, if the secondary insurance plan saved on a patient's demographic becomes the primary insurance, you would then change the plan's sequence to "1" instead of "2." (Select "1.")

i. Confirm that the patient has signed the Assignment of Benefits/Financial Agreement, and select "Yes" from the *Assignment of Benefits* drop-down menu (other options from the drop-down list are "No" or "Patient Refused"). It is imperative that patients sign the Assignment of Benefits authorization so the practice may bill the insurance company for reimbursement.

27. The last field in the *Patient Details* tab is where photos are added. This feature is not active in your student environment. Skip over this field.

28. Prior to navigating to another tab or application, be sure to scroll down and click *Save* to save your entries. Harris CareTracker PM and EMR saves the patient and assigns a unique identification number. The newly registered patient is also pulled into context. After completing the new patient registration activity, you may receive a pop-up alert advising you of missing information (**Figure 3-31**).

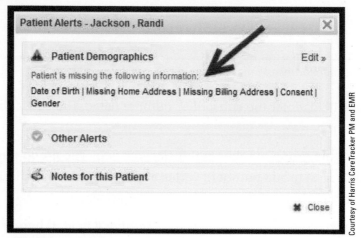

Figure 3-31   *Patient Alerts Pop-up Box*

29. To make further entries to patient demographics, click *Edit* in the Name Bar. Then, at the top of the *Demographics* screen, click on the *Employer* tab, to the right of the *Patient Details* tab.

30. Click on the *+ New Employer* link on the left side of the screen and complete the fields with information from the patient registration form (Source Document 3-1).

   a. A list of the practice's most common patient employers is available from the *Employer* field drop-down list. Select the appropriate employer choice from the drop-down list. When an employer is selected from the list, the employer's work address information will be populated in the *Address* fields.

TIP To Search for an Employer

In this activity, you won't need to search for an employer, but you may need to do so in future activities. To search for an employer:

1. If the patient's employer is not an option in the *Employer* drop-down list, search Harris CareTracker PM's employer database. This can be done by clicking the *Search* 🔍 icon next to the *Employer* field (**Figure 3-32**). This will open the *Search Employers* window. If the employer is not listed, you can click the *+ New Employer* link and add the employer information.

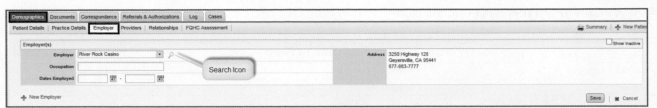

Figure 3-32   *Employer Field in Patient Demographics Screen*   Courtesy of Harris CareTracker PM and EMR

2. Enter the name of the employer in the *Employer Name* field. In addition, you can narrow the search by entering the employer's city and state. Click on the *Search* button to display a list of the employers that match the information entered.

3. By clicking on the appropriate selection, the employer's name, address, phone number, and fax number are entered into the respective fields.

b. The patient's occupation should be entered in the *Occupation* field, for example, "P/T Bookkeeper."

c. Enter the start and end dates in the *Dates Employed* fields as noted on the Patient Registration form (Source Document 3-1) (if any). If the patient is presently an employee, no ending date is entered. A date can be entered into either of the fields manually in MM/DD/YYYY format, or by clicking on the *Calendar* icon and selecting the appropriate date.

d. Click *Save*.

31. Now update the emergency contact information with the following steps:

a. Click on the *Relationships* tab.

b. Click the drop-down next to "Add Relationship."

c. Select *Emergency Contact* and the *Add Emergency Contact* dialog box will appear.

d. Leave the drop-down in the *Patient* field as "-Select Patient-."

e. In the *Non-Patient* field, enter the name of the *Emergency Contact* (Janet Jones).

f. Use the drop-down next to "Relationship" and select the appropriate relationship as noted on the patient registration form (Child).

g. In the "Phone" field, enter the information as noted on the patient registration form (use *Mobile* for the *Phone Type* and enter the phone number listed in the Registration Form).

h. Click "Yes" as "Preferred."

i. Then click *Save*.

32. If necessary, click *Edit* and continue the full registration process for any missing information. It is important to know that all fields should be completed, although they are not required. The pop-up will also alert you to missing information such as primary location (should be "Napa Valley Family Associates [NVFA]"), preferred language, secondary language, ethnicity, race, organ donor status, religion, and more. Click *Save* to save any changes made.

33. (FYI) There are additional tabs in the *Demographics* application that may or may not be used by the practice.

Print the completed *Patient Details* and *Employer* screens, label them "Activity 3-2," and place them in your assignment folder.

Source Document 3-1

Patient Registration Form			NVFHA

Patient's Last Name	First (legal name)	First (Preferred name)	Middle Name
Lyndsey	Jordyn		L

Address (Number, Street, Apt #)		City	State	Zip Code
2455 Currier Place		Fairfield	CA	94533

Mail will be sent to the address listed above, unless patient indicates a different address (leave blank if same as above)

Send mail to Address (Number, Street, Apt #)		City	State	Zip Code

Phone Options	Phone Number	Okay to leave detailed message	Call this number (circle one)
Home	(707) 555 - 4749	Yes __X__ No _____	(1st) 2nd 3rd choice
Cell	( ) -	Yes ____ No _____	1st 2nd 3rd choice
Work	( ) -	Yes ____ No _____	1st 2nd 3rd choice

Would you like to communicate by Email	Yes _X_ No __	Email Address	jllyndsey@email.com

Date of Birth	Sex	Social Security Number
1/17/1952	Female __X__ Male ____	000-00-9118

Marital Status (*circle one*)	What is your preferred language / secondary language
Single / Married / Divorced / (Widowed) / Partner	English

Race (*circle one*)

African American (Black) / Asian / Bi-Multi-racial / Pacific Islander-Hawaiian / Caucasian–White / Native American Eskimo Aleut / Decline to state / Other

Ethnicity (*circle one*)

Hispanic-Latino / (Non-Hispanic-Latino) / Other

Religion	Baptist	Organ Donor	Yes ___X___ No _____

Are you new to our practice	Who referred you to our practice	Who is your Primary Care Physician
Yes __X__ No _____	Amir Raman	Amir Raman

Additional Notes

Emergency Contact

Emergency Contact's Name	Relationship to patient	Phone
Janet Jones	Daughter	(510) 555 - 2246

On-Line Patient Portal Communication via Email

On-Line communication is used for non-urgent message/requests only. NVFHA uses secure technology to protect the privacy and confidentiality of your personal information. Only you, your physician, and authorized staff can read your message.

What is your preferred method of communication	Phone __X__ Letter _____ Patient Portal _____ Email _____

Insurance Information

Subscriber (Insurance Holder) Name	Date of Birth	Relationship to patient	Subscriber Phone Number
Self	/ /		( )

Health Plan Information	Primary Health Plan	Secondary Health Plan
Health Plan Name	Medicare Cengage	
Health Plan Address	PO Box 234434, San Francisco, CA, 94134	
Group Number	CARE 1357	
Subscriber Number	CARE 1357	

Elig Date From	1/17/2017	Copay	N/A

Patient Employer Information

Employer Name & Address (Number, Street, Apt #, City, State, Zip Code)	Employer Phone Number
Carneros Inn	( )

Occupation	P/T bookkeeper	Start Date	6/19/2014

Assignment of Benefits • Financial Agreement

I hereby give lifetime authorization for payment of insurance benefits to be made directly to **Napa Valley Family Health Assoc.,** and any assisting physicians, for services rendered. I understand that I am financially responsible for all charges whether or not they are covered by insurance. In the event of default, I agree to pay all costs of collection, and reasonable attorney's fees. I hereby authorize this healthcare provider to release all information necessary to secure the the payment of benefits.

I further agree that a photocopy of this agreement shall be as valid as the original.

Date: __XX/XX/20XX__ Your Signature: *Jordyn Lyndsey*

Method of Payment: ☐ Cash ☐ Check ☐ Credit Card

Source Document 3-2

NVFHA

NOTICE OF PRIVACY PRACTICES (NOPP)

ACKNOWLEDGEMENT OF RECEIPT

Patient Name: Jordyn L. Lyndsey

(Please Print)

By signing this form, you acknowledge receipt of the Notice of Privacy Practices of NAPA VALLEY FAMILY HEALTH ASSOCIATES. Our Notice of Privacy Practices provides information about how we may use and disclose your protected health information (PHI). We encourage you to read it in full.

Our Notice of Privacy Practices is subjected to change. If we change our notice, we will provide you with the revised notice or you may obtain a copy of the revised notice by accessing our web-site at http://www.nvfha.org or contacting our organizations' customer service department at (707) 555-1212.

If you have any questions about our Notice of Privacy Practices, please contact the Privacy Officials at the medical practice you visit or the Quality Improvement Department at (707) 555-1212.

- -

I acknowledge receipt of the Notice of Privacy Practices of NAPA VALLEY FAMILY HEALTH ASSOCIATES.

Date: XX/XX/20XX

Name: Jordyn L. Lyndsey

(Please Print)

If legal representative give relationship: _____

Inability to Obtain Signature	Date: _____

Why: _____

_____

Provider Representative: _____   Provider Rep Signature: _____

(Print)

As part of your end-of-chapter Case Studies, you will repeat Activity 3-2 (Register a New Patient) and register an additional new patient.

Scan/Attach Insurance Card(s)

In the Harris CareTracker PM and EMR *Demographics* application, patient's insurance cards can be scanned/attached to the patient's medical record. Your student version of Harris CareTracker PM does not have scanning capabilities; however, it is important that you understand the workflow and reasoning for scanning/attaching insurance cards. After a scanned insurance card is saved in Harris CareTracker PM and EMR, you can view the image whenever the patient is pulled into context. This is helpful when questions arise regarding the patient's insurance information and eliminates the need to photocopy the insurance card.

Even though a patient's insurance card is scanned and saved in Harris CareTracker PM and EMR, the insurance information must be manually entered into the insurance fields. A scanner must be attached to your computer to scan documents and images into Harris CareTracker PM and EMR.

FYI Attach an Insurance Card Scan

1. Pull into context the patient for whom you want to attach a scanned insurance card image.

2. Click the *Patient* module and then click the *Demographics/Patient Details* tab. Harris CareTracker PM displays the patient's demographic record.

3. Click *Edit*. Harris CareTracker PM displays the page in edit mode.

4. In the *Insurance Plan(s)* section, click the *Add Insurance Card* icon (**Figure 3-33**). **Note:** You will not be able to scan insurance attachments in your student version of Harris CareTracker and will receive an error message.

5. Close out of the error message box and click *Save* in the lower-right screen of the Patient Details screen.

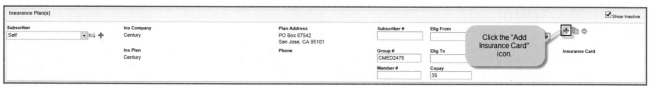

Figure 3-33   Add Insurance Attachment   Courtesy of Harris CareTracker PM and EMR

There are additional features in Harris CareTracker for uploading documents. Although there is no *Document Management* feature in your student version of Harris CareTracker PM, it is best to have an understanding of the functions. Additional information and references to *Document Management* can be found in *Help*.

The steps to attach a photo are similar to attaching documents or insurance cards, but there are slight deviations. **Figure 3-34** shows where you would attach a photo in the *Patient Details* tab of the *Demographics* application. This feature is not functional in your student version of Harris CareTracker and you will receive an error message when attempted.

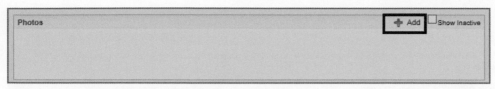

Figure 3-34   *Add Picture Link in Patient Details Screen*
Courtesy of Harris CareTracker PM and EMR

Print Patient Demographics Report

Medical practices may find it useful to print a patient's demographic report for a variety of reasons. Some practices will give a copy of the printed report to a patient at check-in to verify information and to make any necessary corrections/updates. Following this workflow will help identify inconsistencies between the patient information and information stored in your practice management software.

However, for practices that are trying to stay "paperless," you could use the *At-a-Glance* button for quick verification of demographics, balance due, appointments, and so on. To access *At-a-Glance*, click the *Info* icon next to the patient's name to view the patient's demographic information, *Patient Portal* status, primary/secondary insurance information, primary/secondary copayment amounts, previous and pending appointment details, and provider information.

You can generate (print) a *Patient Demographics* report for the patient in context, which includes:

- Some of the detailed demographic information entered in the *Patient Details* tab of the *Patient* module
- The patient's previous four and pending appointments and recalls
- Primary and secondary insurance information
- Provider information

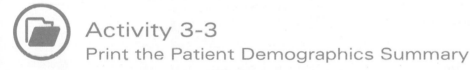

Activity 3-3
Print the Patient Demographics Summary

1. Pull a patient into context (New Patient—Jordyn Lyndsey).

2. Click the *Patient* module. Harris CareTracker PM and EMR displays the *Demographics* tab.

3. Click the *Print* icon to the left of the *Summary* link in the upper-right corner of the *Demographics* application. Harris CareTracker PM displays your printing options, along with a *Patient Summary Printout* screen (**Figure 3-35**). (Note: It may take a little time to generate the report.)

4. Choose a printer listed in the *Print* dialog box to print the patient demographics summary (**Figure 3-36**). (Alternatively, you can close the print prompt box and take a screenshot of the report, or right click on the report and select *Print*.)

📰 **Print the *Patient Demographics* report, label it "Activity 3-3," and place it in your assignment folder.**

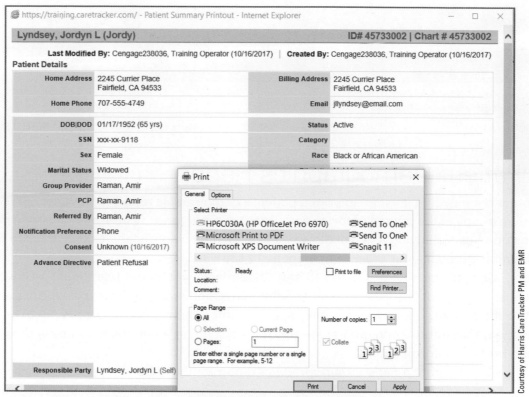

Figure 3-35   Patient Demographics Report for Jordyn Lyndsey

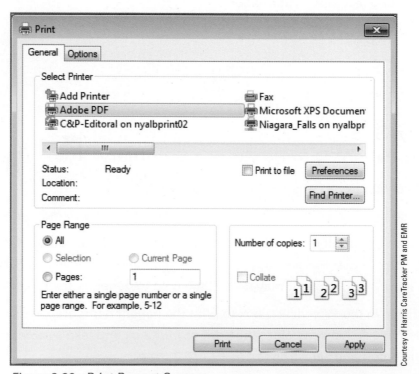

Figure 3-36   Print Prompt Screen

As part of your end-of-chapter Case Studies, you will print the demographics *Summary* (using the instructions in Activity 3-3) for each new patient you register.

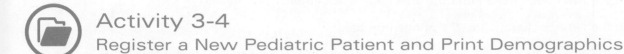

Activity 3-4
Register a New Pediatric Patient and Print Demographics

Register new pediatric patient Francisco Powell Jimenez and print his demographics. Search the existing database to confirm the patient has never been registered. After confirming he is not in the system, click *New* on the *Name Bar*. Harris CareTracker PM displays the *Patient Details* window. Register Francisco Jimenez's demographic information from his patient registration form using the information in Source Document 3-3 (Registration Form), located at the end of this activity. When finished, click *Save* and then print the demographics report. Because Francisco is a new pediatric patient, there will be slight changes in the registration process. Those changes/additions are noted below and reference the step number in Activity 3-2.

1. *Name*: Enter the patient's name.

2. *Address*:

   a. In the *Line 1* box, enter the patient's street address (house number + street name).

   b. In the *Line 2* box, enter the patient's apartment or condominium number, if applicable.

   c. In the *Zip* box, enter the patient's zip code (**Figure 3-37**). Click on the [Match] icon. Harris Care-Tracker PM automatically populates the *City, State,* and *Country* fields based on the zip code.

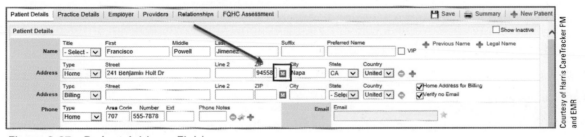

Figure 3-37   Patient Address Fields

   d. Leave the check mark in the "Home Address for Billing" box.

3. *Phone*:

   a. The phone number field will default to the patient's home phone number. Enter the patient's phone number from his Patient Registration form (**Figure 3-38**).

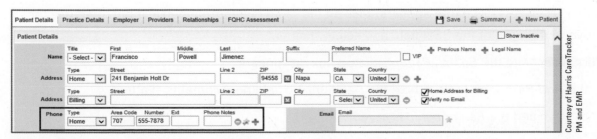

Figure 3-38   Patient Phone Number Fields

b. In the *Area Code* field, enter the area code if not already populated.

c. In the *Number* field, enter the phone number.

d. In the *Phone Notes* field, enter any notes related to the patient's contact information as noted in Source Document 3-3. For example, "Do not leave detailed messages."

e. Click on the *Set as Preferred Contact* ☆ icon at the end of the line.

f. Leave the *Email* field blank. Place a check mark in the "Verify no Email" box to the above and right of the email field.

4. *Date of Birth* (DOB) (Age): Enter the date of birth in 08/31/YYYY format (use last year for the year in this field).

5. *SSN* (Social Security Number): Enter the patient's Social Security number. Do not include dashes.

6. *Sex*: Enter the patient's sex.

7. *Marital Status*: *Marital Status* defaults to "non-declared." Choose the status from the drop-down list.

8. *Group Provider*: Select from the drop-down list the provider listed on the patient registration form.

9. *PCP* (Primary Care Provider): Select the PCP for the patient noted on the registration form from the drop-down list.

10. *Referred By*: From the drop-down list, select the most appropriate. Leave as "-Select-" if no referring provider is noted (do not enter a non-provider in this field for this activity).

11. *Notification Preference*: From the drop-down list, select "phone."

12. *Consent*: From the drop-down box, select from the options: Unknown, Yes, No, or Revoked. Because Francisco is a pediatric patient, select "Unknown."

13. *Advance Directive*: The advance directive field defaults to "No." Because Francisco is a pediatric patient, leave as is.

14. *Responsible Party*: Enter the responsible party information from the patient registration form and insurance card. The only option available from the drop-down list is "Self." Because new patient Francisco is not the Responsible Party, you will follow Step 15.

15. Click on the + icon to the right of the field, the *Add Responsible Party* dialog box will pop up (see **Figure 3-39**), and add the responsible party noted on the patient registration form.

16. Click on the *Search* icon 🔍 in the *Add Responsible Party* box that allows you to search the practice's database. Because Francisco's father, Frank Powell, is the *Responsible Party*, enter his name in the *Search Patients* box and click *Search*.

17. When Frank Powell's name appears, click on the radio dial button to select him, and use the drop-down to the right of the SSN field and select "Father."

18. Click *Select* and the *Search Patients* dialog box disappears.

19. In the *Add Responsible Party* box, the *Relationship* field now contains "Father."

20. Click *Save* and the *Relationship* is saved.

21. *Status*: This field is used to note the patient's status. Choose "Active" for new patients.

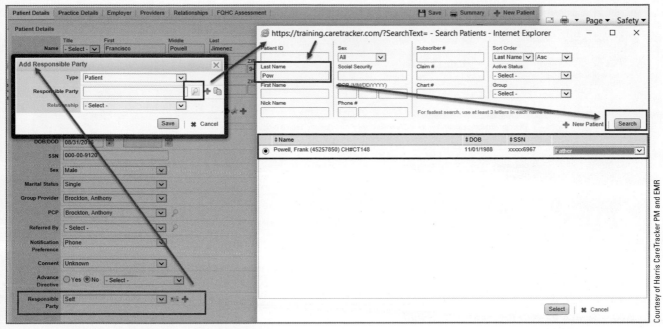

Figure 3-39   Add New Responsible Party

22. *Category*: From the drop-down list, select the most appropriate category (if any). Leave Category as "-Select-" when registering a new patient.

23. *Race*: In the drop-down menu, select the race indicated on his patient registration form.

24. *Ethnicity*: In the drop-down menu, select the ethnicity indicated on his patient registration form. If there is no entry, select "Patient Refusal."

25. *Preferred Lang*: Select the preferred language of the patient from the drop-down menu. If no entry is on the patient registration form, leave this field as "-Select-."

26. *Second Lang*: Select the patient's second language from the drop-down menu, if applicable.

27. *Organ Donor*: Identify whether the patient is an organ donor (if noted on the patient registration form). If there is no entry, leave as "-Select-."

28. *Religion*: Select the patient's religion from the drop-down menu. If there is no entry, leave as "-Select-."

29. *NPP* (Notice of Privacy Practices): Select the radio dial button "No" because Francisco is a pediatric patient.

30. *Notes* (*Practice* or *Clinical*): Enter any notes that you want to include for this patient. For example, enter in the *Practice Notes* "Direct any communications to Mr. Frank Powell, Francisco's father."

31. *Insurance Plan(s)*: Use the scroll feature on the right-hand side of the *Patient Details* window to display the entire *Plan(s)* field.

   a. The Subscriber field defaults to "Self."

   b. Click on the + at the end of the *Subscriber* field to add a new Subscriber (patient's father, Frank Powell).

   c. Harris CareTracker PM displays the *Add Subscriber* window (**Figure 3-40**).

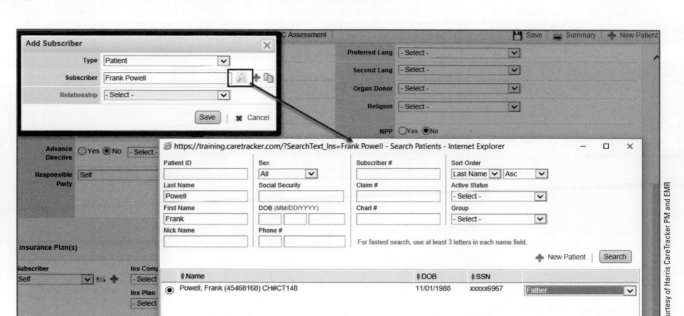

Figure 3-40   Search Icon in the Subscriber Field

d. In the *Add Subscriber* dialog box, you will select the appropriate *Type* (Patient); Enter *Subscriber* (Frank Powell) and, click on the *Search* 🔍 icon. Select "Frank Powell" (by clicking the radio dial button) and then selecting "Father" from the drop-down next to the Social Security number in the *Search Patients* dialog box (see Figure 3-39).

e. Click the *Select* button at the lower right of the *Search Patient* dialog box. The box will disappear.

f. In the *Add Subscriber* dialog box, you will see Frank Powell as the *Subscriber* and "Father" as the *Relationship*. Click on *Save* and Frank Powell is pulled into the *Subscriber* field in the *Insurance Plan(s)* section.

g. *Ins Company* field: Refer back to the patient registration form and using the drop-down, select the insurance information. Once selected the *Ins Plan* will automatically populate.

h. In the *Subscriber* # field, enter the subscriber number listed.

i. (If applicable) Enter the group number in the *Group* # field.

j. (If applicable) Enter the member number in the *Member* # field. (There is no member number for this patient.)

k. In the *Elig From* and *Elig To* fields, enter the patient's birth date (08/31/XX—use last year). The *Elig To* field remains blank until the patient changes insurance plans.

l. Enter the copayment amount in the Copay field. Do not use dollar signs.

m. Leave the Se*quence* field as "1."

n. Confirm that the patient has signed the Assignment of Benefits/Financial Agreement, and select "Yes" from the *Assignment of Benefits* drop-down menu (patient's father, Frank Powell, signed the patient registration form, which includes the Assignment of Benefits/Financial Agreement).

32. The last field in the *Patient Details* tab is where photos are added. Skip this section as this feature is not active in your student environment.

33. Click *Save* to save your entries. **Note:** Once you have hit *Save*, to make further entries in the *Patient Details* screen, you will have to first click *Edit*.

34. Because Francisco is a pediatric patient, you will skip the *Employer* tab information.

35. Now update the emergency contact information contained in the Patient Registration form with the following steps:

    a. Click on the *Relationships* tab.

    b. Click the drop-down next to "Add Relationship."

    c. Select *Emergency Contact* and the *Add Emergency Contact* dialog box will appear.

    d. Next to the *Patient* field, click on the looking glass.

    e. In the *Search Patients* dialog box, enter "Frank Powell" and click *Search*.

    f. Select "Frank Powell" (by clicking on the radio dial button), and then select "Father" from the drop-down next to the Social Security number (SSN) in the *Search Patients* dialog box.

    g. Click the *Select* button at the lower right of the *Search Patient* dialog box. The box will disappear.

    h. The drop-down next to the "Relationship" field will auto-populate with "Father." The "Phone" fields will also auto-populate with the information in the database for Frank Powell. Leave these fields as is.

    i. Click "Yes" as "Preferred."

    j. Click *Save*.

36. (If applicable) Click *Edit* (**Figure 3-41**) and continue the full registration process for any missing information.

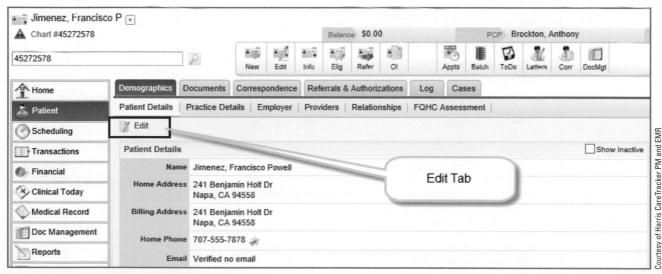

Figure 3-41   Edit Patient Demographics

37. Click the *Print* icon to the left of the *Summary* link in the upper-right corner of the *Demographics* application. Harris CareTracker PM displays your printing options, along with a *Patient Summary Printout* screen (**Figure 3-42**). (Note: It may take a few moments to generate the report.)

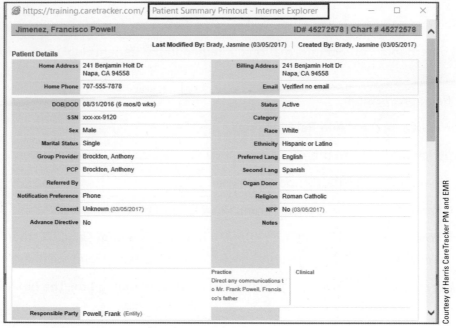

Figure 3-42   *Patient Demographics Report for Francisco Powell Jimenez*

38. Choose a printer listed in the *Print* dialog box to print the patient demographics summary (**Figure 3-43**). (Alternatively, you can close the print prompt box and take a screenshot of the report, or right click on the report and select *Print*.)

📇 Print the *Patient Demographics* report, label it "Activity 3-4," and place it in your assignment folder.

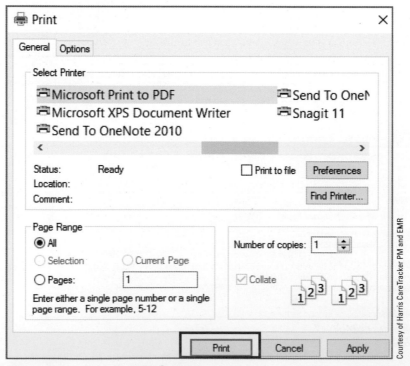

Figure 3-43   *Print Prompt Screen*

Source Document 3-3

Patient Registration Form			NVFHA

Patient Registration Form

Patient's Last Name	First (legal name)	First (Preferred name)	Middle Name
Jimenez	Francisco		Powell

Address (Number, Street, Apt #)	City	State	Zip Code
241 Benjamin Holt Drive	Napa	CA	94558

Mail will be sent to the address listed above, unless patient indicates a different address (leave blank if same as above)

Send mail to Address (Number, Street, Apt #)	City	State	Zip Code

Phone Options	Phone Number	Okay to leave detailed message	Call this number (circle one)
Home	(707) 555 - 7878	Yes ____ No __X__	①st 2nd 3rd choice
Cell	( ) -	Yes ____ No ____	1st 2nd 3rd choice
Work	( ) -	Yes ____ No ____	1st 2nd 3rd choice

Would you like to communicate by Email	Yes ___ No X	Email Address	

Date of Birth	Sex	Social Security Number
8/31/20XX	Female ____ Male __X__	000-00-9120

Marital Status (*circle one*)

(Single) / Married / Divorced / Widow /Partner

What is your preferred language / secondary language

Race (*circle one*)

African American-Black / Asian / Bi-Multi-racial / Pacific Islander-Hawaiian / (Caucasian–White) / Native American Eskimo Aleut / Decline to state / Other

Ethnicity (*circle one*)

(Hispanic-Latino)/ Non-Hispanic-Latino / Other

Religion	Catholic	Organ Donor	Yes ____	No ____

Are you new to our practice	Who referred you to our practice	Who is your Primary Care Physician
Yes __X__ No ____	Frank Powell	Anthony Brookton

Additional Notes

Emergency Contact

Emergency Contact's Name	Relationship to patient	Phone
Frank Powell	Father	(510) 555 - 7878

On-Line Patient Portal Communication via Email

On-Line communication is used for non-urgent message/requests only. NVFHA uses secure technology to protect the privacy and confidentiality of your personal information. Only you, your physician, and authorized staff can read your message.

What is your preferred method of communication	Phone __X__ Letter ____ Patient Portal ____ Email ____

Insurance Information

Subscriber (Insurance Holder) Name	Date of Birth	Relationship to patient	Subscriber Phone Number
Frank Powell	11/1/1988	Father	(707) 555 - 7878

Health Plan Information	Primary Health Plan	Secondary Health Plan
Health Plan Name	Century Medical PPO	
Health Plan Address	PO Box 87542, San Jose, CA, 95101	
Group Number		
Subscriber Number	CMED 2478	

Elig Date From		Copay	$ 35.00

Patient Employer Information

Employer Name & Address (Number, Street, Apt #, City, State, Zip Code)	Employer Phone Number
Frank Powell - Trinchero Family Estates	(707) 257 - 0200
Occupation	Start Date 05/01/2011

Assignment of Benefits • Financial Agreement

I hereby give lifetime authorization for payment of insurance benefits to be made directly to <u>Napa Valley Family Health Assoc.,</u> and any assisting physicians, for services rendered. I understand that I am financially responsible for all charges whether or not they are covered by insurance. In the event of default, I agree to pay all costs of collection, and reasonable attorney's fees. I hereby authorize this healthcare provider to release all information necessary to secure the the payment of benefits.

I further agree that a photocopy of this agreement shall be as valid as the original.

Date: __XX/XX/20XX__   Your Signature: *Frank Powell*

Method of Payment: ☐ Cash   ☐ Check   ☐ Credit Card

EDIT PATIENT INFORMATION

Learning Objective 5: Edit patient information in Harris CareTracker.

It is important to verify accuracy and update (edit) information when a patient schedules an appointment or checks in for an appointment. This makes the treatment process faster and avoids unnecessary complications in billing due to outdated information (**Figure 3-44**).

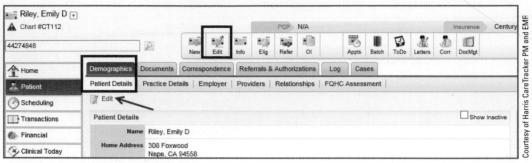

Figure 3-44   Edit Patient Information Tab

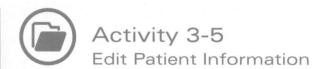

Activity 3-5
Edit Patient Information

1. Pull patient Emily Riley into context and click *Edit* on the *Name Bar*.

2. Harris CareTracker PM displays the *Patient Details* window.

3. Click on the *Employer* tab at the top of the screen.

4. Click the *Edit* link at the top left of the screen.

5. Deactivate Ms. Riley's current employer (Napa State Hospital) by clicking on the *Deactivate Employer* icon.

6. Then, click on the + *New Employer* link at the bottom left of the screen. (**Note:** You may receive a pop-up window asking if you want to leave the page. Click on "Leave this page.")

7. You can select a new employer from the *Employer* drop-down menu. Ms. Riley's current employer, Silverado Resort and Spa in Napa, CA, is not listed in the drop-down menu. Instead, click on the *Search* 🔍 icon, which will open the *Search Employers* window. Enter "Silverado Resort and Spa" in the *Employer Name* field and click *Search*. Click on the appropriate result. The new employer information, including address, will populate in the *Employer* window.

8. Update the *Employer* window with *Occupation* ("Massage Therapist") and *Dates Employed* (use today's date as the start date, and leave the ending date blank) (see **Figure 3-45**).

9. Click *Save*.

10. Click back on the *Patient Details* (Demographics) tab, click *Edit*, change the work address to her new employer just entered and the work phone number to (707)257-0200.

11. Click *Save*.

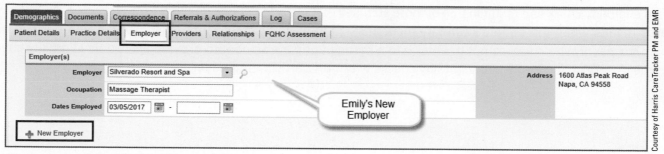

Figure 3-45   *Edited Patient Employer Field*

Print the updated *Demographics/Employer* screen, label it "Activity 3-5," and place it in your assignment folder.

ELIGIBILITY CHECKS

Learning Objective 6: View and perform eligibility checks.

The *Eligibility* application enables you to view a history of eligibility checks. It also enables you to electronically check eligibility with the primary insurance as well as the secondary insurance saved in *Patient Demographics*. Harris CareTracker PM and EMR automatically performs eligibility checks every evening for all patients scheduled for appointments for the next five days. Automated batch eligibility checks are performed for a patient once every 30 days regardless of the number of appointments scheduled for the patient during that month. However, it is sometimes necessary to perform individual eligibility checks periodically throughout the treatment and payment cycle or for any walk-in patients. The eligibility check helps to identify potential payer sources, reducing the number of denied claims or bad debt write-offs, and decrease staff hours required for performing manual eligibility checks.

Your student version of Harris CareTracker PM does not have the electronic eligibility feature active. To perform the simulated workflow of an eligibility check, you would click the *Elig* button on the dashboard, and then access payer website or call the insurance company to verify eligibility when electronic access is not available (**Figure 3-46**).

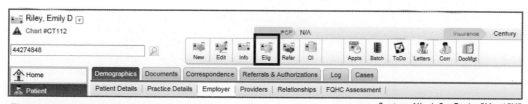

Figure 3-46   *Patient Eligibility Icon*   Courtesy of Harris CareTracker PM and EMR

SPOTLIGHT   If a patient's primary insurance is a non-participating payer and your practice has not signed up to check eligibility for the payers, the *Elig* button is disabled, preventing you çfrom performing electronic checks. This feature is not available on your student version of Harris CareTracker PM.

An eligibility check can result in one of three statuses that include *Eligible, Ineligible,* or *Unknown.* An **unknown status** results when the patient's primary insurance is a non-participating (non-par) payer. A **non-participating** payer is a payer who chooses not to enter into a participating agreement to provide electronic eligibility checks for free. A service fee applies to eligibility checks with non-participating payers.

Activity 3-6
View and Perform Eligibility Check

1. Pull patient Emily Riley into context and then click *Elig* on the *Name Bar.* Harris CareTracker PM displays the *Eligibility History* dialog box. In the live version of Harris CareTracker, this box would contain a list of eligibility checks performed for the patient and additional details about the most recent eligibility check. In your student version of Harris CareTracker, you will receive a message stating "No Eligibility History available for this patient."

2. In a live environment, you would click the *Check Eligibility* button in the top right corner to check eligibility. For this activity, you will have to manually simulate checking for patient eligibility. To do this, click the ☑+ *Add Notes* icon to the left of the *Check Eligibility* button. This will open the *Manual Eligibility* box.

3. Enter information into the *Manual Eligibility* box as shown in **Figure 3-47A**.

   a. *Status*: Select "Eligible."

   b. *Verification*: Enter today's date.

   c. *Mark Reviewed*: Select "No."

   d. *Note*: Enter "Patient is eligible."

   e. Click *Save.*

4. The manual eligibility check will now show in the *Eligibility History* window (**Figure 3-47B**).

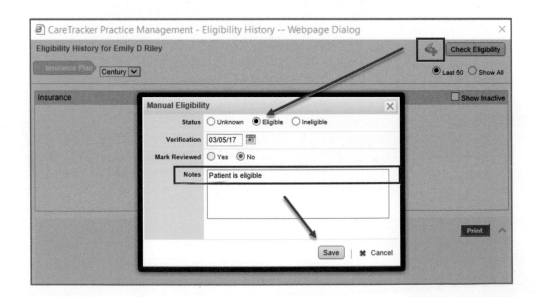

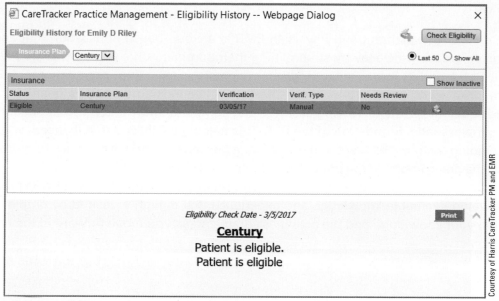

Figures 3-47A and 3-47B   Eligibility Check

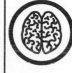 **Print the *Eligibility History* screen, label it "Activity 3-6," and place it in your assignment folder.**

5.   Click "X" in the top right corner of the *Eligibility History* window to close out of it.

CRITICAL THINKING   Now that you have completed your Chapter 3 activities, how did the challenge put forth in the Real-World Connection apply to you? Did you read each activity in its entirety before you started to enter data? Were you accurate in your entries? Did you struggle with any of the activities or steps? If so, which ones? What measures did you take to correct any errors and move forward with the activity, if any?

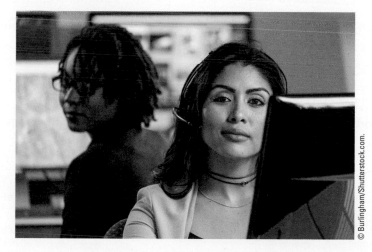

SUMMARY

Harris CareTracker Practice Management and Physician EMR is a cloud-based application that enables physician practices to achieve greater efficiency by streamlining their administrative workflows. The *Patient* module in Harris CareTracker PM and EMR is where you register patients and save important patient information. The information stored in this module includes the patient's basic and detailed demographics, health insurance information, and referrals and authorizations. Having accurate and complete information within patient registration and demographics is the essential foundation of the EHR. This database will lead to enhanced workflows in the medical practice, providing the most efficient and quality care possible, along with maximizing productivity.

Congratulations on having completed the patient registration and demographics portion of Harris CareTracker PM, including completing activities in your live training environment. Understanding and being proficient in the use of an EHR will give you valuable knowledge and experience that is highly desired by employers. You will continue to build upon your knowledge and the activities completed as you move forward in the next chapters.

CHECK YOUR KNOWLEDGE

Select the best response.

_____ 1. A patient who has tertiary insurance would have how many types of coverage?

a. One

b. Two

c. Three

d. None

_____ 2. Which of the following is not one of the applications launched from the *Name Bar*?

a. Eligibility

b. Insurance

c. Edit

d. Add New Patient

_____ 3. Which is not considered patient information that is entered into the *Demographics* application?

a. Social Security number

b. Date of birth

c. Employment information

d. Reason for encounter

_____ 4. When navigating in the *Demographics* application, which key should be used to move between fields?

a. Enter

b. Tab

c. Space

d. Control

_____ 5. Which of the following is a reason for editing patient information?

a. Updating address

b. Recording test results

c. Avoiding unnecessary complications in billing

d. Both a and c.

_____ 6. Eligibility checks help the practice:

a. identify potential payer sources.

b. reduce number of denied claims.

c. increase revenue through improved collection rates.

d. all of the above

_____ 7. When entering the patient's Social Security number, use the _____ key when moving between fields.

a. Enter

b. Tab

c. Space

d. Do not use any keys, hyphen will automatically populate

_____8. Which of the following is not a method to de-identify PHI?

a. Encryption in the electronic record

b. Shredding paper records

c. Blacking out information that would identify a patient.

d. Untethering documents

_____9. The *Patient Alerts* window is divided into four sections. Which of the following is not contained in *Patient Alerts*?

a. Encounter form

b. Eligibility

c. Patient demographics

d. Notes for this patient

_____10. The *Patient Alerts* window will notify you of missing information that must be entered in the *Patient/Details* tab. What required information is listed here?

a. Ethnicity

b. Race

c. Preferred language

d. All of the above

CASE STUDIES

Please note, throughout the textbook, end-of-chapter Case Studies related to new patient James Smith will build upon previously completed case studies. If you do not complete Case Study 3-1, later chapter case studies regarding James Smith will not function. There are other Case Studies provided that do not require completion of prior chapter case studies.

Case Study 3-1

Register new patient James M. Smith. Refer to Source Document 3-4 (Patient Registration Form, provided on the next page) in order to complete this case study. Assume that NPP forms have been signed and requisite consent has been given. Mr. Smith is considered a "VIP." Be sure to note that when entering his demographics. Refer to Activity 3-2 for help.

After you register new patient James Smith, print the Patient Demographics report. Refer to Activity 3-3 for help.

Print the Patient Demographics report, label it "Case Study 3-1," and place it in your assignment folder.

Case Study 3-2

Update patient demographics for the following three patients with the date of death (DOD) as indicated. Note that the *Date of Death* (DOD) field is only enabled when the *Status* field has been changed to "Deceased." Refer to Activity 3-5 for help.

a.   Francine Quigley—DOD 11/17/2017

b.   Cosima Smith—DOD 1/5/2018

c.   Bruce Thomas—DOD 1/17/2018

Print the Patient Demographics report for each patient, label them "Case Study 3-2a, b, and c," and place them in your assignment folder.

Source Document 3-4

Patient Registration Form			NVFHA

Patient's Last Name	First (legal name)	First (Preferred name)	Middle Name
SMITH	JAMES	JIM	M

Address (Number, Street, Apt #)	City	State	Zip Code
2455 E. Front, Apt. 205	Napa	CA	94558

Mail will be sent to the address listed above, unless patient indicates a different address (leave blank if same as above)

Send mail to Address (Number, Street, Apt #)	City	State	Zip Code

Phone Options	Phone Number	Okay to leave detailed message	Call this number (circle one)
Home	(707) 221 - 4040	Yes X No _____	(1st) 2nd 3rd choice
Cell	( ) -	Yes ____ No _____	1st 2nd 3rd choice
Work	(877) 833 - 7777	Yes ____ No X	1st (2nd) 3rd choice

Would you like to communicate by Email Yes X No __	Email Address	Jmsmith@email.com

Date of Birth	Sex	Social Security Number
2/23/1965	Female ____ Male X	000-00-9009

Marital Status (*circle one*)	What is your preferred language / secondary language
(Single)/ Married / Divorced / Widow /Partner	English

Race (*circle one*)	Ethnicity (*circle one*)
African American-Black / Asian / Bi-Multi-racial / Pacific Islander-Hawaiian / (Caucasian–White)/ Native American Eskimo Aleut / Decline to state / Other	Hispanic-Latino / Non-Hispanic-Latino / Other

Religion		Organ Donor Yes _____ No _____

Are you new to our practice	Who referred you to our practice	Who is your Primary Care Physician
Yes X No ____	David Dodgin	Rebecca Ayerick

Additional Notes	No call after 8 pm

Emergency Contact

Emergency Contact's Name	Relationship to patient	Phone
Joan Smith	Mother	(510) 478 - 5151

On-Line Patient Portal Communication via Email

On-Line communication is used for non-urgent message/requests only. NVFHA uses secure technology to protect the privacy and confidentiality of your personal information. Only you, your physician, and authorized staff can read your message.

What is your preferred method of communication	Phone X Letter _____ Patient Portal _____ Email _____

Insurance Information

Subscriber (Insurance Holder) Name	Date of Birth	Relationship to patient	Subscriber Phone Number
James M. Smith	2/23/1965	Self	(707) 221 - 4040

Health Plan Information	Primary Health Plan	Secondary Health Plan
Health Plan Name	Blue Shield Cengage	
Health Plan Address	PO Box 32245, Los Angeles, CA, 90002	
Group Number	BCBS987	
Subscriber Number	BCBS987	

Elig Date From	1/1/2010	Copay	$ 25.00

Patient Employer Information

Employer Name & Address (Number, Street, Apt #, City, State, Zip Code)	Employer Phone Number
River Rock Casino, 3250 Highway 128, Geyserville, CA 95441	(877) 833 - 7777

Occupation	IT Support	Start Date	8/25/2009

Assignment of Benefits • Financial Agreement

I hereby give lifetime authorization for payment of insurance benefits to be made directly to **Napa Valley Family Health Assoc.**, and any assisting physicians, for services rendered. I understand that I am financially responsible for all charges whether or not they are covered by insurance. In the event of default, I agree to pay all costs of collection, and reasonable attorney's fees. I hereby authorize this healthcare provider to release all information necessary to secure the payment of benefits.

I further agree that a photocopy of this agreement shall be as valid as the original.

Date: **XX/XX/20XX**_____ Your Signature: _____ *James M. Smith*

Method of Payment: ☐ Cash   ☐ Check   ☐ Credit Card

BUILD YOUR PROFICIENCY

Proficiency Builder 3-1: Search for a Patient by ID Number

You can search for a patient using various methods. Using the information you obtained for patients in Activity 3-1, search for the same patients by ID number.

1. In the *ID* search box (see Figure 3-3), enter patient Kevin Johnson's ID number (using the ID number obtained from the patient search in Activity 3-1). (**Note:** New ID numbers are assigned to patients for each student version of Harris CareTracker; therefore, patient ID numbers will vary by student.)

2. Hit [Enter]. The patient with the corresponding *ID number* launches into context.

🖫 Print the Search Results screen, label it "BYP Activity 3-1," and place it in your assignment folder.

3. Search for four additional established patients by their ID number, using the information obtained in your Activity 3-1 search.

   a. Jane Morgan

   b. Kirk Johnson

   c. Abby Zuffante

   d. Frank Powell

🖫 Print the Search Results screen for each patient, label it "BYP 3-1a-d," and place it in your assignment folder.

Proficiency Builder 3-2: Search for a Patient by Chart Number

You may also search for a patient by chart number. Typically, the chart number and the Harris CareTracker PM and EMR ID are the same. However, if the practice files paper charts by chart number, Harris CareTracker PM and EMR can assign chart numbers based on your medical record number. In your student version, the chart number and ID number are different for existing patients. New patients will have the same chart number and ID number. (**Note:** If your practice has electronically converted patient demographics to Harris CareTracker PM and EMR from another practice management system, the chart number will be the patient's ID number from your legacy practice management system.)

1. With no patient in context, click the *Search* 🔍 icon; it will take you to the *Patient Search* pop-up box where you will need to enter the patient's *Chart Number* in the *Chart #* field.

2. Enter the chart number of patient Frank Powell (CT148) and click *Search* (Figure 3-48).

🖫 Print the Search Results screen, label it "BYP 3-2," and place it in your assignment folder.

3. Click directly on the patient's name with the corresponding *Chart Number* to launch him or her into context. (**Note:** It may take a few moments for Harris CareTracker to "search" and populate the patient demographics.)

4. Repeat Proficiency Builder Activity 3-2 by searching for four additional established patients using their chart numbers, which were obtained in your Activity 3-1 search.

   a. Kevin Johnson

   b. Jane Morgan

(Continues)

(*Continued*)

    c. Kirk Johnson

    d. Abby Zuffante

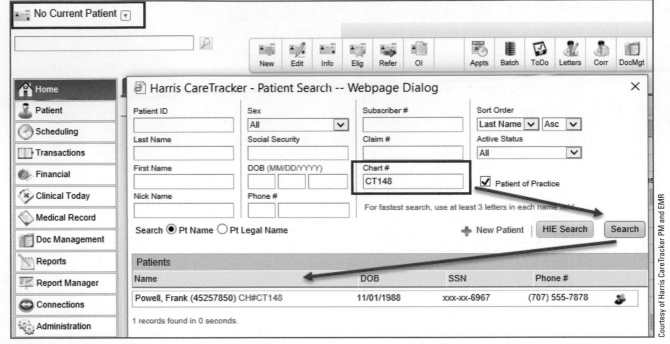

Figure 3-48   Pt Search by Patient Chart Number

🖫 **Print the Search Results screen for each patient, label it "BYP Activity 3-2a-d" and place it in your assignment folder.**

Proficiency Builder 3-3: Search for a Patient by Social Security Number (SSN)

Another method of patient search is by patient Social Security number. Follow the instructions below and search for patients by Social Security number.

1. With no patient in context, click the *Search* 🔍 icon.

2. In the *Patient Search* pop-up, enter the last four digits of patient Frank Powell's Social Security number (6967), obtained in Activity 3-1, and hit [Enter] (or click on the *Search* button).

🖫 **Print the Patient Search pop-up screen, label it "BYP Activity 3-3," and place it in your assignment folder.**

3. Click on the corresponding patient (Figure 3-49). The application pulls the patient into context and launches the *Patient Demographics* application.

4. Repeat Proficiency Builder Activity 3-3 by searching for the four additional established patients using their Social Security numbers obtained in your Activity 3-1 search.

    a. Kevin Johnson

    b. Jane Morgan

    c. Kirk Johnson

    d. Abby Zuffante

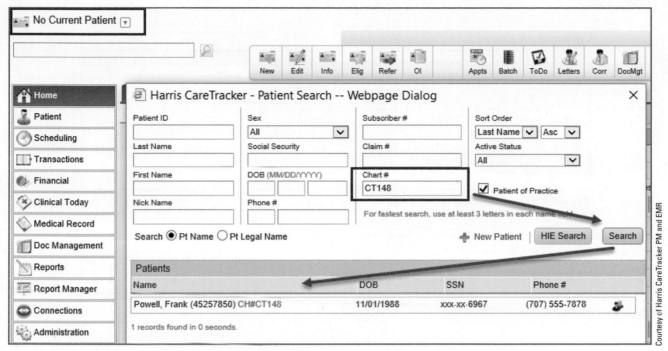

Figure 3-49   Search by Social Security Number

📖 **Print the Patient Search pop-up screen for each patient, label it "BYP 3-3a-d," and place it in your assignment folder.**

Proficiency Builder 3-4: View the VIP Log

As discussed previously in the textbook, there are times when patients are flagged as VIPs. This is done for a variety of reasons. Having previously registered and noted patients as VIPs, you will now run and view the VIP log. (Note: If no patients have been flagged as VIPs, nothing will display.)

1. Click the *Administration* module. Harris CareTracker PM displays the *Practice* tab.

2. Click the *VIP Log* link under the *Security Logs* section. The application displays the *VIP Patient Log* (Figure 3-50) fields.

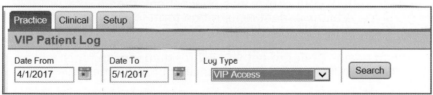

Figure 3-50   VIP Patient Log   Courtesy of Harris CareTracker PM and EMR

3. Select the date range in the *Date From* (select the first day of the month you are working in) and in the *Date To* field select today's date.

4. Select the *Log Type* to view (select VIP Access), which displays operators with *VIP Patient Access* override included in their profile.

5. Click *Search*. Harris CareTracker PM displays the log (Figure 3-51).

6. Click the plus sign next to the patient's name to expand the log and view additional details (Figure 3-52) (if any patients are displaying).

(Continues)

(Continued)

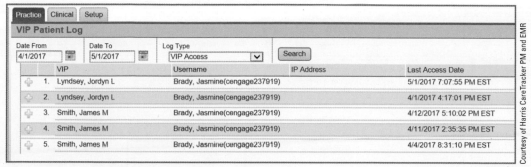

Figure 3-51   *VIP Patient Log Created*

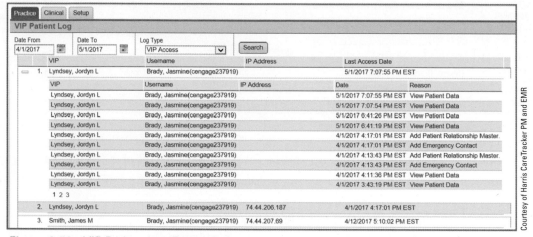

Figure 3-52   *VIP Patient Log Expanded*

🖫 **Print a screenshot of the VIP Log, label it "BYP 3-4," and place it in your assignment folder.**

Proficiency Builder 3-5: Additional Practice Registering a New Patient

Register a fictional patient of your choice as a new patient, then print the patient's demographics. A blank patient registration form is provided for you here (Source Document 3-5). A blank registration form is also available on your student companion website so you can print additional forms for unlimited practice. (If needed, refer to Activity 3-2 for guidance in registering a new patient, and refer to Activity 3-3 for guidance in printing the patient's demographics.)

🖫 **Print the Patient Demographics report, label it "BYP 3-5," and place it in your assignment folder.**

Source Document 3-5

Patient Registration Form   NVFHA

Patient's Last Name	First (legal name)	First (Preferred name)	Middle Name

Address (Number, Street, Apt #)		City	State	Zip Code

Mail will be sent to the address listed above, unless patient indicates a different address (leave blank if same as above)

Send mail to Address (Number, Street, Apt #)	City	State	Zip Code

Phone Options	Phone Number	Okay to leave detailed message	Call this number (circle one)
Home		Yes ____ No _____	1st 2nd 3rd choice
Cell		Yes ____ No _____	1st 2nd 3rd choice
Work		Yes ____ No _____	1st 2nd 3rd choice

Would you like to communicate by Email	Yes __ No __	Email Address

Date of Birth	Sex	Social Security Number
	Female ____ Male ____	

Marital Status (*circle one*)	What is your preferred language / secondary language
Single / Married / Divorced / Widow /Partner	

Race (*circle one*)		Ethnicity (*circle one*)
African American-Black / Asian / Bi-Multi-racial / Pacific Islander-Hawaiian / Caucasian–White / Native American Eskimo Aleut / Decline to state / Other		Hispanic-Latino / Non-Hispanic-Latino / Other

Religion	Organ Donor	Yes _____ No _____

Are you new to our practice	Who referred you to our practice	Who is your Primary Care Physician
Yes _____ No _____		

Additional Notes

Emergency Contact

Emergency Contact's Name	Relationship to patient	Phone

On-Line Patient Portal Communication via Email

On Line communication is used for non-urgent message/requests only. NVFHA uses secure technology to protect the privacy and confidentiality of your personal information. Only you, your physician, and authorized staff can read your message.

What is your preferred method of communication	Phone ____ Letter _____ Patient Portal _____ Email _____

Insurance Information

Subscriber (Insurance Holder) Name	Date of Birth	Relationship to patient	Subscriber Phone Number
	/ /		( )

Health Plan Information	Primary Health Plan	Secondary Health Plan
Health Plan Name		
Health Plan Address		
Group Number		
Subscriber Number		
Elig Date From		Copay

Patient Employer Information

Employer Name & Address (Number, Street, Apt #, City, State, Zip Code)	Employer Phone Number
Occupation	Start Date

Assignment of Benefits • Financial Agreement

I hereby give lifetime authorization for payment of insurance benefits to be made directly to Napa Valley Family Health Assoc., and any assisting physicians, for services rendered. I understand that I am financially responsible for all charges whether or not they are covered by insurance. In the event of default, I agree to pay all costs of collection, and reasonable attorney's fees. I hereby authorize this healthcare provider to release all information necessary to secure the the payment of benefits.

I further agree that a photocopy of this agreement shall be as valid as the original.

Date: _____ Your Signature: _____

Method of Payment: ❑ Cash   ❑ Check   ❑ Credit Card

(*Continued*)

Proficiency Builder 3-6: Enter a Foreign Address in Patient Demographics

Follow the instructions noted below and edit the new fictional patient you registered in Proficiency Builder 3-5 by entering a foreign address. Refer to Activity 3-5 for help. Use the following steps to complete the activity:

1. Open an existing patient's demographic record (select the fictional patient account you created in Proficiency Builder 3-5). Click *Edit* in the *Name Bar*.

2. From the *Type* list in the *Addresses* section, select the type of address you are entering. The default selection is *Home* address. Select "Home."

3. In the Line 1 box enter the patient's house number and street name. Enter fictitious address of "123 Anywhere."

4. In the Line 2 box enter the patient's city and state. Depending on the country, this may be a city/town and province. Enter fictitious address information of "Ensenada."

5. In the *City* box, enter the country in which the patient lives. Enter fictitious address information of "Mexico."

6. From the *Country* list, select the county in which the patient lives. Enter fictitious address information of "Mexico" for the country. This field does not pull onto the claim and that is why it is necessary to enter the country in the *City* field (Figure 3-53).

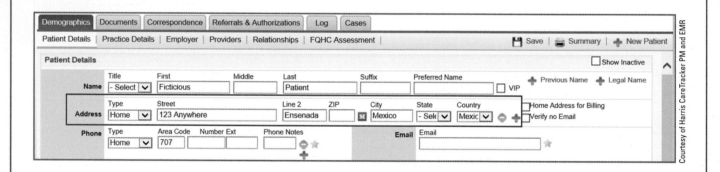

Courtesy of Harris CareTracker PM and EMR

Print the Patient Demographics report, label it "BYP 3-6," and place it in your assignment folder.

Proficiency Builder 3-7: Additional Practice Viewing and Performing an Eligibility Check

Perform an eligibility check on the new fictitious patient account you created in Proficiency Builder 3-5. Enter result of "Ineligible" and "Patient is ineligible per manual check." Refer to Activity 3-6 for help.

Print the Patient Eligibility report, label it "BYP 3-7," and place it in your assignment folder.

Proficiency Builder 3-8: Add Relationships

Access *Help* and locate the *Patient* folder in the *Contents* tab. Click on the *Relationships* folder. Using the instructions found there, add a school and emergency contact for the new fictitious patient account you created using the following information:

a. School: University of New Hampshire; Degree: MBA; Year Graduated 1999.

b. Emergency Contact: Non-patient "Jocynn Gentry"; Relationship: "Sister"; Phone (Home): 707-555-2214; Preferred: "Yes."

💾 **Print the Patient Demographics report, label it "BYP 3-8," and place it in your assignment folder.**

Proficiency Builder 3-9: Deactivate Employer/Add New Employer

Deactivate the employer on the new fictitious patient account you created and add a new employer, following the steps below. For further assistance, access *Help*.

1. Click on the *Employer* tab in *Demographics*.

2. Click *Edit*.

3. If there is no active employer, add G.L. Mezzeta; Occupation: Assembly worker; Dates Employed: Enter beginning date of January 3, 2012.

4. Now *Deactivate* the current employer.

5. Add a New Employer. Add employer "University of Davis," with the address of 101 Main Street, Suite 200, Davis, CA 95618.

6. Click *Save* and then check the box to *Show Inactive*.

7. Click back on the *Patient Details* tab.

8. Click *Edit* and update the Occupation to "Adjunct Instructor" and Dates Employed of start date of January 3, of last year.

9. Click *Save*.

10. Place a check mark in the "Show Inactive" box.

💾 **Print the Patient Demographics report, label it "BYP 3-9," and place it in your assignment folder.**

Proficiency Builder 3-10: Deactivate Address/Activate Address

There are times when it is necessary to deactivate or activate an address, insurance, medication, and so on. Practice deactivating and activating a patient's address using the fictitious patient account you created.

11. Click the *Deactivate* icon at the end of the address line (Figure 3-54). The deactivated address remains in the patient's record but is now grayed out. Additionally, the *Deactivate* icon is changed to *Activate*. Note: If there is both a *Home* and *Billing* address, deactivate both.

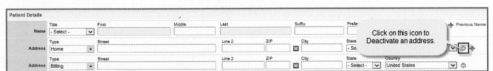

Figure 3-54   Deactivate Patient Address   Courtesy of Harris CareTracker PM and EMR

💾 **Print the Patient Demographics report, label it "BYP 3-10," and place it in your assignment folder.**

12. Click the *Activate* icon next to the deactivated address to reactivate it. The address will no longer be grayed out.

Appointment Scheduling

4

Key Terms

batch
chief complaint (CC)
copayment
history of present illness
  (HPI)
multi-resource
  appointment
nonverbal
  communication
recall
receipt
resource
TeleVox®
verbal communication

Learning Objectives

1. Book, reschedule, and cancel appointments.
2. Schedule non-patient appointments.
3. Add a patient to the *Wait List*.
4. Perform activities managing the daily schedule.
5. Check in patients.
6. Create a batch, accept payments, print patient receipts, run a journal, and post the batch.

Real-World Connection

Answering the phones and scheduling appointments are two of the most challenging tasks in the medical office. These tasks require an individual who is highly organized, can multitask, and has great communication skills.

Imagine holding the key to your provider's home and controlling which guests have the authority to enter the home and at what times. In some respects, this is similar to what you do when scheduling appointments. Instead of holding the key to the provider's house, you hold the key to the provider's workplace. However, this is only half of the scenario; you must also be cognizant of the severity of the patient's symptoms and the time constraints that prevent the patient from taking the "next available" appointment.

You must ask yourself: Do you have the key attributes of a scheduler? Can you handle the fast pace and keep providers on task, all while accommodating your patients? Consider the desired characteristics of a scheduler as you practice scheduling patients using Harris CareTracker PM. The first step to being a good scheduler is becoming familiar with the software! At the end of the chapter, you will be asked to evaluate your experience scheduling patients. Let's begin!

INTRODUCTION

All appointment information is entered and saved in the *Scheduling* module. The *Book* application is where you schedule, reschedule, and cancel both patient and non-patient appointments (e.g., meetings). To find future appointment availability, you can set specific appointment search criteria, for example, provider, location, and day of the week. Conveniently, the *Book* application is set up so that through a patient's scheduled appointment, you can access several other applications and functions in Harris CareTracker PM and EMR. This makes it possible to edit patient demographics, print encounter forms, save visits, and enter patient **copayments** without having to navigate away from the *Book* application.

Appointment history is tracked in Harris CareTracker PM and EMR. Any time an appointment is rescheduled or canceled, the information is saved in the *Scheduling* module. A reason for rescheduling or canceling the appointment must be entered and will always be linked to the appointment. All previous, rescheduled, and canceled appointments can be accessed in the *History* application. In addition, scheduled, rescheduled, and canceled appointments can also be linked to **recalls**. Recalls are reminders to patients that an appointment needs to be booked.

There are a few different ways to view appointments in the *Scheduling* module besides the *Book* application. The *Month* and *Calendar* applications allow you to view all patient scheduled appointments in a calendar, bar chart, or date book format. When a patient is in context, all upcoming appointments for any family member linked to that patient can be viewed in the *Family* application. The list includes the patient's upcoming appointments as well.

Within the *Scheduling* module there are eight applications: *Book, Month, Calendar, Family, Recall, History, Advanced,* and **TeleVox**®, outlined in **Table 4-1**. *TeleVox*® is an optional application of an automated appointment reminder and confirmation system that can be used to notify patients of upcoming appointments.

Table 4-1   Application Summaries

	DESCRIPTION
Book	In this application you will schedule, reschedule, and cancel patient appointments. You can access several other applications and functions within Harris CareTracker PM and EMR through the mini-menu that displays when you click on a patient's appointment.
Month	At a glance, this application displays the number of appointments scheduled for each day of a particular month. You can choose the month, the resource, and the location for which to view a month calendar. In this application you can also view a month's appointments in bar chart format instead of a calendar view. **Resources** can be people, places, or things. Providers are always considered a resource, but an exam room or a piece of equipment can also be considered a resource. Something that requires a schedule is considered a resource because it has specific availability with days and times it can provide certain services. If the resource does not need a set schedule, then it is not considered a "resource" in Harris CareTracker PM and EMR.
Calendar	This application allows you to view appointments in a small date book calendar.
Family	You can view all upcoming appointments for any family members linked to the patient in context and the patient's upcoming appointments are listed in this application as well.
Recall	An appointment recall for the patient in context is entered in this application and any pending recalls for the patient are listed in this application as well.
History	This application shows all pending, previous, canceled, and rescheduled appointments for the patient in context. Canceling a patient's upcoming appointments should be completed from this application as well.
Advanced	This application enables you to book and reschedule appointments in accordance with predetermined parameters and criteria established by your practice. The *Advanced* method of booking appointments prevents overbooking and scheduling conflicts and also maintains consistency in terms of the days and times that different services and procedures are provided. The patient's existing appointments, pending recalls, and referrals are listed in this application as well.
TeleVox®	This is an automated appointment reminder and confirmation system that can be used to notify patients of upcoming appointments. Two major steps are involved in the *TeleVox*® interface: sending an electronic appointment list and viewing the results of the automated calls made by *TeleVox*®. This is an optional feature of Harris CareTracker PM and EMR, but not available in your student environment.

Courtesy of Harris CareTracker PM and EMR

Before you begin the activities in this chapter, refresh your memory on working with Harris CareTracker by referring back to the Best Practices list on page xxiii of this textbook. This list is also posted to the student companion website. Following best practices will help you complete work quickly and accurately.

BOOK APPOINTMENTS

Learning Objective 1: Book, reschedule, and cancel appointments.

Building upon activities in Chapter 3, you will now learn how to book (schedule) appointments. The most common method of initiating an appointment booking is when the patient calls on the phone. At times you will also book appointments while the patient is in the office (commonly when booking a follow-up appointment). You must demonstrate excellent communication skills, both verbal and nonverbal.

Verbal communication is the use of language or actual words spoken. **Nonverbal communication** consists of body language, gestures, eye contact, and expressions to communicate a message. Because most patient appointments are made over the phone, it is important that medical assistants develop positive telecommunication skills. The patient's impression of the practice will be strongly influenced by the medical assistant's phone etiquette.

SPOTLIGHT   Examples of proper phone etiquette:

- Answer promptly (within three rings when possible).
- Speak clearly into the phone (and do not forget to smile). Smiling changes your tone, and patients can tell.
- Identify the medical practice and yourself.
- If you must place a caller on hold, ask permission first, and thank the caller.
- If the wait time is going to be long, it is often better to ask the patient if you can return the call rather than keep the patient on hold. Do not forget to return calls as you promised. Always get the best contact number (and an alternate) and the best time to call, especially if a manager or another team member must return the call.
- Never interrupt the patient while he or she is talking to you.
- Never engage in an argument with a caller or allow an angry or aggressive caller to upset you. Remain calm and composed, and ask for your supervisor's assistance if necessary.
- Maintain privacy. Ensure identity as well (name and date of birth are commonly asked).
- Do not handle an unhappy caller's concern openly at the check-in/check-out desk.
- Be patient, and do not give the impression that you are rushed or unconcerned. Learn how to handle several callers simultaneously with ease and grace.
- Always make collection calls in private and away from the patient flow or public areas.
- Make sure that the caller, or the person called, hangs up first.

Booking appointments in Harris CareTracker PM and EMR takes place in the *Book* application of the *Scheduling* module. Both patient and non-patient appointments (e.g., meetings) are booked in this application. You must have a patient in context in the *Name Bar* to book a patient appointment. Three methods are used to book appointments (**Figure 4-1**):

1. Schedule directly in *Book*: This allows you to book patient and non-patient appointments by manually moving the schedule to a specific day and clicking on a specific time. You can use the *Book* filters to view the schedule for a specific time, day, location, and provider. Scheduling appointments directly from *Book* gives you the advantage of seeing appointment times that can be double-booked.

2. Using *Find*: This allows you to search for the next available appointment time based on specific appointment criteria you set. When searching appointment availability, you can filter your search by provider, location, appointment type, date, day, and time.

3. Using *Force*: This allows you to double-book appointments and to book an appointment during a different appointment-type time slot. Forced appointments appear outlined in blue on the schedule.

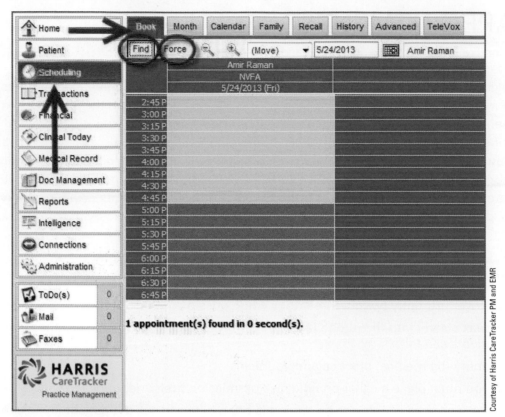

Figure 4-1   Screenshot of Book, Find, Force

Harris CareTracker offers the versatility of customizing appointment types. In your student version, the physician and practice schedules have been built in Harris CareTracker PM and EMR so that only certain appointment types can be scheduled during certain times, at certain locations, or for certain providers. Further customization of *AppointmentTypes* for your practice is done in the *Setup* tab of the *Administration* module. The schedule can also be customized by color coding appointment types. For example, you can assign a color to help quickly identify new patient visits on the schedule. The color is applied to the border of the appointment in the *Book* application. The color assigned to an appointment type overrides the default border colors used to identify appointment conflicts (brown/pink) and forced appointments (blue).

When booking an appointment, there is an option to either select a **chief complaint (CC)** from a list of favorites or manually enter a complaint in a free text field. A chief complaint is the patient's reasons for being seen for the visit in the patient's own words. You can only use one of the fields to enter a chief complaint. The chief complaint is displayed on the schedule and carried over to the progress note for the visit associated with the appointment in certain templates.

If the chief complaint is linked to a progress note template, Harris CareTracker PM and EMR will automatically apply the associated progress note template and select the chief complaint that is linked to the appointment. If the complaint is entered manually, this text will appear on the schedule in brackets [ ] and for a limited amount of templates, the text can be pulled into the CC/HPI (Chief Complaint/**History of Present Illness**) text box (see **Figure 4-2**).

You can create a list of favorite complaints for your group in the *Chief Complaint Maintenance* application in the *Administration* module. HPI is the patient's account of related symptoms for today's visit. The HPI is generated with the use of problem-focused templates, voice dictation, or handwriting and voice recognition (Figure 4-2).

CRITICAL THINKING Identify when and why documenting a chief complaint would be critical in your role as a medical assistant and the importance of accuracy.

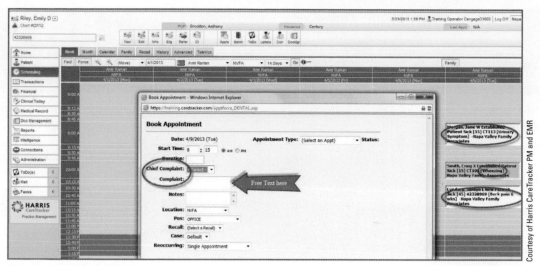

Figure 4-2   Chief Complaint

Using established patients in your database as well as building upon your previously registered new patients (from Chapter 3), schedule an appointment for each of the patients in **Table 4-2** by following the directions in Activity 4-1.

 ALERT! Certain scheduling activities will not function in a past date, and billing activities will not function in a future date. It is important to keep this in mind as you schedule patient appointments. Avoid booking too far in the future because that would affect future patient visits and billing activities.

 Activity 4-1
Book an Appointment

Using the instructions below and the patient data in **Table 4-2**, schedule an appointment for each patient.

1. Pull the patient for whom you are booking an appointment into context on the *Name Bar*.

2. Click the *Scheduling* module. Harris CareTracker PM and EMR opens the *Book* application by default.

3. Display the desired date using one of the following options:

    a. Select an option from the *Move* list to display the schedule for specific time increments such as Next Day, Next Week, 2 Months, and so on.

    b. Manually enter a date in MM/DD/YYYY format or click the *Calendar* 🔲 icon to display the schedule for a specific date.

4. Select the provider, location, and the number of days to display, and then click *Go* (**Figure 4-3**).

5. Click on the *time slot* for which you are booking the appointment. (If the schedule is displayed for multiple providers and locations, be sure to click the *time slot* in the appropriate column.) The application displays the *Book Appointment* window.

✓ **TIP** If the patient has existing appointments scheduled, the application displays the *Existing Appointments* window. Click *Book Appointment* at the bottom of the window to book a new appointment.

Table 4-2 Patient Appointments to Be Scheduled

PATIENT NAME *PROVIDER*	COMPLAINT	TYPE OF APPOINTMENT: RECORD DATE/TIME SELECTED
Jane Morgan *Dr. Raman*	Urinary symptoms	1st available next week/Est. Pt. Sick Date: _____ Time: _____
Ellen Ristino *Dr. Brockton*	Sore throat and nasal congestion	1st available next week/Est. Pt. Sick Date: _____ Timc: _____
Craig X. Smith *Dr. Raman*	Wheezing	1st available next week/Est. Pt. Sick Date: _____ Time: _____
Adam Thompson *Dr. Brockton*	Productive cough	1st available next week/Est. Pt. Sick Date: _____ Time: _____
Francisco Powell Jimenez* *Dr. Brockton* (*Registered in Activity 3-4)	New Patient (CPE). In *Notes* field, enter "New Pediatric Patient"	1st available next week/New Patient CPE Date: _____ Time: _____
Edith Robinson *Dr. Raman*	Back pain, six weeks, discuss possible MRI and referral to orthopedist	1st available next week/Est. Pt. Sick Date: _____ Time: _____

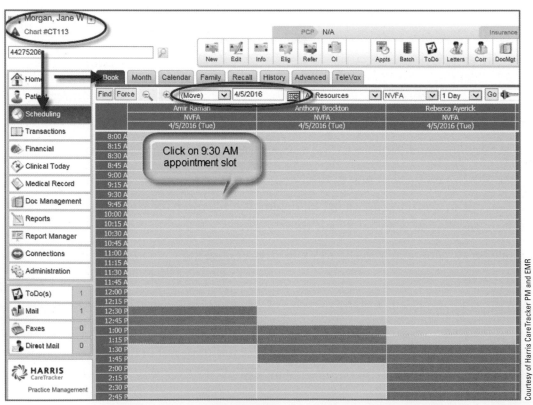

Figure 4-3 Book Appointment for Jane Morgan

6. From the *Appointment Type* list, select the appointment type. When you select an appointment type, Harris CareTracker PM and EMR automatically populates the *Task* and *Duration* fields (**Figure 4-4**).

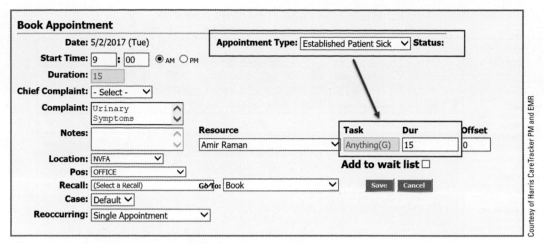

Figure 4-4   Book Appointment Window for Jane Morgan

7. From the *Resource* list, select the resource (i.e., provider) needed for the appointment.

8. There are two options for entering a *Chief Complaint* (you can only use option [a]):

a. Free text the chief complaint (as noted in **Table 4-2**) in the *Complaint* box (see **Figure 4-4**). For example, enter "Urinary Symptoms" for patient Jane Morgan. (The application will display the complaint in brackets [ ] next to the patient's name on the schedule.)

b. (FYI) From the *Chief Complaint* list, select a chief complaint from the drop-down list. This list is populated with the favorite complaints selected in the *Chief Complaint Maintenance* application in the *Administration* module. (This is not available in your student version. You will use the "free text" option.)

SPOTLIGHT If *Chief Complaints* have not been set up for your groups, this list is disabled. If the chief complaint is linked to a progress note template, Harris CareTracker PM and EMR will automatically apply the associated progress note template and select the chief complaint that is linked to the appointment. If the complaint is entered manually, this text will be pulled into the CC/HPI text box in certain templates.

9. In the *Notes* box, enter any notes about the appointment. (Only Francisco Powell Jimenez will need a note entered, as indicated in **Table 4-2**. Notes appear in parentheses next to the patient's name on the schedule and also appear when you move your mouse over the appointment on the schedule.)

TIP Do not use any symbols when entering appointment notes or patient complaints. Using symbols will cause an error when you try to print encounter forms.

10. From the *Location* list, select "NVFA."

11. From the *Pos* (Place of Service) list, select "OFFICE."

12. Do not link the appointment to an open recall for the patient.

13. Do not link the patient's appointment to a specific case.

14. Do not select recurring appointment.

15. Click *Save.* The application schedules the appointment (**Figure 4-5**).

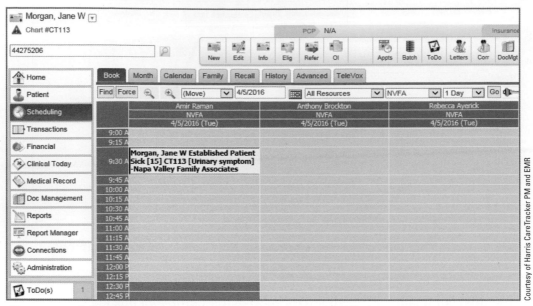

Figure 4-5 *Scheduled Appointment for Jane Morgan*

Print the Schedule/Booking screen for each patient scheduled (from Table 4-2), label them "Activity 4-1," and place them in your assignment folder.

Booking an Appointment Using Find

Often when scheduling an appointment, you will need to find the next available open time slot for that particular encounter (e.g., CPE, same day/urgent, procedure, follow-up). The *Find* feature allows you to search for the next available appointment time based on specific appointment criteria you set. When searching appointment availability, you can filter your search by provider, location, appointment type, date, day, and time.

When using *Find*, Harris CareTracker PM and EMR will search for appointments from the current day forward.

Building upon your previous scheduling practice (see Activity 4-1), schedule an appointment on the most appropriate date for the following patient using the *Find* button (**Table 4-3**). Record the date and time of the appointment scheduled for future reference.

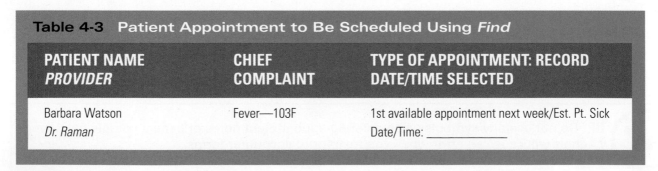

Table 4-3 Patient Appointment to Be Scheduled Using *Find*

PATIENT NAME *PROVIDER*	CHIEF COMPLAINT	TYPE OF APPOINTMENT: RECORD DATE/TIME SELECTED
Barbara Watson *Dr. Raman*	Fever—103F	1st available appointment next week/Est. Pt. Sick Date/Time: _____

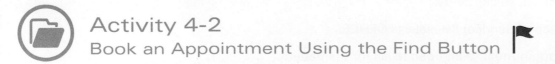

Activity 4-2
Book an Appointment Using the Find Button

1. Pull patient Barbara Watson into context.

2. Click the *Scheduling* module. Harris CareTracker PM displays the *Book* application.

3. Click the *Find* button in the top left corner of the *Book* application. Harris CareTracker PM displays the *Appointment Criteria* window (**Figure 4-6**).

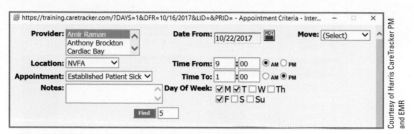

Figure 4-6   *Appointment Criteria Window*

4. Select the parameters of the appointment:

   a. *Provider* (Amir Raman)

   b. *Location* (NVFA)

   c. *Appointment* type (Established Patient Sick)

   d. *Date From* (select first available appointment next week, using the calendar icon or by using *Move*)

   e. *Time From* (select 9:00AM)

   f. *Time To* (select 1:00PM)

   g. *Day of Week* (place check mark by M, T, F only)

 TIP You can select multiple providers by holding down the [Ctrl] key on your keyboard while clicking on each provider name.

---

5. *Find* will default to display the first 20 appointments that match the search criteria. Change the number to "5" and click *Find* (see **Figure 4-6**).

6. To select an available appointment, click in the *Appointment/Task Class* column or anywhere on the row that corresponds to the desired date and time for that particular appointment. Harris CareTracker PM re-displays the *Book* application for the selected appointment date, highlighting the selected time in red (**Figure 4-7**).

7. Click the selected time slot. The application displays the *Book Appointment* window.

8. Select the *Appointment Type* (Established Patient Sick). When you select an *Appointment Type*, the application automatically populates the *Resource, Task,* and *Duration* fields.

9. Enter the *Complaint* by entering the free text description (Fever 103F).

10. From the *Location* list, select the location "NVFA."

11. From the *Pos* list, select the place of service (OFFICE).

12. Click *Save*. The application schedules the appointment (**Figure 4-8**).

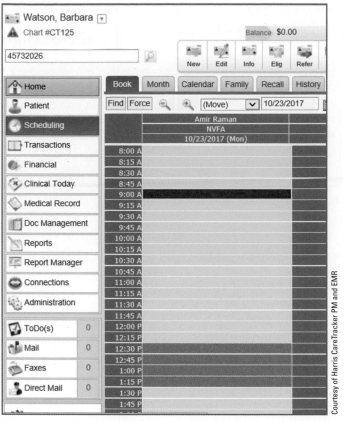

Figure 4-7   Find Appointment—Red Highlight

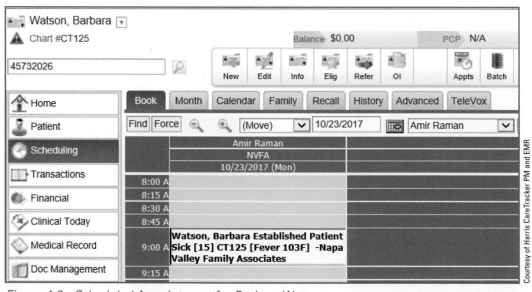

Figure 4-8   Scheduled Appointment for Barbara Watson

⊡ **Print the Booked Appointment screen, label it "Activity 4-2," and place it in your assignment folder.**

Forcing an Appointment

Using *Force* allows you to double-book appointments and to book an appointment during a different appointment-type time slot. You can also double-book appointments by left-clicking on the appointment time slot from the drop-down mini-menu. *Forced* appointments appear outlined in blue on the schedule. Using the patient in **Table 4-4,** force an appointment at the same time slot as the previous patient in Activity 4-2, Barbara Watson.

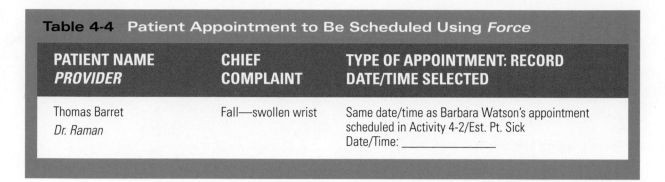

Table 4-4   Patient Appointment to Be Scheduled Using *Force*

PATIENT NAME *PROVIDER*	CHIEF COMPLAINT	TYPE OF APPOINTMENT: RECORD DATE/TIME SELECTED
Thomas Barret *Dr. Raman*	Fall—swollen wrist	Same date/time as Barbara Watson's appointment scheduled in Activity 4-2/Est. Pt. Sick Date/Time: _____

Activity 4-3
Book an Appointment Using the Force Button

1. Before you start, refer back to the appointment you just booked for Barbara Watson in Activity 4-2. You will need the date and time of the appointment to complete this activity. Once you have that information in hand, continue with step 2.

2. Pull patient Thomas Barret into context.

3. Click the *Scheduling* module. Harris CareTracker PM displays the *Book* application.

4. Click the *Force* button in the top left corner of the *Book* application. Harris CareTracker PM displays the *Book Appointment* window.

5. From the *Appointment Type* list, select the appointment type "Established Patient Sick." When you select an appointment type, Harris CareTracker PM automatically populates the *Task* and *Duration* fields (**Figure 4-9**).

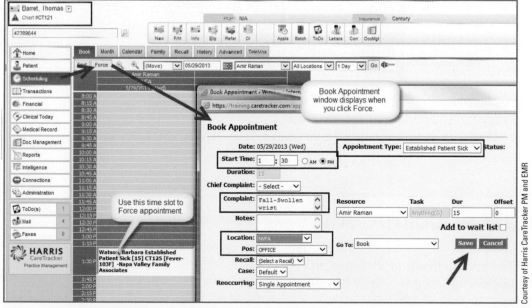

Figure 4-9   Force Appointment for Thomas Barret

6. From the *Resource* list, select the resource needed for the appointment (Dr. Raman).

7. In the *Start Time* field, enter the start time for the appointment. (Use the same date and time as for the patient booked in Activity 4-2, Barbara Watson.)

8. Enter *Complaint* by entering free text (Fall – swollen wrist).

9. From the *Location* list, select "NVFA."

10. From the *Pos* list, select "OFFICE."

11. Click *Save.* The application schedules the appointment (**Figure 4-10**).

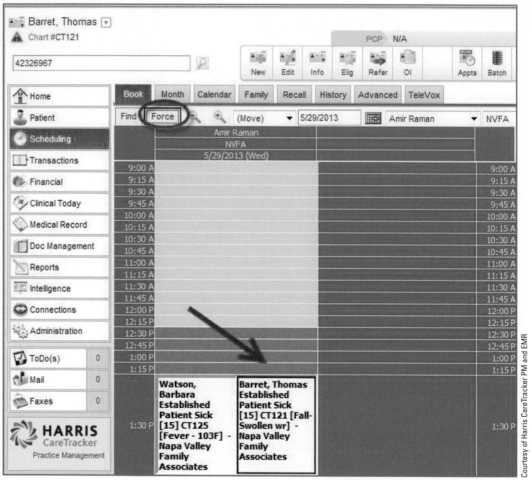

Figure 4-10   Scheduled Appointment Using Force for Thomas Barret

🖨 **Print the Booked Appointment using Force screen, label it "Activity 4-3," and place it in your assignment folder.**

Reschedule Appointments

There are two ways to reschedule patient appointments in the *Book* application: either directly from the schedule or by using the *Find* button. In either instance, the patient needs to be in context so the existing appointments will display. Harris CareTracker PM and EMR saves the rescheduled appointment in the *History* application in the *Scheduling* module.

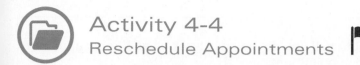

Activity 4-4
Reschedule Appointments

Reschedule an appointment to the following day:

1. Before you start, begin by booking an appointment for patient Galah Piccerelli approximately two weeks from today using the following information (refer to Activity 4-1 if you need help):

   a. *Appointment Type*: Follow up

   b. *Complaint*: Follow up labs

   c. *Resource*: Amir Raman

2. When finished scheduling the appointment in Step 1, with the patient in context, click the *Scheduling* module. The application displays the *Book* application by default.

3. From the date of Galah's current appointment, *Move* to "Next Day," same provider, and same location (**Figure 4-11**).

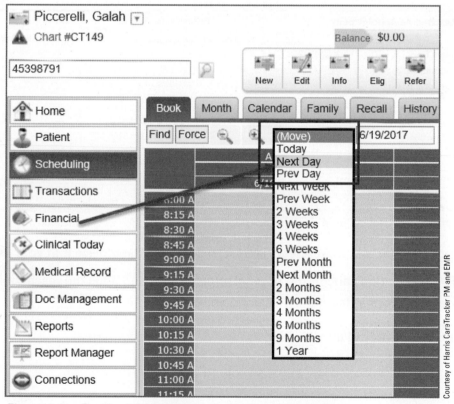

Figure 4-11   *Reschedule Appointment for Galah Piccerelli*

4. Click on the time slot in which you want to reschedule the appointment (same time slot as previous appointment). The application displays the patient's existing appointment(s) (**Figure 4-12**). (**Note:** You cannot reschedule an appointment that has an encounter created or that has already passed.)

5. From the *Action* list, select "Reschedule" and then click *Go*. The application displays the *Reschedule Appointment* window.

> **TIP** Do not click the *Book Appointment* button. If you do, you will book an additional appointment instead of rescheduling the existing appointment.

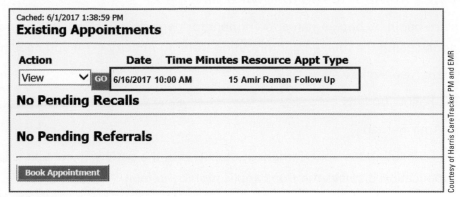

Figure 4-12 Existing Appointments Window

6. From the *Reschedule* list, (*Select a Reason*) for rescheduling the appointment (Figure 4-13). (Select "Entry Error.")

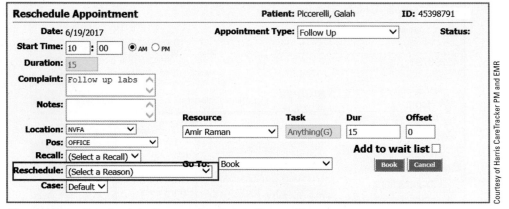

Figure 4-13 Reschedule Reason for Galah Piccerelli

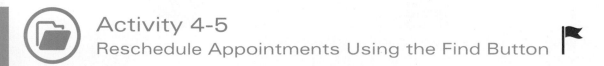 **Print the Rescheduled Appointment screen, label it "Activity 4-4," and place it in your assignment folder.**

7. Click *Book*. The application cancels the original appointment and adds the rescheduled appointment to the calendar. Record the date/time of Galah's appointment here: _____.

As mentioned, the *Find* button can also be used to reschedule an appointment.

Activity 4-5
Reschedule Appointments Using the Find Button ⚑

Using Galah Piccerelli, reschedule the appointment from Activity 4-4 using the *Find* button.

> **ALERT!** If Galah's appointment date has already passed, you will need to first enter a new appointment for the patient scheduled out one week from today, as appointment dates that have already passed cannot be rescheduled.

1. With patient Galah Piccerelli in context, click the *Scheduling* module. Harris CareTracker PM displays the *Book* application by default.

2. Click *Find* in the top left corner of the *Book* application. Harris CareTracker PM displays the *Appointment Criteria* window. Select the search parameters for the appointment you want to find. Select the same provider, location, and appointment type as the patient's original appointment (from Activity 4-4). Change the *Date From* to three (3) weeks from today; leave the *Time From*, *Time To*, and *Day of Week* as is.

3. Click *Find* (**Figure 4-14**). Harris CareTracker PM displays the *Search Results* window containing the first 20 appointments that match the search criteria.

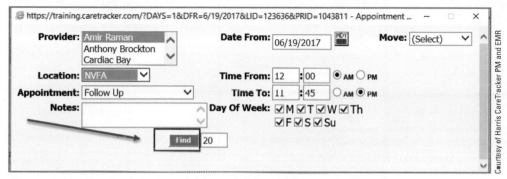

Figure 4-14   *Reschedule Appointment for Galah Piccerelli Using Find*

4. Click on an appointment in the *Appointment\Task Class* column to select it. (Select any time slot for the next available day.) The application then displays the selected appointment in the *Book* application.

5. A red bar on the schedule marks the available appointment time you selected from the *Search Results* list. Click on the red bar in the selected time slot. Harris CareTracker PM displays the patient's existing appointment(s) (**Figure 4-15**).

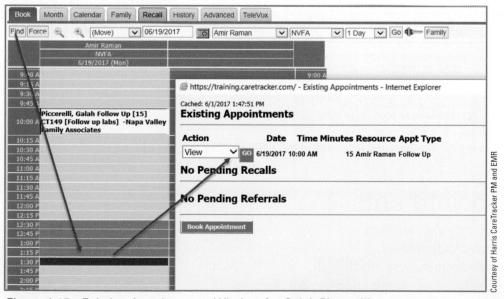

Figure 4-15   *Existing Appointments Window for Galah Piccerelli*

6. From the *Action list* select "Reschedule" and then click *Go.* The application displays the *Reschedule Appointment* window. Do <u>not</u> click the *Book Appointment* button. If you do, you will book an additional appointment instead of rescheduling the existing appointment.

7. From the *Reschedule* list, select a reason for rescheduling the appointment (**Figure 4-16**). (Select "Entry Error.")

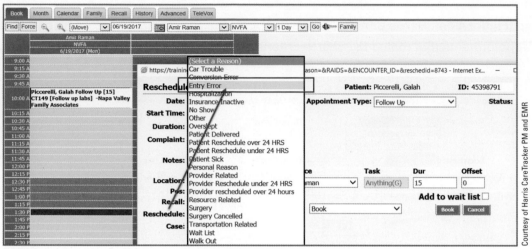

Figure 4-16   Reschedule Reason for Galah Piccerelli

🖨 **Print the Rescheduled Appointment screen, label it "Activity 4-5," and place it in your assignment folder.**

8. Click *Book*. Harris CareTracker PM cancels the original appointment and adds the rescheduled appointment to the calendar (**Figure 4-17**). Record the date/time of Galah's appointment here: _____ .

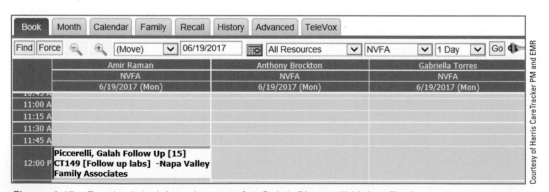

Figure 4-17   Rescheduled Appointment for Galah Piccerelli Using Find

Cancel Appointments

Upcoming appointments are canceled in the *History* application. You can click on the appointment you wish to cancel and select *View Appointment*, and then cancel it from the *Appointment Detail* window that appears. If the patient's canceled appointment was attached to a recall, the recall will become active again once the appointment is canceled. You can also click on the appointment you wish to cancel and select *View Appointment*, and then cancel it from the *Appointment Detail Window* that appears.

Activity 4-6
Cancel Appointments

Using the appointment you scheduled for Thomas Barret in Activity 4-3, cancel the appointment in the *History* application.

1. Pull the patient for whom you are canceling an appointment into context (Thomas Barret).

2. Click the *Scheduling* module and then click the *History* tab (**Figure 4-18**).

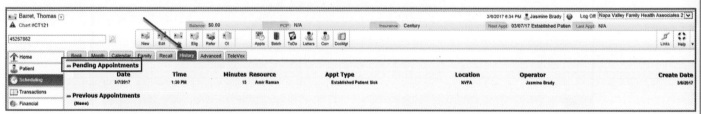

Figure 4-18   *History Tab in Scheduling Module*   Courtesy of Harris CareTracker PM and EMR

3. Under the *Pending Appointments* heading, click on the appointment you want to cancel (the appointment scheduled in Activity 4-3). Harris CareTracker PM displays the *Appointment Detail* window (**Figure 4-19**).

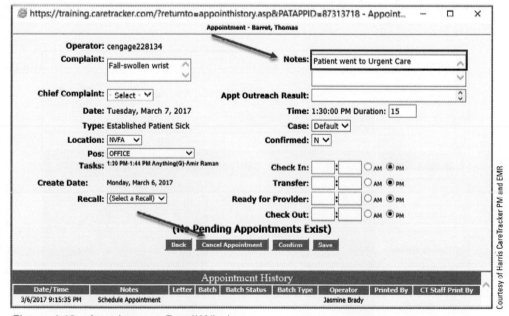

Figure 4-19   *Appointment Detail Window*

4. Enter a note regarding the canceled appointment in the *Notes* box. (Free text note: "Patient went to Urgent Care.")

5. Click the *Cancel Appointment* button.

6. From the *Cancel Reason* list, select the reason for canceling the appointment (**Figure 4-20**). (Select "Hospitalization.")

> **TIP** A note saved in a canceled appointment will always be linked to that cancellation and appears in the *History* application.

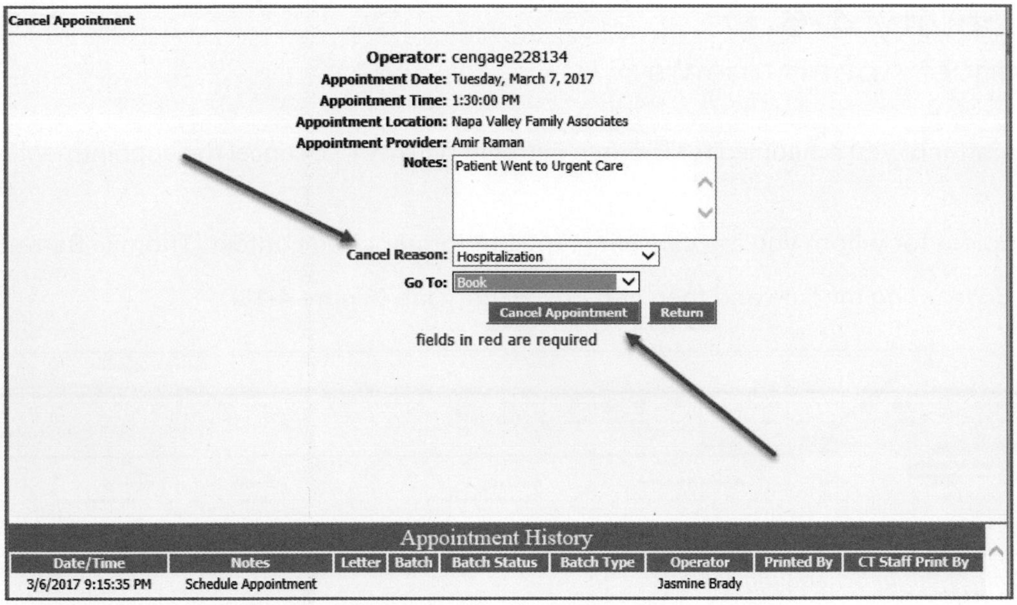

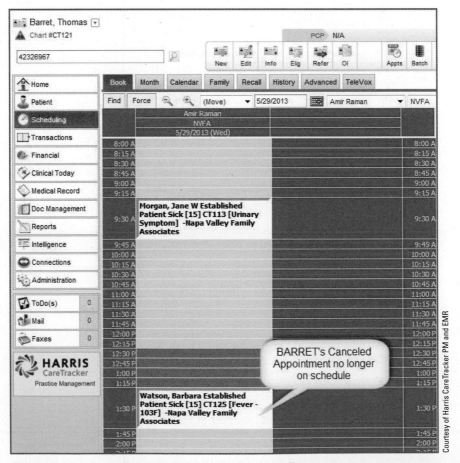

Figure 4-20   Cancel Appointment Window

7. The *Go To* field defaults to "(Select)." From the drop-down menu you can select an application so that when the appointment is canceled, Harris CareTracker PM opens that application. (Select "Book.")

8. Click *Cancel Appointment*. Harris CareTracker PM cancels the appointment and removes it from the schedule (**Figure 4-21**).

Figure 4-21   Canceled Appointment for Thomas Barret

📰 **Print the Canceled Appointment screen, label it "Activity 4-6," and place it in your assignment folder.**

Appointment Conflicts

Other reasons to cancel or reschedule an appointment occur when there is an appointment conflict. Appointment conflicts occur if an appointment is forced or booked into an unavailable time slot, booked at a location where the provider is not scheduled, or if the provider changes his or her schedule. Appointments remain in conflict until they are canceled or rescheduled. The steps to cancel an appointment due to conflict are slightly different than a cancellation by a patient. To view appointment conflicts, click the *Home* module and the *Practice* dashboard. Under *Front Office > Appointments*, click *Appointment Conflicts*. By default, Harris CareTracker PM displays any appointment availability conflicts for all providers at every location with scheduled appointments for the next 30 days. If needed, you can use the filters to select a specific conflict type, time period, provider, or location, and then click *Go*. Harris CareTracker PM displays a list of conflicted appointments. Currently, you should have no appointment conflicts.

NON-PATIENT APPOINTMENTS

Learning Objective 2: Schedule non-patient appointments.

Non-patient appointments, such as meetings or out-of-office times (i.e., provider vacation or training), are scheduled in the *Book* application of the *Scheduling* module. You can book a non-patient appointment with or without a patient in context on the *Name Bar*. A non-patient appointment can be scheduled for multiple providers at one time. However, you cannot search non-patient appointment availability using the *Find* button or the *Advanced* application.

Activity 4-7
Booking a Non-Patient Appointment with No Patient in Context

1. Using the drop-down, select "None" from the *Name* list on the *Name Bar* so that there is no patient in context (**Figure 4-22**).

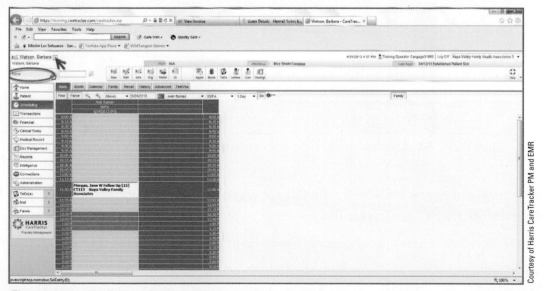

Figure 4-22   No Patient in Context

Courtesy of Harris CareTracker PM and EMR

2. Click the *Scheduling* module. Harris CareTracker PM opens the *Book* application by default.

3. Select "Next Month" (**Figure 4-23**). To display the desired date, use one of the following options:

   a. Select an option from the *Move* list to display the schedule for specific time increments such as Next Day, Next Week, 2 Months, and so on. (Select "Next Month" or do the following.)

   b. Manually enter a date in MM/DD/YYYY format or click the *Calendar* icon 📅 to display the schedule for a specific date.

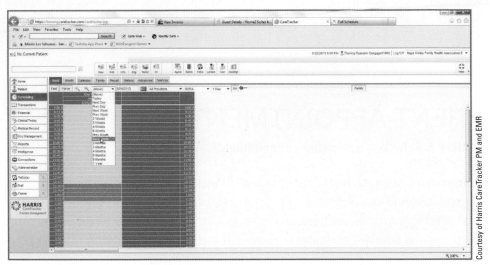

Figure 4-23   Move Schedule to Next Month

4. Select the resources (All Resources), location (All Locations), and the number of days (1 Day) to display and then click *Go* (**Figure 4-24**). If not all providers are showing, move the schedule to the next day until all four provider schedules display.

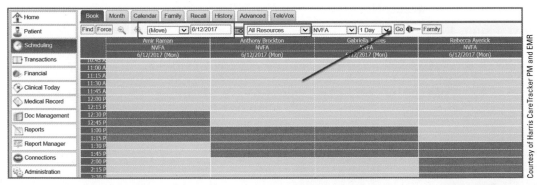

Figure 4-24   Set Schedule for Non-Patient Appointment

5. Click on the time slot in any provider's schedule for which you are booking the appointment (select the 1:00 PM time slot). Harris CareTracker PM displays the *Non-Patient Appointment* window.

6. In the *Description* field, enter a brief description of the appointment. (Enter "Monthly Providers Meeting.")

7. In the *Notes* field, enter any additional information about the appointment. (Enter "Guest Speaker, Cardiology Group.")

8. In the *Resources* field, click on the resource needed for the appointment. You can select multiple resources by holding down the [Ctrl] key on your keyboard and clicking on each resource (select all providers: Amir Raman, Anthony Brockton, Gabriella Torres, and Rebecca Ayerick). If you select *All*, you will include all resources such as lab, cardiac bay, and so on.

9. The *Location, Date,* and *Time* fields are automatically populated.

10. The *Duration* defaults to 30 minutes but you can change the duration as needed (change to 60 minutes) (Figure 4-25).

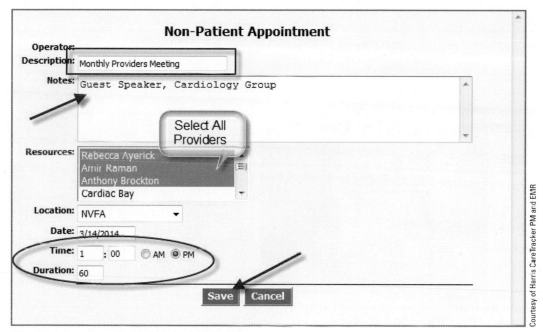

Figure 4-25   Non-Patient Appointment Window

11. Click *Save.* The application schedules the appointment for all of the selected resources.

📧 **Print the Book screen with the non-patient appointment scheduled, label it "Activity 4-7," and place it in your assignment folder.**

ADD PATIENT TO THE WAIT LIST

Learning Objective 3: Add a patient to the Wait List.

Patients who would like an appointment with a provider sooner than their currently scheduled appointment can be added to the *Wait List* in Harris CareTracker PM and EMR. A patient must have a currently scheduled appointment in Harris CareTracker PM and EMR to be added to the *Wait List*.

When adding a patient to the *Wait List*, you must provide information about the appointment the patient needs, such as the appointment type, provider, and location. Harris CareTracker PM and EMR will only flag available appointments that match the appointment criteria selected for the patient.

There are several places you can add a patient to the *Wait List* in Harris CareTracker PM and EMR:

- From the scheduling mini-menu in the *Book* application (see **Figure 4-26** and Activity 4-8)

- From the *Book Appointment* window in the *Book* application (**Figure 4-27**)

- From the *Appointments* tab in *Clinical Today, Actions* menu in the *Appointment List* (**Figure 4-28**)

The *Wait List* is managed in the *Wait List* application accessed from the *Wait List* link under the *Appointment* section of the *Dashboard* (**Figure 4-29**). The *Wait List* identifies any patient on the *Wait List* and any available appointments that match the appointment criteria. From the *Wait List*, you can reschedule a patient's appointment or remove the patient from the *Wait List* after his or her scheduled appointment date has passed.

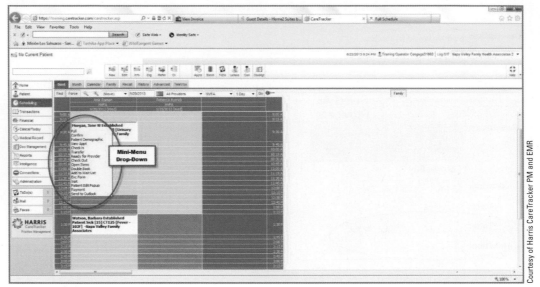

Figure 4-26   Scheduling Mini-Menu

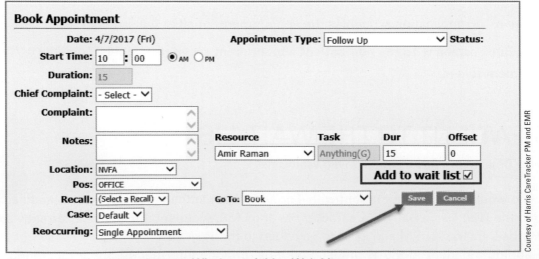

Figure 4-27   Book Appointment Window—Add to Wait List

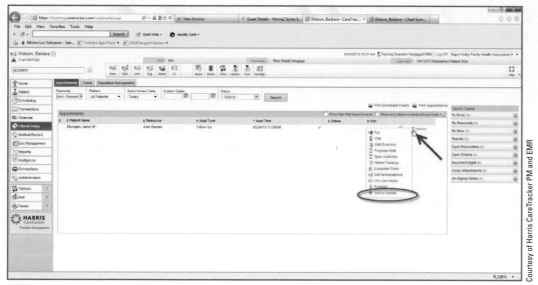

Figure 4-28   Appointments tab in Clinical Today, *Appointments Actions Drop-Down*

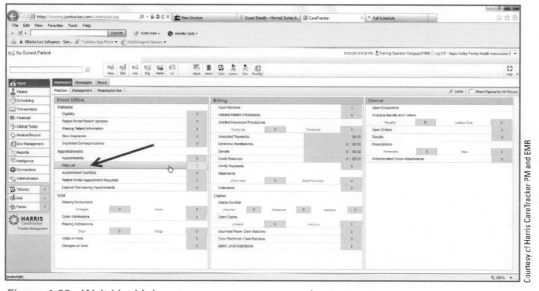

Figure 4-29   *Wait List Link*

Mini-Menu

When you left-click on a patient's name in the schedule, Harris CareTracker PM displays a convenient mini-menu (**Figure 4-26**) that contains a list of shortcuts. From this menu you can access several applications in Harris CareTracker PM and EMR that help create a more efficient workflow.

After you left-click on a patient's name, the mini-menu displays on the screen for only eight seconds. If the mini-menu disappears before you make your selection, left-click on the patient's name again.

SPOTLIGHT   In the *Scheduling* module, *VIP* patient appointments are visible to all operators, but an operator cannot use the scheduling mini-menu for a *VIP* patient unless the operator's profile contains either the "VIP Patient Access" or the "VIP Patient Access Break Glass" override.

Activity 4-8
Add Patient to the Wait List from the Mini-Menu

1. Before beginning this activity, refer back to the appointment date and time you scheduled for Galah Piccerelli in Activity 4-5. You will need this information on hand to complete this activity; then proceed to step 2.

> **(!) ALERT!** If Galah's appointment date has already passed, you will need to first enter a new appointment for the patient scheduled out one week from today, as appointment dates that have already passed cannot be wait listed.

2. Click the *Scheduling* module. Harris CareTracker PM displays the *Book* application by default.

3. *Move* the schedule to display the appointment for the patient you want to add to the wait list (select the appointment you created for Galah Piccerelli in Activity 4-5). This can be done by manually entering the date in the *Date* box by clicking the *Calendar* 🔲 icon, or by selecting a time period from the *Move* list.

4. Left-click on the appointment and select *Add to Wait List* from the mini-menu. The application displays the *Appointment Wait List* window (**Figure 4-30**).

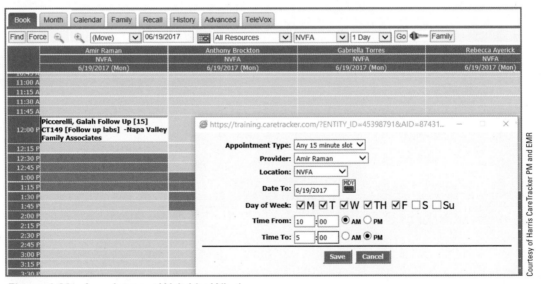

Figure 4-30   Appointment Wait List Window

5. From the *Appointment Type* list, select the type of appointment the patient needs or select "Any 15 minute slot" to book the first available appointment type. (Select "Any 15 minute slot.")

6. From the *Provider* list, select the provider the patient wants to see (select Amir Raman). You would select "Any Provider" to book the first available provider.

7. From the *Location* list, select the location where the patient wants to be seen. (Select "NVFA.")

8. In the *Date To* field, click the *Calendar* MDY icon and select the last date before which the appointment must fall. Select the day the appointment was scheduled for patient Galah Piccerelli in Activity 4-5.

9. In the *Day of Week* field, select the checkbox next to each day the patient is available for an appointment (select Monday through Friday, unchecking the other days).

10. In the *Time From* and *Time To* fields, select the desired time for the appointment. (Select "10:00 AM" through "5:00 PM.")

11. Click *Save.* The application adds the patient to the *Wait List.* (The *Wait List* is managed from the *Wait List* link in the *Front Office* section of the *Dashboard,* under *Appointments.*)

12. Return to the *Dashboard* (*Home* module) and click on the *Wait List* link (under the *Appointments* header) (see **Figure 4-29**).

13. Select *Resource* (Amir Raman).

14. Review the *Date From* and *Date To* displayed. Enter today's date in the *Date From* field. Enter a date approximately four weeks from today in the *Date To* field.

15. Then click *Go.*

16. The wait-listed appointment will appear with a *Possible Match* (**Figure 4-31**). **Note**: A possible match will not display if there are no dates that meet the specified criteria.

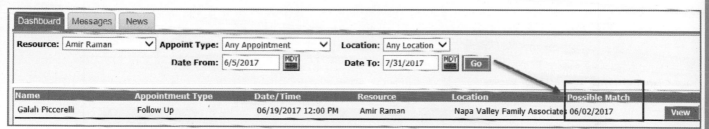

Figure 4-31   Wait List Dashboard Display

Courtesy of Harris CareTracker PM and EMR

🖨 **Print the Patient Wait List screen, label it "Activity 4-8," and place it in your assignment folder.**

DAILY SCHEDULE

Learning Objective 4: Perform activities managing the daily schedule.

Now that you have completed the *Book* activities, you can further manage the daily schedule using the other seven applications in the *Scheduling* module: *Month, Calendar, Family, Recall, History, Advanced,* and *TeleVox®.*

Month Application

The *Month* application displays at a glance the number of appointments scheduled for each day of a particular month and for a particular resource. This is a useful application for quickly viewing the number of scheduled appointments. You can choose the month, resource, and location for which to view the *Month* calendar, or you can choose to view the month's scheduled appointments as a bar chart.

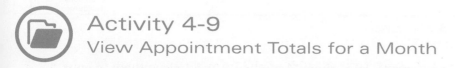

Activity 4-9
View Appointment Totals for a Month

1. Click the *Scheduling* module. Harris CareTracker PM opens the *Book* application by default. This can be done with or without a patient in context.

2. Click the *Month* tab. Harris CareTracker PM displays the *Month* application.

3. Select the month. (Choose the month you have entered appointments for in this chapter.)

4. Select a *Resource* for which to view appointments. (Select "Amir Raman.")

5. The *Location* field defaults to "(Locations)," which displays appointment totals for all the resource locations. You can also select a specific location. (Select "NVFA.")

6. (Display Options): The default display is *Calendar* format. (You also have the option of selecting *Bar Chart*.)

   a. Click *Go*.

   b. Repeat the activity for both *Calendar* (**Figure 4-32**) and *Bar Chart* (**Figure 4-33**) display formats.

   c. Harris CareTracker PM displays the appointment totals for each day of the month.

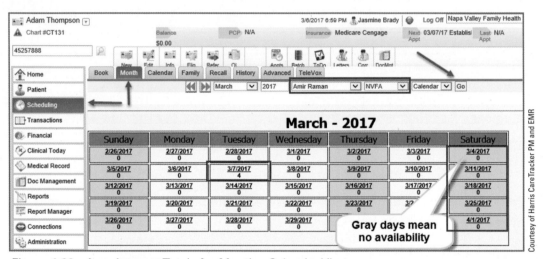

Figure 4-32   Appointment Totals for Month—Calendar View

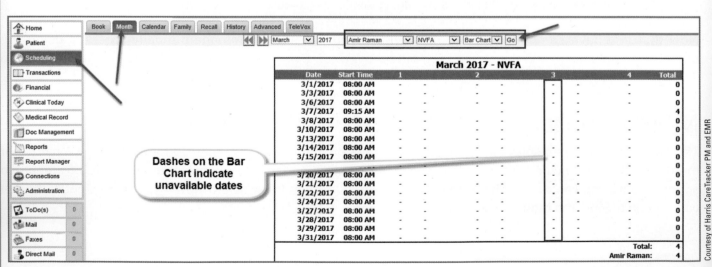

Figure 4-33   Appointment Totals for Month—Bar Chart View

💾 **Print both the Calendar and Bar Chart screens, label them "Activity 4-9," and place them in your assignment folder.**

Calendar Display

On the *Calendar* screen (in the *Month* tab), gray days represent days on which the provider has no availability at the location selected (see **Figure 4-32**). In the *Calendar* format, you can drill down into any day of the month by clicking on the *Date Link* for that day.

The *Calendar* application allows you to view appointments in the format of a small date book calendar. The *Date Book* is more concise than the schedule in the *Book* application but contains fewer appointment details. For each scheduled appointment, the *Calendar* shows the appointment time, the patient's name, his or her Harris CareTracker ID number, the appointment type, duration, and any saved patient complaint. *Calendars* can be generated for multiple providers for either one day or one week.

Bar Chart Display.

Unavailable days on the *Bar Chart* (in the *Month* application) are indicated with dashes rather than the name of the resource. You cannot access the schedule from the *Bar Chart* format (see **Figure 4-33**).

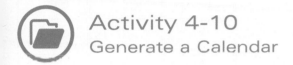

Activity 4-10
Generate a Calendar

1. Before beginning this activity, refer back to the appointments you scheduled in Activity 4-1. You will need the date of the appointments scheduled in hand before moving to step 2.

2. Click the *Scheduling* module. Harris CareTracker PM opens the *Book* application by default.

3. Click the *Calendar* tab. Harris CareTracker PM displays the *Calendar* application.

4. In the *Date* field, enter the date in MM/DD/YYYY format for which you want to generate a calendar (select the date for the appointments you scheduled in Activity 4-1) or click the *Calendar* MDY icon and select the date.

5. From the *Display* list, select either a one day or one week calendar. (Select "1 week.")

6. In the *Resource* field, select the resources(s) for which you want to generate a calendar. (Select "All.")

7. By default, the appointment information will display in multiple lines. Select the *1 Line* checkbox to display the appointment information in a single line.

8. From the *Location* list, select the location for which you want to generate a calendar. (Select "All.") (**Figure 4-34**).

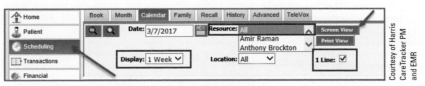

Figure 4-34   Generate Calendar—Screen View

Courtesy of Harris CareTracker PM and EMR

9. To view the calendar on the screen, click *Screen View* (see **Figure 4-34**). Harris CareTracker PM displays the calendar (**Figure 4-35**).

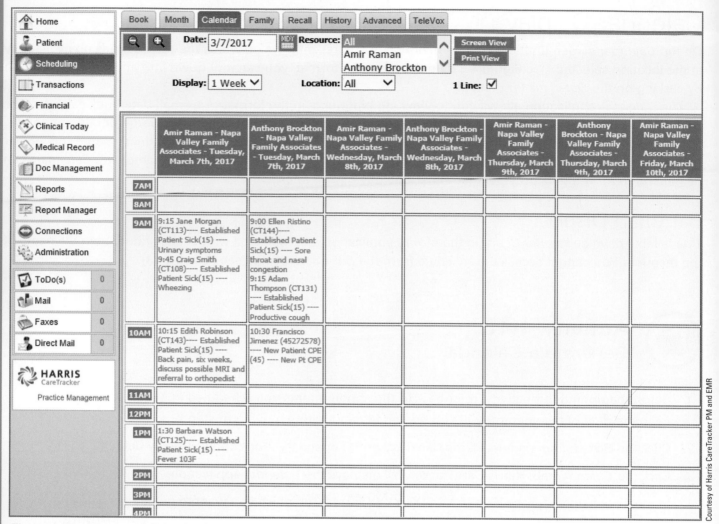

Figure 4-35 *Generated Calendar for All Providers*

Courtesy of Harris CareTracker PM and EMR

10. To *Print* the calendar:

    a. Click *Print View*. Harris CareTracker PM displays the calendar (**Figure 4-36**).

    b. Right-click on the calendar and select *Print* from the shortcut menu (**Figure 4-37**).

Figure 4-36 *Generate Calendar—Print View*

Courtesy of Harris CareTracker PM and EMR

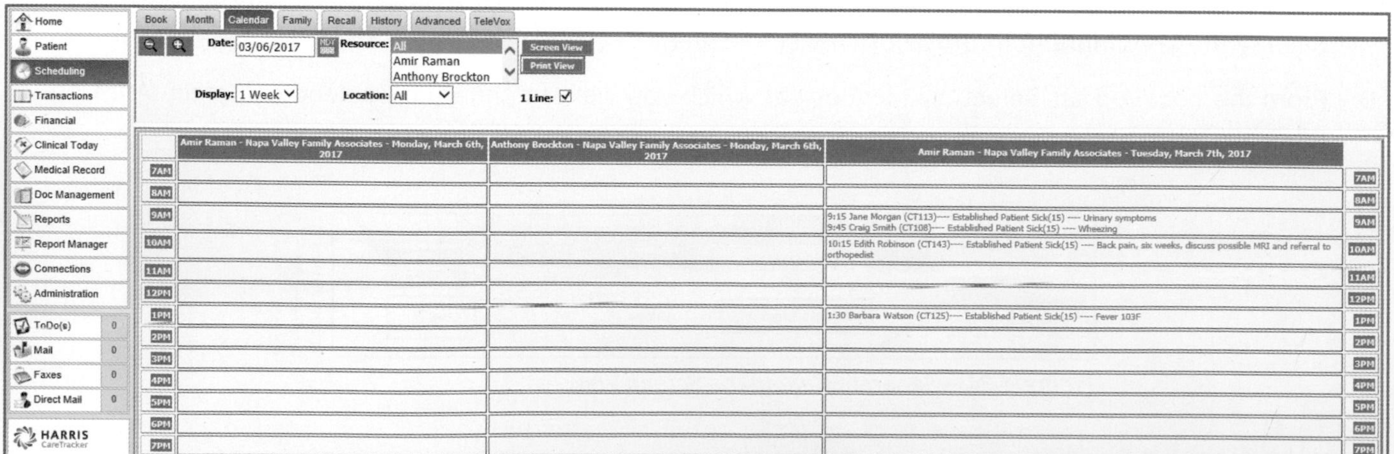

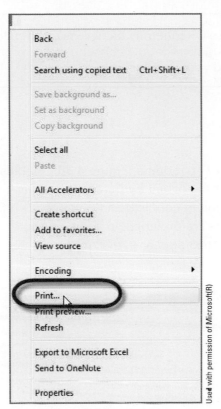

Figure 4-37   Right-Click to Print

💾 **Print the Calendar screen, label it "Activity 4-10," and place it in your assignment folder.**

Family

When multiple family members see the same provider, it is common for them to request appointments on the same day. The *Family* tab in the *Scheduling* module lists all upcoming appointments for family members as well as for the patient in context. With a patient in context, you can access the *Book* application from the *Family* tab by clicking on the appointment line.

The *Family* application is used to store the patient's family information and emergency contacts and link the patient's family members. This is especially useful in family billing situations, such as a pediatric practice, because multiple patients can be linked to one responsible party. When a common responsible party is indicated, Harris CareTracker PM and EMR generates one statement for all the patients linked to the responsible party. In addition, when in the *Scheduling* module, you can view upcoming appointments for all family members that are linked together.

In Activity 3-4, you successfully linked new patient Francisco Powell Jimenez with his father, Frank Powell. In Activity 4-1, you created an appointment for Francisco. Because family members are linked in the system, you can see his appointment by pulling his father Frank into context, clicking the *Scheduling* module, and clicking the *Family* tab.

Deleting and Editing Family Members.

At times it may be necessary to delete or edit a family member from a patient's record. To delete a family member, you would select the checkbox in the *Delete* column next to the family member you want to remove and then click *Update*. To edit a family member, click the *Edit* button next to the family member you want to edit.

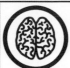

CRITICAL THINKING   List times when it may be necessary to delete or edit a family member from a patient's record and why. Explain what the consequences might be for not deleting or editing the record and how you reached your conclusion.

Advanced

The *Advanced* application in the *Scheduling* module (**Figure 4-38**) enables you to book appointments in accordance with predetermined parameters established by the practice. The *Advanced* method of booking appointments prevents overbooking and scheduling conflicts and helps to maintain consistency in terms of the days and times when services and procedures are provided. In addition, the existing appointments, pending recalls, and active referrals for the patient in context appear in the *Advanced* screen.

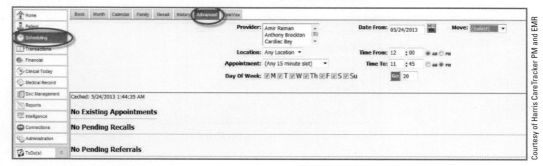

Figure 4-38   Advanced Application in the Scheduling Module

The use of the *Advanced* application is recommended if your practice books **multi-resource appointments**. A multi-resource appointment is an appointment that requires two or more resources. For example, if a patient is to be seen by a provider but also needs an ultrasound at the same visit, the *Advanced* application allows you to book one appointment for both resources.

You can also reschedule and cancel existing patient appointments in the *Advanced* application. When you reschedule an appointment in the *Advanced* application, you can search future appointment availability and be assured that you are rescheduling the appointment with the same criteria as the original appointment. If necessary, additional appointment search parameters can be added or removed from the *Advanced* fields. Canceling an appointment from the *Advanced* application functions the same way as when canceling an appointment from *Book*. Before you are allowed to cancel an existing appointment, you are required to select a reason for the cancellation. Any scheduled, rescheduled, or canceled appointment made in the *Advanced* application is saved in the patient's record and can be viewed in the *History* application of the *Scheduling* module.

Recalls

Recalls are reminders to patients that an appointment needs to be booked. Rather than scheduling a future appointment, a recall (reminder) date is set for the appointment. You can generate patient recall letters for any recall tracked in Harris CareTracker PM and EMR.

You can manually link an appointment to recalls when booking the appointment. In the case where a recall already exists, and a patient schedules an appointment for the same type as the existing recall, this recall will also be linked to the appointment. After a recall is linked to an appointment, it becomes inactive rather than open, but should the patient cancel the appointment, the recall becomes open again.

TIP You can access the *Recalls* application from one of the following locations:

1. *Scheduling* module > *Recall* tab

2. *Medical Record* module > *Recall* link on the *Clinical Toolbar* (Figure 4-39)

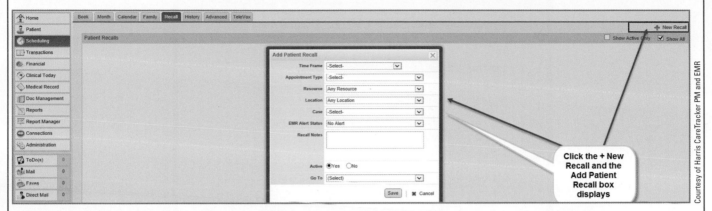

Figure 4-39   *Patient Recalls in the Visit Window via Recalls Link*

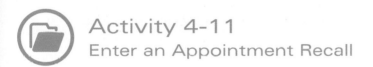

Activity 4-11
Enter an Appointment Recall

1. Pull patient Edith Robinson into context.

2. Click the *Scheduling* module and then click the *Recall* tab.

3. Click *+ New Recall*. Harris CareTracker PM displays the *Add Patient Recall* box (see **Figure 4-40**).

4. Select the time frame for the recall from the *Time Frame* list (select "1 Year"). When Days, Weeks, Months, or Years is selected, you must also enter a numeric value to correspond to the selected time unit.

5. Select the type of appointment from the *Appointment Type* list. (Select "Lab.")

6. Select the provider from the *Resource* list. (Select "Amir Raman.")

7. Select the location from the *Location* list. (Select "Napa Valley Family Associates.")

8. If the recall appointment needs to be linked to a case, select the appropriate case from the *Case* list (not applicable here).

9. Select an alert type from the *EMR Alert Status* list. (Select "Soft Alert.")

10. Enter a note about the recall in the *Recall Notes* field. (Free text note: "Annual CPE Labs.")

11. Leave the *Active* field "Yes."

12. Leave the *Go To* field as (Select).

13. Click *Save* (**Figure 4-40**).

14. When you receive the "Success" box, click on "X" to close.

Courtesy of Harris CareTracker PM and EMR

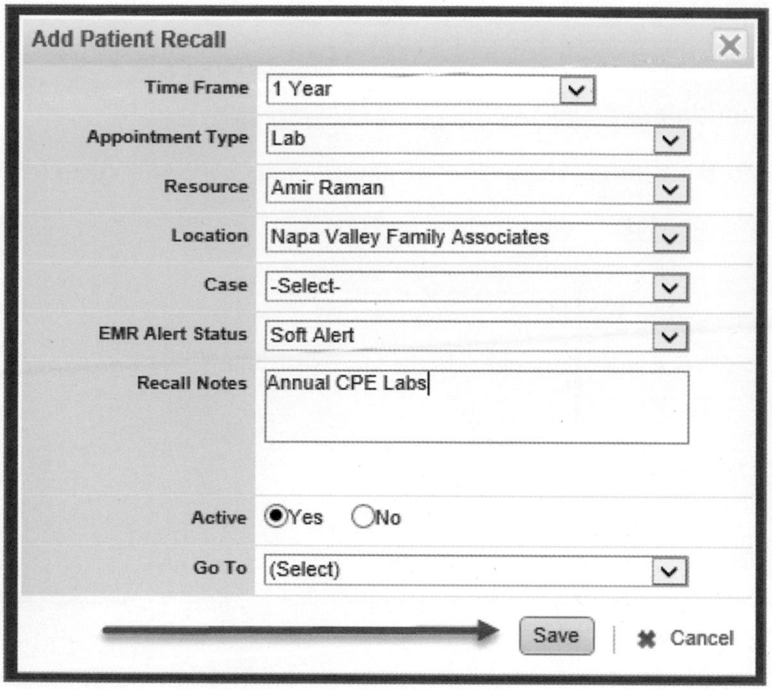

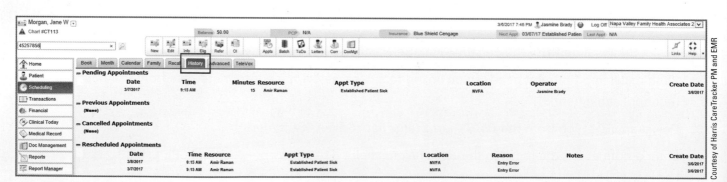

Figure 4-40 Entering an Appointment Recall

Print the Patient Recalls screen, label it "Activity 4-11," and place it in your assignment folder.

There are times when you need to inactivate an appointment recall. Conversely, there are times you may need to activate an appointment recall you had previously inactivated. You can practice this function in the end-of-chapter Proficiency Builders 4-1 and 4-2.

History

Harris CareTracker PM and EMR maintains a detailed history of all appointments, including those that are canceled or rescheduled, in the *History* tab of the *Scheduling* module. The *History* tab has four different sections: *Pending Appointments, Previous Appointments, Cancelled Appointments,* and *Rescheduled Appointments* (**Figure 4-41**).

Courtesy of Harris CareTracker PM and EMR

Figure 4-41 Appointment History

Pending appointments display from oldest to newest to keep them in chronological order. You can view the *Appointment Details* dialog box (date, time, location provider, etc.) by clicking on the *Appointment Line.* Upcoming appointments are canceled in the *History* application. If the patient's canceled appointment was attached to a recall, the recall will become active again once the appointment is canceled.

TeleVox®

Missed appointments are a significant concern for medical practices. Not only is revenue lost for the missed appointment, but continuity of care may be compromised. In addition, missed appointments do not afford the opportunity for another patient to be seen in that time slot. Therefore, most practices have initiated some form of appointment reminder system. In Harris CareTracker, *TeleVox*® is an optional application of automated appointment reminder and confirmation system that can be used to notify patients of upcoming appointments. There are two main steps involved in using *TeleVox*®:

- Sending an electronic appointment list to *TeleVox*®
- Viewing the results of the automated calls made by *TeleVox*®

When the appointment list is received at *TeleVox*®, reminder phone calls are transmitted during calling hours that are chosen by your practice. If the reminder call does not go through to a patient, answering machine, or voice mail, *TeleVox*® continues to try and reach the patient.

You can review the *TeleVox*® results the day after the appointment list was sent. From the results list, you can either confirm or cancel patient appointments, depending on the result of the call. There are nine *TeleVox*® call results. The practice is only charged for calls that go through (any status except Called-No Answer and Invalid Phone Number). The practice will be charged a standard rate per successful call as stated in the contract.

It is important to know that multiple calls are restricted when using *TeleVox*®. This means that *TeleVox*® cannot call two people who have the same phone number and have an appointment on the same date of service (such as siblings, parent/child, spouses, etc.).

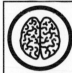 **CRITICAL THINKING**   Identify issues that a missed patient appointment causes for a medical practice. What steps can and should be taken to avoid missed appointments?

Appointment Reminder System

If a patient does not want to get a confirmation call from *TeleVox*®, you must update his or her demographic information on the *Patient Details* tab in the *Patient* module/*Demographics* tab by updating the patient's *Notification Preference* field to "Patient Refusal." You will remove a patient from the call list and change to Patient Portal notification in the end-of-chapter Proficiency Builder 4-3.

 TIP   A patient must be activated in the *Patient Portal* to receive *Patient Portal* email notifications.

Viewing *TeleVox*® Call Results.

As a best practice, you should review the call results list the day after you sent the appointment list to *TeleVox*®; however, your student version of Harris CareTracker is not enrolled in the *TeleVox*® feature so you will be unable to use this function.

CHECK IN PATIENTS

Learning Objective 5: Check in patients.

For a patient encounter to be generated in the electronic medical record (EMR), the patient must be checked in when he or she arrives for an appointment. Checking in a patient changes his or her Harris CareTracker PM and EMR status to "Checked in," and Harris CareTracker PM and EMR verifies that the patient's billing and demographic information is complete. Harris CareTracker PM and EMR will display the *Patient Alert* dialog box if the patient is missing important billing or demographic data.

 TIP *Patient Alerts* will only display if the *Show Alerts* feature is activated in your batch.

You can check in a patient in Harris CareTracker PM and EMR in the following places:

- In the *Book* application of the *Scheduling* module, using the mini-menu drop-down feature (see **Figure 4-42**)
- From the *Appts* button in the *Name Bar*
- From the *Appointments list* on the *Dashboard*
- From the *Appointments* tab in *Clinical Today*

 ## Activity 4-12
Check in Patient from the Mini-Menu

1. You will check in the following patients in this activity:

   a. Francisco Powell Jimenez (**Note:** This is the new patient you registered in Activity 3-4.)

   b. Craig X. Smith

   c. Jane Morgan

   d. Ellen Ristino

   e. Adam Thompson

   f. Edith Robinson

   g. Barbara Watson

   Before you begin this activity, refer back to the dates of the appointments you scheduled for each of them in Activities 4-1 and 4-2. If you did not record their appointment dates, pull the patient into context, click on the *Scheduling* module, and click on the *History* tab. All of the patient's appointments will be displayed. Once you have the patients' appointment dates in hand, continue to step 2.

2. Click the *Scheduling* module. Harris CareTracker PM opens the *Book* application by default.

3. With or without the patient in context, move the schedule to display the appointment for the patient you want to check in. This can be done by manually entering in the date in the *Date* box, by clicking the *Calendar* icon, or by selecting a time period from the *Move* list. Be sure that "All Resources" and "All Locations" display. If not, use the drop-down, change the parameters and click *Go*.

4. Left-click the name of the patient you want to check in and select *Check In* from the mini-menu (see **Figure 4-42**). Harris CareTracker PM and EMR changes the patient's status to "Checked In" and highlights the patient's appointment in green in both the *Book* application and the *Appointments* link in the *Front Office* section of the *Dashboard* (*Home* module). Checking in a patient from the mini-menu will pull the patient into context. **FYI:** Harris CareTracker PM and EMR records the check-in time and displays the patient's wait time in the *Appointments* link (**Figure 4-43**). For all the

patients to appear in the *Appointments* link, be sure to change the *Resource* to *All*, enter the date you want to check status for, and select *All* from the *Status* drop-down.

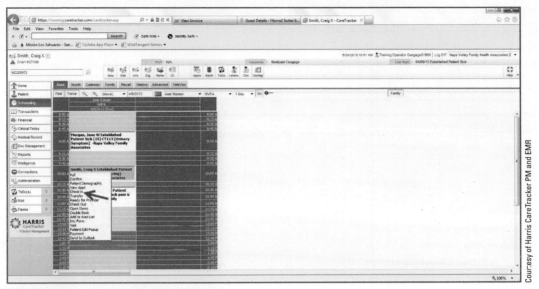

Figure 4-42   Mini-Menu Check-In

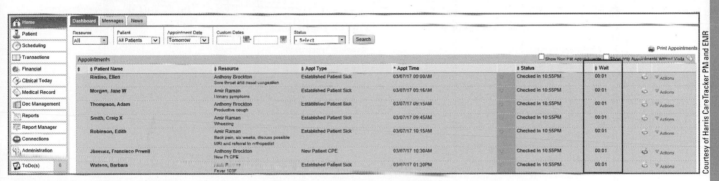

Figure 4-43   Check-in Wait Time Noted in the Dashboard, Appointments link.

5. Repeat steps 2 through 4 until you have all patients from step 1 checked in.

📖 Print the Schedule screen for each day that patients were checked in, label it/them "Activity 4-12," and place it/them in your assignment folder.

Harris CareTracker PM and EMR allows you to view the patient tracking log that tracks the progress of the patient's appointment. You can track the progress by logging an entry each time the patient's status changes and each time a patient is moved to a different location. The log displays a time stamp next to each activity and calculates the total time of the visit, beginning at check-in and ending at check-out. You can view the tracking log by following the steps outlined in your end-of-chapter Proficiency Builder 4-4.

CREATE A BATCH

Learning Objective 6: Create a batch, accept payments, print patient receipts, run a journal, and post the batch.

The *Batch* application is used for setting defaults for both "Financial" and "Clinical" components. The "Financial" portion of the **batch** establishes defaults and assigns a name to a batch (group) of financial transactions you will be entering into Harris CareTracker. A new financial batch is created daily to enter financial transactions into

Harris CareTracker; for example, charges, payments, and adjustments. This helps identify transactions linked to the batch, the date of each transaction, and the operator who entered it into the system. Setting up the financial batch helps identify a group of charges or payments and helps run reports to balance against the actual charges or payments entered.

The "Clinical" batch settings are typically set up only once and are used to set preferences and prepopulate fields common to your workflow (**Figure 4-44**). The "Clinical" batch settings are in the middle and lower sections of the *Operator Encounter Batch Control* dialog box. Setting the defaults here can speed up scheduling by having default *Resource* and *Location* defined.

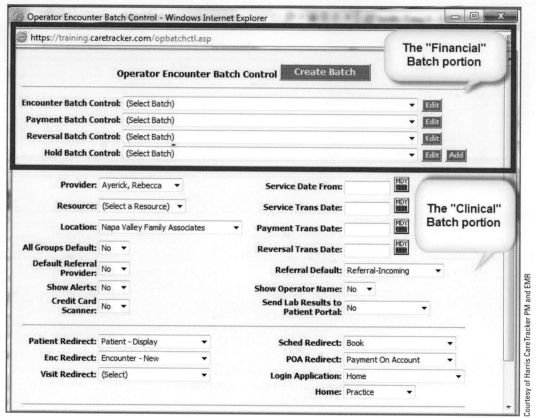

Figure 4-44   *Financial and Clinical Components of a Batch*

For this learning objective, you will create a batch, accept copays, and print a **receipt**. Once you have created your batch, you will run a journal to verify your batch information, click the link to view all open batches, and then post your batch (a later activity) into the system. Posting a batch permanently stores all financial transactions linked to it in Harris CareTracker. The application is updated in real time. Receipts in Harris CareTracker PM can identify a patient's previous balance, the activity of charges and payments for that date of service, and the new patient balance.

Setting Operator Preferences

The *Batch* application enables you to set up operator preferences based on the workflow for your role. This reduces the number of clicks required to get from one application to the other, making navigation through Harris CareTracker PM and EMR easy.

The first time you log in to Harris CareTracker you will be prompted to create a batch. Activities related to searching for a patient or scheduling a patient do not require that a batch be created and you may simply close out the batch prompt. For the activities related to financial and clinical workflows, you will need to have a batch open. You begin by setting your operator preferences (Activity 4-13).

The available batch redirects are described in **Table 4-5**. These are located in the lower section of the *Operator Encounter Batch Control* dialog box (**Figure 4-45**).

Table 4-5 Batch Redirects

REDIRECTS *FIELD*	DESCRIPTION
Patient Redirect	Launches the selected application after editing a *Demographic* record in the *Patient* module. You can also change this setting in the *Demographic* application if necessary.
Enc Redirect	Launches the selected application after saving a *Charge* in the *Transactions* module.
Visit Redirect	Launches the selected application after a visit is saved in the *Visit* application.
Sched Redirect	Launches the selected application after an appointment is booked via the *Book* application of the *Scheduling* module.
POA (Payment on Account) Redirect	Launches the selected application after a payment is entered via the *Payment on Account* application of the *Transaction* module.
Login Application	Launches the selected application when you log in to Harris CareTracker PM and EMR.
Home	If the *Log in Application* is set to "Home," you can select which *Home* module application to display by default. For example, the *Management, Meaningful Use, Messages,* or *News* applications.
When finished with redirects, click *Save*	Your screen will be saved with selections made.

Courtesy of Harris CareTracker PM and EMR

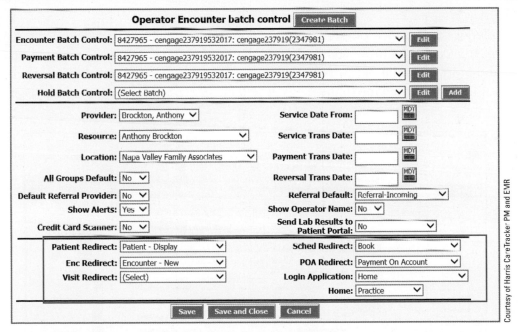

Figure 4-45 *Operator Encounter Batch Control*

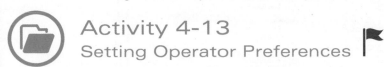

Activity 4-13
Setting Operator Preferences 🚩

1. With no patient in context, click on the *Batch* icon on the *Name Bar*. Harris CareTracker PM and EMR displays the *Operator Encounter Batch Control* dialog box.

2. If there is an open batch, by default the batch will display. Harris CareTracker PM and EMR assigns redirects, making it easy to navigate from different applications within Harris CareTracker PM and

EMR. The default redirects are based on the most commonly used workflow. Redirect means to change the path or direction; for example, changing a redirect allows the operator to select the most efficient workflow.

3. Click *Edit* if the fields are grayed out. Otherwise, enter (or confirm if already populated) the information for each of the fields in the *Operator Encounter Batch Control* dialog box (see **Figure 4-45**) as follows:

    a. Patient Redirect: (Select "Patient – Display")

    b. Enc Redirect: (Select "Encounter – New")

    c. Visit Redirect: (Select "Select")

    d. Sched Redirect: (Select "Book")

    e. POA (Payment on Account) Redirect: (Select "Payment on Account")

    f. Login Application: (Select "Home")

    g. Home: (Select "Practice")

4. Click *Save*. Screen will be saved with selections made.

5. Click *Close* to close out the batch control box.

💾 **Print the Operator Encounter Batch Control screen, label it "Activity 4-13," and place it in your assignment folder.**

A provider's paperless desk is incorporated in the *Clinical Today* module. Therefore, selecting the *Clinical* module from the *Login Application* list takes you directly to the *Clinical Today* module each time you log in to Harris CareTracker PM and EMR, streamlining workflow (**Figure 4-46**). When you begin clinical activities in Chapter 6, you will change your *Login Application* to the *Clinical* setting.

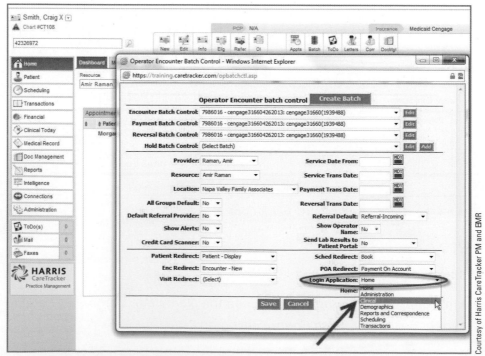

Figure 4-46   Login Application—Clinical

Table 4-6 outlines the fields and related instructions to complete your batch details. You will finish creating a batch in Activity 4-14, referencing instructions in **Table 4-6**. After entering the copayments as assigned in Activity 4-15, you will print a receipt (see Activity 4-16), run a journal (see Activity 4-18), and post your batch (see Activity 4-19). Posting a batch permanently stores all financial transactions linked to it in Harris CareTracker PM and EMR. The application is updated in real time.

Table 4-6 Batch Details Field and Instructions

BATCH DETAILS FIELD	INSTRUCTIONS
Provider	From the *Provider* list, select the name of the billing provider associated with the batch. **Note:** The *Admissions* application accessed via the *Dashboard* and the *Charges* application in the *Transaction* module display the billing provider set up in the batch.
Resource	From the *Resource* list, select the servicing provider. In most instances, the billing provider and the resource are the same. **Note:** The *Book* application in the *Scheduling* module and the *Appointment* application in the *Clinical Today* module display the resource set up in the batch.
Location	From the *Location* list, select the location associated with the batch. **Note:** The *Admissions* application accessed via the *Dashboard* and the *Book* application in the *Scheduling* module display the location set up in the batch.
All Groups Default	By default, the *All Groups Default* list is set to "No." Change the list to "Yes" if necessary. This displays patient financial information for the current group or all groups in the practice based on the setting selected. If *Yes* is selected, you can only see the financial transactions for the groups that you have access to as an operator. This setting mostly benefits multi-group practices and also determines the default value in the *Open Items* application of the *Financial* module and *Edit* application of the *Transactions* module.
Default Referral Provider	By default, the *Default Referral Provider* list is set to "No." Change the field to "Yes" if there is no referring provider in the patient's demographics or if there is no active referral/authorization for the patient. This sets the billing provider as the referring provider.
Show Alerts	In the *Show Alerts* field, select "Yes" to enable Harris CareTracker PM to display the *Patient Alert* window; otherwise select "No." The *Patient Alerts* window notifies users when key information is missing from a patient's demographics or when there are other issues with a patient's account.
Credit Card Scanner	The *Credit Card Scanner* field is set to "No" by default. Your student version of Harris CareTracker will NOT have this feature. In a real practice setting, select "Yes" if your group uses a credit card scanner to process payments by credit card.
Service Date From	Click the *Calendar* icon 🗓️ **MDY** and select the start of the service dates included in the batch.
Service Trans Date	Click the *Calendar* icon 🗓️ **MDY** and select the service transaction date included in the batch.
Payment Trans Date	Click the *Calendar* icon 🗓️ **MDY** and select the payment transactions date included in the batch.
Reversal Trans Date	Click the *Calendar* icon 🗓️ **MDY** and select the reversal transactions date included in the batch.
Referral Default	By default, the *Referral Default* list is set to "Referral-Incoming." Select a referral type based on your practice specialty. The selected option will display as the default option when the *Ref/Auth* application is accessed via the *Name Bar* or *Patient* module.

(*continues*)

Table 4-6   Batch Details Field and Instructions *(continued)*

BATCH DETAILS FIELD	INSTRUCTIONS
Show Operator Name	Select "Yes" to display the operator's name on the Harris CareTracker PM and EMR interface. Select "No" if you do not want the operator's name displayed.
Click *Save*. The batch information is saved.	
Note: Click *Edit* to make changes if necessary.	
Click *X* on the right-hand corner to close the dialog box.	

Courtesy of Harris CareTracker PM and EMR

Having set up your operator preferences in the *Operator Encounter Batch Control* in Activity 4-13, you will now create a batch. Reference the instructions in **Table 4-6** when creating your batch.

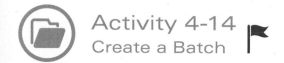

Activity 4-14
Create a Batch

1. Before creating a batch, make sure your fiscal period and fiscal year are open for the month(s) in which patient appointments are scheduled (refer to Activities 2-5 and 2-6 if you need to refresh your memory). For example, if Jane Morgan's appointment is in March 2017, make sure the fiscal period March 2017 is open. Once you have confirmed the fiscal period and year are open, proceed to step 2. **Note:** If you are working at the month's end and are booking appointments in the following month, you would need to open the current <u>and</u> next month in fiscal period. This would also apply to the fiscal period selected in your batch.

2. Click on the Batch icon on the Name Bar. Then click *Edit* and then click *Create Batch*. The *Batch Master* dialog box displays (**Figure 4-47**).

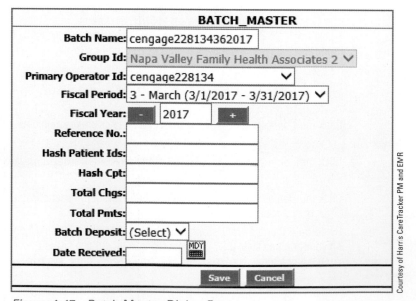

Figure 4-47   Batch Master Dialog Box

3. By default, the *Batch Name* box displays a batch identification name. The name consists of your user name followed by the current date. (**Note:** You can edit the batch name if necessary and change the batch name to identify the types of financial transactions associated with the batch; for example, "copayment5132017.") Do not use symbols when editing the name. Change the Batch Name to "FrontOffice Copayment" (**Figure 4-48**).

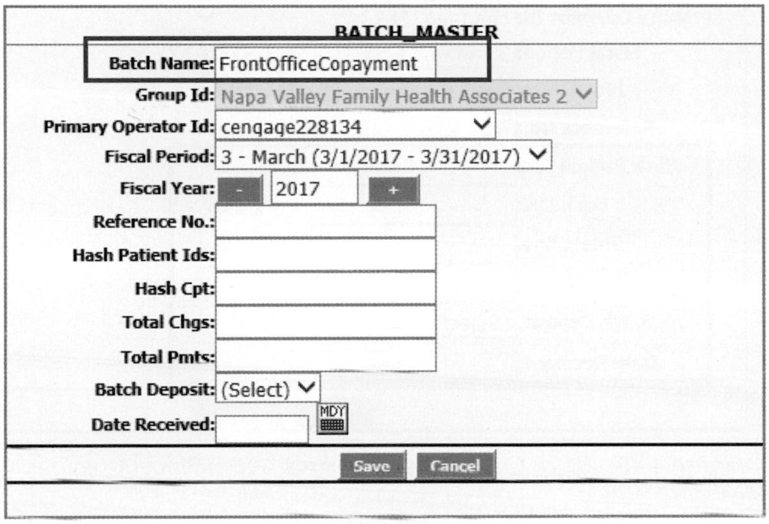

BATCH_MASTER

Batch Name: FrontOfficeCopayment
Group Id: Napa Valley Family Health Associates 2 ∨
Primary Operator Id: cengage228134 ∨
Fiscal Period: 3 - March (3/1/2017 - 3/31/2017) ∨
Fiscal Year: − 2017 +
Reference No.:
Hash Patient Ids:
Hash Cpt:
Total Chgs:
Total Pmts:
Batch Deposit: (Select) ∨
Date Received: [MDY]

Save   Cancel

Figure 4-48   Rename Batch FrontOfficeCopayment

4. By default, the *Group Id* displays the name of your group.

5. By default, the *Primary Operator Id* displays your user name.

6. In the *Fiscal Period* field, click the month in which patients from Activity 4-1 have appointments. The list will only display fiscal periods that are currently open.

7. By default, the *Fiscal Year* displays the current financial year set up for your company in Activity 2-5.

8. *Hash Patient Ids* box—Leave blank for this activity. **FYI:** The *Hash Patient Ids* box is where the person entering the batch data would enter the sum of all patient Harris CareTracker PM and EMR ID numbers pertaining to the charges associated with the batch. This is to ensure that a charge is entered for all patients associated with the batch.

9. *Hash Cpt* box—Leave blank for this activity. **FYI:** The *Hash Cpt* box is where you enter the sum of all CPT® codes pertaining to the charges associated with the batch. This is to ensure that a charge is entered for all procedures. Example: If two patients are seen for the day, and the CPT® codes selected on the encounter form for the first patient are 71101 and 99213, and the second patient are 71101 and 99203, calculate the *Hash CPT* by adding 71101+ 99213+ 71101+ 99203 = 340618.

10. *Total Chgs* box—Leave blank for this activity. **FYI:** The *Total Chgs* box is where you enter the sum of all charges that are associated with the batch.

11. *Total Pmts* box—Leave blank for this activity. **FYI:** The *Total Pmts* box is where you enter the sum of check(s) that are associated with the batch.

12. *Batch Deposit* list—Leave blank for this activity. **FYI:** The *Batch Deposit* list is where you would select the *Deposit ID* to link to a deposit number, if using the *Batch Deposit* application. (This feature is not active in your student version.)

13. *Date Received* box—Leave blank for this activity. **FYI:** You could enter the date the encounter was received in MM/DD/YYYY format or click the *Calendar* icon MDY and select the date. (**Figure 4-49**).

Courtesy of Harris CareTracker PM and EMR

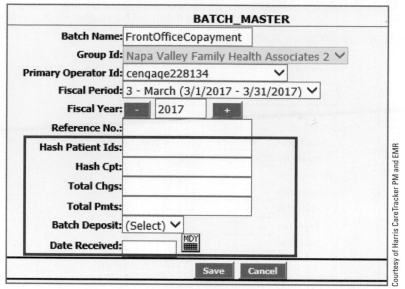

Figure 4-49 Batch Master Selections for "FrontOfficeCopayment" Batch

14. Click *Save*. You may receive a message box asking if you are sure you want to select the fiscal period. After confirming the correct fiscal period is displaying, click *OK*. Harris CareTracker PM and EMR displays the *Operator Encounter Batch Control* dialog box with the new batch information (**Figure 4-50**).

Courtesy of Harris CareTracker PM and EMR

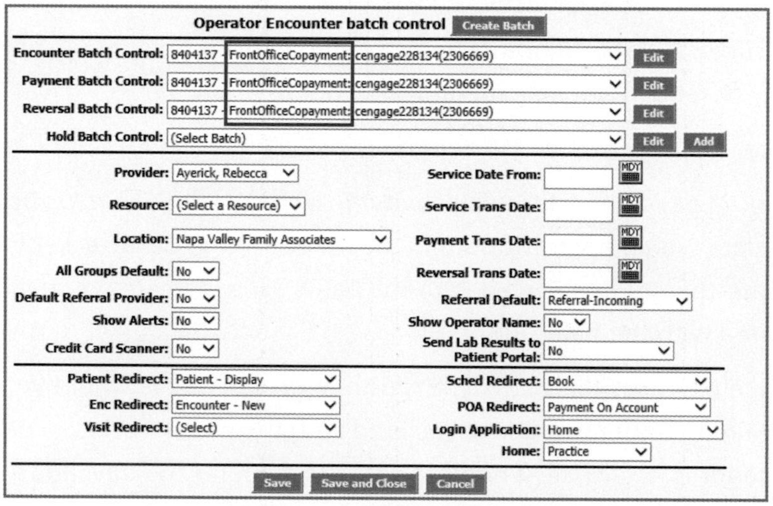

Figure 4-50 Operator Encounter Batch Control Dialog Box

15. Now, further edit your batch by updating the provider, resource, location, and so on (the middle section of the *Operator Encounter Batch Control box*). Select the *Provider* (Amir Raman), *Resource* (Amir Raman), and *Location* (Napa Valley Family Associates).

16. Click *Save*.

17. Write down your "Encounter Batch Control No." for future reference. (Should include "FrontOfficeCopayment") ______________________.

Print the Batch screen, label it "Activity 4-14," and place it in your assignment folder.

18. Click "X" in the right-hand corner to close the *Batch* dialog box.

Accept a Payment

In Harris CareTracker PM and EMR, there are many ways to record both patient and insurance payments. Payments may be processed electronically or manually. All payments entered into Harris CareTracker PM and EMR must be associated with a batch and should be verified using a journal before the batch is released for posting. All payments entered are associated with a billing period for financial reporting purposes.

Entering Payments on Account.

The *Payments on Account (Pmt on Acct)* application is used to record patient payments. The application also shows any outstanding balance, unapplied credits, and unposted payments accrued from previous visits. After a patient's visit is saved in Harris CareTracker PM and EMR, that visit must be turned into a charge and the patient's payment must be applied to the charge.

Accessing Payments on Account.

You can access the *Payments on Account* application from locations within practice management, as outlined below.

- *Scheduling* module > *Book* tab > left-click on a patient's *appointment* to display the Mini-Menu > Select *Payment* link
- *Name Bar* > *Appts* button > *Actions* menu > *Payment* link
- *Transactions* module > *Pmt on Acct* tab
- *Transactions* module > *Charge* tab

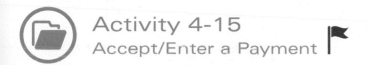

Activity 4-15
Accept/Enter a Payment

1. Pull patient Jane Morgan into context.

2. In the *Transactions* module, click on the *Pmt on Acct* tab.

3. From the drop-down list at the top of the screen, select whether the payment is being made by the *Patient* or *Responsible Party*. (Select "Patient.")

4. If a patient is paying a portion of his or her balance (or copayment), enter the dollar amount of the payment in the *Amount* box. (Enter "$20.00.")

   (FYI) If the patient was paying his or her entire balance, you would click *Pay Bal*. Harris CareTracker PM and EMR automatically pulls the patient's balance into the *Amount* box.

5. From the *Payment Type* list, select the payment method. (Select "Payment - Patient Check.") **Note:** If the payment type was a credit card, you would select the *Process Credit Card* checkbox.

6. If the payment method is a check, enter the check number in the *Reference #* box. (Enter "5013" as the check number.) The reference number will print on the patient's receipt.

7. From the *Method* list, select how to apply the payment to the patient's account:

   a. If you are collecting a copayment for a patient who does not have an outstanding balance, select only "Force Unapplied." Harris CareTracker PM and EMR creates an unapplied balance for the patient that is applied to the patient's private pay balance when their charges are saved.

   b. Because Ms. Morgan has a scheduled appointment, select "Force Unapplied" and check the *Copay?* box.

   (FYI) If the patient has an outstanding balance you would:

- Select *Today's First* in the *Method* field to apply the money starting with the most current balance and then back toward the oldest date of service for which the patient has an outstanding balance.

- Select *Oldest to Newest* in the *Method* field to apply the money to the oldest date of service for which the patient has an outstanding balance and then forward toward the most current date of service.

8. In the *Trans. Date* box, enter the transaction date to which you want to link the payment. Because you are entering a copayment for a patient visit, select the date of the patient's appointment. (You scheduled Jane Morgan's appointment in Activity 4-1.) **Note:** If you had selected dates in your batch defaults when you set up your batch, they would prepopulate. **Hint:** If you are working at the month's end and are booking appointments in the following month, you would need to open both the current and next month in fiscal period. This would also apply to the fiscal period selected in your batch.

   (FYI) The following are the various Transaction Date Defaults:

- If a transaction date was selected when you created your batch, Harris CareTracker PM and EMR pulls that date into the *Trans. Date* box.

- If a transaction date was not selected, the transaction date defaults to the date in your batch name.

- If there is no date in your batch name, the transaction date defaults to the date the payment is entered in Harris CareTracker PM and EMR.

9. Because this is a copay:

   a. Select the *Copay?* checkbox.

   b. In the *Appt* field, select the appointment date to which the copay applies (the appointment scheduled in Activity 4-1), if possible. (**Note:** You cannot link a copay to a future appointment date. If your appointment is in the future, you won't be able to select it, and you can skip this step.)

   c. **FYI:** The *Plan Name* and *Copay Amt* fields display the insurance plan and copay amount saved in the patient's demographics, if applicable. These fields are read-only.

10. The *Go To* field defaults to the redirect option selected in the operator's batch. You can select a different option if needed (**Figure 4-51**). (Select "Payment on Account.")

11. To view a summary of the transaction prior to saving, click *View Trans* (**Figure 4-52**).

   Note: If you do not need to view the transaction, you can click directly on *Quick Save* to save the transaction.

12. After clicking *View Trans*, then click *Save*. Harris CareTracker PM and EMR saves the payment information and launches the application selected in the *Go To* field. (You selected the *Go To* of *Payment on Account*, which brings you back to the original *Pmt on Acct* tab.)

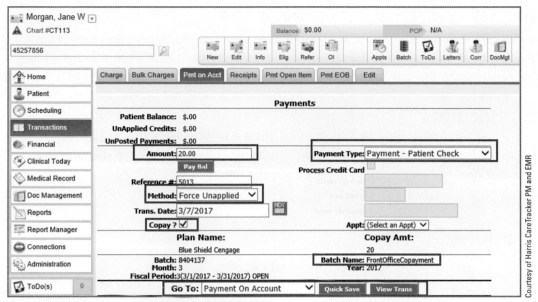

Figure 4-51   Enter Payment on Account

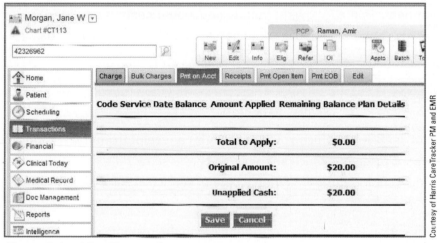

Figure 4-52   View Transaction

! **ALERT** Do <u>NOT</u> post the batch.

---

13. Click on the *Home* module and the *Open Batches* link under the *Billing* header on the *Dashboard* (**Figure 4-53**) to view your batch with the payment recorded. **Note:** Only view the batch, do not post it.

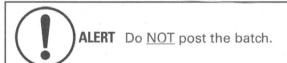

Figure 4-53   Open Batches

Courtesy of Harris CareTracker PM and EMR

14. You will later print a receipt from the *Receipts* tab in the *Transactions* module (Activity 4-16).

📃 **Print the Open Batch screen, label it "Activity 4-15," and place it in your assignment folder.**

Copayment

A copayment is a predetermined (flat) fee that an individual pays for health care services in addition to what the insurance covers. For example, some HMOs require a $10 "copayment" for each office visit, regardless of the type or level of services provided during the visit. Copayments are not usually specified by percentages.

Print Patient Receipts

After entering the payment information in Activity 4-15, print a receipt from the *Receipts* tab in the *Transaction* module. Receipts in Harris CareTracker PM and EMR identify a patient's previous balance, the activity of charges and payments for that date of service, and the new patient balance.

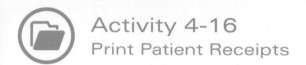

Activity 4-16
Print Patient Receipts

1. With the patient in context (Jane Morgan), click the *Transactions* module. **Note:** You will still be working in the *Batch* you created in Activity 4-14. **Hint:** If you are working at the month's end and are booking appointments in the following month, you would need to open the current <u>and</u> next month in fiscal period. This would also apply to the fiscal period selected in your batch.

2. When the *Transactions* module opens, click on the *Receipts* tab.

3. From the drop-down list at the top of the screen, select who you would like to view the receipt from, *Patient* or *Responsible Party*. (Select "Patient.")

4. Select the date of service for which you need to print a receipt from the *Receipts* list. (Select the date of the payment received, which should also be the same date as your batch and the date that matches the patient's appointment.) When a date of service is selected, the receipt displays on the screen.

5. Click on the *Print* button (**Figure 4-54**), or right-click on the receipt.

   When you right-click, a gray pop-up menu appears; select *Print*, and the receipt will print.

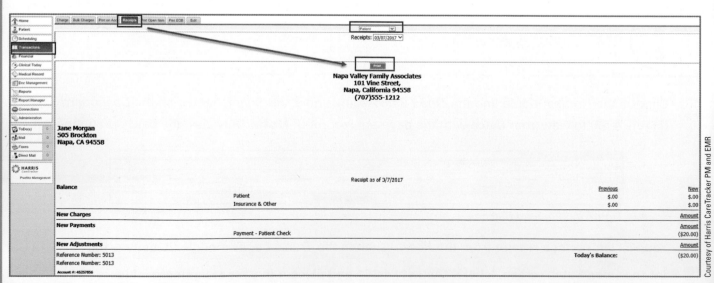

Figure 4-54   Print Patient Receipt

📧 **Print the Patient Receipt, label it "Activity 4-16," and place it in your assignment folder.**

Activity 4-17
Accept/Enter a Payment and Print Receipt

1. Using the information below and steps 2 through 17, accept/enter a payment and print a receipt for each of the following patients:

   a. Ellen Ristino; $20.00 copay paid by CHECK # 4452.

   b. Barbara Watson; $20.00 copay paid by CHECK # 11247.

2. Pull patient into context.

3. In the *Transactions* module, click on the *Pmt on Acct* tab.

4. From the drop-down list at the top of the screen, select whether the payment is being made by the *Patient* or *Responsible Party*. (Select *Patient*.)

5. Enter the amount of copay for each patient listed in steps 1a and 1b.

6. From the *Payment Type* list, select the payment method listed in steps 1a and 1b.

7. If the payment method is a check, enter the check number in the *Reference #* box.

8. From the *Method* list, select how to apply the payment to the patient's account. For this activity, select "Force Unapplied" and check the *Copay?* box for each of the patient's noted in steps 1a and 1b.

9. In the *Trans. Date* box, enter the transaction date to which you want to link the payment. Select the date of the appointment you scheduled previously in the chapter for each patient. (**Note:** This date must be a date within the fiscal period of the batch you created in Activity 4-14.)

10. In order to record or override the copayment amount noted in the patient's demographic record for a specific appointment:

    a. Select the *Copay?* checkbox.

    b. In the *Appt* box, select the appointment date to which the copay applies. If possible, select the appointment date for the patient(s) you created previously in the chapter. **Note:** This is not an option for an appointment date that is after the date you are completing this activity.

11. In the *Go To* field, select "Payment on Account" (see **Figure 4-51**).

12. Click *Quick Save*. Harris CareTracker PM and EMR saves the payment information and launches the application selected in the *Go To* field of the batch.

13. With the patient in context, click the *Transactions* module.

14. When the *Transactions* module opens, click on the *Receipts* tab.

15. From the drop-down list at the top of the screen, select "Patient" or "Responsible Party" as noted in step 4.

16. Select the date of service for which you need to print a receipt from the *Receipts* list. (Select the date of the payment received, which should be the same as the date of the patients' appointments scheduled previously in the chapter.)

17. Click on the *Print* button (see **Figure 4-54**), or right-click on the receipt. When you right-click, a gray pop-up menu appears; select *Print*, and the receipt will print.

📧 **Print the Patient Receipt for each of the patients, label them "Activity 4-17," and place them in your assignment folder.**

Now that you have entered copayments, you will complete the process by running a journal and posting your batch as part of your "end-of-day" workflow.

Journals

You must run a journal prior to posting your batch to verify that you have entered all the financial transactions correctly in Harris CareTracker PM and EMR. Once you have verified your balance with your journal, post the batch. Journals provide a summary of financial transactions, for example, charges, payments, and adjustments. Typically, each operator who enters financial transactions into Harris CareTracker should run a journal for his or her batch before posting to review and audit only the transactions that he or she entered.

It is important to identify any errors before a batch is posted. Once a batch has been posted, the transactions linked to it are locked in the system and cannot be changed. To be corrected, the charges must be reversed. Posted errors can only be corrected by reversing the transaction on the patient's account, which occurs in the *Edit* application of the *Transaction* module. It is highly recommended as a best practice, that you run a journal before posting your batch to make sure that your transactions for the day are correct and balance.

Harris CareTracker PM and EMR offers multiple drill-down options that allow you to run a journal that fits certain criteria. Open batches are easily chosen from the list of filters. Posted batches are accessible at any time so you can always access an old journal from the *Historical Journals* link (**Figure 4-55**) under the *Financial Reports* section of the *Reports* application, which alleviates the need to save paper copies of journals.

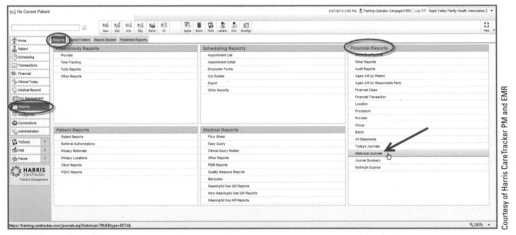

Figure 4-55   Historical Journals Link

✓ **TIP** For a quick "totals only" view of a batch, the *Open Batches* link on the *Dashboard* displays the total amount of payments, charges, and unapplied money entered into that batch. If the total amount of money collected equals the *Payments Match* or *Unapplied* column, you do not need to run a journal (**Figure 4-56**).

Figure 4-56   Money Collected Equals Payments Match or Unapplied Column

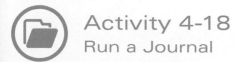

Activity 4-18
Run a Journal

1. Click the *Reports* module.

2. Click the *Todays Journals* link under the *Financial Reports* section (**Figure 4-57**). Harris CareTracker PM displays the *Todays Journal Options* screen (**Figure 4-58**). All of your group's open batches are listed in the *Todays Batches* box.

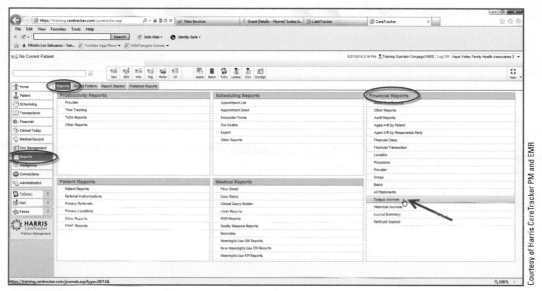

Figure 4-57 Todays Journals Link

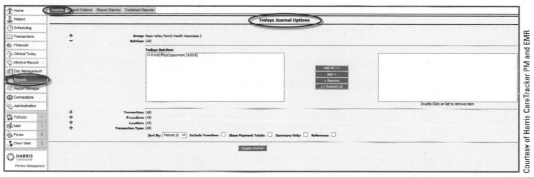

Figure 4-58 Todays Journal Options

3. Select a batch to include in the journal either by double-clicking on the batch name or by clicking on the batch and then clicking *Add* (**Figure 4-59**). Harris CareTracker PM and EMR adds the selected batches to the box on the right. (Add batch "FrontOfficeCopayment.")

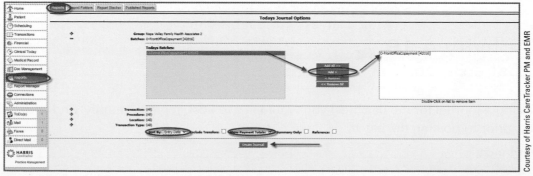

Figure 4-59 Select a Batch for the Journal

4. From the *Sort By* list drop-down, select "Entry Date."

5. Select the *Show Payment Totals* checkbox (see **Figure 4-59**).

6. Click *Create Journal*. Harris CareTracker PM generates the journal (**Figure 4-60**).

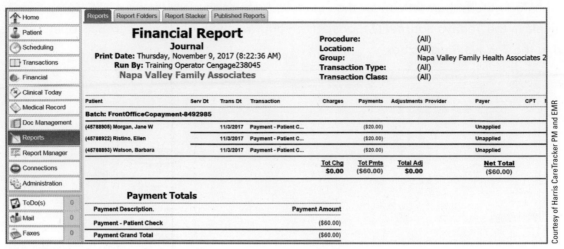

Figure 4-60   Create Journal

7. To print, right-click on the journal and select *Print* from the shortcut menu.

 Print the Journal screen, label it "Activity 4-18," and place it in your assignment folder.

After reviewing the transactions in your journal for accuracy, you will post your open batch (Activity 4-19). Batches should only be posted after a journal has been generated and you have verified your journal balances. Posting batches locks the transactions permanently in Harris CareTracker. All transactions will show on reports generated in Harris CareTracker, and any corrections to posted transactions must be made via the *Edit* application in the *Transactions* module. *Open Batches* can also be viewed and posted by clicking on the *Open Batches* link under the *Billing* section of the *Dashboard* on the *Home* page.

TIP

- As a best practice, you should close out (post) your batch at the end of each day; however, <u>wait</u> until instructed to do so in a particular activity in this text.

- All transactions must be posted before running any *Month End* report in Harris CareTracker, and *Periods* cannot be closed with open batches linked to them, however, <u>wait</u> until instructed to do so in a particular activity in this text.

- A password may be required to post a coworker's batch.

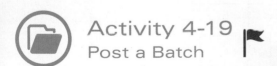

Activity 4-19
Post a Batch

After generating a journal for the batch(es) you would like to post, review, identify, and correct transactions errors, if any, prior to posting the batch.

To post your batch:

1. Click the *Administration* module. The application opens the *Practice* tab (**Figure 4-61**).

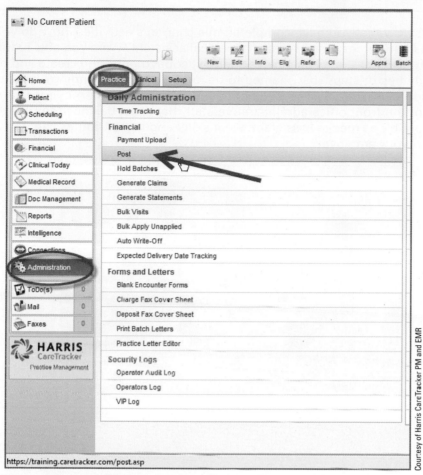

Figure 4-61   Post Link from Admin Practice Tab

2. Click the *Post* link under the *Daily Administration > Financial* header (see **Figure 4-61**). Harris CareTracker PM displays a list of all open batches for the group.

3. Select the checkbox next to the batch you want to post. (Select batch "FrontOfficeCopayment.")

🖳 **Print the Post Batch screen, label it "Activity 4-19," and place it in your assignment folder.**

4. Click *Post Batches* (**Figure 4-62**).

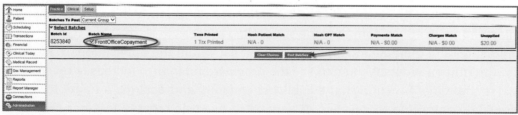

Figure 4-62   Post Batches

Courtesy of Harris CareTracker PM and EMR

An alternative way of posting batches is via the *Open Batches* link on the Home > *Dashboard*, under the *Billing* header. Although not required, it is recommended to only post a batch after a journal has been generated and balances verified. The total number of open batches for your group displays next to the *Open Batches* link.

CRITICAL THINKING Now that you have completed this chapter's activities, how do you feel about the scheduling and financial responsibilities of a medical assistant? Were you able to follow instructions and accurately schedule patients, receive and post copayments, and create and post a batch? Were there any activities or steps that seemed to be difficult and challenging? If so, which ones? What measures did you take to accurately complete the activities and move forward? What are your impressions of the front office administrative staff that must balance their responsibilities? If you become a front office medical assistant, what skills and key attributes can you comfortably say you can offer to your employer?

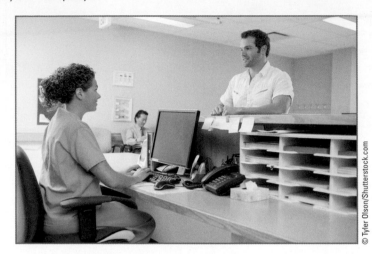

© Tyler Olson/Shutterstock.com

SUMMARY

This chapter wraps up the patient scheduling module of front office/practice management responsibilities in Harris CareTracker that are required before the clinical application of the EHR can be used. Mastering the various methods of scheduling, rescheduling, and canceling appointments lays the foundation for the patient visit and billing activities.

Other duties associated with managing the appointment schedule include appointment reminders (*TeleVox*®) and the effect on the practice and patients; scheduling non-patient appointments, which are vital to prevent appointment conflicts with a provider's schedule; and creating a wait list. There are many reasons an appointment would need to be canceled or rescheduled and this happens frequently in today's busy medical practice. You are now familiar with the steps to complete the scheduling process in Harris CareTracker PM and EMR, and the importance of creating and maintaining an effective wait list within the application. These functions help to fill open time slots with other patients waiting to see the provider and in turn increases revenue to the practice.

Creating a batch is the initial function that establishes defaults and assigns a name to a batch (group) of financial transactions you enter into the system. A new batch must be created to enter financial transactions. You have completed activities that include setting operator batch preferences, accepting a payment, generating a patient receipt, running a journal, and posting the batch. These front office activities related to the batch links the patient visit to the Billing module, which is covered in Chapters 9 and 10. You will continue to refer to batch activities throughout this book and when completing many future activities.

CHECK YOUR KNOWLEDGE

Select the best response.

_____ 1. Booking non-patient appointments must be done directly from the:

      a. Dashboard
      c. Schedule

      b. Administration module
      d. None of the above

_____ 2. How do you access the mini-menu?

      a. Left-click on patient's name in the schedule
      c. In the batch setup

      b. Click on the *Dashboard Schedule*
      d. None of the above

_____ 3. How long does the mini-menu schedule display on the screen?

      a. As long as you are operating in the *Schedule* module
      c. As long as the patient is in context

      b. 8 minutes
      d. 8 seconds

_____ 4. Which of the following is NOT one of the key reason(s) a Batch is used?

      a. To print a receipt for patient copays and monthly statements
      c. To assign a name and defaults to a group of financial transactions

      b. To set up workflow preferences (e.g., administrative or clinical activities)
      d. To be able to run reports that identify a group of charges or payments

_____ 5. When a patient is to be seen by a provider but also needs an ultrasound at the same visit, what feature do you use?

      a. ALT
      c. Multi-resource

      b. Tab
      d. Ctrl

_____ 6. You can select multiple providers by holding the _____ key while clicking on the provider names.

      a. Tab
      c. F1

      b. Ctrl
      d. Either a or c

_____ 7. If a patient does not want to get a confirmation call from *TeleVox*®, you must update his or her _____ on the *Patient Details* tab in the *Patient* module/*Demographics* tab.

      a. notification preference
      c. privacy practices

      b. phone number
      d. All of the above

_____ 8. When rescheduling an existing appointment, which button must you use to avoid creating an additional appointment?

      a. Go
      c. Tab

      b. Book Appointment
      d. Search

_____ 9. The *Hash Cpt* box of the batch is where you enter the sum of all CPT® codes pertaining to the charges associated with the batch. If three patients are seen for the day with the first patient CPT® codes of 99212 and 71101, second patient CPT® codes of 99215 and 93000, and third patient CPT® codes of 99203 and 99173, what is the number you would enter into *Hash Cpt*?

      a. 2
      c. 297630

      b. 4
      d. 560904

_____ 10. To enter/accept a payment on account from a patient with no outstanding balance (in the *Payments* screen of the *Transaction* module, *Pmt on Acct* tab), select:

a. Method >Today's First

c. Method > Oldest to Newest

b. Method > Force Unapplied

d. Copay?

CASE STUDIES

To complete Case Study 4-1, you must have completed Case Study 3-1 in Chapter 3. If you have not completed Case Study 3-1, you may use Case Study 4-2 instead. For Case Studies 4-1 and 4-2, you will not be able to link the copay to a visit if the appointment you booked is on a future date. For example, if you are entering data on the weekend and the first available appointment was scheduled on Monday, you will not be able to link the copay to a "future visit date" but you will be able to complete the rest of the steps as instructed.

Case Study 4-1

1. Book the following appointment for James M. Smith. Refer to Activity 4-1 for help.

   • Provider: Dr. Ayerick

   • Time: Book today or first available (Record date/time here: _____)

   • Appointment Type: Follow Up

   • Complaint: Follow-up exam/consultation; review lab and EKG

2. Check in patient James Smith from the mini-menu. Refer to Activity 4-12 for help.

3. Create a batch. Name the batch "CaseStudyCopayment4-1." Refer to Activity 4-14 for help.

4. Accept/Enter a cash payment for James Smith. Refer to Activity 4-15 for help. (**Hint**: Look in his patient demographics to confirm the amount of his copay.)

5. Print the patient receipt for James Smith. Refer to Activity 4-16 for help.

6. Run a journal for the "CaseStudyCopayment4-1" batch created in this case study. Refer to Activity 4-18 for help.

7. Post the batch "CaseStudyCopayment4-1" created in this case study. Refer to Activity 4-19 for help.

   Print the Post Batch Screen, label it "Case Study 4-1," and place it in your assignment folder.

Case Study 4-2

1. Book an Appointment for Kimberly Johnson using the following criteria. Refer to Activity 4-1 for help.

   • Provider: Dr. Ayerick

   • Time: Book today or first available (Record date/time here: _____)

   • Appointment Type: Follow Up

   • Complaint: Follow-up exam/consultation; review lab and EKG

2. Check in patient Kimberly Johnson from the mini-menu. Refer to Activity 4-12 for help.

3. Create a batch. Name the batch "CaseStudyCopayment4-2." Refer to Activity 4-14 for help.

4. Accept/Enter a payment by check# 4478 for Kimberly Johnson. (**Hint**: look in her patient demographics to confirm the amount of her copay). Refer to Activity 4-15 for help.

5. Print a patient receipt for Kimberly Johnson. Refer to Activity 4-16 for help.

6. Run a journal for the "CaseStudyCopayment4-2" batch created in this case study. Refer to Activity 4-18 for help.

7. Post the batch "CaseStudyCopayment4-2" created in this case study. Refer to Activity 4-19 for help.

🖶 **Print the Post Batch Screen, label it "Case Study 4-2," and place it in your assignment folder.**

BUILD YOUR PROFICIENCY

Proficiency Builder 4-1: Inactivate an Appointment Recall

Recalls are reminders to patients that an appointment needs to be booked. Rather than scheduling a future appointment, a recall (reminder) date is set for the appointment. After a recall is linked to an appointment, it becomes inactive rather than open, but should the patient cancel the appointment, the recall becomes open again. You have the ability to activate and inactivate recalls in Harris CareTracker. (**Note:** You must have completed Activity 4-11 in order to complete this Proficiency Builder.)

1. Pull patient Edith Robinson into context.

2. Open the *Scheduling* module and click the *Recall* tab.

3. Click the *Edit* icon next to the appointment recall you want to inactivate (**Figure 4-63**). In the *Edit Patient Recall* box, change the *Active* status to "No" and click *Save*. Harris CareTracker PM changes the recall status from Active to Inactive.

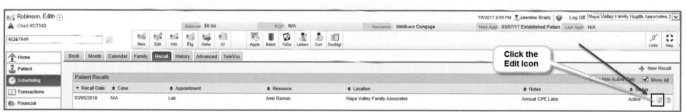

Figure 4-63   Pending Recall

Courtesy of Harris CareTracker PM and EMR

🖶 **Print the Inactive Appointment Recall Screen, label it "BYP 4-1," and place it in your assignment folder.**

4. In the "Success" box, click the "X" to Close.

Proficiency Builder 4-2: Activate an Appointment Recall Previously Inactivated

1. After completing Proficiency Builder 4-1, pull patient Edith Robinson into context.

2. Open the *Scheduling* module and click the *Recall* tab.

(Continues)

(Continued)

3. Click *Show All*. Harris CareTracker PM displays all active and inactive appointment recalls.

4. Click the *Edit* icon in the *Status* column to open the *Edit Patient Recall* box (**Figure 4-64**). Change the *Active* status to "Yes" and click *Save*.

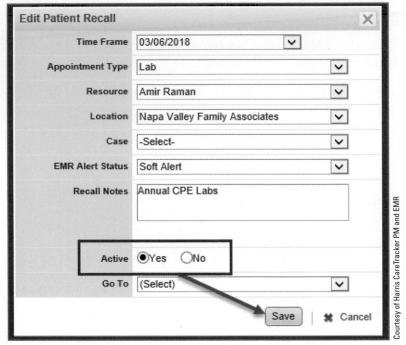

Figure 4-64   Activate Recall

5. In the "Success" box, click on the "X" to Close.

6. The *Status* is now updated to "Active" again.

📁 **Print the Active Appointment Recall Screen, label it "BYP 4-2," and place it in your assignment folder.**

Proficiency Builder 4-3: Update Patient Notification Preference

Patients will often request that the method of notification be changed. For example, in years past, a written letter might be the preferred contact method. That later evolved to telephone messaging, and now the added options of text messaging and notifications via patient portals are widely used.

1. Pull patient Edith Robinson into context.

2. Click the *Patient* module, which will default to the *Demographics/Patient Details* tab.

3. Click *Edit*.

4. Scroll down to the *Notification Preference* field. Click on the drop-down menu and select "Patient Portal" (**Figure 4-65**).

5. Scroll down and click *Save*. The patient's notification preference is now listed as "Patient Portal" (**Figure 4-66**).

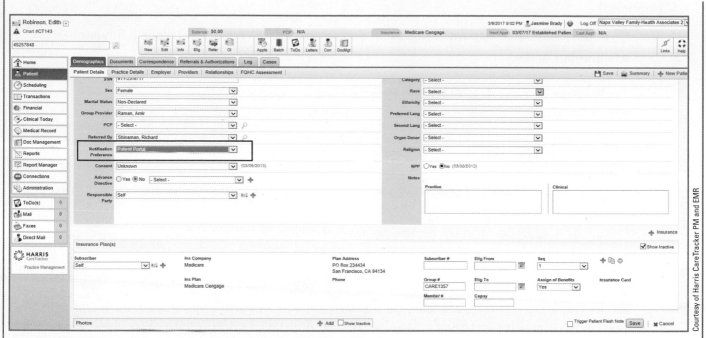

Figure 4-65   Update Patient's Notification Preference

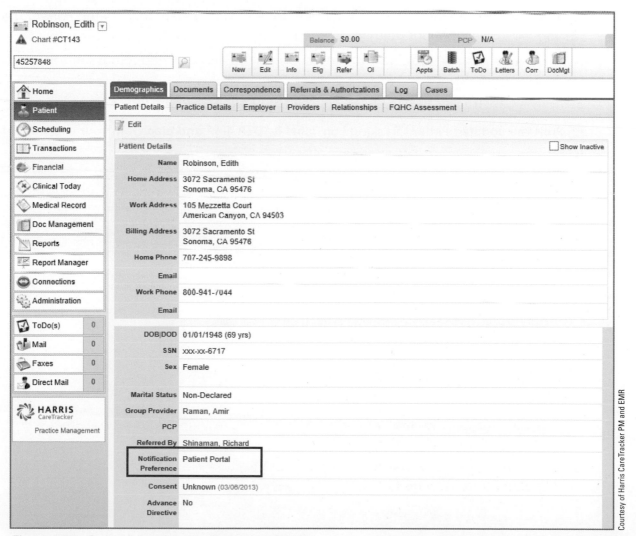

Figure 4-66   Patient's Notification Preference Saved

(Continues)

(*Continued*)

📧 **Print the updated Patient Notification Screen, label it "BYP 4-3," and place it in your assignment folder.**

Proficiency Builder 4-4: View the Patient Tracking Log

Harris CareTracker allows you to view the patient tracking log that tracks the progress of the patient's appointment. You can track the progress by logging an entry each time the patient's status changes and each time a patient is moved to a different location. The log displays a time stamp next to each activity and calculates the total time of the visit, beginning at check in and ending at check out.

1. With patient Edith Robinson in context, access the *Appointments* application from one of the following locations:

    a.   The *Appts* button 🗓 on the *Name Bar*

    b.   The *Appointments* link on the *Practice* tab of the *Dashboard*

    c.   The *Appointments* tab in the *Clinical Today* module

2. In the *Appointments* list, change the *Resource* to *All*, and enter the *Custom Dates* to 12 months prior to today's date (beginning date) and ending date of today.

3. In the *Status* field, use the drop-down and select *All*.

4. Click *Search* and locate the appointment for which you want to view the *Patient Tracking log.* (Select patient Edith Robinson.)

5. Click the *Arrow* ▼ icon next to the *Actions* menu along the appointment row, and click *Patient Tracking*.

6. Harris CareTracker PM and EMR displays the *Patient Tracking* log.

📧 **Print the updated Patient Tracking Log, label it "BYP 4-4," and place it in your assignment folder.**

MODULE 3
Clinical Skills

This module includes:

- Chapter 5: Preliminary Duties in the EMR
- Chapter 6: Patient Work-Up
- Chapter 7: Completing the Visit
- Chapter 8: Other Clinical Documentation

As a health care professional, you may use Harris CareTracker PM and EMR to perform clinical duties. Once a patient is registered in the database and has an appointment scheduled, you will perform the steps to activate care management registries, check in and track patients throughout their visits, record vital signs, update the patient's medical record, create progress notes, and capture the visit to create a billable encounter. All the activities you complete in this module mimic a real-world setting using the clinical features of electronic health records.

QUICK START

Because Harris CareTracker is a live EMR, you will need to complete several tasks to simulate a live clinic where patient accounts are ready for a clinical work-up. The following activities are required in order to complete the activities in this module. **If you have been following along in this book from the beginning and have completed all Required ⚑ activities as you've moved sequentially through the text, then you have already completed the activities below and can move forward. If you are beginning with this module, then you will need to complete the activities below *before* you can complete any other activities in this Module.**

Be sure you are working in a supported browser (Internet Explorer 11 or Safari for iPad) before you begin. Other browsers (such as Chrome and Firefox) are not supported. Review Best Practices, included on page xxiii of this text.

- ❑ Activity 1-1: Disable Toolbars
- ❑ Activity 1-2: Set Up Tabbed Browsing
- ❑ Activity 1-3: Turn Off Pop-Up Blocker
- ❑ Activity 1-4: Change Page Setup
- ❑ Activity 1-5: Add Harris CareTracker to Trusted Sites
- ❑ Activity 1-6: Clear Your Cache
  - *Note: Remember that you should clear your cache each time before you being working in CareTracker.*

❑ Activity 1-8: Disable Download Blocking
  • *Note: Once you have completed the system set-up requirements (Activities 1-1, 1-2, 1-3, 1-4, 1-5, and 1-8), you will not need to repeat these activities unless you change the device you are using or the settings automatically default back to prior settings.*

❑ Activity 1-9: Register Your Credentials and Create Your Harris CareTracker PM and EMR Training Company
  • *Note: It will take up to 24 hours for your CareTracker "Student Company" to be created. Plan accordingly.*

❑ Activity 2-1: Log in to Harris CareTracker PM and EMR
  • *Note: Be sure to write down your new password inside the front cover of your book for easy reference.*

❑ Activity 2-5: Open a New Fiscal Year
  • *Note: Every January 1, you will need to open a new fiscal year.*

❑ Activity 2-6: Open a Fiscal Period
  • *Note: Every first of the month, you will need to open a new fiscal period.*

❑ Activity 3-1: Searching for a Patient by Name
  • *Complete steps 1 and 2 only.*
  • *Note: You will search for patients throughout the text using the steps in Activity 3-1.*

❑ Activity 3-4: Register a New Pediatric Patient and Print Demographics
  • *You can complete only steps 1 through 6, 31, and 33. However, if you complete Chapter 3 later in your studies, you should complete the rest of the steps in Activity 3-4 by editing the patient's demographics.*

❑ Activity 4-1: Book an Appointment
  • *The directions for this activity state to book the appointment for one week from today. Instead, book the appointment for today (the day you are working). If no appointments are available today, then book the appointment for a day within the past week.*
  • *Also book an "Established Patient Sick" appointment for today for Barbara Watson with Amir Raman. Her chief complaint is "Fever—103F".*

❑ Activity 4-12: Check in Patient from the Mini-Menu
❑ Activity 4-14: Create a Batch
  • *Note: At various times throughout the activities, you will be directed to create batches.*

❑ Activity 4-15: Accept/Enter a Payment
❑ Activity 4-17: Accept/Enter a Payment
  • *Complete steps 1 through 12 only. You do not need to print receipts for this activity at this time.*

❑ Activity 4-19: Post a Batch
  • *Note: At various times throughout the activities, you will be directed to post batches.*

Once you have completed these activities as part of this Quick Start, you will not need to complete them again if you come across the activities while working in Chapters 1–4.

PREREQUISITES FOR CASE STUDIES

In addition to the activities listed in the Quick Start, you will need to complete these case studies if you plan to complete case studies in the Clinical Module:

❑ Case Study 3-1
  • *You can complete an abbreviated registration by only entering the patient's name, address, phone number, date of birth, social security number, sex, and insurance information.*

❑ Case Study 4-1
  • *You may complete steps 1 and 2 only.*

Preliminary Duties in the EMR

Key Terms

American Recovery and
  Reinvestment Act
  (ARRA)
attestation period
Certification Commission
  for Health Information
  Technology (CCHIT®)
encounter

Health Information
  Technology for
  Economic and Clinical
  Health (HITECH) Act
interoperable
lot
meaningful use

Learning Objectives

1. Define meaningful use and list its stages.
2. Describe tools within Harris CareTracker PM and EMR that assist with meaningful use.
3. View the meaningful use dashboard in Harris Care-Tracker PM and EMR.
4. Activate the care management registries in Harris CareTracker PM and EMR.
5. Navigate throughout the Medical Record module.
6. View the patient's encounter information, medications, allergy information, and problem list.
7. State the three types of alerts in Harris CareTracker PM and EMR.
8. View, change, and print a chart summary in Harris CareTracker EMR.
9. Perform routine maintenance functions in Harris CareTracker PM and EMR such as adding a room, editing a room, adding a custom resource, and managing immunizations.

Real-World Connection

In the first four chapters, you learned a great deal about the practice management side of the Harris CareTracker software. This chapter introduces you to the EMR component. This chapter focuses on the utilization of EMRs in ambulatory care settings. For providers to obtain full reimbursement from governmental agencies such as Medicare and Medicaid, they must be in full compliance with specific guidelines set forth by those agencies.

EMRs have been in use for the past couple of decades, but their widespread adoption skyrocketed largely due to Medicare and Medicaid financial incentives offered by the federal government for practices that meet meaningful use as well as the penalties that come about for not instituting and meaningfully using the EMR. As you work in this chapter, keep in mind how your position as a medical assistant may be impacted by meaningful use, and how you will be able to assist both providers and patients in meeting these goals.

INTRODUCTION

This chapter introduces you to the Harris CareTracker EMR—a fully integrated, CCHIT®-certified, cloud-based EHR solution guaranteed to help providers meet meaningful use requirements, a term you will learn more about later in the chapter. The abbreviation **CCHIT®** stands for **Certification Commission for Health Information Technology**, an organization appointed by the Department of Health and Human Services (HHS) to certify electronic medical record software. Professionals using Harris CareTracker Physician EMR can access electronic health records seamlessly from any location through a secure and centralized gateway. Combining clinical and business workflows into one comprehensive system helps providers save staff time, enhance practice productivity, and simplify administrative workflows. Harris CareTracker Physician EMR is a cloud-based system that provides secure, one-click access to patient charts, refill requests, and lab results from any Internet-connected computer and is fully integrated with Harris CareTracker's Practice Management.

Learning to use the robust functionality of Harris CareTracker software will prepare you to use any EMR software on the market. In this chapter, you will learn the basics of electronic medical records and how to navigate throughout the *Medical Record* module within Harris CareTracker EMR.

> Before you begin the activities in this chapter, refresh your memory on working with Harris CareTracker by referring back to the Best Practices list on page xxiii of this textbook. This list is also posted to the student companion website. Following best practices will help you complete work quickly and accurately.

ELECTRONIC MEDICAL RECORDS

Learning Objective 1: Define meaningful use and list its stages.

In Chapter 1, you learned that electronic medical records (EMRs) are patient records in digital format. EMRs can be found in all health care environments, but this chapter focuses on the utilization of EMRs in ambulatory care settings. For providers to obtain full reimbursement from governmental agencies such as Medicare and Medicaid, they must be in full compliance with specific guidelines set forth by those agencies. EMRs assist providers with meeting those guidelines.

Background of Meaningful Use

The **Health Information Technology for Economic and Clinical Health (HITECH) Act** was signed into law on February 17, 2009, to promote the adoption and meaningful use of health information technology. HITECH was enacted as part of the **American Recovery and Reinvestment Act (ARRA)**, also known as the "stimulus bill." HITECH provides the Department of Health and Human Services (HHS) with the authority to establish programs to improve health care quality through the promotion of health information technology. Components of HITECH have been promoted through incentives paid to providers for complying with the act. If providers are not compliant, they will face penalties through payment reductions.

Meaningful Use

EMRs have been in use for the past couple of decades and come in a variety of forms and from a wide array of companies that develop the technology. Harris CareTracker PM and EMR is one of the widely used EMRs today. HealthIT.gov describes **meaningful use** as using certified electronic health record technology to:

- Improve quality, safety, efficiency, and reduce health disparities
- Engage patients and family
- Improve care coordination, and population and public health outcomes
- Maintain privacy and security of patient health information

Meaningful use is the way in which EHR technologies must be implemented and used for a provider to be eligible for the EHR Incentive Programs and to qualify for incentive payments. These incentives specify three components of meaningful use:

- The use of a certified EHR in a meaningful manner
- The use of certified EHR technology for electronic exchange of health information to improve quality of health care
- The use of certified EHR technology to submit clinical quality and other measures

The purpose of meaningful use is to not only institute the adoption of EMRs but also establish that practices use their EHR software to its fullest. Benefits of meaningful use include complete and accurate medical records, better access to information, and patient empowerment. One of the major goals of meaningful use is to make medical records **interoperable** so that immediate access can be given to any provider who works with the patient. Interoperability "refers to the architecture or stands that make it possible for diverse EHR systems to work compatibly in a true information network" (HealthIT.gov). Three stages are associated with meaningful use.

Stage 1: Data Capture and Sharing Stage

This stage focuses on the following:

- Electronic capturing of health information in a coded format
- Using electronically captured health information to track key clinical conditions and communicate information for care coordination purposes
- Implementing clinical decision support tools to facilitate disease and medication management
- Reporting information for quality improvement and public health information

Two sets of objectives must be met to prove attestation for this stage: core and menu. All of the core objectives are required; however, eligible providers may choose which menu set objectives to follow. Eligible providers (EPs) must be credentialed with Medicare and may be a doctor of medicine or osteopathy, doctor of dental surgery or medicine, doctor of podiatric medicine, doctor of optometry, or a chiropractor. Medicaid EPs include physicians, dentists, certified nurse-midwives, nurse practitioners, and physician assistants. Providers in the health care setting can only apply for attestation with either Medicare or Medicaid but not both.

Meaningful Use Criteria for Eligible Professionals. Meaningful use criteria require providers to meet 14 core objectives, 5 out of 10 menu set objectives, and 6 total clinical quality measures. **Figures 5-1A** and **5-1B** illustrate what is included in the core and menu set objectives. (In **Figure 5-1A**, please note that core objective C-12 was required through 2013, but will not be a requirement moving forward.) Stage 1 was implemented in 2011 and 2012.

Stage 2: Advance Clinical Processes

This stage focuses on expanding on Stage 1 criteria to encourage the use of health information technology (HIT) for continuous quality improvement at the point of care and the exchange of health information in the most structured format possible. Criteria for Stage 2 include:

- More rigorous health information exchange (HIE)
- Increased requirements for e-prescribing and incorporating lab results
- Electronic transmission of patient care summaries across multiple settings
- More patient-controlled data

The final rule for Stage 2 was released in October 2012 and was implemented in 2014. Modified Stage 2 must be demonstrated by 2017. In Stage 2, eligible providers must meet 17 core objectives and 3 of 6 menu objectives. **Figures 5-2A** and **5-2B** illustrate the objectives for Stage 2 meaningful use.

Refer to the *Meaningful Use* tab in the *Contents* section of *Help* in Harris CareTracker for the most current information available on meaningful use.

List of Core Requirements - Final Regulation

ARRA EHR MEANINGFUL USE STAGE 1 REQUIREMENTS

CT #	CORE REQUIREMENTS (must meet all of these)
C 1	Record demographics as structured data for preferred language, race, ethnicity, date of birth, and gender (50 percent requirement).
C 2	Record and chart changes in vital signs (BP, height, weight, & display BMI); additionally, plot and display growth charts for children age 2 to 20 including BMI (50 percent requirement).
C 3	Maintain an up-to-date problem list of current and active diagnoses based on ICD-9-CM or SNOMED CT (80 percent of all unique patients admitted have at least one entry or an indication of "no problems are known" recorded as structured data).
C 4	Maintain active medication list with at least one entry or indication of "no currently prescribed medications" as structured data (80 percent requirement).
C 5	Maintain active medication allergy list with at least one entry or indication of "no known medication allergies" as structured data (80 percent requirement).
C 6	Record smoking status for patients 13 years old or older as structured data (50 percent requirement).
C 7	Provide patient with clinical summary for patients for each office visit within 3 business days (more than 50 percent for all office visits).
C 8	Provide patients with electronic copy of their health information (problems, medication, medication allergies, diagnostic test results) upon request (50 percent of patients must receive electronic copy within three days).
C 9	Generate and transmit permissible prescriptions electronically — eRx (40 percent requirement, does not apply to hospitals)
C 10	Use CPOE for medication orders directly entered by any licensed healthcare professional who can enter orders into the medical record per state, local, and professional guidelines. (30 percent for patients with at least one medication ordered through CPOE)
C 11	Implement drug-drug and drug-allergy interaction checks (functionality is enabled for these checks for the entire reporting period)
C 12	Implement capability to electronically exchange key clinical information among providers and patient authorized entities (Perform at least one test of EHR's capacity to exchange information)
C 13	Implement one clinical decision support rule relevant to specialty or high clinical priority along with and ability to track compliance for that rule.
C 14	Protect electronic health information created or maintained by the certified EHR technology through the implementation of appropriate technical capabilities (conduct or review a security risk analysis in accordance with the requirements and implement security updates as necessary)
C 15	Report ambulatory clinical quality measures to CMS or states (For 2011, provide aggregate numerator, denominator, and exclusions through attestation, 2012 submit electronically).

© Ingenix, Inc. 6

INGENIX.

Courtesy of Harris CareTracker PM and EMR

Figure 5-1A   Stage 1 List of Core Requirements

The Menu Set Requirements – Final Regulation

ARRA EHR MEANINGFUL USE STAGE 1 REQUIREMENTS

CT #	MENU SET (must meet 5 of these)
M 16	Implement drug-formulary checks (generate at least one report for entire reporting period).
M 17	Incorporate clinical lab-test results into EHR as structured data (40 percent of all tests ordered with results in a positive/negative or numerical format).
M 18	Generate lists of patients by specific conditions to use for quality improvement, reduction of disparities, research, and outreach (generate at least one report with a list of patients with a specific condition)
M 19	Use certified EHR to identify patient-specific education resources and provide to patient if appropriate (10 percent requirement).
M 20	The eligible provider who receives a patient from another setting of care or provider of care or believes an encounter is relevant should perform medication reconciliation (50 percent requirement).
M 21	The eligible provider who transitions there patient to another setting of care or provider of care or refers their patient to another provider of care should provide summary care record for each transition of care and referral (50 percent requirement).
M 22	Capability to submit electronic data to immunization registries or Immunization Information Systems and actual submission in accordance with applicable law and practice (perform at least one test if the registry has the capability to receive electronically). NOTE: EP must complete one of Immunization or Syndromic Surveillance unless has an exception for both.
M 23	Capability to submit electronic syndromic surveillance data to public health agencies and actual transmission in accordance with applicable law and practice (perform at least one test unless public health agencies to not have the capacity to receive electronically) NOTE: Must complete one of Immunization or Syndromic Surveillance unless EP has an exception for both.
M24	Send appropriate reminders to patients per patient preference for preventative/follow up care during the 90 day reporting period for patients 65 and older or 5 years and younger (20 percent requirement).
M 25	Provide patients with timely electronic access to their health information, including laboratory results, problem list, medication list, and medication allergies within four business days of the information being available to the eligible provider (10 percent requirement).

INGENIX.

Courtesy of Harris CareTracker PM and EMR

Figure 5-1B   Stage 1 Menu Set Requirements

Eligible Professionals

Report on all 17 Core Objectives:
1. Use computerized provider order entry (CPOE) for medication, laboratory and radiology orders
2. Generate and transmit permissible prescriptions electronically (eRx)
3. Record demographic information
4. Record and chart changes in vital signs
5. Record smoking status for patients 13 years old or older
6. Use clinical decision support to improve performance on high-priority health conditions
7. Provide patients the ability to view online, download and transmit their health information
8. Provide clinical summaries for patients for each office visit
9. Protect electronic health information created or maintained by the Certified EHR Technology
10. Incorporate clinical lab-test results into Certified EHR Technology
11. Generate lists of patients by specific conditions to use for quality improvement, reduction of disparities, research, or outreach
12. Use clinically relevant information to identify patients who should receive reminders for preventive/follow-up care
13. Use certified EHR technology to identify patient-specific education resources
14. Perform medication reconciliation
15. Provide summary of care record for each transition of care or referral
16. Submit electronic data to immunization registries
17. Use secure electronic messaging to communicate with patients on relevant health information

Courtesy of CMS.gov

Figure 5-2A   Stage 2 List of Core Requirements

Report on 3 of 6 Menu Objectives:
1. Submit electronic syndromic surveillance data to public health agencies
2. Record electronic notes in patient records
3. Imaging results accessible through CEHRT
4. Record patient family health history
5. Identify and report cancer cases to a State cancer registry
6. Identify and report specific cases to a specialized registry (other than a cancer registry)

Courtesy of CMS.gov

Figure 5-2B   Stage 2 Menu Set Requirements

Stage 3: Improved Outcomes

This stage focuses on the following:

- Promoting improvements in quality, safety, and efficiency
- Clinical decision support for national high-priority conditions
- Patient access to self-management tools
- Improving population health

This stage is expected to be implemented in 2017.

Tools within Harris CareTracker to Assist Providers with Meaningful Use

Learning Objective 2: Describe tools within Harris CareTracker PM and EMR that assist with meaningful use.

Learning Objective 3: View the meaningful use dashboard in Harris CareTracker PM and EMR.

The *Meaningful Use Dashboard* within Harris CareTracker PM tracks a provider's progress toward meeting the Medicare and Medicaid EHR Incentive Program reporting requirements for the core and menu set items. The dashboard displays a progress bar next to each of the measures that has a reporting requirement. **Figure 5-3A** illustrates a graphing screen of the core requirements for Dr. Olivia Sherman and **Figure 5-3B** illustrates the

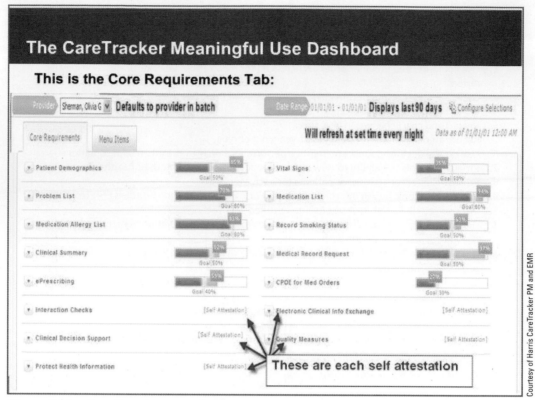

Figure 5-3A   Core Requirements for Dr. Olivia Sherman

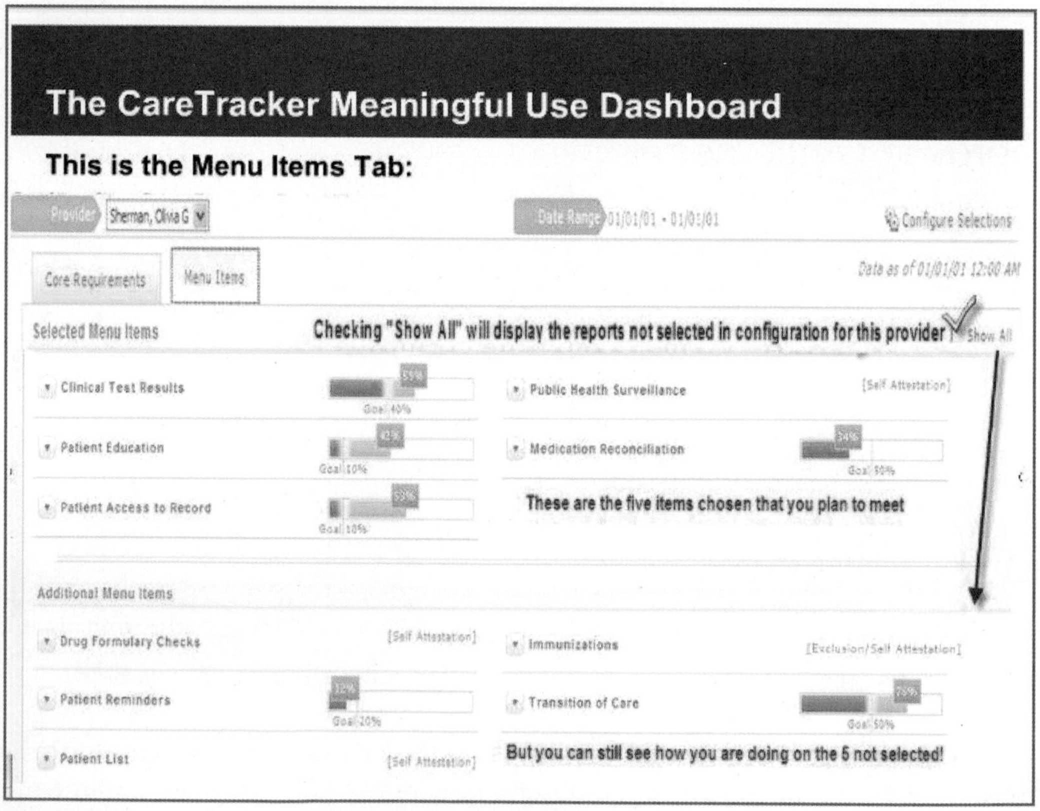

Figure 5-3B   Menu Requirements for Dr. Olivia Sherman

graphing features of the menu set requirements for Dr. Olivia Sherman. (Dr. Sherman is not a provider in our NVFHA environment.)

The dashboard's default date range is determined by when the provider begins the **attestation period**, or the date that begins the 90-day reporting period of meeting the core and menu measures listed previously. The dashboard calculates these measures over the previous 90 days.

From the dashboard, you can

- customize the requirements displayed on the dashboard for each participating provider,
- view a status of a provider's progress for the last 90 days (percentages updated nightly),
- hover over the percentage bar to review the data used to calculate the provider's percentage,
- click the *Menu Items* tab and then the drop-down arrow to download reference documents or run Key Performance Indicator (KPI) reports.

Activity 5-1
Viewing the *Meaningful Use Dashboard*

Note: Any time you are working in the EMR side of Harris CareTracker, you need to make sure that "Compatibility View" is turned off in your Internet Explorer browser. If you experience any functionality issues, please check your settings. (Refer to Best Practices for help.)

1. Click the *Home* module.

2. Click the *Meaningful Use* tab under the *Dashboard* tab (**Figure 5-4**). Harris CareTracker PM displays the *Meaningful Use Dashboard.*

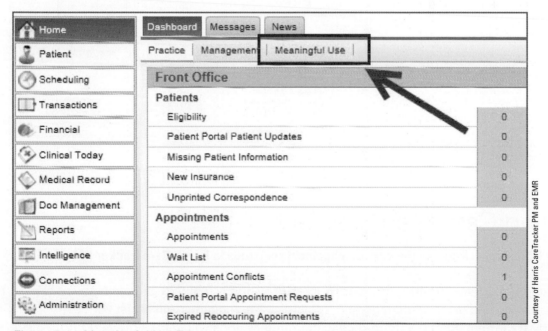

Figure 5-4   Meaningful Use Tab

3. From the *Provider* list, select the name of the provider whose data you want to view. In this case, click on "Brockton, Anthony." Harris CareTracker PM displays the provider's percentages on the *Core Requirements* tab (**Figure 5-5**).

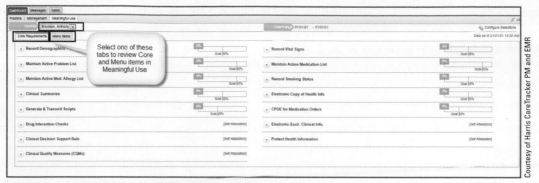

Figure 5-5   Dr. Brockton's Core Requirements

💾 **Print the Core Requirements screen, label it "Activity 5-1A," and place it in your assignment folder.**

4. Click the *Menu Items* tab to view the *Menu Items* requirements. On the *Menu Items* tab, select the *Show All* checkbox on the right-hand side of the screen to view any excluded requirements.

💾 **Print the Menu Items screen, label it "Activity 5-1B," and place it in your assignment folder.**

Because this is a training environment, you are only able to see the shell; no meaningful use statistics are available. **Figure 5-6** illustrates what a *Core Requirements* tab looks like in a fully functional environment.

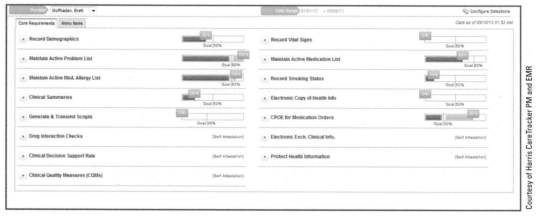

Figure 5-6   Core Requirements in a Fully Functional Environment

Activating Care Management

Learning Objective 4: Activate the care management registries in Harris CareTracker PM and EMR.

The *Care Management* feature in Harris CareTracker PM and EMR allows practices to set clinical measures for health maintenance and disease management registries. The registries will assist with early identification of disease and early treatment. Keeping up-to-date with immunizations will help to prevent future disease and control costs associated with those diseases. This feature also assists in meeting some of the standards of meaningful use.

By default, clinical measures are turned off in Harris CareTracker PM and EMR. You need to activate the registries and measures you want to make available to the providers in your group. As you will observe, these registries will check to determine if the patient is up-to-date with preventive testing and immunizations. After activation, the registries and measures selected are included in the *Pt Care Management* application of the *Medical Record* module and the *Care Management* application of the *Clinical Today* module. Registries are repopulated with the *Clinical Today/Population Management* tab. Once activation occurs, anytime you open the patient's chart, you can see where he or she falls within the registries and help the patient to come into compliance with testing or procedures.

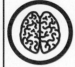

Activity 5-2
Activating Care Management Items

1. Click on the *Administration* module and then click the *Clinical* tab.

2. Click the *Care Management Activation* link under the *Maintenances* heading (**Figure 5-7A**). Harris CareTracker PM and EMR launches the *Care Management Activation* application.

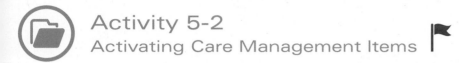

Figure 5-7A   Care Management Activation Link

3. Select all of the measures and registries listed by selecting/clicking on all of the boxes. The check boxes are dynamic and will auto-save on a single click. (A green "Saved" message appears briefly when each box is clicked to indicate the settings are saved [**Figure 5-7B**].)

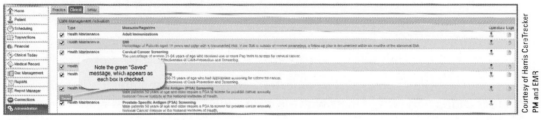

Figure 5-7B   Care Activation Measures and Registries

Print the Care Management Activation screen, label it "Activity 5-2," and place it in your assignment folder.

CRITICAL THINKING As a clinical medical assistant, it will be your job to help patients stay current with prevention measures and disease management goals. This not only helps the practice stay in compliance with meaningful use, but also promotes improved overall health for the patient. Review **Figure 5-8** and identify the patient's overdue test(s).

Outline an action plan to assist the patient in getting back on track with overall health prevention and maintenance. Share the action plan with the patient, and, if possible, schedule any necessary future appointments during the current visit to help the patient reach his or her overall goals. Submit your action plan to your instructor for class discussion.

(Continues)

(Continued)

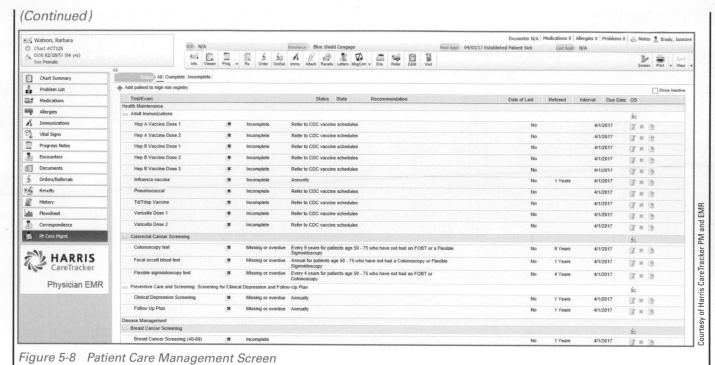

Figure 5-8   *Patient Care Management Screen*

Courtesy of Harris CareTracker PM and EMR

NAVIGATING THE MEDICAL RECORD MODULE

Learning Objective 5: Navigate throughout the Medical Record module.

The *Medical Record* module is designed to mimic a paper chart and to follow the provider's normal workflow, facilitating effective EHR documentation for a patient. The module is accessed by pulling the patient into context on the *Name Bar* and then clicking the *Medical Record* module. If a patient has an appointment scheduled, you can click the patient name in the *Appointments* application (tab) of the *Clinical Today* module to launch the *Medical Record* module. You will learn more about the *Clinical Today* module in Chapter 6. Some of the primary advantages of the *Medical Record* module in Harris CareTracker PM and EMR are as follows:

- Reduces or eliminates chart supply and storage, transcription costs, malpractice premiums, and other costs
- Replaces paper charts and file cabinets with electronic files and minimizes space required to store paper charts
- Maximizes revenue with effective patient services, improves documentation capabilities, improves coding accuracy through use of templates, and enhances charge capturing
- Increases clinical and staff efficiency through reduced data entry, high-quality documentation, patient education, and more
- Includes multitasking capability to work on a number of patient records simultaneously
- Provides a user-friendly interface that helps customize the electronic paper chart to suit user needs

The *Medical Record* module consists of four main components: *Patient Detail Bar, Patient Health History* pane, *Clinical Toolbar,* and *Chart Summary.* **Table 5-1** provides a brief description of each component.

Patient Detail Bar

The *Patient Detail Bar* (**Figure 5-9**) can be found at the top of the window once you open the patient's medical record. **Table 5-2** describes the components of the *Patient Detail Bar.* When working in the patient's *Medical Record* module (clinical side), the *Patient Detail* bar displays the patient's picture along with a summary of demographic, appointment, and clinical information. Additionally, the operator's name (your name) displays reflecting who is currently accessing the patient's medical record. Having the patient's picture display each time you access his or her medical record helps to quickly identify the patient.

Table 5-1 *Medical Record* Module Components

COMPONENT	DESCRIPTION
Patient Detail Bar	Provides a summarized view of demographic, appointment, and clinical information pertinent to the patient
Patient Health History Pane	A series of panes reviewing, entering, and editing historical patient information such as allergies, problem list, medications, and more
Clinical Toolbar	A series of tool buttons used as a workflow tool during a patient's appointment to record information such as progress notes, medications, immunizations, *Message Center,* visits, and more
Chart Summary	Provides an overview of a patient's medical record

Courtesy of Harris CareTracker PM and EMR

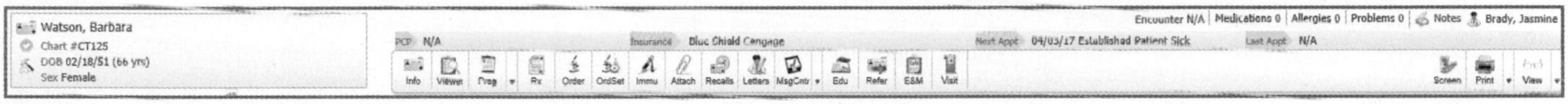

Figure 5-9   Patient Detail Bar

Table 5-2 Patient Detail Bar Components in the *Medical Record* Module

COMPONENT	DESCRIPTION
Patient Information	Located just to the left of the patient's name and includes the patient's name, address, telephone numbers, provider's name, appointment information, and more.
Patient Alert	When working in the *Medical Record* module, the *Patient Alert* box appears as a red triangle below the *Patient Information Bar* and contains three types of alerts: clinical alerts, patient care management alerts, and clinical notes. The red triangle appears both inside and outside of the patient's record once the patient's name is brought into context. If the patient does not have any clinical alerts, a blue check mark appears in the space where the red triangle would normally appear to illustrate that there are no clinical concerns at this time.
Patient's Chart Number	Located beside the *Patient Alert* and identifies the chart number assigned to the patient.
Break the Glass	The hammer (if displayed), located below the *Patient Alert* icon indicates "Break the Glass." This allows users to review *VIP* patient charts, and patient charts from other groups when the practice has more than one group. Even though the user is not in the specified group, by breaking the glass, the user is able to review the contents of the patient's chart for that session. Users who have "Break the Glass" privileges must provide a reason for breaking the glass.
Patient's DOB and Age	This is located beside the hammer (if displayed) and lists the patient's birth date and age.
Sex	Located just below the patient's DOB and states the patient's sex.
PCP	Located just above the clinical tool bar and lists the patient's primary care provider.

(*Continues*)

Table 5-2   **Patient Detail Bar Components in the *Medical Record* Module** (*Continued*)

COMPONENT	DESCRIPTION
Insurance	Located to the right of the PCP and lists the patient's insurance provider.
Next Appointment Date	Located just to the right of the insurance information. Displays the patient's next scheduled appointment.
Last Appointment Date	Located to the right of the next appointment information. Lists when the patient's last appointment took place.
Encounter	Located above and to the right of the next appointment information. This is the area that you click on when you want to review dates of previous encounters or to create a new encounter.
Medications	Located beside encounter information and lists how many medications the patient is taking. By clicking on "Medications," you can see the names of the medications the patient is taking and their doses.
Allergies	Located by the medication information and lists the number of allergies the patient has. By clicking on "Allergies," you can see a listing of the patient's allergies.
Problems	Located beside the allergy information. This lists the number of diagnoses or problems that are considered current. By clicking on "Problems," you can see a list of diagnoses and ICD codes for the patient.
Notes	Located beside the problems. This lists any notes about the patient such as what the patient wants to be called, reminder information, etc.
Training Operator	Should include your sign-in name.

Courtesy of Harris CareTracker PM and EMR

Activity 5-3
Viewing a Summary of Patient Information

1. In the *ID* search box on the *Name Bar*, enter "tol" (for the last name "Tolman" and hit [Enter]. The *Patient Search* dialog box displays with a list of patients matching the search criteria you entered.

2. Click on Gabby Tolman's name to bring her record into context (**Figure 5-10**).

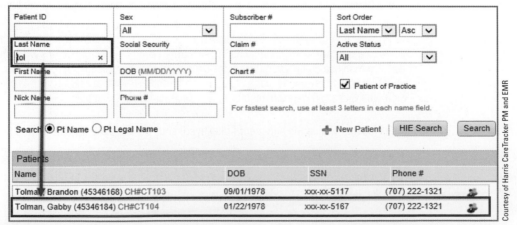

Figure 5-10   Click on Gabby Tolman's Name to Bring Up Her Medical Record

3. Click on the *Patient* module, which will open the *Demographics* tab.

4. You will notice that in Gabby's demographics window, no primary care provider (PCP) has been selected. Click on *Edit*, then scroll down to *PCP*, click on the drop-down list, and select "Anthony Brockton" as her PCP.

5. Scroll down and click *Save*. The *Patient Alerts* dialog box will display after saving. Close out of the *Patient Alerts* dialog box. You will see the update you made to the patient's PCP in her *Patient Details* screen.

6. Click on the *Medical Record* module.

7. A clinical alert comes up alerting you that the patient is allergic to codeine. Click on *Close* to exit the box.

8. To view Gabby's summary information, click the *Patient Information* icon 🖼️ to the left of the patient's name. **Figure 5-11** illustrates what the summary looks like once you click on the *Patient Information* icon.

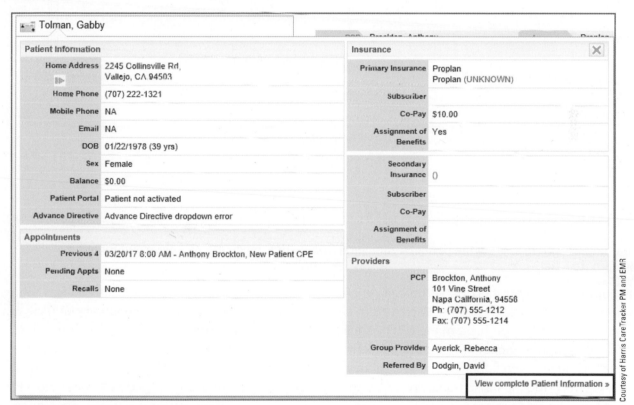

Figure 5-11   Patient Information Screen

9. To view additional patient information details, click the *View complete Patient Information* link on the lower right of the window. **Figure 5-12** illustrates what the window should like once you click on the *View complete Patient Information* link.

10. Close out of the *Complete Patient Information* screen by clicking "X" on the browser window.

💾 **Print the View complete Patient Information screen by right-clicking on the screen and selecting the Print function. Label it "Activity 5-3" and place it in your assignment folder.**

11. Close out of Gabby Tolman's *Chart Summary* by clicking "X" on the browser window.

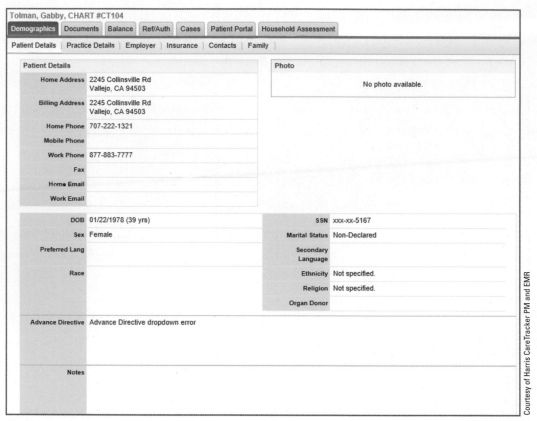

Figure 5-12   *View Complete Patient Information Link*

Viewing Encounter Information

Learning Objective 6: View the patient's encounter information, medications, allergy information, and problem list.

An **encounter** is an interaction with a patient on a specific date at a specific time and includes visits, phone calls, renewal requests, results, and more. Each patient can have many encounters, each encounter can have many services, and each service can have many CPT® codes associated with it. You must review, capture visit information, transcribe, sign, and bill appointment-based patient "visit"-type encounters, something you will learn more about in subsequent chapters. Additionally, you must capture visit information and bill custom encounters that are flagged as "Billing Required." You must also transcribe and sign notes for encounters that are flagged as "Signed Note Required."

In addition, the *Encounters* application enables you to view the primary diagnosis pertaining to an encounter and sort encounters based on specific diagnoses. This makes it easy to review data for a specific diagnosis when seeing patients for a recurring problem.

Activity 5-4
Viewing the Encounters Application, Active Medications, Allergies, and Problems

1. Pull patient Gabby Tolman into context.

2. Click on the *Medical Record* module. The *Clinical Alerts* dialog box will display. Close out of the *Clinical Alerts* dialog box and proceed with the activity.

3. To view Gabby Tolman's encounter information, click on the word *Encounter* (which appears blue) in the detail bar (at the top right of the screen). A box with a listing of the patient's previous encounters will pop up as well as an option to create a new encounter (**Figure 5-13**). Make a note of the date of the patient's only encounter that displays in your screen: _____.

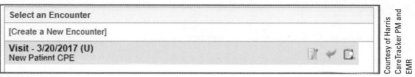

Figure 5-13   *Creating a New Encounter*

4. Close the encounter window by clicking on the "X" in the top right corner of the window.

5. View clinical information for the patient, such as the active medications, allergies, and problems, by clicking the corresponding link in the *Patient Detail* bar (located in the upper-right portion of your screen on the same line following *Encounter*) and record this information.

📰 **On a blank sheet of paper write down the date of the patient's only encounter, a listing of the patient's active medications, and any problems listed for the patient. Label the page "Activity 5-4" and place it in your assignment folder.**

6. Close out Gabby Tolman's chart summary by clicking "X" on the *Medical Record* browser window.

Viewing Patient Alerts.

Learning Objective 7: State the three types of alerts in Harris CareTracker PM and EMR.

In Chapter 3, you learned about patient alerts. This chapter expands on the clinical components of this feature. You can view clinical alert information for a patient by clicking on the *Alert* ⚠ icon next to the chart number in the *Medical Record* module. Harris CareTracker PM and EMR displays the *Clinical Alerts* dialog box with three patient alert types. **Table 5-3** describes each alert type.

Table 5-3 Alert Types	
ALERT	**DESCRIPTION**
Clinical Alerts	Alerts with important information related to the patient's health. The clinical alerts are categorized to display alerts for patient allergies, medications, diagnoses, and more.
	Additionally, for OB/GYN practices, the clinical alerts provide you the ability to view estimated gestational age (EGA) alerts.
Patient Care Management Alerts	Alerts for overdue important patient health maintenance and disease management items.
Clinical Notes	Clinical notes entered in the *Demographic* application of the *Patient* module.

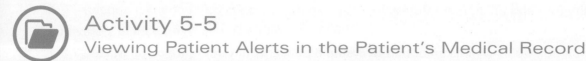

Activity 5-5
Viewing Patient Alerts in the Patient's Medical Record

1. Pull patient Gabby Tolman into context.

2. Click on *Medical Record.*

3. When you open the *Medical Record*, the alert box automatically pops up. Review the information in the box before closing it out. Close out of the box by clicking on *Close*.

4. Click on the *Alert* ⚠ icon to the left of the chart number. Notice that the information that pops up here is the same clinical alert information that popped up when you opened the medical record.

💾 **Write down any alerts listed for Gabby on a piece of paper. Label the page "Activity 5-5" and place it in your assignment folder.**

5. Click *Close* on the *Clinical Alerts* box.

6. Close Gabby Tolman's *Chart Summary* screen by clicking "X" on the *Medical Record* browser window.

Patient Health History Pane

The *Patient Health History* pane (**Figure 5-14**) is a series of panes located to the left of the *Chart Summary* content in the *Medical Record* module that you can use to access different applications for reviewing, entering, and editing patient information such as diagnoses, medications, and more. The function of each pane is described in **Table 5-4**.

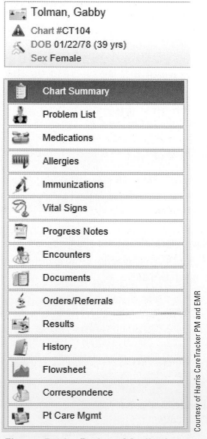

Figure 5-14 Patient Medical History Pane

Courtesy of Harris CareTracker PM and EMR

Table 5-4   Patient Health History Panes

PATIENT HEALTH HISTORY PANE	FUNCTION
Chart Summary	A view-only window displaying a summary of patient medical information. The *Chart Summary* is customizable based on the layout and level of detail you want to see.
Problem List	A list of chronic and ongoing patient problems. The *Problem List* application helps you to add and edit patient diagnoses including conditions managed by other physicians.
Medications	Displays all prescribed medications for the patient. The *Medications* application is where you add and edit routine and over-the-counter (OTC) medications, medications provided by other providers, and also renew existing prescriptions.
Allergies	A list of patient allergies. The *Allergies* application is where you add and edit allergies and other types of sensitivities. It is important to keep all allergy information updated, especially medication allergies, for screening purposes.
Immunizations	A list of immunizations given to the patient. The application provides access to child and adult immunization schedules and is where you record any immunizations refused by the patient.
Vital Signs	Displays patient statistics such as height, weight, and blood pressure taken during each office visit or at home. The *Vital Signs* application is where you record vital signs for each "visit" type encounter. Harris CareTracker PM and EMR supports graphing of vital signs that assists in identifying trends.
Progress Notes	Displays information about patient visits documented via quick text, point and click, dictation, or a combination of methods. It is important to review and sign notes taken during a visit.
Encounters	Displays all patient encounters. These encounters can vary from a telephone conversation to an office visit.
Documents	Displays all scanned or uploaded documents and voice recordings for the patient; for example, clinical documents, insurance cards, or identification cards. You can open the documents in the *Document Viewer* to add annotations, edit, delete, and sign.
Orders/Referrals	Displays test orders and referrals for the patient. The *Orders* application works simultaneously with the *Results* application to provide quick access to test results of completed orders, enabling entering of manual results and linking to lab results received electronically. The *Referrals* application is where you manage the process of patient movement between primary care providers, specialists, and institutions.
Results	Displays patient test results. Abnormal results display in red to help identify issues needing immediate attention. The *Results* application works simultaneously with the *Orders* application, enabling you to view the order associated with the result.
History	Displays patient information such as the family, past medical and social history. The application enables recording more information for existing and additional family members when necessary.
Flowsheet	Displays clinical measures, allowing you to track several aspects of a patient's health at one time. *Flowsheets* are most commonly used for tracking vital statistics, diabetic insulin dosages, pain assessment, lab results, blood pressure, medication start and stop dates, physical assessment, and drug frequency. It is also a good solution for pediatric growth charts and prenatal recordings.
Correspondence	Displays all *To Do*(s) for the patient and other communications such as patient education, recall, or collection letters provided or mailed to the patient.
Pt Care Mgmt	Displays a list of overdue preventive or maintenance items such as screening plans that need to be completed for the patient.

Courtesy of Harris CareTracker PM and EMR

To familiarize yourself with these panes, go into Gabby Tolman's medical record, click out of the alert box, and click on each of the panes in the *Patient Health History Pane* (e.g., click on *Chart Summary, Problem List, Medications*). You will learn the specifics of each pane in future activities.

Clinical Toolbar

The *Clinical Toolbar* (**Figure 5-15**) is a convenient workflow tool that you can use to record information during a patient appointment. The toolbar can be found in *Medical Record* module and contains a series of tool buttons. The function of each button is described in **Table 5-5**.

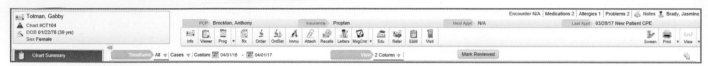

Figure 5-15   Clinical Toolbar
Courtesy of Harris CareTracker PM and EMR

Table 5-5   The Clinical Toolbar

CLINICAL TOOL BUTTON	FUNCTION
Patient Information (Info)	The *Patient Information* window provides access to a patient's demographic, appointment, and other information. The information is grouped into categories and is accessible by clicking the specific tab. You can also view a picture of the patient, if available. For information on the *Patient Information* window, see *Name Bar > Info* in the *Help* system.
Chart Viewer (Viewer)	The *Chart Viewer* provides a quick and easy way to access other applications when documenting a clinical encounter at the point of care. Each section corresponds to data saved in Harris CareTracker PM and EMR for the patient.
Progress Note (Prog)	The *Progress Notes* application helps you document the patient visit in various methods that include diagnosis-specific guidelines, provider-specific templates, quick-pick templates, dictation, or a combination of all. Harris CareTracker PM and EMR supports a variety of data entry methods including quick text, pen-tablets with handwriting recognition, voice recognition, or point-and-click mechanism.
Prescriptions (Rx)	The *Rx Writer* application (Surescripts® certified for prescription routing), uses the Surescripts® network to transmit electronic prescriptions directly to a selected pharmacy. A medication is always screened for interactions before it is prescribed. Additionally, the application provides a dosing calculator to view dosage recommendations for medications based on weight and age.
Order	The *Orders* application enables you to enter new orders and process orders by printing and sending to a clinical lab or by sending electronically via the Health Level 7 (HL7) interface. Orders sent electronically provide speed and efficiency for processing and reduces the amount of time spent filling in the lab requisition and related paperwork.
Order Set (OrdSet)	The *Order Set* application enables you to group patient orders for a specific diagnosis or condition. This promotes efficiency during the clinical decision-making process, standardizes the patient care processes, expedites the process of order entry, and reduces delays due to inconsistent or incomplete orders. The *Order Set* application helps create, modify, and manage order sets, making it available among all providers.

(*Continues*)

CLINICAL TOOL BUTTON	FUNCTION
Immunizations (Immu)	The *Immunization* application facilitates documenting immunizations administered during a patient visit. Additionally, the application helps administer vaccinations from a "lot" and helps you manage information on immunization lots that pertain to the group. **Lot** is defined by the U.S. Food and Drug Administration as a collection of primary containers or units of the same size, type, and style manufactured or packed under similar conditions and handled as a single unit of trade.
Attachments (Attach)	The *Document Management Upload* application helps upload or scan documents that include anything from a letter to a medical report for the patient. Examples of documents include lab results, radiology reports, dictations, photographs, and insurance cards. In addition, you can record audio files with information about the patient. For example, you can record a voice mail message that you left for the patient regarding a treatment process.
Recalls	The *Recall* application helps create patient reminders and letters for events such as annual physical exams, follow-up consultations, and lab tests. This feature helps the office to keep track of patients and ensure that proper medical care is provided.
Letters	The *Letters* application helps generate and print anything from a letter to a label for a patient by extracting information from the patient medical record. For example, referral letters, surgery consent letters, and appointment letters.
Message Center (MsgCntr)	The *Messages* application facilitates patient-related communications with patients (if the patient is registered in Harris CareTracker's Patient Portal), office staff, and Harris CareTracker PM and EMR Support Department staff without having to pull or file a chart. For example, a provider can send a *ToDo* to the front office staff to call the patient. There are three components in the Message Center: (1) New ToDo, (2) New Fax, and (3) New Mail.
Patient Education (Edu)	The *Patient Education* application gives you access to a comprehensive library of education material provided by Krames StayWell (the largest provider of interactive, print and mobile patient education solutions, consumer health information, and population health management communications in the country). This is useful to view and print disease-specific educational information you can give to a patient. The application also provides links to clinical websites (such as Medline Plus) and specialty-specific associations.
Referral (Refer)	The *Referral* application helps manage inbound and outbound referrals and authorizations. This helps manage the process of patient movement among primary care providers, specialists, and institutions.
E&M Evaluator (E&M)	The *E&M Evaluator* application helps identify the most appropriate E&M procedure (CPT®) code to use when charging for office visits and consultations. The code is calculated based on the information documented during the visit. Additionally, the application helps you apply either the 1995 or the 1997 E&M Documentation Guidelines issued by the American Medical Association (AMA) and the Centers for Medicare and Medicaid Services (CMS) to identify the correct code for the level of service provided.
Visits (Visit)	The *Visits* application helps capture information such as CPT® and ICD codes for the patient encounter. The electronic format supports a paperless information capturing system for submitting claims to the corresponding insurance companies in an expedited manner, that in turn increases the practice cash flow.
Screen	The *Screen* feature enables you to check for drug interactions in real time for the patient in context. This complete screening is for informational purposes only and includes interactions based on active diagnoses, medications and allergies, patient's age and weight, duplicate therapy, food interactions, and precaution screening.

(Continues)

Table 5-5   The Clinical Toolbar (*Continued*)

CLINICAL TOOL BUTTON	FUNCTION
Print 🖨	The *Print* feature exports patient data into a PDF format in one- or two-column layout. Additionally, you can print the chart summary, formal medical record, visit summary, and also print reports pertaining to each section in the patient's medical record. For example, you can access the *Medications* application, then click *Print* on the *Clinical* toolbar to print the Medication Summary Report.
View 👓	The *View* feature enables you to view the Clinical Log and the Continuity of Care Document (CCD) of the patient. Additionally, the feature displays interfaces active for your company. However, you can access the interface only if data is available for the patient in context.

Courtesy of Harris CareTracker PM and EMR

You will be using these tools throughout your training activities.

Chart Summary

Learning Objective 8: View, change, and print a Chart Summary in Harris CareTracker EMR.

The *Chart Summary* is a paperless format of a patient's medical record. It is a proprietary display that serves as a medical and legal record of a patient's clinical status, care history, and caregiver involvement.

The information on the *Chart Summary* is taken from various applications within Harris CareTracker PM and EMR. Information available in the *Chart Summary* includes contact and personal information, problem and medication lists, lab results, patient history, and other information. You can access the *Chart Summary* by clicking on the *Medical Record* module.

Activity 5-6
Accessing a Patient Chart Summary Using the Name Bar

1. Pull patient Gabby Tolman into context.

2. Click the *Medical Record* module.

3. Review the *Clinical Alerts* dialog box and then close.

4. By default, the *Chart Summary* tab displays from the *Patient Health History* pane. (Your screen should look like **Figure 5-16**.) Review all of the categories in the *Chart Summary* by scrolling up and down using the scroll bar.

5. To change the look of the *Chart Summary*, find the gray *View* tab in the middle of the page, just below the *Clinical Toolbar* (**Figure 5-17**). Click on the drop-down arrow next to the *View* tab and change the view to "3 Column."

💾 **Click on the drop-down arrow next to the Printer 🖳 icon and select "Print Chart Summary." Label the printed chart summary "Activity 5-6" and place it in your assignment folder.**

6. Now change the *View* using the drop-down arrow and change the view to "1 Column."

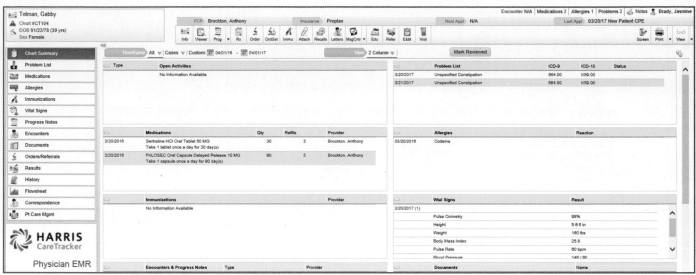

Figure 5-16   *Chart Summary*   Courtesy of Harris CareTracker PM and EMR

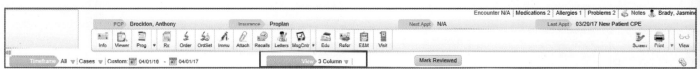

Figure 5-17   *View Column Drop-Down Menu*   Courtesy of Harris CareTracker PM and EMR

7. Change the *View* again using the drop-down arrow and selecting "Chronological."

8. Change the *View* back to the original "2 Column" view as originally set.

9. Close Gabby Tolman's *Chart Summary* screen by clicking "X" on the *Medical Record* browser window.

MAINTENANCE FUNCTIONS THAT AFFECT HARRIS CARETRACKER EMR

Learning Objective 9: Perform routine maintenance functions in Harris CareTracker PM and EMR such as adding a room, editing a room, adding a custom resource, and managing immunizations.

We have finished our navigation of the *Medical Record* module and are ready to make other adjustments in the PM side of Harris CareTracker. These adjustments will affect available options and other features displayed on the EMR side. There are several maintenance options in Harris CareTracker; however, we only spotlight a few features that impact the EMR.

Room Maintenance

It is important to have an efficient appointment workflow to better serve the patient during an appointment. The *Room Maintenance* feature helps you set up rooms to keep track of a patient appointment by updating a patient's location during his or her stay at your office. Building upon room maintenance activities completed in Chapter 2, continue with Activity 5-7, which illustrates how to add and name rooms within the system.

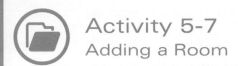

Activity 5-7
Adding a Room

1. Click the *Administration* module and then click the *Setup* tab.

2. Click the *Room Maintenance* link at the bottom of the *Scheduling* section (**Figure 5-18**).

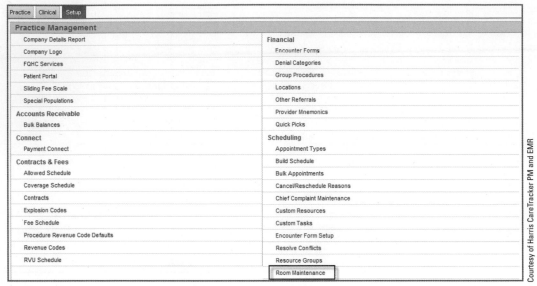

Figure 5-18   Room Maintenance Link

3. Click the drop-down menu beside (*Select*) to see what rooms are already in the system. (You will notice that there are two rooms listed for our environment: "Exam Room # 1" and "Exam Room # 2." You added "Exam Room # 2" in Activity 2-13. Note: If you began your work with the Clinical Module Quick Start, you will not have added Exam Room # 2, and it will not display.)

4. Click *Add* beside the (*Select*) drop-down menu.

5. Enter "Exam Room # 3" in the *Room Name* box (**Figure 5-19**).

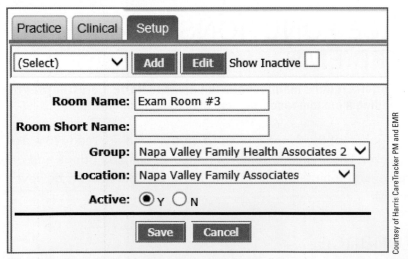

Figure 5-19   Add Exam Room #3

6. A "Room Short Name" field is available, which is not necessary to complete unless a short version or acronym of the room name is often used (leave blank).

7. Select "Napa Valley Family Health Associates 2" from the *Group* list.

8. Select "Napa Valley Family Associates" from the *Location* list. (These lists are useful for multilocation practices.)

9. By default, the *Active* field is set to "Y." This means the room is active.

10. Click *Save.* The application adds the room.

11. Click on the drop-down menu. "Exam Room # 1," "Exam Room # 2," and "Exam Room # 3" should appear in the drop-down list.

12. Now repeat the same procedure, adding the following rooms: "Triage Room" and "Cardiac Bay" with the same *Group* and *Location* as in Steps 7–8.

13. Click on the (*Select*) drop-down menu. All the rooms you added should appear in the drop-down list.

14. Click on the "Cardiac Bay" room listing.

🖫 **If you have a screenshot application with a "10-second delay" feature, you will be able to capture the drop-down list. If not, print the information from the Cardiac Bay field to illustrate that it was added to the list. Label it "Activity 5-7" and place it in your assignment folder.**

After a room is created you can edit the room's name, group, or location. You can also activate or deactivate a room. In a Build Your Proficiency activity at the end of the chapter, you will learn to edit rooms.

Custom Resources

There may be times where you will need to add *Resources* to the system. Resources can be people, places, or things. Providers are always considered a resource, but an exam room or a piece of equipment can also be considered a resource. Something that requires a schedule is considered a resource because it has specific availability with days and times it can provide certain services. If the resource does not need a set schedule then it is not considered a "resource" in Harris CareTracker PM and EMR.

After a resource is entered in the system, you can customize the resource, assign it to resource classes, and assign it to a resource group for scheduling purposes. Building upon the activities you completed in Chapter 2, add a custom resource (Activity 5-8).

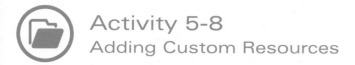

Activity 5-8
Adding Custom Resources

1. Click the *Administration* module and then click the *Setup* tab.

2. Click the *Custom Resources* link (**Figure 5-20**) under the *Scheduling* section. Harris CareTracker PM displays the *Schedule Resource* page. All providers and resources in the practice are listed as *Available Resources*.

3. Click *New* to the right of the *Available Resources* list. Harris CareTracker PM displays a dialog box, prompting you to enter a name for the resource.

4. In the dialog box, enter "Accent Laser Machine" (**Figure 5-21**).

5. Click *OK.* The application adds the resource to the *Available Resources* list (**Figure 5-22**).

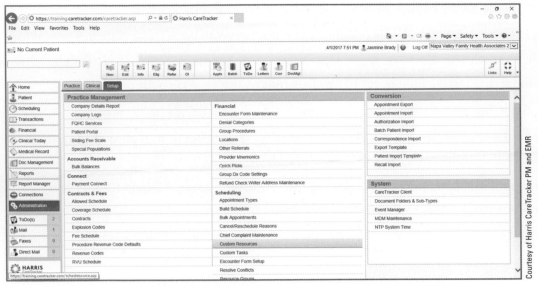

Figure 5-20   Custom Resources Link

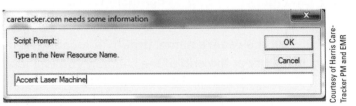

Figure 5-21   Add an Available Resource

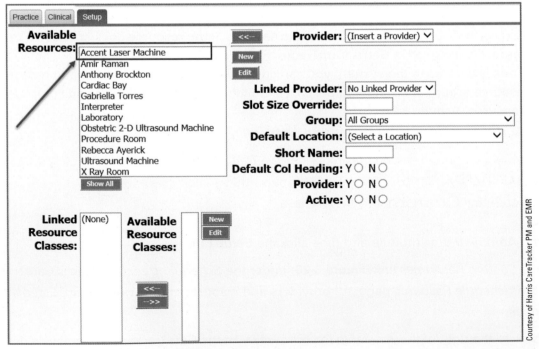

Figure 5-22   Available Resources List

Print a copy of the Available Resources screen, indicating that the Accent Laser Machine is now in the Available Resources box. Label it "Activity 5-8" and place it in your assignment folder.

Favorite Lab Maintenance

Every medical clinic has a few select labs they work with. Napa Valley Family Health Associates has its own lab, but some insurance companies require patients to go to a lab that they contract with. This is known as an "In Network" lab. The lab agrees to do testing for a fraction of the usual charge in exchange for the increased volume of patients. This results in a win for both the insurance company and the lab. Another lab may also be used when a test is requested that is not available through the Napa Valley lab. Having favorite labs available to be selected by the drop-down list and global database expedites the ordering process by avoiding the need to go through a long list of facilities supported by Harris CareTracker PM and EMR each time you create a lab order.

Favorite Labs can be managed through the *Administration* module, *Clinical* tab. In the *Daily Administration* section, you would click *Favorite Labs*. On the *Favorite Lab Maintenance* application, you can add new labs or modify or delete existing labs. This function is normally reserved for your site administrator, and therefore you will not complete *Favorite Lab* activities while using this book.

Manage Immunization Lots

The *Manage Immunization Lots* application enables you to manage immunization lots that pertain to groups. When immunizations are received, you can add the lot information for the immunizations to the system. After an immunization lot is added, the system keeps track of the inventory and deducts administered immunization from the quantity in the lot. Tracking inventory ensures that required immunizations can be reordered in a timely manner.

The *Manage Immunization Lots* application also enables you to modify lots, make lots inactive, and delete lots as necessary. You can also add and manage immunization lots via the *Add Immunization Lot* and *Edit Immunization Lot* dialog boxes accessed via the *Immunization* application in the *Clinical Toolbar*. Immunization lots are practice-specific and not determined by the provider selected in the *Admin Provider* list. Therefore, lot details recorded display in the *Lots* list for all providers.

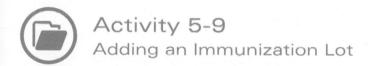

Activity 5-9
Adding an Immunization Lot

1. Click the *Administration* module, and then click the *Clinical* tab.

2. Click the *Manage Immunization Lots* link under the *Daily Administration* header. Harris CareTracker PM and EMR displays the *Immunization Lots* application, which displays existing immunization lots that have not yet been exhausted.

3. Click *+ Add Immunization Lot* (**Figure 5-23**) located to the far right of your screen. Harris CareTracker displays the *Add Immunization Lot* dialog box (**Figure 5-24**).

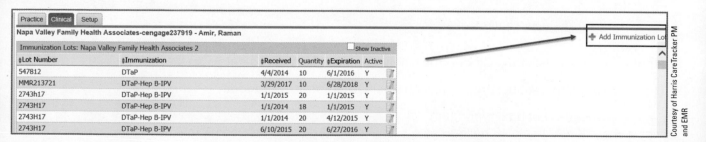

Figure 5-23   Adding an Immunization Lot

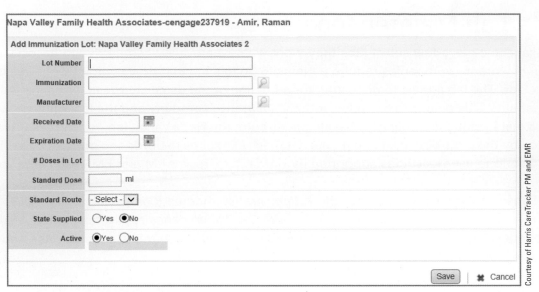

Figure 5-24   Add Immunization Lot Dialog Box

4. In the *Lot Number* box, enter "MMR" followed by your operator number. (For example, if your login username (operator number) is "cengage59290," you would enter the lot number "MMR59290".)

5. In the *Immunization* box, type "MMR" and then click the *Search* 🔍 icon.

6. Click on the word "MMR" under *Search Results* (**Figure 5-25**).

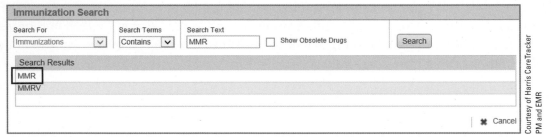

Figure 5-25   Select MMR in the Immunization Search Box

7. In the *Manufacturer* box, type the word "MedImmune" and then click the *Search* 🔍 icon. Select the radio dial (**Figure 5-26**) next to "MedImmune" under *Search Results*.

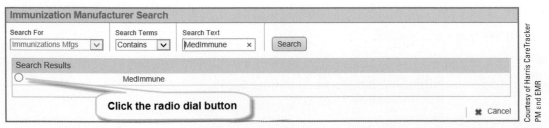

Figure 5-26   Radio Button

8. In the *Received Date* box, click on the calendar and select today's date.

9. In the *Expiration Date* box, type in a date that is 15 months from today's date.

10. In the *# Doses in Lot* box, type "10."

11. In the *Standard Dose* box, type "0.5."

12. In the *Standard Route* box, click the drop-down menu and select "SC" for "subcutaneous."

13. In the *State Supplied* category, click "No."

14. In the *Active* category, select "Yes."

15. Your dialog box should look like **Figure 5-27**. Click on *Save.*

Napa Valley Family Health Associates-cengage237919 - Amir, Raman

Add Immunization Lot: Napa Valley Family Health Associates 2

Lot Number	MMR237919
Immunization	MMR
Manufacturer	MedImmune
Received Date	04/01/2017
Expiration Date	07/01/2018
# Doses in Lot	10
Standard Dose	0.5 ml
Standard Route	SC
State Supplied	◯Yes ◉No
Active	◉Yes ◯No

Save | ✖ Cancel

Figure 5-27   Completed Add Immunization Lot Box

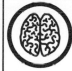 **Print the screen listing the Immunization Lots for NVFA to illustrate that the vaccine has been added to the list. Label it "Activity 5-9" and place in your assignment folder. (Hint: In order to find the lot you entered, you may need to scroll down the list in the "Lot Number" column, or it may help to sort the list by "Received" date.)**

CRITICAL THINKING   At the beginning of this chapter, you were asked to keep in mind how your position as a medical assistant may be impacted by meaningful use, and how you will be able to assist both providers and patients in meeting these goals. Having completed your studies and activities, describe how you see your role in the practice as an advocate for both the provider and patients. How will you incorporate meaningful use and patient care management in your daily activities?

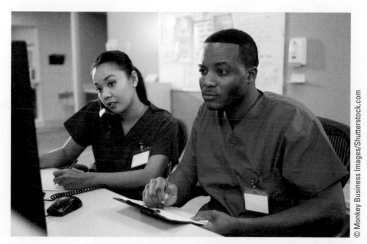

© Monkey Business Images/Shutterstock.com

SUMMARY

The electronic medical record consists of a wide range of capabilities. In this chapter, you learned some of the basic functions of Harris CareTracker EMR. The concept of meaningful use was introduced, and the stages of meaningful use were discussed. For providers to collect the financial incentives associated with Stage 1 meaningful use, they must go through a rigorous 90-day attestation period where they demonstrate that they have met the core and menu requirements. The provider must demonstrate attestation for a full year during the second year of the program. Meaningful Use Stage 2 requires two full years of attestation in order to receive financial incentives.

Meaningful use standards and the financial incentives created by the federal government for EMR implementation and has a substantial impact on the breadth and scope of EMR use. With most practices using electronic medical records, the need for medical professionals to be familiar with them and to be proficient in their use is critical.

Most of the activities in this chapter were designed to introduce you to the clinical side of Harris CareTracker and how to navigate in the EMR. Performing basic functions such as viewing the patient's medical record, adding rooms, and managing immunization lots will prepare you for working in the electronic medical record. As you begin your career in health care, this basic knowledge of electronic medical records will be essential to your success.

CHECK YOUR KNOWLEDGE

Select the best response.

_____ 1. Which of the following is the acronym for the commission that certifies electronic medical records?

    a. CBHAT   c. HICCT

    b. CCHIT®   d. CCMIT

_____ 2. Which stage of meaningful use is considered the "Improved Outcome" stage?

    a. Stage 1   c. Stage 3

    b. Stage 2   d. Stage 4

_____ 3. How many core objectives are associated with Stage 2 meaningful use?

    a. 5   c. 14

    b. 10   d. 20

_____ 4. How long is the attestation period for Stage 1 meaningful use, during the first year of the program?

    a. 90 days   c. 180 days

    b. 120 days   d. 220 days

_____ 5. What tool within Harris CareTracker helps to measure meaningful use?

    a. *Clinical Toolbar*   c. *Meaningful Use* toolbar

    b. *Care Management* dashboard   d. *Meaningful Use* dashboard

_____ 6. The red triangle icon represents what in Harris CareTracker PM and EMR?

    a. Patient's chart number   c. Break the glass

    b. Patient alerts   d. Drug interactions

_____ 7. Where in the *Patient Health History* panes can you track vital statistics, diabetic insulin dosages, pain assessment, and other useful tracking information?

        a. Results   c. Flowsheet

        b. History   d. Patient Care Management

_____ 8. Where can you find the E&M evaluator in Harris CareTracker?

        a. *Clinical Toolbar*   c. *Administration* module

        b. *Chart Summary*   d. *Patient Health History* pane

_____ 9. What is the name of the Rx writer in Harris CareTracker EMR?

        a. CompleteScripts   c. Rx Scripts

        b. ElectronicScripts   d. Surescripts®

_____ 10. Once you open up the patient's medical record, where can you find the name of the patient's primary care provider?

        a. The *Patient Detail* bar   c. *Clinical Toolbar*

        b. The *Patient Health History* pane   d. *Chart Summary*

CASE STUDIES

Case Study 5-1

Access Donald Schwartz's chart using the *Name Bar*. Change the view of the chart summary to *Chronological* view. For help completing this activity, refer to Activity 5-6.

💾 **Print the screen with Donald Schwartz's chronological chart view, label it "Case Study 5-1," and place it in your assignment folder.**

Case Study 5-2

Add two new rooms to Harris CareTracker: *X-Ray* and *Laboratory*. For help completing this activity, refer to Activity 5-7.

💾 **Print a copy of the screens that illustrate you added the rooms. Label the *X-Ray* screenshot "Case Study 5-2A" and the *Laboratory* screenshot "Case Study 5-2B." Place each one in your assignment folder.**

BUILD YOUR PROFICIENCY

Proficiency Builder 5-1: Access the *Patient Care Management* Screen

The *Patient Care Management* application is used as a proactive reminder tool to improve the care management process. The application helps manage the recurring preventive care items pertinent to a patient by evaluating and moving to registries, flagging overdue items, processing order sets, and more. The registries include:

- *Health Maintenance*: This section displays all tests/exams that a patient is due for in the *Health Maintenance* registries.

(Continues)

BUILD YOUR PROFICIENCY (*Continued*)

- *Disease Management.* This section displays all tests/exams that a patient is due for OR is required according to disease management measures. You can click the *Expand* icon in the *Disease Management* section to view all items that are part of the disease management measure.

Important: A patient is placed into a disease management measure only if the patient has an active diagnosis that triggers the ICD code rule.

To access the *Patient Care Management* application:

1. Pull patient Jane Morgan into context.

2. Click on the *Medical Record* pane.

3. Click on the *Pt Care Mgmt* pane and the patient's health maintenance record will display.

4. The red "x" in the status column indicates that the patient is overdue for the test/exam recommendations.

5. You can also sort the status by clicking on "All," "Complete," or "Incomplete" in the *Status* row at the top of the page.

🖬 **Print the screen with Jane Morgan's *Patient Care Management*, label it "BYP 5-1," and place it in your assignment folder.**

Proficiency Builder 5-2: Edit a Room

There are times when the practice moves office locations, brings on new providers, converts one type of room to another use, etc. In these instances, it is required to change (edit) the existing room references. This Proficiency Builder will give you practice in performing this function. *(Note: You must have completed Activity 5-7 to be able to complete this activity.)*

1. Click the *Administration* module and then click the *Setup* tab.

2. Click the *Room Maintenance* link at the bottom of the *Scheduling* section.

3. (Optional) If you want to view all rooms created in Harris CareTracker PM and EMR including inactive rooms, select the *Show Inactive* checkbox. (All of our rooms are active.)

4. Select "Exam Room # 3" from the drop-down menu and then click *Edit.*

5. Change the name of the room to "Procedure Room" and click *Save.*

6. Click back on the *Administration* module.

7. Click on the *Setup* tab and then select the *Room Maintenance* link at the bottom of the *Scheduling* section.

8. Click the drop-down menu beside (*Select*). Make certain that "Exam Room # 3" is no longer an option and that "Procedure Room" is now an option. (If your changes did not go through, start again from step 2.)

🖬 **Print a copy of the window that illustrates you changed the name of the room to "Procedure Room." Label it "BYP 5-2" and place it in your assignment folder.**

Patient Work-Up

6

Key Terms

advance directive
anthropometric
contraindication
encounter
family history
flowsheet template
growth chart
iteration
open encounter

open order
patient history
progress note
sensitive information
SIG
Surescripts®
ToDo
transfer
unsigned note

Learning Objectives

1. Set operator preferences in your Batch applications.
2. List major applications of the Clinical Today module.
3. View daily appointments in Clinical Today.
4. Perform check-in duties and track patients throughout their visits.
5. Describe basic tasks of the medical assistant when working in Clinical Today.
6. View prescription renewals and new prescriptions within Clinical Today.
7. Retrieve the patient's EMR and update sections within the patient health history panes.
8. Record vital signs and document the patient's chief complaint.
9. View and create Flowsheets within Harris Care-Tracker EMR.
10. Create and print a growth chart.
11. Update the Patient Care Management application.
12. Create and print a Progress Note.

Real-World Connection

In this chapter, you are going to learn a great deal about working in the patient's electronic medical record (EMR). You are very fortunate to enter the medical field at a time when technology is flourishing. Electronic medical records organize the patient's information so that you know exactly where each item is stored within the patient's chart. EMRs also help medical assistants stay on task and keep up with lab reports and prescription renewals. Your challenge is to embrace the training in this chapter so that you are able to fully navigate the patient's medical record in Harris CareTracker EMR.

INTRODUCTION

As a medical assistant working in a clinical capacity, you will be responsible for completing the patient's work-up and documenting your findings; however, this is only a small portion of your responsibilities. You will also be responsible for screening patient phone calls, handling prescription requests, tracking lab results, and responding to messages from providers and other staff members within the practice. The *Clinical Today* module within Harris CareTracker PM and EMR helps to categorize and organize these tasks, improving quality and efficiency throughout the day. As a result, providers and staff members are continuously in sync with one another, enhancing communications, and, ultimately, patient care. This chapter introduces you to the *Clinical Today* module and provides activities representative of those you will perform in the industry.

This chapter also focuses on how to build the patient's electronic health record. As a student medical assistant working in the Harris CareTracker system, you will learn how to track patients throughout the visit, record vital signs and chief complaints, enter medication and history information, and transcribe physical and diagnostic findings from the provider. These activities comprise the front end of the clinical portion of the visit; the back end of the patient visit is discussed in Chapter 7.

> Before you begin the activities in this chapter, refresh your memory on working with Harris CareTracker by referring back to the Best Practices list on page xxiii of this textbook. This list is also posted to the student companion website. Following best practices will help you complete work quickly and accurately.

SETTING OPERATOR PREFERENCES IN THE BATCH APPLICATION

Learning Objective 1: Set operator preferences in your Batch applications.

As discussed in previous chapters, the *Batch* application in Harris CareTracker PM and EMR enables you to set operator preferences based on the workflow for your role. This reduces the number of clicks required to get from one application to the other, making navigation through Harris CareTracker easy. As a medical assistant working in a clinical capacity, you will want your screen to open in the *Clinical Today* module each time you log in to Harris CareTracker. Selecting the appropriate setting from the *Login Application* in your *Batch* preferences will take you directly to the *Clinical Today* module after logging in. Activity 6-1 will assist you in making the appropriate changes to your preferences. Changing your batch settings now is highly recommended to improve workflow.

 ## Activity 6-1
Setting Operator Preferences in Your Batch Application

1. To set up operator preferences, click *Batch* on the *Name Bar*. Harris CareTracker PM and EMR displays the *Operator Encounter Batch Control* dialog box.

2. Click on the *Edit* button.

3. Click on the drop-down arrow beside *Provider* and select "Dr. Raman," if he has not already been selected.

4. Click on the drop-down arrow beside *Resource* and select "Dr. Raman," if he has not already been selected.

5. Click on the drop-down arrow beside *Show Alerts* and select "Yes."

6. In the *Login Application* box, click on the drop-down arrow and select "Clinical."

7. Click on *Save*. Now every time you log in to Harris CareTracker, you will be taken directly to the *Clinical Today* module.

8. Click "X" in the right-hand corner to close the dialog box.

OVERVIEW OF THE CLINICAL TODAY MODULE

Learning Objective 2: List major applications of the Clinical Today module.

Within Harris CareTracker EMR, the *Clinical Today* module is the area where most medical assistants working in a clinical capacity spend their time. The *Clinical Today* module works as an electronic desk. It organizes and helps manage tasks by displaying items to be worked on daily. It also automates a large number of routine tasks, thereby increasing productivity. In addition, the module helps track patient workflow efficiently by displaying information about scheduled appointments and patient movements within the clinic. The application helps track the care of one or more patients in the practice and provides instant access to a patient's medical record that includes test results, clinical information, and more. The *Clinical Today* module consists of three main applications: *Appointments*, *Tasks*, and *Population Management*. This chapter focuses on the *Appointments* and *Tasks* applications.

Appointments

Learning Objective 3: View daily appointments in Clinical Today.

The *Appointments* application (**Figure 6-1**) consists of patient and nonpatient appointments scheduled via the *Book* application in the *Scheduling* module. The application mimics most features in the *Scheduling* module, enabling you to manage appointments and the appointment workflow. You can use the application to update, confirm and cancel appointments, update the appointment status, access the patient's medical record, view the patient's open activities, capture visit information, and more.

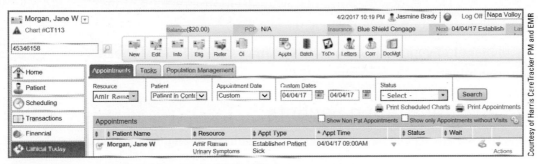

Figure 6-1   Appointment Screen in Clinical Today

Viewing Appointments in Clinical Today.

At the start of each day, you will review the patient appointment list for the current workday. Some workers like to make copies of the schedule and have it close by for easy referencing; however, with Harris CareTracker PM and EMR, this information is just a screen away.

In Chapter 4, you scheduled nine patients for future appointments and cancelled one, leaving eight patients with appointments. Now you will pull up some of these patients in *Clinical Today* and start working in the EMR portion of their records.

> **ALERT!** When you click on *Clinical Today*, the screen automatically defaults to the patients scheduled for the current date. For Activity 6-2, you will need the dates of the appointments you scheduled for patients in Chapter 4.

Activity 6-2
Viewing Appointments

1. Click on *Clinical Today*.

2. Click on the drop-down arrow under *Resource* and select "All."

3. Click on the drop-down arrow under *Patient* and select "All Patients."

4. Click on the drop-down arrow under *Appointment Date* and select "Custom."

5. Click on the calendar beside the first box under *Custom Dates* and select the date you scheduled Jane Morgan's appointment in Chapter 4.

6. Click in the second box to the right of the calendar under *Custom Dates*. The date that you inserted in the first box should automatically populate in this box.

7. In the status box, click on the drop-down arrow and select "All" (**Figure 6-2**). **Note:** You may have to click back on the body of the *Status* box field for the drop-down to disappear.

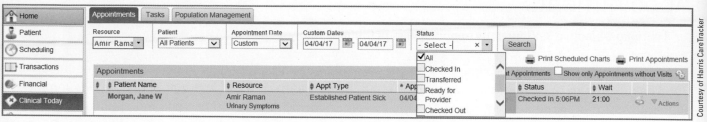

Figure 6-2   Select All

8. Click on *Search*. (The appointment screen with Ms. Morgan's appointment should now appear along with any other appointments scheduled on this day.)

📷 **Print a screenshot of your Appointment screen from Clinical Today. Label it "Activity 6-2" and place it in your assignment folder.**

Checking In and Transferring Patients

Learning Objective 4: Perform check-in duties and track patients throughout their visits.

In Chapter 4 (Activity 4-12), you practiced checking in patients. Patients are typically checked in upon arrival. This cues the clinical staff that the patient is ready to be taken back to the exam room. Once the patient has been transferred to the exam room, this will alert the staff of the patient's current status. Activity 6-3 describes how to change a patient's status from "Checked In" to "Transferred." **Transfer** refers to the status of a patient when he or she has been taken to an exam room.

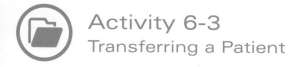

Activity 6-3
Transferring a Patient

1. Click on *Clinical Today*.

2. Match the search parameters to those set in Activity 6-2. Click *Search*.

3. Jane Morgan's appointment should be listed in the *Appointments* window. Her current status is green, which means that she has already been checked in. (**Note:** A row highlighted in red means the patient has been checked out. If you completed billing activities prior to this activity, the status would be red.)

4. Change her status by clicking on the drop-down arrow in her *Status* column and selecting "Transfer."

5. The *Patient Location* box will pop up. Select the radio button next to "Exam Room # 1."

6. Click *Select* (**Figure 6-3**). (**Note:** If the there is nothing listed in the *Patient Location* box, review your Compatibility View setting (refer to Best Practices) and try again.)

7. Ms. Morgan's entry line should now be blue, indicating that she has been transferred to the exam room. The appropriate exam room number will now appear in the *Status* column (**Figure 6-4**).

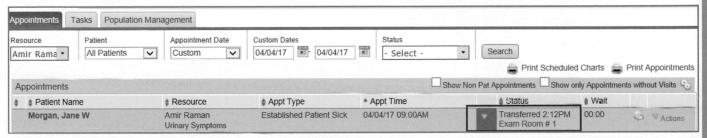

Figure 6-3   Patient Location Box

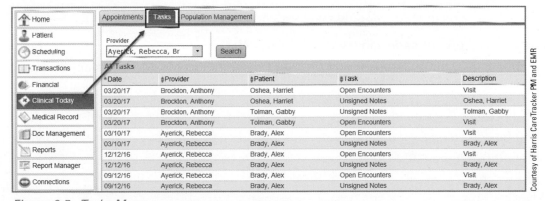

Figure 6-4   Exam Room Status Column

Courtesy of Harris CareTracker PM and EMR

Print a screenshot of the Exam Room Status Column. Label it "Activity 6-3" and place it in your assignment folder.

Tasks Menu

Learning Objective 5: Describe basic tasks of the medical assistant when working in Clinical Today.

The *Tasks* menu (**Figure 6-5**) displays an up-to-date number of any outstanding activities, such as lab results pending review, incomplete encounters, documents pending review, and more for all providers. Clicking on a specific task category will direct you to the list of items that requires attention. An **encounter** is an interaction with a patient on a specific date and time. Encounter types include visits, phone calls, referrals, results of a test, and more.

Figure 6-5   Tasks Menu

Courtesy of Harris CareTracker PM and EMR

TIP Currently there are only a few tasks populated within the *Tasks* application of *Clinical Today*. This environment will become populated with the activities that you will perform throughout the book. As you progress in completing activities, you will use this application frequently. In this section of the chapter, you will go through the steps of viewing clinical tasks, even though there are only a few tasks that are retrievable.

The *Tasks* application provides an integrated view of all open and active tasks that require attention. The tasks list helps you to efficiently manage routine tasks occurring throughout the practice and provide improved patient services. The tasks list provides the capability to manage the following:

- Complete all daily tasks in a timely manner.

- Create, reply, and transfer *ToDo*(s), mail, and fax messages. A **ToDo** is Harris CareTracker's internal messaging system.

- Review and sign unsigned test results.

- Review **open orders** (diagnostic tests that have been ordered but have no results).

- Efficiently manage prescription renewal requests.

- Efficiently manage patient documents.

- Resolve notes that must be transcribed.

- Resolve **open encounters** by entering visit information and signing notes. An open encounter is documentation of a patient visit that took place that was never completed.

- Resolve unmatched attachments.

SPOTLIGHT To leave at your regularly scheduled time each day, it is vital that you work on tasks between patients as well as the beginning and end of the day. There are usually two to three steps for each task: reviewing the task, alerting the provider, and following up with the patient when applicable. Not only will you need to be efficient, but you may need to keep your provider on course as well. When you observe visits that are incomplete, lab results not reviewed, or prescription requests unanswered, gently remind the provider that there are tasks waiting for his or her attention.

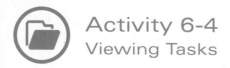

Activity 6-4
Viewing Tasks

1. Click on the *Clinical Today* module.

2. Click on the *Appointments* tab (see Figure 6-1). (**Note:** You may need to reset the *Resources* to "All," the *Patient* field to "All," and enter a *Custom Date* to reflect Ms. Morgan's appointment [see Activity 6-2].)

3. Find the *Quick Tasks* heading all the way over on the right side of the window. Click on the drop-down menu beside *Open Encounters*. (**Note:** You may need to scroll down in the tab to view all the *Open Encounters* [Figure 6-6].) *Quick Tasks* will populate as you work in Harris CareTracker entering patient data.

4. All open tasks can be reviewed by selecting the *Tasks* tab in *Clinical Today* (Figure 6-7). In the *Provider* box, click on the drop-down arrow and select "All." Click the *Search* button. The screen will populate with a list of all open and active tasks pertaining to patients for all providers (Figure 6-8).

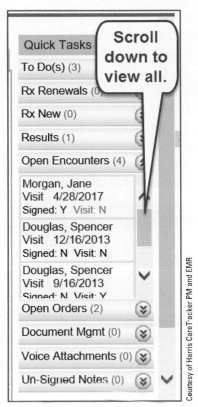

Figure 6-6   Open Encounters

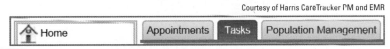

Figure 6-7   Tasks Tab in Clinical Today

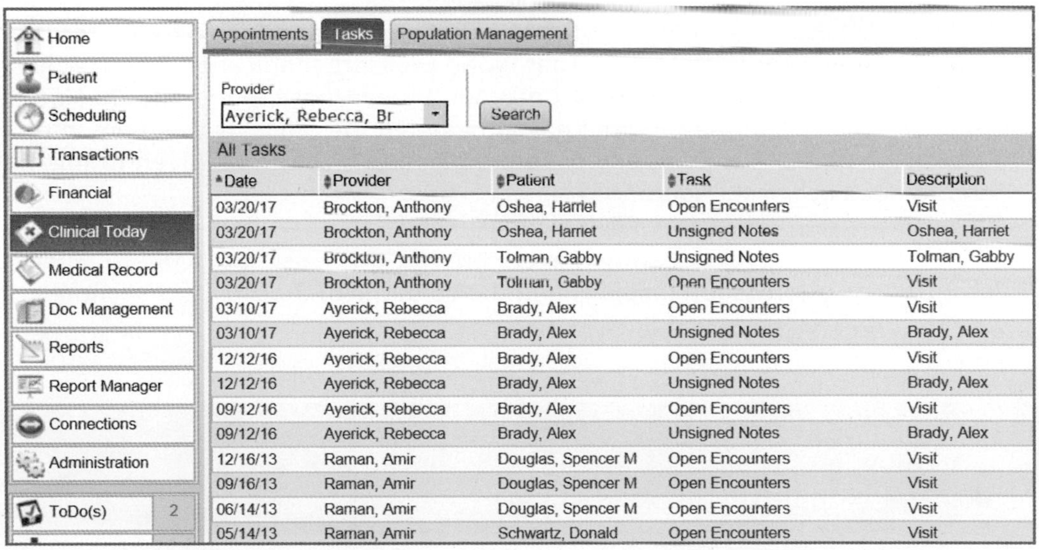

	Appointments	Tasks	Population Management		
Home					
Patient	Provider				
Scheduling	Ayerick, Rebecca, Br ▾	Search			
Transactions	All Tasks				
Financial	▲Date	⬍Provider	⬍Patient	⬍Task	Description
Clinical Today	03/20/17	Brockton, Anthony	Oshea, Harriet	Open Encounters	Visit
	03/20/17	Brockton, Anthony	Oshea, Harriet	Unsigned Notes	Oshea, Harriet
Medical Record	03/20/17	Brockton, Anthony	Tolman, Gabby	Unsigned Notes	Tolman, Gabby
Doc Management	03/20/17	Brockton, Anthony	Tolman, Gabby	Open Encounters	Visit
	03/10/17	Ayerick, Rebecca	Brady, Alex	Open Encounters	Visit
Reports	03/10/17	Ayerick, Rebecca	Brady, Alex	Unsigned Notes	Brady, Alex
	12/12/16	Ayerick, Rebecca	Brady, Alex	Open Encounters	Visit
Report Manager	12/12/16	Ayerick, Rebecca	Brady, Alex	Unsigned Notes	Brady, Alex
Connections	09/12/16	Ayerick, Rebecca	Brady, Alex	Open Encounters	Visit
	09/12/16	Ayerick, Rebecca	Brady, Alex	Unsigned Notes	Brady, Alex
Administration	12/16/13	Raman, Amir	Douglas, Spencer M	Open Encounters	Visit
	09/16/13	Raman, Amir	Douglas, Spencer M	Open Encounters	Visit
ToDo(s) 2	06/14/13	Raman, Amir	Douglas, Spencer M	Open Encounters	Visit
	05/14/13	Raman, Amir	Schwartz, Donald	Open Encounters	Visit

Figure 6-8   Open and Active Tasks

🖥 **Print a screenshot of your Open and Active Tasks screen from Clinical Today. Label it "Activity 6-4" and place it in your assignment folder.**

Tasks that display in the *Tasks* tab pertain to the provider associated with the operator. If you are not a provider, or not associated with a specific provider, the *All Tasks* list in the center of the screen displays tasks only for the provider listed in your batch. However, the tasks you can view and access are based on the security settings assigned to your role in Harris CareTracker PM and EMR. The only tasks that are loaded in the training environment thus far are *Open Encounters* and *Unsigned Notes*. An **unsigned note** is a progress note that was never signed. As you complete more activities, you will see more tasks populate in this window.

To review a particular task, click on the line item that corresponds with the task you want to review. Harris CareTracker PM and EMR opens the task in a new window. The window that opens is determined by the type of the task. **Figure 6-9** illustrates an unsigned note that needs to be completed by the provider, and **Figure 6-10** illustrates the open order screen (no orders have yet been entered).

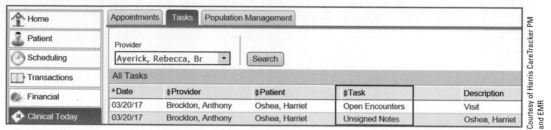

Figure 6-9 Unsigned Note That Needs Completion

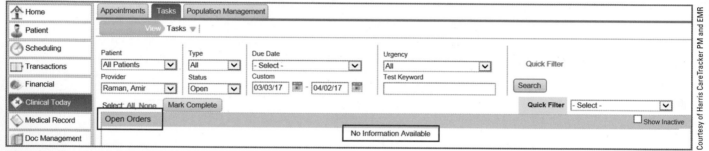

Figure 6-10 Open Orders

 CRITICAL THINKING One of your patients called early this morning for a prescription request. She stated that she is completely out of her blood pressure medication. The task is showing up in the prescription renewal column, but it does not appear that the provider has addressed it yet. It is now closing time and the provider has already left the office. Is there anything that can be done to assist the patient? Is there any patient education that can be given to this patient so that this scenario does not occur again?

Table 6-1 describes the information displaying in the columns of the *All Tasks* section of the *Tasks* tab. Refer back to Figure 6-8 as you review this table.

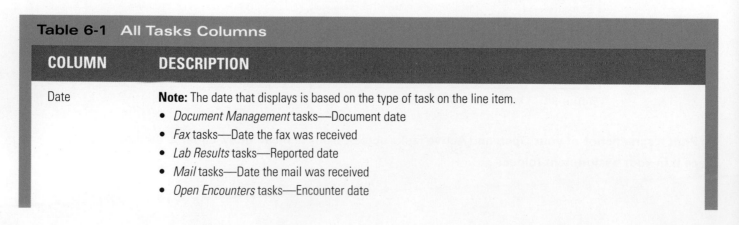

Table 6-1	All Tasks Columns
COLUMN	**DESCRIPTION**
Date	**Note:** The date that displays is based on the type of task on the line item. • *Document Management* tasks—Document date • *Fax* tasks—Date the fax was received • *Lab Results* tasks—Reported date • *Mail* tasks—Date the mail was received • *Open Encounters* tasks—Encounter date

COLUMN	DESCRIPTION
	• *Open Orders* tasks—Due date for the order • *Rx New* tasks—Original date of the prescription • *Rx Renewals* tasks—Written date of the Rx • *ToDo* tasks—Last modified date • *Unsigned Notes* tasks – Encounter date • *Untranscribed Notes*—Encounter date • *Voice Attachments*—Document date
Provider	Displays the provider associated with the task
Patient	Displays the patient associated with the task
Task	Displays the task name
Description	**Note:** The description is based on the type of task on the line item. • *Document Management* tasks—Document name • *Fax* tasks—Where the fax was sent from • *Lab Results* tasks—Report status and test name • *Mail* tasks—Where the mail message was received from • *Open Encounters* tasks—Note (signed or not signed) • *Open Orders* tasks—Test description • *Rx New* tasks—Medication name • *Rx Renewals* tasks—Medication name • *ToDo* tasks—Subject line on the *ToDo* • *Unsigned Notes* tasks—Patient name • *Untranscribed Notes* tasks—File name (.wav) • *Voice Attachments* tasks —File name (.wav)

Viewing Prescription Renewals

Learning Objective 6: View prescription renewals and new prescriptions within Clinical Today.

The *Rx Renewals* application displays a list of renewal requests sent electronically by the pharmacy and patient to the provider set up in your batch. The *Rx Renewal* application can be accessed via the *Tasks* tab in the *Clinical Today* module. If you were working for a provider using Harris CareTracker EMR, your practice would need to first enroll in the **Surescripts**® network—a network used by thousands of physicians nationwide to prescribe medications without the use of paper, pens, or fax. Surescripts® is the largest network of its kind and provides electronic connectivity between pharmacies and physician offices. Once enrolled in the Surescripts® network, the practice would be required to send five new prescriptions to receive renewal requests, and accept or deny the request within 48 hours. Surescripts® monitors and requires at least a 90 percent response rate. If the response rate falls below 90 percent for more than four weeks, Surescripts® terminates the ability to electronically receive renewal requests. As a clinical medical assistant, you will need to work with the provider to keep the response rate above 90 percent.

To receive prescription renewal requests (**Figure 6-11**) electronically from a patient, the practice must enroll the patient in the Harris CareTracker *Patient Portal* application supported by Harris CareTracker PM and EMR. All requests made by a patient using the Harris CareTracker *Patient Portal* application are saved in the *Rx Renewals* application (*Tasks* tab in *Clinical Today*) for the medical assistant to review. The *Patient Portal* is not active in your student version of Harris CareTracker (**Figure 6-12**).

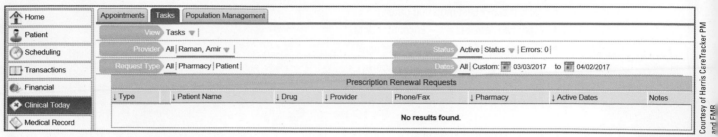

Figure 6-11   Prescription Renewal Requests

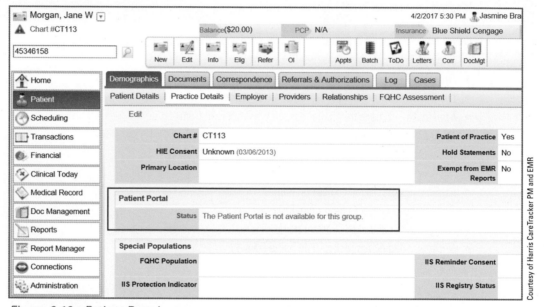

Figure 6-12   Patient Portal

 CRITICAL THINKING You notice that your provider's Surescripts® response rate is at 88 percent. It has been below 90 percent for the last two weeks. Two of your provider's partners recently retired and the practice is interviewing new providers to take their place. This process may take up to three months. In the meantime, the workload has been overwhelming. At this point, only your provider has the authority to approve renewals. You do not want your provider's Surescripts® contract to be terminated. Is there anything that you can do to help improve the Surescripts® response rate?

Table 6-2 describes the information displaying in the *Rx Renewals* application. Refer back to Figure 6-11 as you review this table.

Table 6-2	Rx Renewal Columns
COLUMN	**DESCRIPTION**
Type	Where the renewal request initiated from. Renewal requests can be initiated by a patient or a pharmacy.
Patient Name	The name of the patient associated with the renewal request.

COLUMN	DESCRIPTION
Drug	The name of the medication that requires a refill.
Provider	The name of the provider who originally issued the prescription.
Phone/Fax	The pharmacy phone and fax numbers.
Pharmacy	The name of the pharmacy where the prescription was filled previously. You can click on the line item to view the pharmacy address information.
Active Dates	The date and time Harris CareTracker EMR received the renewal request.
Notes	Notes entered by the pharmacy or patient when creating the renewal request.

Courtesy of Harris CareTracker PM and EMR

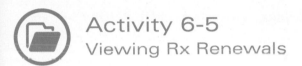

Activity 6-5
Viewing Rx Renewals

1. Click on the *Clinical Today* module.

2. Select the *Tasks* tab.

3. View the *Tasks* panes on the right side of the window.

4. Click on the *Rx Renewals* link (**Figure 6-13**) in the *Tasks* pane.

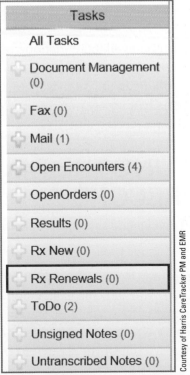

Courtesy of Harris CareTracker PM and EMR

Figure 6-13   Rx Renewals Link in Tasks Pane

5. To set your parameters, click on the word "All" beside *Provider*.

6. Click on the word "All" for *Request Type*.

7. For *Status*, click on "Active."

8. Click on "All" beside the *Dates* tab (**Figure 6-14**). Setting the parameters to "All" in the *Rx Renewals* application allows you to review all active prescription renewals for all providers in the practice.

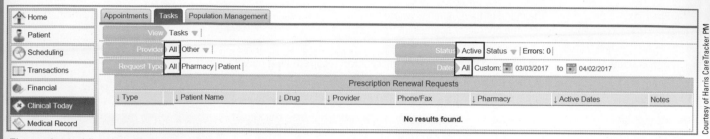

Figure 6-14   *Viewing Rx Renewals Tab*

💾 **Print this screen, even though it does not show any prescription renewals. Label it "Activity 6-5" and place it in your assignment folder.**

Viewing New Prescriptions

The *Rx New* application displays a list of prescriptions that are not transmitted electronically, printed, or failed transmission that you must review and resolve on a daily basis. Additionally, you can view details for each prescription listed and reorder a prescription, eliminating the need to reenter redundant information, view interactions, and more. Along with prescription renewals, new prescriptions can be viewed from the *Tasks* tab in *Clinical Today*. Instead of clicking on the *Rx Renewal* link, click on *Rx New* on the right-hand side of the screen and follow the prompts.

This chapter has just briefly touched on a few of the available functions in the *Clinical Today* module. Harris CareTracker PM and EMR provides users with an assortment of tools to streamline and organize information so that important tasks are never overlooked. When working in the medical field, you should review electronic tasks throughout the workday and resolve unsettled items in a timely manner.

RETRIEVING AND UPDATING THE PATIENT'S ELECTRONIC MEDICAL RECORD

Learning Objective 7: Retrieve the patient's EMR and update sections within the patient health history panes.

Once the patient has been checked in and transferred to an exam room, you are ready to bring up his or her electronic medical record (EMR). In the case of Jane Morgan, she is an established patient. Napa Valley Family Health Associates has transitioned from paper records to Harris CareTracker PM and Physician EMR. Because Ms. Morgan has not been seen since the practice converted to electronic health records, her chart has not yet been converted. You will need to build her electronic chart from scratch in this chapter's activities.

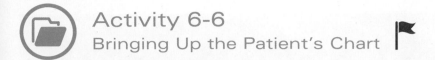

Activity 6-6
Bringing Up the Patient's Chart

1. Click on *Clinical Today.*

2. In the *Appointments* screen within *Clinical Today*, bring up the date of Jane Morgan's appointment. Be sure that *Resource* reflects "All." **Hint:** If you don't recall the date of the appointment, with the patient in context, click on the *History* tab in the *Scheduling* module to locate the patient's appointment. Do not create a new encounter for this visit, only use the appointment/encounter previously scheduled.

3. Click on Ms. Morgan's name. The patient's *Chart Summary* will open in a new window (**Figure 6-15**).

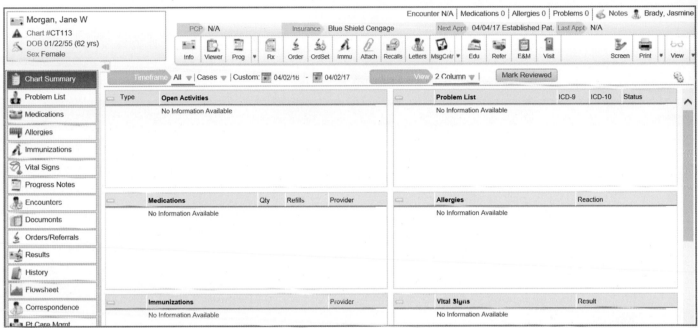

Figure 6-15   *Chart Summary in New Window*   Courtesy of Harris CareTracker PM and EMR

Print a screenshot of the Chart Summary in new window. Label it "Activity 6-6" and place it in your assignment folder.

The order in which you complete activities in the patient's chart is purely subjective. Some medical assistants start by entering the vital signs and chief complaint, and then adding new medications, allergies, and history information. The order really does not matter as long as you complete the process. We are going to start the process by creating the patient's current medication list.

Updating the Patient's Medication List

In the patient's *Chart Summary*, the *Medications* application allows you to manually update the patient's medication list. New prescriptions can also be added here; however, you will only enter the patient's current medications at this time. **Table 6-3** describes all medication status categories within the *Medications* application. It is important to ensure that all active medications are recorded to screen for interactions when prescribing new medications.

Table 6-3 Medication Status Categories

STATUS	DESCRIPTION
Active	A medication the patient is currently taking.
Inactive	A medication the patient is not taking at the present time.
Discontinued	A medication discontinued for the patient.
Erroneous	A medication entered in error for the patient.
Completed	A medication the patient has completed by taking the full recommended dosage.
Medication Refused	A medication the provider recommended, but the patient refused to take. **Note:** All patients with a Medication Refused status and an active diagnosis of asthma are excluded from the Asthma Pharmacologic Therapy (NQF 0047) quality measure report.
Failed	A medication that the patient did not respond well to.

Courtesy of Harris CareTracker PM and EMR

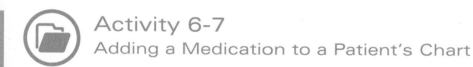

Activity 6-7
Adding a Medication to a Patient's Chart

1. Following the steps used in Activity 6-6, bring up Jane Morgan's patient chart using the *Clinical Today* module:

   • Click on *Clinical Today*.

   • In the *Appointments* screen within *Clinical Today*, bring up the date of Jane Morgan's appointment. Be sure that *Resource* reflects "All." **Hint:** If you don't recall the date of the appointment, with the patient in context, click on the *History* tab in the *Scheduling* module to locate the patient's appointment. Do not create a new encounter for this activity; use only the appointment/encounter previously scheduled.

   • Click on Ms. Morgan's name. The patient's *Chart Summary* will open in a new window (refer to Figure 6-15).

2. In the *Patient Health History* pane, click on the *Medications* link (**Figure 6-16**). The *Medications* window displays.

3. Click *+ Patient Med*, which is located at the top right side of the screen (**Figure 6-17**). The *Medication* dialog box will display (**Figure 6-18**).

4. In the *Provider* drop-down list, select the patient's provider "Amir Raman." The *Provider* list displays the group providers first, followed by the referring providers.

5. By default, the *Status* list is set to "Active" (**Figure 6-19**), but you can change to another applicable status if necessary. Refer to Table 6-3 for a complete listing of medication statuses. (Leave the *Status* as "Active.")

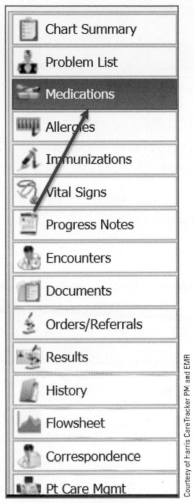

Figure 6-16   Medications Link

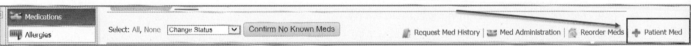

Figure 6-17   Add a Patient Medication

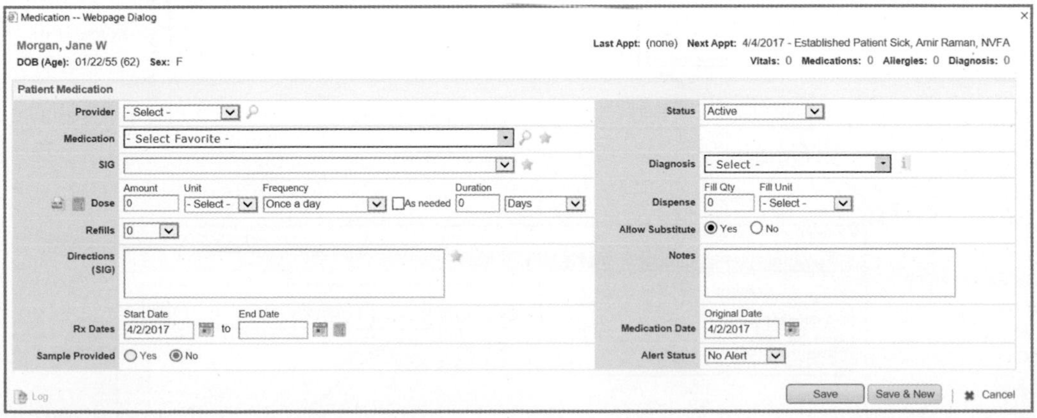

Courtesy of Harris CareTracker PM and EMR

Figure 6-18   Medication Dialog Box

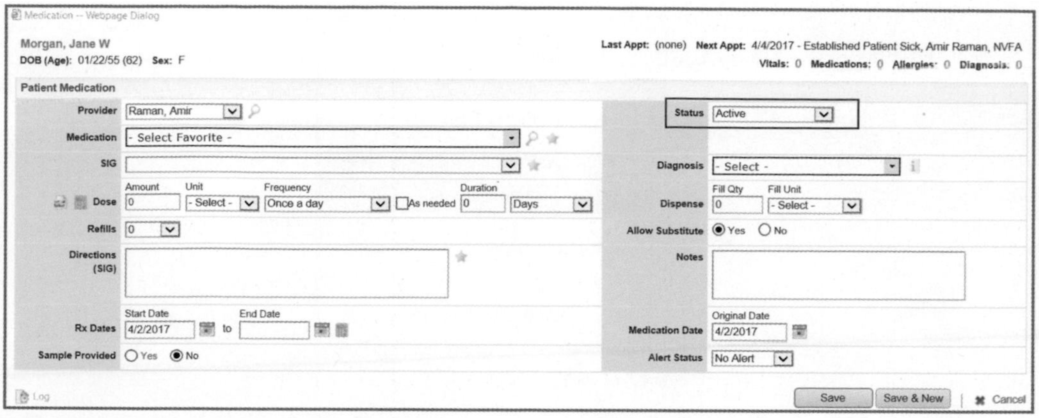

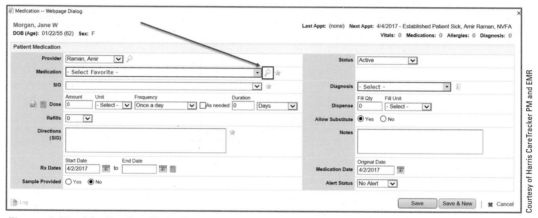

Figure 6-19   Status List Set to Active

6. In the *Medication* field, click on the search icon 🔍 (**Figure 6-20**). The *Medication Search* dialog box opens. In the *Search Text* box, type in "Boniva" and click on *Search* (**Figure 6-21**). The various options display. Click on "Boniva Oral Tablet 150 MG." (Ms. Morgan is currently taking Boniva to help slow down her osteoporosis.) An *Interaction Screening* box will pop up (**Figure 6-22**).

Figure 6-20   Medication Field Search Icon

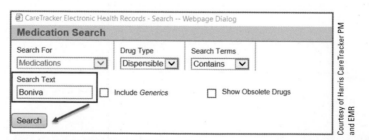

Figure 6-21   Medication Search Text

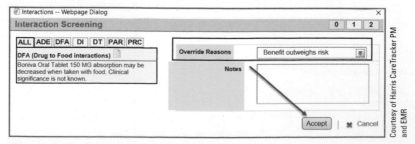

Figure 6-22   Interaction Screening Dialog Box

ALERT! Selected medications are screened for possible **contraindications** in regard to the patient's active medications, allergies, and problems. A contraindication is something (a symptom or condition) that makes a particular treatment or procedure inadvisable. The *Interaction Screening* box alerts you if the interaction is higher than the severity level set in your configurations. If the screening triggers an interaction that is higher than the severity settings set for the provider in the batch, the *Interaction Screening* dialog box displays.

7. Acknowledge the screening by selecting one or more *Override Reasons* and entering notes. Using the drop-down, select "Benefit outweighs risk" (see Figure 6-22). **Note:** If you click *Cancel* in the *Interaction Screening* dialog box before accepting an override reason, you may receive an error message.

8. Click *Accept* (see Figure 6-22).

9. You will skip over the SIG box for now. Refer to the FYI box below. Once a SIG is saved as a favorite, you will be able to select it from the manage favorites icon. **SIG** is an abbreviation for *signa* in Latin (meaning "label" or "sign"). SIG refers to specific dosage instructions that are given when prescribing medications.

 FYI The drop-down selections only display if a SIG is associated as a favorite to the medication selected and auto-populates in the specific fields. Because this is a live (educational) version of Harris CareTracker, multiple previous entries may display. To avoid duplication, you will proceed and enter the *Dose* information manually.

10. Enter the dosage information in the *Dose* boxes. Enter "1" in the *Amount* box, "Tablet" in the *Unit* box, and "Once every month" in the *Frequency* box, and "6" in the *Duration* box (**Figure 6-23**). As you enter the *Dose* information, the *Directions* (SIG) will populate.

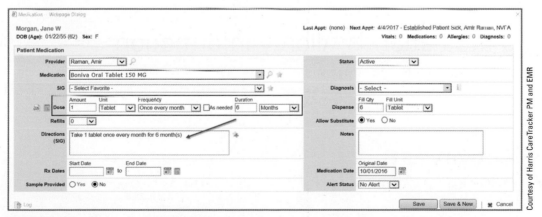

Figure 6-23   Dose—Amount, Unit, Frequency

11. Tab down to the *Rx Dates* field. Because the medication is not being renewed, remove any dates that appear in the *Start Date* box. Leave the *End Date* box blank as well.

12. The patient states that she started taking the medication on October 1 of last year. Insert this information in the box titled *Medication Date/Original Date* on the right side of the screen (**Figure 6-24**).

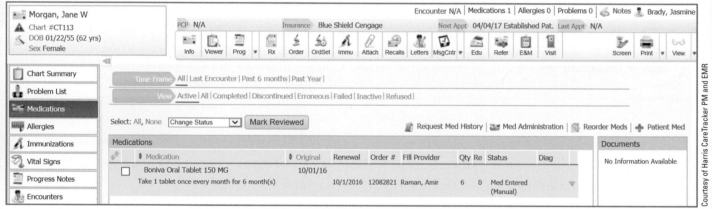

Figure 6-24   Original Date

13. Because you are not creating a new prescription, no other information needs to be entered. Click *Save*.

14. "Boniva Oral Tablet 150 MG" should now appear in the *Medications* box of the *Patient Health History* pane (**Figure 6-25**).

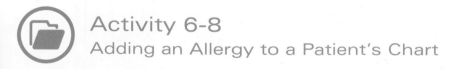

Figure 6-25   Boniva Oral Tablet Added to Medications Window

Updating the Patient's Allergy Information

The *Allergies* application is where you add new and existing allergies to a patient's medical record. It is important to ensure that all active allergies are recorded for accurate drug–allergy contraindication checks when prescribing medications and ordering immunizations.

Activity 6-8
Adding an Allergy to a Patient's Chart

1. If you are not in Jane Morgan's medical record, access it by using the following steps:

   - Click on *Clinical Today*.

   - In the *Appointments* screen within *Clinical Today*, bring up the date of Jane Morgan's appointment. Be sure that *Resource* reflects "All." **Hint:** If you don't recall the date of the appointment, with the patient in context, click on the *History* tab in the *Scheduling* module to locate the patient's appointment. Do not create a new encounter for this activity; use only the appointment/encounter previously scheduled.

   - Click directly on the patient's name under *Appointments*, and the *Patient Health History* pane will appear. (**Note:** Close out of the *Clinical Alerts* dialog box if displaying.)

2. In the *Patient Health History* pane, click on *Allergies*. Harris CareTracker EMR displays the *Allergies* window.

3. Click + *Add Allergy* (**Figure 6-26**). Harris CareTracker EMR displays the *Patient Allergy* dialog box (**Figure 6-27**).

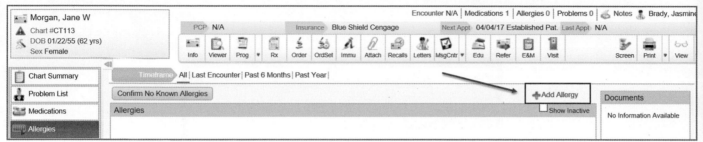

Figure 6-26   Add Allergy   Courtesy of Harris CareTracker PM and EMR

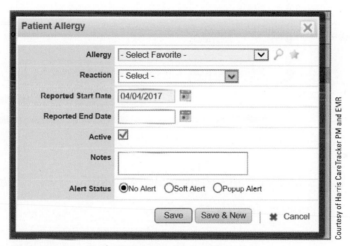

Figure 6-27   Patient Allergy Dialog Box

4. Ms. Morgan is allergic to codeine, so this information will need to be entered in her electronic chart. Search for codeine by clicking on the *Search* 🔍 icon next to the *Allergy* field. (**Note:** If codeine has been previously entered as a favorite in the system, it will appear in the drop-down *Allergy* list. We will mimic searching for it as though it were not saved as a favorite.)

5. In the *Search Text* box, type "Codeine." Click the *Search* button.

6. A list of several medications will pop up that include the word "codeine." If "Codeine" is already on the favorites list, it will be indicated by the *On Favorites* ⭐ icon.

7. Click on the search result "Codeine Phosphate." The *Patient Allergy* window will reappear with "Codeine Phosphate" listed beside *Allergy*.

8. In the *Reaction* box, click on the drop-down arrow and select "Anaphylaxis." (**Note:** Click on the drop-down arrow again to minimize the drop-down list. "Anaphylaxis" is now selected.)

9. In the *Reported Start Date* box, enter the date of onset for the allergy in MM/DD/YYYY format or click the *Calendar* 📅 icon to select the date. Enter a start date of April 1 of last year.

10. Leave the *Reported End Date* blank.

11. By default, the *Status* is set to *Active* to indicate that the allergy is an active allergy. (**Note:** The active checkbox is read only and is updated based on *Reported End Date* status.)

12. In the *Notes* box, enter additional comments, if necessary. (Leave this section blank.)

13. By default, the *Alert Status* is set to "No Alert." Due to the seriousness of this patient's allergy, click on "Popup Alert" (**Figure 6-28**). The pop-up alert will now pop up whenever Ms. Morgan's medical record is launched and will stop displaying when the alert is closed. You can also click the Alert ⚠ icon next to the patient's chart number on the *Patient Detail* bar to view both soft alerts and pop-up alerts.

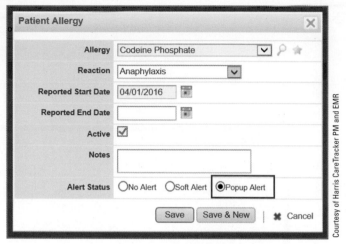

Figure 6-28   Patient Allergy Popup Alert

14. Click *Save & New* to save and add another allergy without exiting the *Patient Allergy* dialog box.

15. Add "Peanuts" as a new allergy for Ms. Morgan.

   a. In the *Reaction* box, scroll down the list and select both "Diarrhea" and "Vomiting."

   b. Click back on the *Reaction* field drop-down arrow to close the list of options.

   c. In the *Reported Start Date* box, enter a date that is 10 years prior to the date of the appointment.

   d. Leave the *Reported End Date* box blank.

   e. In the *Notes* section, type the following: "The reported start date is just an estimate. Patient doesn't know the actual day or year she had the reaction."

   f. Select "Soft Alert" in the *Alert Status* category.

16. Click *Save.* "Peanuts" and "Codeine" will now be listed in the *Allergies* pane (**Figure 6-29**).

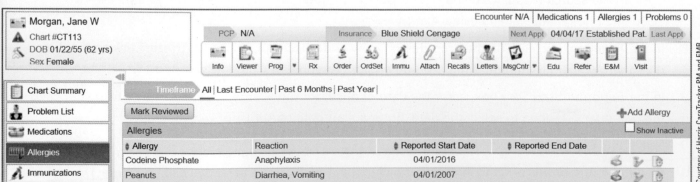

Figure 6-29   Allergies Pane

CRITICAL THINKING Why do you think that Ms. Morgan's peanut allergy was only flagged as a soft alert instead of the pop-up alert that was selected for Ms. Morgan's codeine allergy?

Updating the Patient's Immunization Status

The *Immunizations* module allows you to enter history information regarding the patient. It also allows you to enter immunizations you administer in your office. Activity 6-9 describes how to enter a patient's past immunizations.

 ## Activity 6-9
Entering Past Immunizations in a Patient's Chart

1. If you are not in Jane Morgan's medical record, access it by using the following steps:
   - Click on *Clinical Today.*
   - In the *Appointments* screen within *Clinical Today*, bring up the date of Jane Morgan's appointment. Be sure that *Resource* reflects "All." **Hint:** If you don't recall the date of the appointment, with the patient in context, click on the *History* tab in the *Scheduling* module to locate the patient's appointment. Do not create a new encounter for this activity; use only the appointment/encounter previously scheduled.
   - Click on Ms. Morgan's name. The patient's *Chart Summary* will open in a new window (refer to Figure 6-15).

2. In the *Patient Health History* pane, click on *Immunizations*. Harris CareTracker EMR displays the *Immunizations* window.

3. Click on the + *Add Past/Refused Immunization* link (**Figure 6-30**).

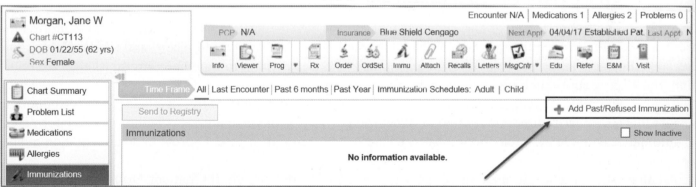

Figure 6-30   *Add Past/Refused Immunization Link*

Courtesy of Harris CareTracker PM and EMR

4. Type in the word "Tetanus" in the *Immunization* field and then click on the *Search* 🔍 icon.

5. An *Immunization Search* dialog box will pop up. Click on "tetanus toxoid, adsorbed" under *Search Results.* The selected immunization will now appear in the *Immunization* field.

6. Because Ms. Morgan's tetanus immunization was not administered at Napa Valley Family Health Associates, the only other information that can be entered is when she received the immunization and where she received it. Ms. Morgan stated that she received the shot on March 3 of last year. Type this information in the *Admin Date* box.

7. Enter a description in the *Administration Notes* field. Ms. Morgan stated that she received the tetanus shot at America's Urgent Care. Enter the following description: "Pt. received Tetanus shot at America's Urgent Care after stepping on a nail."

8. Click *Save*. Your *Immunizations* pane should match **Figure 6-31**.

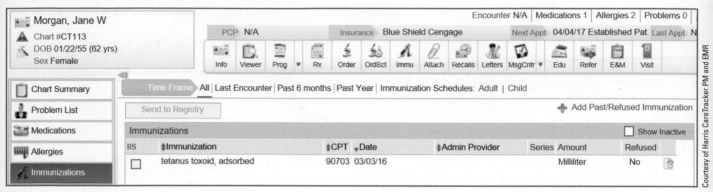

Figure 6-31   *Immunizations Pane*

 Print your chart summary using the following instructions, which will illustrate the work you did in the last three activities.

- Click on *Chart Summary* in the *Patient Health History* pane.
- Click on the drop-down arrow beside the printer 🖨 icon in the upper-right corner of the screen.
- Click on *Print Chart Summary*. A new window will pop up.
- Click the *Print* button. Label this "Activities 6-7, 6-8, and 6-9" and place it in your assignment folder.
- After printing, close out of the *Formal Health Record* screen.

Accessing the History Application

The *History* application helps capture and review a patient's past medical, family, and social history information from one central location using different data entry methods. It is important to record and review history data because they enable the provider to form a diagnosis and treatment plan together with the clinical examination. The *History* application provides quick and easy data entry methods, such as checkboxes, drop-down lists, text boxes, and more, to record information. In addition, you can also click *Mark Reviewed* for each category to ensure that historical information presented is reviewed to provide better analysis in diagnoses. This information is automatically made available in the *History* section of each progress note, improving documentation quality and patient care.

    An alternative method to document history information is directly via the patient *Progress Note*. History information recorded here is also recorded in the *History* application, including addition of family members to the *Family History* section.

> ✓ **TIP**   By default, Harris CareTracker EMR displays both the date and time stamp when updates are made to the *History* section.

Table 6-4 describes information found in the *History* application.

Table 6-4   History Application Descriptions

TYPE	DESCRIPTION
Patient History	By default, the *History* window displays the **patient history**, which consists of past medical and social history information. Past medical history includes details such as any operations, illnesses, and accidents. Social history includes information on tobacco and alcohol usage.
Sensitive Info	This displays **sensitive information** such as a patient's human immunodeficiency virus (HIV) or sexually transmitted disease (STD) statuses and information on overuse of alcohol and/or chemicals.
Family History	**Family history** displays part of a patient's medical history in which questions are asked in an attempt to find out whether the patient has hereditary tendencies toward particular diseases. Family history is to be present in all patients' charts, including children.
Advance Directives	**Advance directives** are the legal documents, such as the living will, durable power of attorney, and health care proxy that allow people to convey their decisions about end-of-life care ahead of time. Advance directives provide a way for patients to communicate their wishes to family, friends, and health care professionals and to avoid confusion later on, should they become unable to do so. Ideally, the process of discussing and writing advance directives should be ongoing, rather than a single event. Advance directives can be modified as a patient's situation changes. Even after advance directives have been signed, patients can change their mind at any time.
Attachments	In addition to capturing health history information electronically, you can scan or attach health history forms filled by a patient via the *Document Management Upload* application. All history forms assigned as type "Clinical" and subtype "History" display under this tab. You can edit, delete, or annotate documents if necessary.
Log	The log displays a history of all activities performed in the *History* section of the patient's medical record.
Preview	Preview displays a summary view of all history information recorded for the patient. In addition, the preview displays the specific date an item is recorded or updated in the patient's medical record.

Courtesy of Harris CareTracker PM and EMR

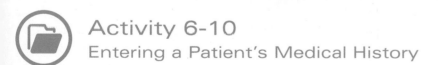

Activity 6-10
Entering a Patient's Medical History

1. If you are not in Jane Morgan's medical record, access it by using the following steps:

   - Click on *Clinical Today*.

   - In the *Appointments* screen within *Clinical Today*, bring up the date of Jane Morgan's appointment. Be sure that *Resource* reflects "All." **Hint:** If you don't recall the date of the appointment, with the patient in context, click on the *History* tab in the *Scheduling* module to locate the patient's appointment. Do not create a new encounter for this activity; use only the appointment/encounter previously scheduled.

   - Click on Ms. Morgan's name. The patient's Chart Summary will open in a new window (refer to Figure 6-15).

2. Click on the *History* tab in the *Patient Health History* pane. Harris CareTracker EMR displays the *History* window (**Figure 6-32**).

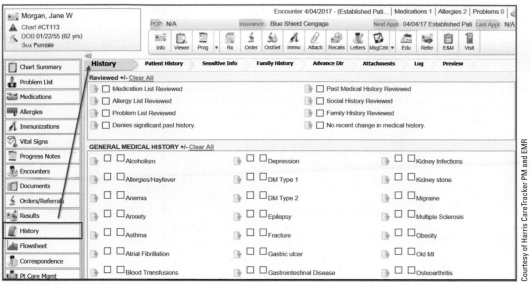

Figure 6-32   History Window

3. In the *General Medical History* section of the *Patient History* screen, click on "Y" (for "Yes") on the conditions listed in Table 6-5. Click on the *Finding Details* icon to the left of the "Y" boxes and follow the instructions in Table 6-5 regarding information to insert in the *Comments* box (Figure 6-33). Click the "X" on the top right of the *Comments* box to close and save each comment. (**Note:** It may take a few moments for the dialog box to activate to be able to enter text.)

Table 6-5 General Medical History Information for Jane Morgan	
CONDITION	**DETAILS**
Allergies/Hay Fever	*Comment:* Usually occurs in the spring of each year. Onset: During childhood. Doesn't know the year. Takes OTC allergy relief medication during flare-ups. (Refer to Figure 6-33.)
Asthma	Under *Severity*, click the box beside "mild." *Comment:* Diagnosed 10 years ago. Has had 2–3 attacks in the past 10 years. Last attack approximately five years ago. Not taking any meds for this condition.
Depression	*Comment:* Has not been formally diagnosed. Has periods of sadness and crying. Doesn't want to do anything during these bouts. Onset: About one year. Occurs a couple of times a month and lasts for a few days.
Joint Pain	*Comment:* Intermittent pain (flare-ups approx. 2–3 times per year). Never been formally diagnosed. Mainly in fingers and toes. Onset date approx. three years ago.

Courtesy of Harris CareTracker PM and EMR

4. Enter the following information in the *Hospitalizations* box:

a. Tonsillectomy at age 3. Doesn't know which hospital.

b. Hospitalized for the birth of her three children at County General. No complications.

c. Left breast lumpectomy in May 2010. Negative for cancer cells.

d. No other hospitalizations.

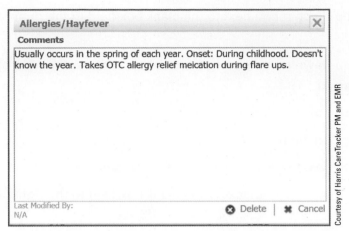

Figure 6-33   Allergies/Hay Fever Comments Box

5. Enter the following information in the *Other Medical History* box: "Five-year history of UTIs. Approximately 1–2 episodes/year. Treatment: Antibiotics."

6. In the *Tobacco Assessment* section, click on the drop-down menu next to the blank box/field to the right of *Smoking Status* and select "Never Smoker." Beside *Tobacco User* click on the "N" for No. Leave everything else in this section blank. (Note that the *Tobacco Assessment* section supports Stage 1 Meaningful Use.)

7. Enter the following information in the *Social History* section:

    a. Click on the drop-down menu next to the blank box/field to the right of *Alcohol Use* and select "Non-Drinker."

    b. Click on the drop-down menu next to the blank box/field to the right of *Caffeine Use* and select "2 servings per Day." Click on the *Finding Details* icon next to *Caffeine Use* and put a check mark beside "coffee" and "tea" in the "Type" column. In the *Comments* box state the following: "Drinks 1 cup of coffee and 1 glass of iced tea daily." Click the "X" to close out of the box.

    c. *Drug Use*: Click on the "N" for No.

    d. *Sun Protection*: Click on the "Y" for Yes. Click on the *Finding Details* icon. Place a check mark in the "sunglasses" and "sunscreen" boxes. Click on *SPF* and select the "30" box. Click the "X" to close out of the *Sun Protection* box.

    e. *Tattoos*: Click on the "N" for No.

    f. *Sexually Active*: Click on the "Y" for Yes.

    g. Click on the drop-down menu next to the blank box/field to the right of *Race* and select "Caucasian."

    h. Click on the drop-down menu next to the blank box/field to the right of *Native language* and select "English."

    i. *Physical Abuse*: Click on the "N" for No.

    j. *Domestic Violence*: Click on the "N" for No.

    k. Click on the drop-down menu next to the blank box/field to the right of *Education Level* and select "Bachelor's Degree."

    l.   Click on the drop-down menu next to the blank box/field to the right of *Marital Status* and select "Married."

    m. Click on the drop-down menu next to the blank box/field to the right of *Exercise Habits* and select "moderate >3 x/wk."

    n.   *Seatbelts*: Click on the "Y" for Yes.

    o.   *Body Piercings*: Click on the "N" for No.

    p.   *Birth Control Method*: Leave all boxes blank in this section.

    q.   Click on the drop-down menu next to the blank box/field to the right of *Religion* and select "Christian."

    r.   *Occupation*: Enter "Nurse."

    s.   *Other Social History* box: Leave blank.

8. In the *Depression Screening* section, click on the drop-down box next to the blank box/field beside the "*Little interest or pleasure in doing things*" line and select "Occasionally." Click on the drop-down box next to the blank box/field beside *Feeling down, depressed*, or *hopeless* and select "Occasionally." Leave the *Date of Last Depression Screening* field blank.

9. Enter the following information in the *OB/GYN History* section:

    a.   *LMP:* Leave blank.

    b.   *Menopause has occurred*: Click on the "Y" for Yes.

    c.   *History of abnormal pap smears*: Click on the "N" for No.

    d.   *Sexually Active*: Click on the "Y" for Yes.

    e.   *Ectopic Pregnancy*: Click on the "N" for No.

    f.   *Menarche Age*: Enter "13."

    g.   *Birth Control:* Leave these boxes blank.

10. Enter the following information in the *Pregnancy Summary* section:

    a.   *Gravida*: Select "4" from the drop-down menu next to the blank box/field.

    b.   *Term:* Select "2" from the drop-down menu next to the blank box/field.

    c.   *Preterm*: Select "1" from the drop-down menu next to the blank box/field.

    d.   *AB:* Skip over this category.

    e.   *Live Children*: Select "3" from the drop-down menu next to the blank box/field.

    f.   *Miscarriage*: Select "1" from the drop-down menu next to the blank box/field.

11. Leave the *Other OB/GYN History* box blank.

12. In the *Surgical/Procedural* section, select the box for *Breast Lumpectomy* and click on the associated *Finding Details* ⯆ icon. In the *Breast Lumpectomy* box, select "left" for the *Location*. In the *Comments* section, enter: "Had lumpectomy in May of 2010. Biopsy negative for cancer cells." Click the "X" to close out of the box. Leave all other boxes in this section blank.

13. Leave the *Other Surgical History* box blank.

14. Enter the following information in the *Preventive Care* section (for all dates, use the previous year unless otherwise indicated):

    a. *Colonoscopy:* Enter 03/12/20XX

    b. *Dilated Eye Exam:* Enter 01/04/20XX

    c. *Flu Vaccine:* Enter 10/12/20XX

    d. *Mammography:* 05/12/20XX

    e. *Pap Smear:* 05/15/20XX (three years ago)

15. In the *Self-Management Goal* box, enter: "Lose 10 pounds this year and start exercising 3x/week."

16. Click *Save*.

 Go to the top right of the History pane. Click on the drop-down arrow beside the Print icon. Click on Print Patient History. When the box opens, you should see the patient's history form. Print this form, label it "Activity 6-10A," and place it in your assignment folder.

> **SPOTLIGHT** There are times a patient will refuse to answer questions outlined on the template. If so, leave the field blank. Do not check "Y" or "N." There is no option of "patient refused," but you could free text a comment in the notes box by clicking the *Finding Details* icon.

17. Click on the *Sensitive Info* tab. Your screen should match **Figure 6-34** (though no selections will have been made yet).

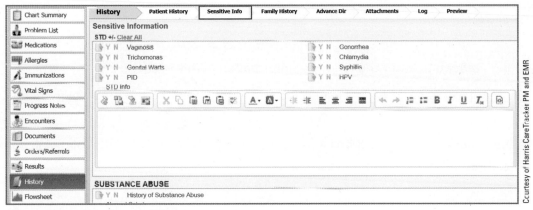

Figure 6-34   Sensitive Info Tab

18. In the *STD* section, click "N" for each disease listed. (**Note:** An easy way to mark all categories with the same response is to click on the [+/−] sign between *STD* and *Clear All*. For this scenario, click on the [−] sign. All diseases should now have a red "X" [indicating "No"] beside their names.)

19. Ms. Morgan has no history of substance abuse, so click on the "N" beside *History of Substance Abuse*.

20. Ms. Morgan is not seeing any mental health providers, so click on the "N" beside *Seeing mental health provider*.

21. Ms. Morgan has never had an HIV test. Enter the following comment in the text box below *HIV Status*: "Patient has never had an HIV test but states that she has been in a monogamous relationship with her husband over the past 30 years."

22. Leave the *Medicare High Risk Criteria* section blank because Ms. Morgan is not enrolled in Medicare.

23. Click *Save*.

🖶 **Click on the drop-down arrow beside the Print icon. Select Print Sensitive Information. When the box opens, you should see the Sensitive Information Form. Print this form and label it "Activity 6-10B." Place it in your assignment folder.**

24. Click on the *Family History* tab.

25. Select the *Mother* tab (**Figure 6-35**). Enter the following information in this section:

    a. Ms. Morgan's mother is still alive. Click on the drop-down menu next to the blank box/field to the right of *Status* and select "Alive."

    b. In the *Age* box, enter "85."

    c. Select the checkbox next to *In good health* to indicate the general health status of Ms. Morgan's mother.

    d. Ms. Morgan's mother suffers from GERD and hypertension. Click on the "Y" for Yes next to these two diseases.

    e. Click *Save*.

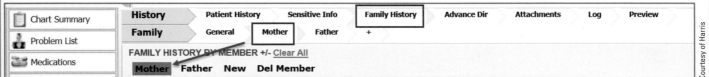

Figure 6-35   Family History/Mother Tab

26. Select the *Father* tab. Enter the following information in this section:

    a. Ms. Morgan's father died in a car accident at age 40. Click on the drop-down menu next to the blank box/field to the right of *Status* and select "Deceased."

    b. In the *Other conditions* text box at the bottom of the screen, enter the following comment: "Ms. Morgan's father died in a car accident at the age of 40."

    c. Click *Save*.

🖶 **Click on the drop-down arrow beside the Print icon. Select Print Family History. When the box opens, you should see the Family History By Family Member form. Print this form, label it "Activity 6-10C," and place it in your assignment folder.**

Recording a Patient's Vital Signs and Chief Complaint

Learning Objective 8: Record vital signs and document the patient's chief complaint.

The *Vital Signs* application allows you to record the patient's vital data at every encounter in the office and includes the patient's blood pressure, temperature, pulse rate, respiration, height, weight, oxygen saturation reading, and pain level. This helps to guide clinical decisions about treatment and to identify the need for additional diagnostic measures. Activity 6-11 describes how to record a patient's vital signs.

Activity 6-11
Recording a Patient's Vital Signs

1. If you are not in Jane Morgan's medical record, access it by using the following steps:

   - Click on *Clinical Today*.

   - In the *Appointments* screen within *Clinical Today*, bring up the date of Jane Morgan's appointment. Be sure that *Resource* reflects "All." **Hint:** If you don't recall the date of the appointment, with the patient in context, click on the *History* tab in the *Scheduling* module to locate the patient's appointment. Do not create a new encounter for this activity; use only the appointment/encounter previously scheduled.

   - Click on Ms. Morgan's name. The patient's Chart Summary will open in a new window (refer to Figure 6-15).

2. In the *Patient Health History* pane, click on *Vital Signs*. Harris CareTracker EMR displays the *Vital Signs* window with vital data taken during the current and past encounters at the office or at home. Because this is Ms. Morgan's first visit since the EMR was instituted, no vital signs have been entered yet.

3. Click on *Record Vital Signs* in the lower-left pane of the screen (**Figure 6-36**). If an encounter is in context, the *Record Vital Signs* dialog box will display.

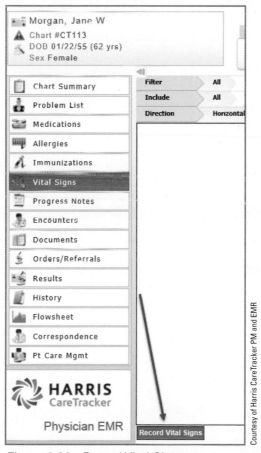

Figure 6-36   Record Vital Signs

TIP If an encounter is not in context, the Select Encounter dialog box displays (**Figure 6-37**), and you must create an encounter. Use the encounter that already exists for this patient because you previously scheduled an appointment and went in through the Appointment application in Clinical Today; however, if the patient was not coming in for an appointment, but rather just stopping by to have his or her vital signs monitored, you would need to create an encounter to record your measurements.

(*continues*)

(Continued)

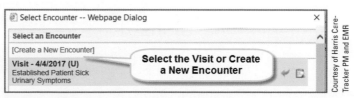

Figure 6-37   Select Encounter Dialog Box

Proceed with step 4 if you do not see the *Select Encounter* dialog box.

4. Using the information in **Table 6-6**, enter the appropriate values in the *Record Vital Signs* dialog box (**Figure 6-38**).

Table 6-6   Vital Signs for Jane Morgan

MEASUREMENT CATEGORY	READING
Height	5 ft 6 in
Weight	160 lb
Body Mass Index	This will automatically populate.
Blood Pressure	146/90
Pulse Rate	84 bpm
Temperature	98.4°F
Respiratory Rate	16
Pulse Oximetry	97%
Pain Level	7/10

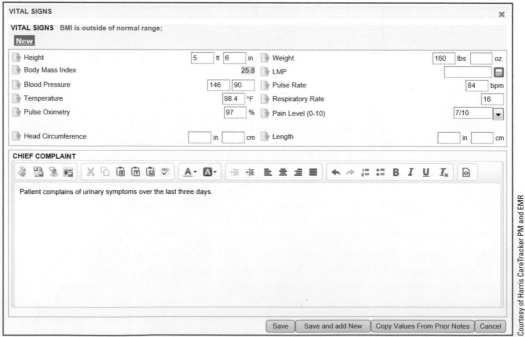

Figure 6-38   Record Vital Signs Dialog Box

5. In the *Chief Complaint* box, type the following: "Patient complains of urinary symptoms over the last three days."

6. Click *Save*. The vital data automatically update the vital grid with the measurements and the date the vitals are recorded. (**Note:** The vital data automatically update the progress note for the same encounter and display the data in the corresponding narrative.)

CRITICAL THINKING   Did you notice how the Body Mass Index field turned orange and the note "BMI is outside of normal range" (see **Figure 6-38**)? Because the patient's blood pressure is "outside of the normal range" it displays in pink once you record and save the vital measurements (see **Figure 6-39**). What should the medical assistant do when the patient's vital signs are elevated?

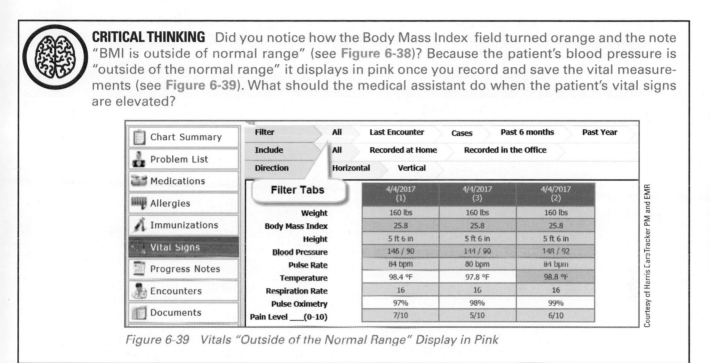

Figure 6-39   Vitals "Outside of the Normal Range" Display in Pink

7. If previously checked to display, the *Clinical Alerts* dialog box will display, including the *Health Maintenance* items (**Figure 6-40**). Close out of the *Clinical Alerts* dialog box by clicking on the "X" in the upper-right hand-corner.

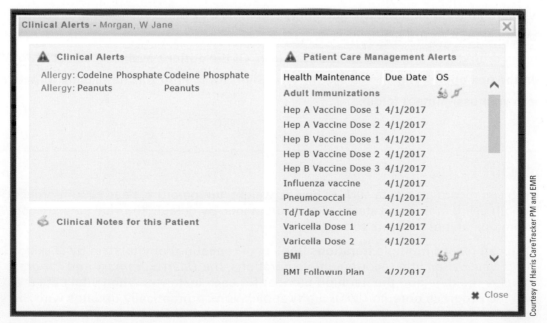

Figure 6-40   Clinical Alerts

8. In Activity 6-13, you are going to be working with flowsheets, which graph a variety of different measurements. Because we can add multiple iterations in one visit for vital signs, click back on *Record Vital Signs* at the bottom-left corner of the window pane.

9. Click on *New*. Using the information in **Table 6-7**, record two more sets of readings so that you can graph your results in the flowsheet activity (Activity 6-11).

Table 6-7   Additional Vital Sign Readings for Jane Morgan

MEASUREMENT CATEGORY	SECOND READING	THIRD READING
Height	5 ft 6 in	5 ft 6 in
Weight	160 lb	160 lb
Body Mass Index	This should automatically populate.	This should automatically populate.
Blood Pressure	148/92	144/90
Pulse Rate	84 bpm	80 bpm
Temperature	98.8°F	97.8°F
Respiratory Rate	16	16
Pulse Oximetry	99%	98%
Pain Level	6/10	5/10

10. Click *Save and add New* to add the additional reading.

11. Once you are finished with the two additional readings, click on *Save*. Now all three measurements should appear (see Figure 6-39).

Click on the drop-down arrow beside the Print icon. Of the options available, select "Print Vital Signs Form." When the box opens, you should see the Vital Signs form. Print this form, label it "Activity 6-11," and place it in your assignment folder.

SPOTLIGHT

- You can record vital data such as height, weight, temperature, head circumference, and length using metric and standard measurements. By default, the vital data are converted from one unit of measure to another.

- You can record multiple **iterations** (the act of repeating) of vital data by clicking *Save and Add New*. When you record multiple iterations, the *Chart Summary* and *Progress Note* display the date and the iteration number for each instance. When vital data are recorded via the progress note, the *Vital Signs* application automatically updates with the same data.

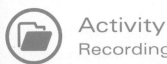 Activity 6-12
Recording a Pediatric Patient's Vital Signs

Note: You must have completed Activity 3-4 (steps 1-6 and 33) and booked an appointment for Francisco Powell Jimenez in Activity 4-1 prior to completing this activity. If you have not already completed those activities, complete them now, before beginning this activity.

1. If you are not in Francisco Powell Jimenez's medical record, access it by using the following steps:
   - Click on *Clinical Today*.
   - In the *Appointments* screen within *Clinical Today*, bring up the date of Francisco's appointment. Be sure that *Resource* reflects "All." Hint: If you don't recall the date of the appointment, with the patient in context, click on the *History* tab in the *Scheduling* module to locate the patient's appointment. Do not create a new encounter for this activity; use only the appointment/encounter previously scheduled.
   - Click on Francisco's name. The patient's *Chart Summary* will open in a new window (refer to Figure 6-15).

2. In the *Patient Health History* pane, click on *Vital Signs*. Because this is Francisco's first visit at NVFHA, no vital signs have been entered yet.

3. Click on *Record Vital Signs* in the lower-left pane of the screen (see Figure 6-36).

4. Using the information in Table 6-8, enter the values in the *Record Vital Signs* dialog box (see Figure 6-37).

Table 6-8   Vital Signs for Francisco Powell Jimenez

MEASUREMENT CATEGORY	READING
Height	2 ft 0 in
Weight	18 lb 3 oz
Body Mass Index	This will automatically populate.
Blood Pressure	
Pulse Rate	112 bpm
Temperature	98.3°F
Respiratory Rate	34
Pulse Oximetry	
Pain Level	

5. In the *Chief Complaint* box, type the following: "Well-Baby checkup."

6. Click *Save.*

▣ Click on the drop-down arrow beside the Print icon. From the options, select "Print Vital Signs Form." When the box opens, you should see the Vital Signs form. Print this form, label it "Activity 6-12," and place it in your assignment folder.

Filtering Vital Data

The *Vital Signs* application enables you to filter vital data based on the location the vitals are monitored and the date the vitals are recorded. Additionally, you can filter to view vitals pertaining to a specific case.

To filter vital data:

- Access the *Medical Record* module using one of the following methods:
  - Pull the patient into context, and click the *Medical Record* module.
  - If the patient has an appointment, click the patient's name in the *Appointments* tab of the *Clinical Today* module.

- In the *Patient Health History* pane, click *Vital Signs*. Harris CareTracker EMR displays the *Vital Signs* window with vital data taken during the current and past encounters at the office or at home.

- Do one of the following:
  - To filter vitals based on the location recorded, click either the *Recorded at Home* or the *Recorded in the Office* tabs.
  - To filter vitals based on the date the vitals are recorded, click on the *Last Encounter*, *Past 6 months*, or *Past Year* tabs (see Figure 6-39).

- To filter vitals pertaining to a specific case, click the *Cases* tab. In the *Select Cases* dialog box, select the checkbox for the case you want and click *Select*.

Viewing Flowsheets

Learning Objective 9: View and create Flowsheets within Harris CareTracker EMR.

The *Flowsheet* application provides electronic management of clinical data entry and review of patient progress over time using different flowsheet templates. A **flowsheet template** is a profile with selected items. Data in a patient medical record can be pulled into a flowsheet, eliminating the need for double entry. It accommodates multidisciplinary documentation requirements and is linked to *Progress Notes*, *Vital Signs*, and *Results* applications. The application displays patient information that includes lab results, medications, vitals, and other medical data in a table or graph view.

The table view includes two formats: vertical grid (**Figure 6-41**) and horizontal grid. In a vertical grid, the columns represent vitals taken, and rows represent an interval of time. The horizontal grid represents the data in the reverse layout. The different formats enable you to analyze data over time from a variety of viewpoints on a single display screen.

Filter	All	Last Encounter	Cases	Past 6 months	Past Year			
Include	All	Recorded at Home	Recorded in the Office					
Direction	Horizontal	Vertical						

	Weight	Body Mass Index	Height	Blood Pressure	Pulse Rate	Temperature	Respiration Rate	Pulse Oximetry	Pain Level ___(0-10)
4/4/2017 - 4/4/2017 (1)	160 lbs/72.57 kg	25.8	5 ft 6 in / 167.6 cm	146/90	84 bpm	98.4 °F/36.9 °C	16	97%	7/10
4/4/2017 - 4/4/2017 (3)	160 lbs/72.57 kg	25.8	5 ft 6 in / 167.6 cm	144/90	80 bpm	97.8 °F/36.6 °C	16	98%	5/10
4/4/2017 - 4/4/2017 (2)	160 lbs/72.57 kg	25.8	5 ft 6 in / 167.6 cm	148/92	84 bpm	98.8 °F/37.1 °C	16	99%	6/10

Figure 6-41   *Vital Signs Vertical Grid*

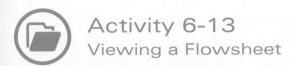

Activity 6-13
Viewing a Flowsheet

1. If you are not in Jane Morgan's medical record, access it by using the following steps:

   - Click on *Clinical Today*.

   - In the *Appointments* screen within *Clinical Today*, bring up the date of Jane Morgan's appointment. Be sure that *Resource* reflects "All." **Hint:** If you don't recall the date of the appointment, with the patient in context, click on the *History* tab in the *Scheduling* module to locate the patient's appointment. Do not create a new encounter for this activity; use only the appointment/encounter previously scheduled.

   - Click on Ms. Morgan's name. The patient's *Chart Summary* will open in a new window (refer to Figure 6-15).

2. In the *Patient Health History* pane, click on *Flowsheet*. Harris CareTracker EMR displays the *Flowsheet* window.

3. Generally, you can select a template from the *Saved Views* drop-down list, but the template you will need for this activity has not been saved yet. Click the *Search* 🔍 icon to the right of *Saved Views* (**Figure 6-42**). Harris CareTracker EMR displays the *Manage Flowsheet Templates* dialog box.

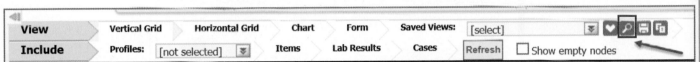

Figure 6-42   Saved Views

4. Enter "Vital Signs" in the *Template* box, and then click on the plus sign (**Figure 6-43**).

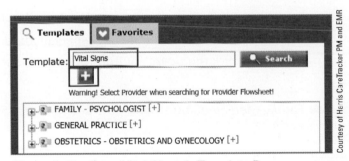

Figure 6-43   Enter Vital Signs in Template Box

5. The *Flowsheet Template* dialog box will appear. In the *Name* box, type "Vital Signs."

6. In the *Specialty* box, click on the drop-down arrow and select "FAMILY MEDICINE."

7. In the *View* box, click on the drop-down arrow and select "Chart."

8. Next to the *Scope* box, click on the drop-down arrow and select "COMPANY."

9. Click on the checkbox next to *In Favorites* to make this a favorite you can select for further activities.

10. Click on the drop-down arrow in the *Flowsheet Profile* box, scroll down, and select "Vital Signs."

11. A list of flowsheet items comes up that you can select for your profile (**Figure 6-44**). Click on the checkboxes next to *Blood Pressure*, *Body Mass Index*, *Height*, *Pain Level*, *Pulse Oximetry*, *Pulse Rate*, *Respiration Rate*, and *Weight*. **Note:** You will need to scroll down the screen to view all options of the *Flowsheet Profile*.

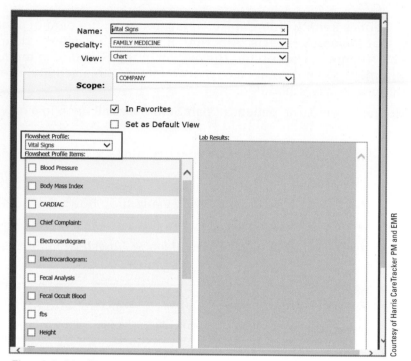

Figure 6-44   Flowsheet Profiles

12. Click *OK*.

13. For the *Manage Flowsheet Template*s application to pop up, you may need to click on the *Favorites* tab and then back on the *Templates* tab and then the new specialty heading *Family Medicine*. (**Note:** Alternatively, you may need to click the *Search* button for your screen to refresh with the new template.)

14. Click on the [+] sign beside *Family Medicine*. You should now see the *Vital Signs* heading (**Figure 6-45**).

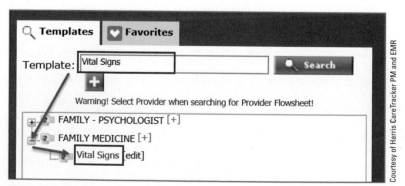

Figure 6-45   Vital Signs Heading

15. Click on the *Vital Signs* heading, which will take you back to the original *Flowsheet* application box (**Figure 6-46**).

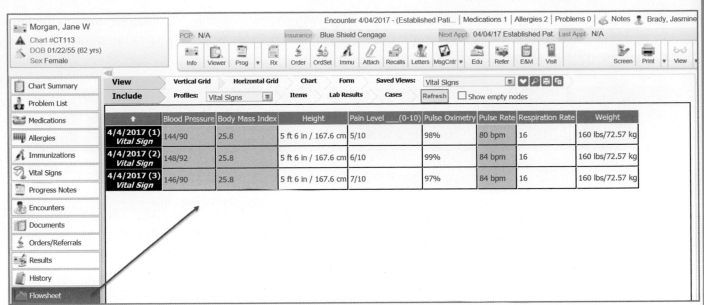

Figure 6-46   Flowsheet Application Showing Vital Signs

16.   Change the view by clicking on the *Horizontal Grid* tab.

Click on the Print icon In the top right corner of the screen. Select Flowsheet. The vital signs flowsheet should open. Print this flowsheet, label it "Activity 6-13," and place it in your assignment folder.

17.   Click "X" to close out of the *Vital Signs Flowsheet*.

Pediatric Growth Chart

Learning Objective 10: Create and print a growth chart.

According to the U.S. Department of Health and Human Services, **growth charts** provide a graphical method to compare a child's achieved growth with that of children of the same age and sex from a suitable reference population. For clinical use, such charts show selected percentiles of **anthropometric** variables such as weight, height, or body mass index (BMI) plotted against age or weight plotted against height. Anthropometric refers to a measurement or description of the physical dimensions and properties of the body, especially on a comparative basis; typically, it is used on upper and lower limbs, neck, and trunk.

Harris CareTracker EMR allows users to create, view, and print pediatric growth charts from the *Flowsheet* application in the patient's EMR. **Table 6-9** illustrates the units of measure for specific age groups.

Table 6-9 Pediatric Growth Chart Units of Measure for Age	
AGE	**UNITS OF MEASURE**
Birth to 6 days	Age is measured in days and is indicated with a "d."
7 days to 1 month	Age is measured in weeks and days and is indicated by "wks" or "wk/d."
1 month to 36 months	Age is measured in months and weeks and is indicated by "mos," "mo/wks," or "wk."
3 years to 21 years	Age is measured in years and months and is indicated by "yrs," "yr/mos," or "mo."

Harris CareTracker PM and EMR houses the standard growth charts available from the Centers for Disease Control and Prevention (CDC) and World Health Organization (WHO). **Table 6-10** highlights the different growth charts available in Harris CareTracker EMR.

Table 6-10 Types of Growth Charts in Harris CareTracker EMR	
GROWTH CHARTS FOR BOYS	**GROWTH CHARTS FOR GIRLS**
Boys HC/WT for Length 0–36 mos	Girls HC/WT for Length 0–36 mos
Boys Length/Weight for Age 0–36 mos	Girls Length/Weight for Age 0–36 mos
Boys BMI for Age 2–20 years	Girls BMI for Age 2–20 years
Boys Stature/Weight for Age 2–20 yrs	Girls Stature/Weight for Age 2–20 yrs

Courtesy of Harris CareTracker PM and EMR

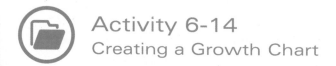

Activity 6-14
Creating a Growth Chart

1. Pull patient Alex Brady into context.

2. Click on the *Medical Record* module.

3. Click on the *Flowsheet* tab in the *Patient Health History* pane.

4. Click on the drop-down arrow beside *Profiles* and select "Boys Length/Weight for Age 0–36 months" (**Figure 6-47**).

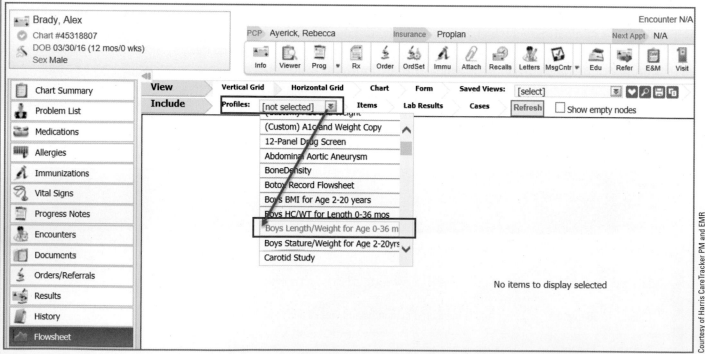

Figure 6-47   *Flowsheet Profiles*

Courtesy of Harris CareTracker PM and EMR

5. Click on the *Items* tab (Figure 6-48).

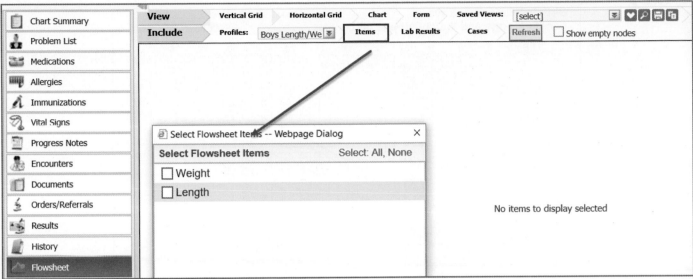

Figure 6-48   Flowsheet Items Tab

Courtesy of Harris CareTracker PM and EMR

6. The *Select Flowsheet Items* box displays. Check the boxes for "Weight" and "Length" and then click on *Select*.

7. Notice that three different weights and lengths are already entered for Alex at different age intervals. The current view is set on *Vertical Grid*. Click on *Horizontal Grid* (Figure 6-49).

8. To bring up Alex Brady's growth chart, click on the *Chart* tab in the *View* row. **Note:** If you receive an error when you click on the *Chart* tab, then print a *Horizontal Grid* view of the flowsheet instead and see Figure 6-50 for an example of what the chart would look like.

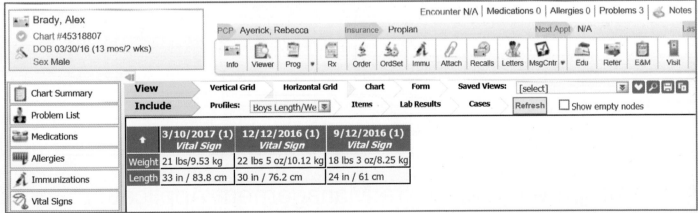

Figure 6-49   Horizontal Grid

Courtesy of Harris CareTracker PM and EMR

📠 **Click on Print in the View row. Label the growth chart "Activity 6-14" and place it in your assignment folder.**

CRITICAL THINKING Where was Alex on the growth chart for all three visits? Is there cause for concern about Alex? Why or why not? See **Figure 6-50**.

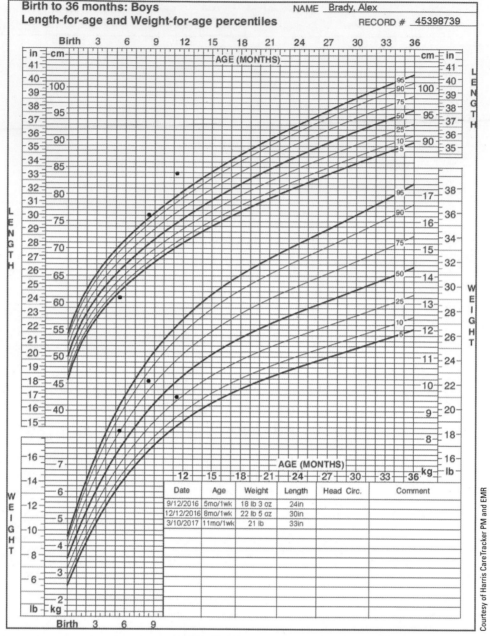

Date	Age	Weight	Length	Head Circ.	Comment
9/12/2016	5mo/1wk	18 lb 3 oz	24in		
12/12/2016	8mo/1wk	22 lb 5 oz	30in		
3/10/2017	11mo/1wk	21 lb	33in		

Courtesy of Harris CareTracker PM and EMR

Figure 6-50   Alex Brady Growth Chart

Accessing the Patient Care Management Application

Learning Objective 11: Update the Patient Care Management application.

The *Patient Care Management* application is used as a proactive reminder tool to improve the care management process. The patient is evaluated and moved to specific health maintenance and disease management registries based on measures that are activated within your group. The application helps manage the recurring preventive care items pertinent to a patient, flags overdue items, enables you to manually move the patient to a high-risk registry, and more. Additionally, you can view a list of care management items that are complete and pending for the patient by clicking the *Pt Care Mgt* link on the *Patient Health History* pane of the *Medical Record* module.

The care recommendations in the *Health Maintenance* and *Disease Management* registries are based on CDC and National Committee for Quality Assurance/Healthcare Effectiveness Data and Information Set (NCQA/ HEDIS) guidelines.

Table 6-11 provides a description of each section within the *Patient Care Management* application. **Table 6-12** provides a further description of each column within the application.

Table 6-11   Sections within the Patient Care Management Application

SECTION	DESCRIPTION
Health Maintenance	This section displays all tests/exams that a patient is due for that are part of *Health Maintenance* registries.
Disease Management	This section displays all tests/exams that a patient is due for OR is required to have according to disease management measures. Click the *Expand* icon in the *Disease Management* section to view all items that are part of the disease management measure.

Courtesy of Harris CareTracker PM and EMR

Table 6-12   Columns within the Patient Care Management Application

COLUMN	DESCRIPTION
Test/Exam	The Test/Exam for which the patient qualifies.
Status	Indicates the status of the Test/Exam. • Indicates that the Test/Exam is complete. • Indicates that the Test/Exam is missing or overdue. • Indicates that the patient refused the Test/Exam.
State	Indicates how well a disease management item is controlled. (**Note:** This is available only in the *Disease Management* section.)
Recommendation	The recommendation for having the specific Test/Exam performed.
Date of Last	The last date the Test/Exam was done.
Refused	The date the patient refused the Test/Exam. However, if the Test/Exam belongs to a series, the due date for the next Test/Exam will display under the *Due Date* column based on the interval set for the Test/Exam.
Interval	The duration between the last and next Test/Exam.
Due Date	The date the patient is due for the specific Test/Exam.
OS (Order Set)	If a *Patient Care Management* (PCM) item is associated with an order set, you can click on the *Order Set* icon to open the order set in a new window. If the PCM items are associated with multiple order sets, you can point to the *Order Set* icon to view the list of order sets. The order sets are grouped under provider, group, and company categories allowing you to click and open in a new window.
Actions (Edit, Activate/ Deactivate/Log)	Provides you the ability to edit, activate and deactivate, and view the log pertaining to the care management item.

Courtesy of Harris CareTracker PM and EMR

The *Patient Care Management* application enables you to update information, such as the due date or interval for a Test/Exam, and flag a Test/Exam that is refused by a patient. Additionally, you can remove a care management item that is due for a patient or move the patient to a high-risk registry if necessary. In Activity 6-15, you will access and update the *Patient Care Management* screen.

Activity 6-15
Accessing and Updating Patient Care Management Items

1. If you are not in Jane Morgan's medical record, access it by using the following steps:
   - Click on *Clinical Today*.
   - In the *Appointments* screen within *Clinical Today*, bring up the date of Jane Morgan's appointment. Be sure that *Resource* reflects "All." **Hint:** If you don't recall the date of the appointment, with the patient in context, click on the *History* tab in the *Scheduling* module to locate the patient's appointment. Do not create a new encounter for this activity; use only the appointment/encounter previously scheduled.
   - Click on Ms. Morgan's name. The patient's *Chart Summary* will open in a new window (refer to Figure 6-15).

2. In the *Patient Health History* pane, click on the *Pt Care Mgmt* tab. Harris CareTracker EMR displays the *Patient Care Management* window with all health maintenance and disease management items for the patient (**Figure 6-51**). The list includes both pending and completed items. **Hint:** You must have completed Activity 5-2 for this feature to display.

Morgan, Jane W	Encounter 4/04/2017 - (Established Pati...	Medications 1	Allergies 2	Problems 0	Notes	Brady, Jasmine
Chart #CT113	PCP N/A	Insurance Blue Shield Cengage	Next Appt 04/04/17 Established Pat...	Last Appt N/A
DOB 01/22/55 (62 yrs)			
Sex Female	Info Viewer Prog Rx Order OrdSet Immu Attach Recalls Letters MsgCntr Edu Refer E&M Visit Screen Print View

Status All | Complete | Incomplete

Add patient to high risk registry ☐ Show Inactive

Test/Exam		Status	State	Recommendation	Date of Last	Refused	Interval	Due Date	OS
Adult Immunizations									
Hep A Vaccine Dose 1	✖	Incomplete		Refer to CDC vaccine schedules		No		4/1/2017	
Hep A Vaccine Dose 2	✖	Incomplete		Refer to CDC vaccine schedules		No		4/1/2017	
Hep B Vaccine Dose 1	✖	Incomplete		Refer to CDC vaccine schedules		No		4/1/2017	
Hep B Vaccine Dose 2	✖	Incomplete		Refer to CDC vaccine schedules		No		4/1/2017	
Hep B Vaccine Dose 3	✖	Incomplete		Refer to CDC vaccine schedules		No		4/1/2017	
Influenza vaccine	✖	Incomplete		Annually		No	1 Years	4/1/2017	
Pneumococcal	✖	Incomplete		Refer to CDC vaccine schedules		No		4/1/2017	
Td/Tdap Vaccine	✖	Incomplete		Refer to CDC vaccine schedules		No		4/1/2017	
Varicella Dose 1	✖	Incomplete		Refer to CDC vaccine schedules		No		4/1/2017	
Varicella Dose 2	✖	Incomplete		Refer to CDC vaccine schedules		No		4/1/2017	

Chart Summary / Problem List / Medications / Allergies / Immunizations / Vital Signs / Progress Notes / Encounters / Documents / Orders/Referrals / Results / History / Flowsheet / Correspondence / Pt Care Mgmt

Figure 6-51 Patient Care Management Window

3. As you are reviewing the registry, note that the information collected during the history phase automatically populated in this section, such as the dates of the patient's last colonoscopy and Pap test. While reviewing the registry information with Ms. Morgan, she states that she just remembered that she received an influenza vaccine on October 12 of last year. The patient received the immunization at America's Urgent Care. Click the *Edit* icon in the row in which Influenza appears. Harris CareTracker EMR displays the *Edit Test/Exam* dialog box (**Figure 6-52**).

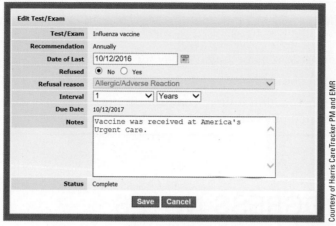

Figure 6-52   Edit Test/Exam Dialog Box

4. In the *Edit Test/Exam* box, enter October 12 of last year in the *Date of Last* field.

TIP By default, the date is auto filled in the *Date of Last* box based on the information available in Harris CareTracker EMR. However, you can change the date if necessary. Additionally, you can update the interval between the last and the next, mark a test that a patient has refused with the refusal reason, and enter additional notes. The due date and the status of the Test/Exam are automatically calculated based on the last date the exam was performed and the interval.

---

5. Leave the other fields blank because the vaccine was not administered at the Napa Valley Family Health Associates facility. Type the following in the *Notes* box: "Vaccine was received at America's Urgent Care."

6. Click *Save.* (**Note:** You may have to close out of the *Patient Care Management* window and reopen it before the influenza entry is updated on the screen. Click on *Status*, which will update as "Complete.")

🖬 **Print the updated Patient Care Management list, label it "Activity 6-15," and place it in your assignment folder.**

Many of the new "Pay for Performance" health care models require the medical assistant to review patient Health and Disease Management registries prior to the scheduled appointment. Following review, the medical assistant writes a plan, establishing steps that will be taken to bring the patient into compliance. The provider reviews the plan and makes necessary adjustments. Electronic orders are placed in the EMR prior to the appointment so that the "Catching Up" process can be performed throughout the visit. If the patient refuses any of the items listed in the plan, the medical assistant will click on the *Edit* 📝 icon and signify that the patient refused the item. The reason for refusal is then entered in the *Notes* section of the dialog box. Sharing this information with the provider prior to patient examination gives the provider an opportunity to encourage those prevention or maintenance items that the patient refused.

You can remove a patient care management item from the list by clicking the *Deactivate* ✖ icon. The inactive item appears dimmed and you can select the *Show Inactive* checkbox to view the item.

CRITICAL THINKING Review the items that Ms. Morgan is behind on and write a plan listing the following:

- Immunizations that may be given today
- Screenings that should be scheduled prior to patient departure

What are some reasons that patient may refuse these items? What can you do as a health care advocate to assist patients who are refusing due to financial constraints?

CREATING PROGRESS NOTES

Learning Objective 12: Create and print a Progress Note.

Progress notes are the heart of the patient record. They serve as a chronological listing of the patient's overall health status. Data pertaining to the findings from the visit are entered into the progress note. Most EMR software programs, including Harris CareTracker EMR, have progress note templates, copy and paste features, and automatic population tools, which make creating progress notes simplistic and efficient. The software also assists in promoting consistency from one provider to the next.

The *Progress Notes* application displays a list of notes recorded during each patient appointment and is required for medical, legal, and billing purposes. The note includes information such as the patient's history, medications, and allergies as well as a complete record of all that occurred during the visit. The application provides a quick and easy way to review and sign notes and helps identify notes that must be signed by a cosigner.

Progress Note Templates

Each predefined specialty and condition specific template available in Harris CareTracker EMR simplifies the process of documenting a patient encounter at the point of care. Harris CareTracker EMR provides several template types, each offering a specific layout and custom options. These options allow providers to select the template that best suits their documenting needs. Staff members can also pull in sections of a prior note and insert documents and images into templates if necessary. Standard templates can be broken down by specialty and template styles. **Table 6-13** describes the standard templates available in Harris CareTracker EMR.

Table 6-13 Progress Note Templates	
TEMPLATE	**DESCRIPTION**
Option 1	This template consists of two tabs and is recommended for providers who prefer using a simple version of a template with quick text or dictation. One tab consists of text boxes for Chief Complaint and History of Present Illness (CC/HPI), History (HX), Review Of Systems (ROS), Physical Exam (PE), Tests, Procedures (Proc), and Assessment and Plan (A&P). The second tab consists of structured data elements that link to the Quality Measure reports in Harris CareTracker PM and EMR.
Option 2	This template consists of eight tabs and is recommended for providers who prefer using a simple version of a template with quick text or dictation. Seven tabs consist of text boxes to document the Chief Complaint and History of Present Illness (CC/HPI), History (HX), Review of Systems (ROS), Physical Exam (PE), Tests, Procedures (Proc), and Assessment and Plan (A&P) in each tab. The last tab consists of structured data elements that link to the Quality Measure reports in Harris CareTracker PM and EMR.

TEMPLATE	DESCRIPTION
Option 3	This template consists of eight tabs and is recommended for providers who are using the structured option or combination of structure and quick text to document a note. The template provides data elements in one screen and additional elements in a pop-up window to be used as necessary. This option allows for no scrolling within the template.
Option 4	This is recommended for providers who are using the structured option or combination of structure and quick text to document a note. All data elements are organized in one screen, enabling you to scroll through to document patient information.

Courtesy of Harris CareTracker PM and EMR

Activity 6-16
Accessing and Updating the Progress Notes Application

Note: Updating the *Progress Note* is typically a provider's responsibility and function; however, it is in the medical assistant's best interest to have knowledge and understanding of the *Progress Note*. Some practices use scribes. It is entirely possible that the medical assistant will then be responsible for recording the provider's findings. Although the entire activity is not required, the creation of the *Progress Note* (steps 1–6) is required and must be completed in order to complete later activities.

1. If you are not in Jane Morgan's medical record, access it by using the following steps:
   - Click on *Clinical Today*.
   - In the *Appointments* screen within *Clinical Today*, bring up the date of Jane Morgan's appointment. Be sure that *Resource* reflects "All." **Hint:** If you don't recall the date of the appointment, with the patient in context, click on the *History* tab in the *Scheduling* module to locate the patient's appointment. Do not create a new encounter for this activity; use only the appointment/encounter previously scheduled.
   - Click on Ms. Morgan's name. The patient's *Chart Summary* will open in a new window (refer to Figure 6-15).

2. In the *Clinical Toolbar*, click the drop-down in the *Progress Notes* tab and select the encounter in context. If an encounter is in context, which in this case it is, Harris CareTracker EMR displays the *Progress Notes* template window (**Figure 6-53**). (**Note:** If documenting a progress note that is not based on an appointment, the *Encounter* dialog box displays, enabling you to create a new encounter. If you are getting an *Encounter* dialog box, it means that you did not have an encounter in context. Repeat step 1 if necessary.)

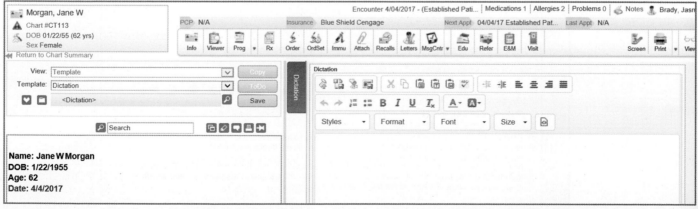

Figure 6-53 Progress Notes Template Window

Courtesy of Harris CareTracker PM and EMR

3. Alternatively, if the *Progress Notes* template window does not display, click on the date of the *Encounter* you want to make a progress note for. Then, beneath the *Progress Note* window, click *Edit*.

4. By default, the *View* field displays "Template." (Skip this box at this time.)

5. In the *Template* field, click on the drop-down arrow and select "IM OV Option 4 (v4) w/A&P" (**Figure 6-54**). Complete the note by navigating through each tab. (The provider would ordinarily work in the progress note, but because the provider is not available or you are the designated scribe, you will be entering the information for the provider.)

6. All the information you entered regarding Ms. Morgan's medical history, allergy information, medication list, vital signs, and preventive care are now populated within the progress note. The *CC/HPI* tab

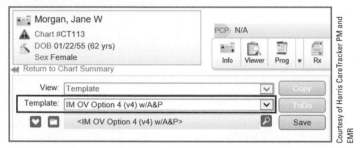

Figure 6-54   IM OV Option 4 (v4) w/A&P Template

will be showing on the right side of the screen (Figure 6-54). Review the note you wrote regarding the patient's chief complaint. The provider will expand a bit on the complaint by developing the History of Present Illness (HPI). Scroll down to the *History of Present Illness* box and type the following:

"Patient has a five-year history of UTIs (1–2 infections/year). Current episode includes frequency, urgency, and pain upon urination (7/10). Pt. denies fever, blood, or pus in urine, or the presence of vaginal symptoms. No back or abdominal pain. Patient drinks very little water and has at least two beverages per day which include caffeine. Last UTI was approximately three months ago. Treatment included a 10-day treatment of Bactrim DS. Patient states that she completed the treatment and was free of urinary symptoms. Patient did not follow up for a post check."

Your documentation should match **Figure 6-55**.

7. Click on *Save*, located in the template box in the middle of the screen (**Figure 6-56**).

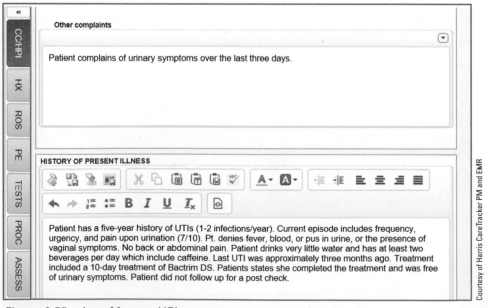

Figure 6-55   Jane Morgan HPI

8. Click on the *HX* tab on the right side of the progress note (center of screen). Review the information

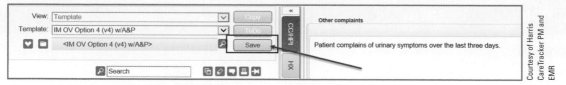

Figure 6-56   Save Button for Template Screen

that you entered while collecting the patient history. Because you are acting as the provider or the scribe in this section, indicate that you reviewed each section of the history by clicking on the plus sign [+] next to *Reviewed* at the top of the screen. Check marks will now appear next to each box in the *Reviewed* section (**Figure 6-57**).

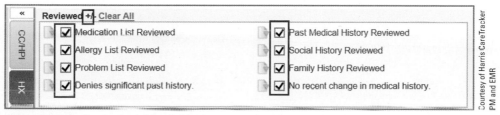

Figure 6-57   Reviewed Check Marks

9. Click on *Save* to update the note.

10. Click on the *ROS* tab. Refer to **Table 6-14** to complete this section of the progress note.

Table 6-14	Completing the ROS Tab
SECTION	**ENTRY**
Constitutional	Check the box beside *No constitutional symptoms.*
Eyes	Check the box beside *No eye symptoms.*
ENMT	No entry.
Neck	Check the box beside *No neck symptoms.*
Breasts	No entry.
Respiratory	Check the box beside *No respiratory symptoms.*
Cardiovascular	Click on the minus symbol so that *N* for No is selected for each box. Now click on the *Y* beside "cold hands or feet."
Gastrointestinal	Check the box beside *No GI symptoms.*
Genitourinary	Select *Y* for Yes for the following categories: "dysuria," "burning on urination," "urgency," and "frequency." Select *N* for No for all other genitourinary (GU) symptoms.
Skin	No entry.
Musculoskeletal	No entry.

(continues)

Table 6-14 (*continued*)

SECTION	ENTRY
Neurological	No entry.
Psychiatric	Select *Y* for Yes for depression and *N* for No for all other symptoms.
Hematologic	No entry.
Endocrine	No entry.

11. Click *Save* to update the progress note with the ROS findings.

12. Click on the *PE* tab. Use Table 6-15 to complete this portion of the note.

Table 6-15 Completing the PE Tab

SECTION	ENTRY
General	Click the plus sign beside *General* so that a check mark is placed beside each box in the section.
HEENT	*Head*: Check the box beside *Negative head exam*. *Eyes*: Click on the *Y* for Yes next to "PERRL." Click on the *N* for No next to "EOMI" and "scleral icterus." *ENT*: No entry.
Neck	Check the box beside *Negative neck exam*.
Lymphatics	No entry.
Chest	*Chest*: Check the box beside *Negative chest exam*. *Breasts*: No entry. *Lungs*: Check the box beside *Negative lung exam*.
Heart	Check the box beside *Negative heart exam*.
Abdomen	Click on the minus sign beside *Abdomen* so that a red "X" is placed beside each box in the section. Click the *Y* for Yes beside "soft" and "tenderness". In the *Other abdomen findings* section, enter: "The abdomen was soft with minimal tenderness to palpation in the left periumbilical and left lower quadrant. There was no guarding or rebound."
Genitourinary	Check the box beside *Negative genitourinary exam*.
Musculoskeletal	No entry.
Neurological	No entry.
Mental Status Exam	No entry.
Skin	No entry.

13. Click *Save* to update the progress note with the PE findings.

14. Skip the *TESTS* and *PROC* tabs.

15. Click on the *ASSESS* tab. By default, the *ASSESS* tab defaults to "Template." The other quick view tabs are the "Problem List" tab and the "Visit" tab (**Figure 6-58**).

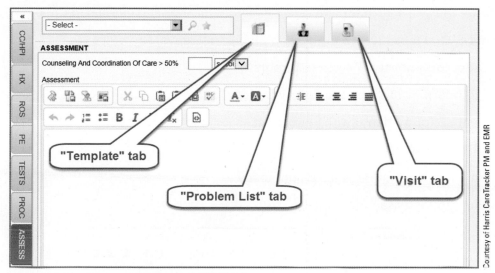

Figure 6-58   Progress Note ASSESS Tab Icons

16. It was discovered during the exam that the patient has hypertension. The provider also diagnosed the patient with a urinary tract infection (UTI) and dysuria. You will be selecting only ICD-10 codes associated with the provider's diagnoses, as directed in steps 17 through 19.

17. Click on the *Search* icon to the right of the *-Select-* drop-down menu at the top of the screen. In the *Diagnosis Search* window that pops up, enter "urinary tract infection" in the *Search Text* field and click the *Search* button. Click on "urinary tract infection" (ICD-10 code N39.0) in the results section of the *Diagnosis Search* window (note that it may have already been marked as a favorite diagnosis).

18. Search for and select "essential hypertension" (ICD-10 code I10).

19. Search for and select "recurrent and persistent hematuria" (ICD-10 code N02.9) and "dysuria" (ICD-10 code R30.0) as well. After selecting each diagnosis, scroll down to the bottom of the *ASSESS* tab, and see all selected codes listed under *Today's Selected Diagnosis*. Both the ICD-9 and ICD-10 versions of the code are listed (**Figure 6-59**).

	Today's Selected Diagnosis	ICD-9	ICD-10	PL	OS
✔	Diagnosis				
✔	Urinary tract infection	599.0	N39.0	✔	
✔	Essential hypertension	401.9	I10	✔	
✔	Recurrent and persistent hematuria	581.9	N02.9	✔	
✔	Dysuria	788.1	R30.0	✔	

Figure 6-59   Today's Selected Diagnosis

20. Click *Save* to update the progress note with the *Assessment* information.

21. Click on the *PLAN* tab to record the provider's plans. Document the following in the *Additional Plan Details* box (**Figure 6-60**):

    a. Stat lab test—"Urinalysis dipstick panel by Automated test strip"

    b. Send urine out for lab test "Urinalysis microscopic panel [#volume] in urine by automated count"

    c. Give patient educational handouts (1) Urinary Tract Infections in Women, and (2) What is Hematuria? (**Note:** You will search for and select Patient Educational handouts in Chapter 7, Activity 7-10.)

    d. Bactrim DS Oral Tabs (80–160 mg), Sig 1 tab bid for 5 days, No refills

    e. Enter Order for 3-phase CT cystourethrogram

    f. Patient to return in 10 days for a Follow-Up UA

    g. Set patient up for a referral with a urologist

        PREVENTION GOALS

    a. Patient to have her first Hepatitis B shot today

    b. Set patient up for a mammogram

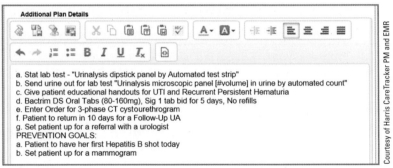

Figure 6-60   *Additional Plan Details Box*

22. Click *Save*.

 Click the orange Print icon in the middle of the screen. The Clinical Note dialog box will open. Click the Print button and select your printer to print a copy of the progress note. Label it "Activity 6-16" and place it in your assignment folder.

23. Close out of the Printed Progress Note by clicking on the "X" in the upper-right-hand corner.

24. Click on the *Return to Chart Summary* link (in blue) at the top left of the screen just under the patient's name and chart number to return to the patient's medical record.

 ## Activity 6-17:
Creating a Progress Note with Pediatric Template (abbreviated version only)

1. If you are not in Francisco Powell Jimenez's medical record, access it by using the following steps:

    - Click on *Clinical Today*.

    - In the *Appointments* screen within *Clinical Today*, bring up the date of Francisco's appointment. Be sure that *Resource* reflects "All." **Hint:** If you don't recall the date of the appointment, with the patient in context, click on the *History* tab in the *Scheduling* module to locate the patient's appointment. Do not create a new encounter for this activity; use only the appointment/encounter previously scheduled.

- Click on Francisco's name. The patient's *Chart Summary* will open in a new window (refer to Figure 6-15).

2. In the *Clinical Toolbar*, click the drop-down in the *Progress Notes* ▤ tab and select the encounter in context. If an encounter is in context, Harris CareTracker EMR displays the *Progress Notes* template window (**Figure 6-61**). (**Hint:** Be sure the encounter is displaying above the name bar for the appointment you booked in Chapter 4.) (**Note:** If documenting a progress note that is not based on an appointment, the *Encounter* dialog box displays, enabling you to create a new encounter. If you are getting an *Encounter* dialog box, it means that you did not have an encounter in context. Repeat step 1 if necessary.)

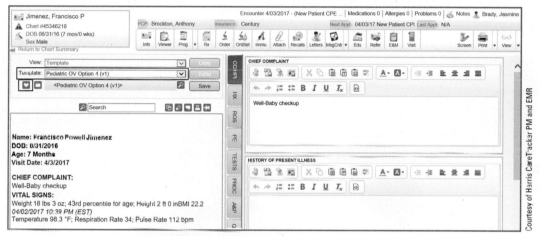

Figure 6-61   Pediatric Progress Note Template

3. Alternatively, if the *Progress Notes* template window does not display, click on the date of the *Encounter* you want to make a progress note for. Then, beneath the *Progress Note* window, click *Edit*.

4. By default, the *View* field displays "Template." (Skip this box at this time.)

5. Below the *Template* field, click on the *Search* icon. The *Search Template* dialog box will display.

6. Scroll down and click on the + sign next to PEDIATRICS.

7. Scroll down and select "Pediatric OV Option 4 (v1)" by clicking on the template.

8. Click on the *Favorite* icon (the heart) to save this template as a favorite.

9. Complete the note by navigating through each tab. **Note:** Because you are only creating an "abbreviated" progress note, you will not be entering additional information at this time.

10. Any information you would have entered regarding Francisco's medical history, allergy information, medication list, vital signs, and preventive care would now be populated within the progress note.

11. The *CC/HPI* tab will be showing on the right side of the screen. Review the note you wrote regarding the patient's chief complaint. The provider will expand a bit on the complaint by developing the History of Present Illness (HPI).

12. Scroll down to the *History of Present Illness* box and type the following:

    "Patient here for Well-Baby Check."

13. Click on *Save*, which is located in the template box in the middle of the screen.

Click the orange Print **icon in the middle of the screen. The Clinical Note dialog box will open. Click the Print button and select your printer to print a copy of the progress note. Label it "Activity 6-17" and place it in your assignment folder.**

14. Close out of the printed progress note.

15. Click on the *Return to Chart Summary* link (in blue) at the top left of the screen to return to the patient's medical record.

CRITICAL THINKING   At the beginning of this chapter, you were challenged to embrace the EMR training in this chapter so that you are able to fully navigate the patient's medical record in Harris CareTracker EMR. Now that you have completed many detailed clinical tasks, did you find the transition from administrative to clinical duties seamless? Were there any particular activities that were challenging? What steps did you take to work through the tasks? Does the amount of information needed to accurately record patient information and patient care help with your understanding of the roles of health care providers and the health care system overall? Explain your thoughts and conclusions.

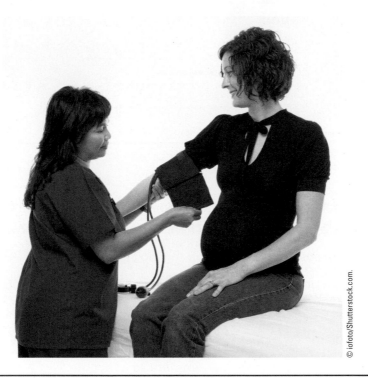

© iofoto/Shutterstock.com.

SUMMARY

In this chapter you learned about the patient's EMR. Electronic medical records help organize the chart and keep the office running efficiently. Harris CareTracker PM and EMR provides users with many tools to keep up with clinical documentation and tasks.

It is your job to work on electronic tasks throughout the day and to help your provider stay on task as well. It is important to remember that even though Harris CareTracker EMR provides all this robust technology, the patient is always your first priority. Do not get trapped behind the technology during the visit. Always remember to look up from the computer so that you can study the patient's face and body language. Treat your patient the way that you would want to be treated.

CHECK YOUR KNOWLEDGE

Select the best response.

_____ 1. Electronic tasks should be checked:

      a. Before patients arrive   c. Before departing for the day

      b. Between patients   d. All of the above

_____ 2. What is considered the heart of the patient record?

      a. The patient's medication list   c. The allergy list

      b. Progress notes   d. The patient's medical history

_____ 3. What application in Harris CareTracker EMR features information regarding prevention and disease management measures?

      a. *Task* menu   c. *Patient Care Management* application

      b. *Clinical Toolbar*   d. None of the above

_____ 4. An unsigned note in Harris CareTracker EMR refers to which of the following?

      a. A prescription that has not been signed   c. A message that has not been signed

              d. A progress note that has not been signed

      b. A fax that has not been signed

_____ 5. Once enrolled in Surescripts®, the practice is required to send a minimum of how many prescriptions within 48 hours to receive renewal requests and to accept or deny requests?

      a. 1   c. 10

      b. 5   d. 15

_____ 6. In the *History* application, which Tab contains information such as a patient's human immunodeficiency virus (HIV) or sexually transmitted disease (STD) statuses and information on overuse of alcohol and/or chemicals recorded?

      a. Patient History   c. Sensitive Info

      b. Family History   d. Advance Directive

_____ 7. An encounter is an interaction with a patient and includes all of the following except:

      a. Visits   c. ICD codes

      b. Payments   d. CPT® codes

_____ 8. Transfer status means that a patient has been transferred to:

      a. The examination room   c. Radiology

      b. Checkout   d. Another provider

_____ 9. Selected medications are screened for possible contraindications in regard to:

      a. The patient's active medications   c. The patient's problems

      b. The patient's allergies   d. All of the above

_____ 10. When a patient is allergic to a medication, what type of alert would be most appropriate?

      a. Pop-up alert   c. No alert

      b. Soft alert   d. There is no set standard

CASE STUDIES

Case Study 6-1

Recheck the quick tasks list for Dr. Raman. (Use the steps in Activity 6-4 for guidance and make sure that Dr. Raman is selected as the provider in your clinical batch.)

1. How many open encounters do you have?

2. How many unsigned notes do you have?

3. How many open orders do you have?

▣ Write the answers down on a separate sheet of paper. Label this "Case Study 6-1" and place it in your assignment folder.

Case Study 6-2

(**Note:** You must have completed all of the prior chapter Case Studies for patient James Smith in order to complete this activity. If you have not previously completed the James Smith case studies, skip to Case Study 6-3.)

Using the steps you learned throughout this chapter and the information packet for James Smith, update Mr. Smith's medical record and create a progress note. See the steps below for more information.

1. Click on *Clinical Today*.

2. In the *Appointments* screen within *Clinical Today*, bring up the date of James Smith's appointment scheduled in Chapter 4. Be sure that *Resource* reflects "All." **Hint:** If you don't recall the date of the appointment, with the patient in context, click on the *History* tab in the *Scheduling* module to locate the patient's appointment. Do not create a new encounter for this activity; use only the appointment/encounter previously scheduled.

3. Click on Mr. Smith's name. The patient's *Chart Summary* will open in a new window (refer to Figure 6-15).

4. Complete the following activities/entries using information from **Table 6-16**:

   • Add medications (refer to Activity 6-7 for help). **Note:** Select "Benefit outweighs risk" in the *Interaction Screening* dialog box when entering medication(s).

Table 6-16	James Smith: CC, Medications, Allergies, and Immunizations
CC for Visit	Follow-up exam/consultation; review lab and EKG
Medication	(1) Atorvastatin Calcium Oral Tablet 20 mg by mouth every night (2) Lasix Oral Tablet 20 mg by mouth every morning
Allergy	No known drug allergies
Past Immunization	Influenza vaccine October 1 of last year

- Add an allergy, if applicable. Refer to Activity 6-8 for help.
- Enter past immunizations to the patient's chart. Refer to Activity 6-9 for help.

5. Enter the patient's medical history using Source Document 6-1, located at the end of this case study. Refer to Activity 6-10 for help.

6. Record the patient's vital signs noted in **Table 6-17**. Refer to Activity 6-11 for help.

Table 6-17   James Smith: Vital Signs

Height	6 ft 2 in
Weight	201 lbs
BMI	(automatically calculates)
Blood Pressure	149/93
Pulse Rate	77
Temperature	98.6°F
Respiratory Rate	16
Pulse Oximetry	99%
Pain Level (0–10)	0 / 10

7. Create a progress note for Mr. Smith using the "IM OV Option 4 (v4) w/A&P" template. Complete the progress note using the information provided in Source Document 6-1, located at the end of this case study. Refer back to Activity 6-16 for guidance if needed.

📠 **After entering all of the information provided in the packet, print a chart summary (label it "Case Study 6-2A") and progress note (label it "Case Study 6-2B"), and place them in your assignment folder.**

(continues)

Source Document 6-1

James M. Smith DOB: 2/23/1965

Patient History

Reviewed

☑ Medication List Reviewed	☑ Past Medical History Reviewed
☑ Allergy List Reviewed	☑ Social History Reviewed
☐ Problem List Reviewed	☑ Family History Reviewed
☐ Denies significant past history.	☐ No recent change in medical history.

GENERAL MEDICAL HISTORY

☐ Alcoholism	☐ Depression	☐ Kidney Infections
☐ Allergies/Hayfever	☐ DM Type 1	☐ Kidney stone
☐ Anemia	☑ DM Type 2	☐ Migraine
☐ Anxiety	☐ Epilepsy	☐ Multiple Sclerosis
☐ Asthma	☐ Fracture	☐ Obesity
☐ Atrial Fibrillation	☐ Gastric ulcer	☐ Old MI
☐ Blood Transfusions	☐ Gastrointestinal Disease	☐ Osteoarthritis
☐ CAD	☐ GERD	☐ Osteoporosis
☐ Cancer	☐ Gestational Diabetes	☐ Pneumonia
☐ Cardiac Pacer	☐ Glaucoma	☐ Progressive Neurological Disorder
☐ Cardiovascular Disease	☐ Heart Murmur	☐ Pulmonary Disease
☐ CHF	☐ Hepatitis	☐ Rheumatic Fever
☐ Cirrhosis	☐ High Cholesterol	☐ Rheumatoid Arthritis
☐ Colitis	☐ Hyperlipidemia	☐ STD
☐ COPD	☐ Hypertension	☐ Terminal Illness
☐ CRF	☐ Hyperthyroidism	☐ Thyroid Disease
☐ Crohn's Disease	☐ Hypothyroidism	☐ TIA
☐ CVA	☑ Joint Pain	☐ Tuberculosis

HOSPITALIZATIONS

OTHER MEDICAL HISTORY

Tobacco Assessment

This section supports Stage 1 Meaningful Use
Smoking Status Current Everyday Smoker   ☒ Tobacco User
pack-years **25**   Date quit smoking
☐ Counseling on tobacco cessation
☐ Rx therapy for tobacco cessation
☑ Discussed Smoking/Tobacco Use Cessation Strategies

Social History

Alcohol Use Occasional	Educational level
Caffeine Use 2 servings per Day	Marital Status Single
☒ Drug Use	Exercise Habits moderate >3 x/wk
☒ sun protection	☑ seatbelts
☒ Tattoos	☐ Body piercings
☒ sexually active	birth control method
Race White	Birth Control Device insertion date
Native language	Birth Control Device removal date
☒ physical abuse	Religion
☒ domestic violence	Occupation **IT Support**
Other Social History	

Depression Screening

☐ Patient Refused
Little interest or pleasure in doing things At no time
Feeling down, depressed, or hopeless

Date of Last Depression Screening/PHQ-2
PHQ-2 Score **PHQ2 Score: 1**

OB/GYN HISTORY

LMP

Frequency of menstrual cycle   Days menstrual cycle

☐ Menopause has occurred

☐ History of abnormal pap smears

☐ Sexually Active   Birth Control
                                                              Birth Control Device insertion date
                                                              Birth Control Device removal date
☐ ectopic pregnancy

PREGNANCY SUMMARY

Gravida

Term

Preterm   Miscarriage
AB   Elective Abortion
Live children   C-Section:

OTHER OB-GYN HISTORY

SURGICAL / PROCEDURAL

☐ No prior surgical history

☐ Appendectomy   ☐ Endometrial Ablation   ☐ Laparoscopy
☐ Breast Lumpectomy   ☐ Gall Bladder   Mastectomy
☐ Cataract Surgery   ☐ Heart Surgery   ☐ Myomectomy

Location:

Location:

☐ Colectomy   ☐ Hemorrhoids   ☐ Oophorectomy
☐ Cone Biopsy   ☐ Hernia   ☐ Tonsil/Adenoidectomy
☐ D&C   ☐ Hysterectomy   ☐ Tubal Ligation

OTHER SURGICAL
HISTORY

PREVENTIVE CARE

A1c %   HPV Test
Air Contrast Barium Enema   HPV Vaccine
Ankle Brachial Index   Last Complete Physical Exam
Blood Glucose   Lipids
Bone Density   Mammography
Chest X-Ray   Pap Smear
Chlamydia Screening   Pneumovax
Colonoscopy 10/14/2016   PSA   02/10/2017
Dilated Eye Exam 04/17/2017   Pulmonary Function Tests
DTaP Vaccine (90700)   Routine Eye Exam
Echocardiogram   Stool Occult Blood
Electrocardiogram   Stress Test
Flexible Sigmoidoscopy   Td
Flu Vaccine 10/09/2017   Tdap Vaccine, Adult
Foot Exam Date   Tuberculin PPD
HIV Test Date   Varicella
                                             Zoster Vaccine (90736)
Self-Management Goal

(continues)

James M. Smith DOB: 2/23/1965

Sensitive Information

STD

☒ Vaginosis		☒ Gonorrhea	
☒ Trichomonas		☒ Chlamydia	
☒ Genital Warts		☒ Syphilis	
☒ PID		☒ HPV	

STD Info

SUBSTANCE ABUSE

☒ History of Substance Abuse

Abused Substances

MENTAL HEALTH

☒ Seeing mental health provider

Mental Health Provider Name

Mental Health Condition(s)

HIV Status

HIV Status

HIV Test Date

HIV Notes

Has never had an HIV test.

Courtesy of Harris CareTracker PM and EMR

James M Smith DOB: 2/23/1965

Family History

GENERAL FAMILY HISTORY

☐ Adopted	☐ Denial of any knowledge of significant family history	
☐ Unknown Paternal Hx	☐ Unknown Maternal Hx	
☐ Alcoholism	☐ Congenital Anomaly	☑ Hypertension
☐ Anemia	☐ COPD	☐ Hypothyroidism
☐ Anxiety	☐ Crohn's Disease	☑ Kidney Disease
☐ Asthma	☐ Depression	☐ Liver Disease
☐ Birth Defects	☑ Diabetes	☐ Multiple Births
☐ CAD	☐ Epilepsy	☐ Osteoarthritis
☐ Cardiovascular Disease	☑ GERD	☐ Osteoporosis
☐ CHF	☐ Hypercholesterolemia	☐ Pulmonary Disease
Cancer	☑ Hyperlipidemia	☐ Stroke
Other conditions	....	

Courtesy of Harris CareTracker PM and EMR

Case Study 6-3

Update Mr. Thompson's medical record and create a progress note. See the steps below for more information.

1. Click on *Clinical Today*.

2. In the *Appointments* screen within *Clinical Today*, bring up the date of Adam Thompson's appointment scheduled in Chapter 4. Be sure that *Resource* reflects "All." **Hint:** If you don't recall the date of the appointment, with the patient in context, click on the *History* tab in the *Scheduling* module to locate the patient's appointment. Do not create a new encounter for this activity; use only the appointment/encounter previously scheduled.

3. Click on Mr. Thompson's name. The patient's *Chart Summary* will open in a new window (refer to Figure 6-15).

4. Complete the following activities/entries using information from **Table 6-18**:

    *   Add medications. Refer to Activity 6-7 for help. **Note:** Select "Benefit outweighs risk" in the *Interaction Screening* dialog box when entering medication(s).

    *   Add an allergy. Refer to Activity 6-8 for help.

    *   Enter past immunizations to the patient's chart. Refer to Activity 6-9 for help.

Table 6-18   Adam Thompson: CC, Medications, Allergies, and Immunizations

CC for Visit	productive cough
Medication	(1) Atorvastatin Calcium Oral Tablet 20 mg by mouth every night (2) Micardis Oral Tablet 40 mg by mouth every night (3) Potassium Chloride Extended-Release Oral Capsules 10 mEq by mouth every morning (4) NEXIUM Delayed-Release Capsule 20 mg by mouth every morning one hour before food (5) Lasix Oral Tablet 20 mg by mouth every morning
Allergy	Penicillin V Potassium (reaction: anaphylaxis). Use date January 1, 1990
Past Immunization	(1) Influenza vaccine September 1 of last year (2) Pneumococcal vaccine September 1 of last year

5. Enter the patient's medical history using information from Source Document 6-2, located at the end of this case study. Refer to Activity 6-10 for help.

6. Record the patient's vital signs from **Table 6-19**. Refer to Activity 6-11 for help.

(continues)

CASE STUDIES *(continued)*

Table 6-19   Adam Thompson: Vital Signs

Height	5 ft 8 in
Weight	197
BMI	(automatically calculates)
Blood Pressure	151/87
Pulse Rate	62
Temperature	100.6°F
Respiratory Rate	19
Pulse Oximetry	95%
Pain Level (0–10)	4/10

7. Create a progress note for Mr. Thompson using the "IM OV Option 4 (v4) w/A&P" template. Complete the progress note using the information provided in Source Document 6-2 (located at the end of this case study). Refer back to Activity 6-16 for guidance if needed.

🖥 **After entering all of the information provided in the packet, print a chart summary (label it "Case Study 6-3A") and progress note (label it "Case Study 6-3B"), and place them in your assignment folder.**

Source Document 6-2

Adam Thompson DOB: 1/1/1942

Patient History

Reviewed

☑ Medication List Reviewed		☑ Past Medical History Reviewed
☑ Allergy List Reviewed		☑ Social History Reviewed
☐ Problem List Reviewed		☑ Family History Reviewed
☐ Denies significant past history.		☐ No recent change in medical history.

GENERAL MEDICAL HISTORY

☐ Alcoholism	☐ Depression	☐ Kidney Infections
☐ Allergies/Hayfever	☐ DM Type 1	☐ Kidney stone
☐ Anemia	☐ DM Type 2	☐ Migraine
☐ Anxiety	☐ Epilepsy	☐ Multiple Sclerosis
☐ Asthma	☐ Fracture	☐ Obesity
☐ Atrial Fibrillation	☑ Gastric ulcer	☐ Old MI
☐ Blood Transfusions	☐ Gastrointestinal Disease	☑ Osteoarthritis
☐ CAD	☑ GERD	☐ Osteoporosis
☐ Cancer	☐ Gestational Diabetes	☐ Pneumonia
☐ Cardiac Pacer	☐ Glaucoma	☐ Progressive Neurological Disorder
☑ Cardiovascular Disease	☐ Heart Murmur	☐ Pulmonary Disease
☐ CHF	☐ Hepatitis	☐ Rheumatic Fever
☐ Cirrhosis	☐ High Cholesterol	☐ Rheumatoid Arthritis
☐ Colitis	☐ Hyperlipidemia	☐ STD
☐ COPD	☑ Hypertension	☐ Terminal Illness
☐ CRF	☐ Hyperthyroidism	☐ Thyroid Disease
☐ Crohn's disease	☐ Hypothyroidism	☐ TIA
☐ CVA	☐ Joint Pain	☐ Tuberculosis

HOSPITALIZATIONS   Cardiac Pacemaker Placement 02/15/2011. Overnight stay at Napa Valley Medical Center. No complications

OTHER MEDICAL HISTORY

Tobacco Assessment

This section supports Stage 1 Meaningful Use	
Smoking Status Former smoker	
# pack-years **20**	☐ Tobacco User
☐ Counseling on tobacco cessation	Date quit smoking **03/14/1990**
☐ Rx therapy for tobacco cessation	
☐ Discussed Smoking/Tobacco Use Cessation Strategies	

Social History

Alcohol Use Occasional	Educational level
Caffeine Use 2 servings per Day	Marital Status
☒ Drug Use	Exercise Habits
☒ sun protection	☑ seatbelts
☒ Tattoos	☐ Body piercings
☒ sexually active	birth control method
Race	Birth Control Device insertion date
Native language	Birth Control Device removal date
☐ physical abuse	Religion
☐ domestic violence	Occupation
Other Social History	

Depression Screening

☐ Patient Refused
Little interest or pleasure in doing things
Feeling down, depressed, or hopeless

Date of Last Depression Screening/PHQ-2
PHQ-2 Score **PHQ2 Score: incomplete**

(continues)

CASE STUDIES *(continued)*

OB/GYN HISTORY

LMP	Menarche Age
Frequency of menstrual cycle	Days menstrual cycle
☐ Menopause has occurred	
☐ History of abnormal pap smears	
☐ Sexually Active	Birth Control
	Birth Control Device insertion date
	Birth Control Device removal date
☐ ectopic pregnancy	

PREGNANCY SUMMARY

Gravida	
Term	
Preterm	Miscarriage
AB	Elective Abortion
Live children	C-Section:
OTHER OB-GYN HISTORY	

SURGICAL / PROCEDURAL

☐ No prior surgical history		
☐ Appendectomy	☐ Endometrial Ablation	☐ Laparoscopy
☐ Breast Lumpectomy	☐ Gall Bladder	Mastectomy
☐ Cataract Surgery	☐ Heart Surgery	☐ Myomectomy
☐ Colectomy	☐ Hemorrhoids	☐ Oophorectomy
☐ Cone Biopsy	☐ Hernia	☐ Tonsil/Adenoidectomy
☐ D&C	☐ Hysterectomy	☐ Tubal Ligation

OTHER SURGICAL HISTORY   Cardiac Pacemaker in 2011

PREVENTIVE CARE

A1c %	HPV Test
Air Contrast Barium Enema	HPV Vaccine
Ankle Brachial Index	Last Complete Physical Exam
Blood Glucose	Lipids
Bone Density	Mammography
Chest X-Ray	Pap Smear
Chlamydia Screening	Pneumovax
Colonoscopy 10/01/2008	PSA
Dilated Eye Exam	Pulmonary Function Tests
DTaP Vaccine (90700)	Routine Eye Exam
Echocardiogram	Stool Occult Blood 05/10/2010
Electrocardiogram	Stress Test 10/10/2013
Flexible Sigmoidoscopy	Td
Flu vaccine 09/15/2013	Tdap Vaccine, Adult
Foot Exam Date	Tuberculin PPD
HIV Test Date:	Varicella
	Zoster Vaccine (90736) 03/22/2007
Self-Management Goal	

Adam Thompson DOB: 1/1/1942

Sensitive Information

STD

☒ Vaginosis	☒ Gonorrhea
☒ Trichomonas	☒ Chlamydia
☒ Genital Warts	☒ Syphillis
☒ PID	☒ HPV
STD Info	

SUBSTANCE ABUSE

☒ History of Substance Abuse
Abused Substances

MENTAL HEALTH

☒ Seeing mental health provider
Mental Health Provider Name
Mental Health Condition(s)

HIV Status

HIV Status
HIV Test Date
HIV Notes

Medicare High Risk Criteria

Age when became sexually active
☐ More than five sexual partners in lifetime
☐ DES history in mother
Pap Smear
☐ History of abnormal pap smears

Adam Thompson DOB: 1/1/1942

Family History

GENERAL FAMILY HISTORY

☐ Adopted	☐ Denial of any knowledge of significant family history	
☐ Unknown Paternal Hx	☐ Unknown Maternal Hx	
☐ Alcoholism	☐ Congenital Anomaly	☑ Hypertension
☐ Anemia	☑ COPD	☐ Hypothyroidism
☐ Anxiety	☐ Crohn's Disease	☐ Kidney Disease
☑ Asthma	☐ Depression	☐ Liver Disease
☐ Birth Defects	☑ Diabetes	☐ Multiple Births
☐ CAD	☐ Epilepsy	☐ Osteoarthritis
☑ Cardiovascular Disease	☐ GERD	☐ Osteoporosis
☐ CHF	☐ Hypercholesterolemia	☐ Pulmonary Disease
Cancer lung	☐ Hyperlipidemia	☑ Stroke
Other conditions		

Courtesy of Harris CareTracker PM and EMR

BUILD YOUR PROFICIENCY

Proficiency Builder 6-1: Additional Practice Transferring Patients
Transfer the rest of the patients you scheduled in Activity 4-12 (each of the patient's noted in step 1 below) to Exam Room # 1. Refer to Activity 6-3 for guidance.

1. Click on the *Clinical Today* module. Match the search parameters to those set in
   Activity 6-2 for each of the following patients and transfer each patient:

   a. Craig X. Smith

   b. Ellen Ristino

   c. Adam Thompson

   d. Edith Robinson

   e. Barbara Watson

   f. Francisco Powell Jimenez

   If you have completed the cases studies for patients James Smith and Kimberly Johnson, check them in and transfer at this time as well.

2. Click *Search.*

3. The patient's current status should be green, which means that he or she has already been checked in. Change the patient's status by clicking on the drop-down arrow in his or her *Status* column and selecting "Transfer."

4. The *Patient Location* box will pop up. Select the radio dial button next to "Exam Room # 1." Click *Select* (**Figure 6-62**). (**Note:** If the there is nothing listed in the *Patient Location* box, review your *Compatibility View* setting [refer to Best Practices] and try again.)

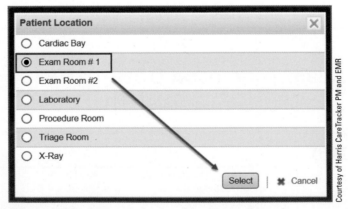

Figure 6-62   Patient Location Box (Exam Room)

5. The patient's entry line should now be blue, indicating that he or she has been transferred to the exam room selected. The appropriate exam room number will now appear in the *Status* column.

6. Repeat for each of the patients listed in step 1. Your screen should look like **Figure 6-63**.

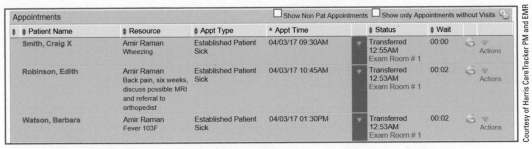

Figure 6-63   Patient Status in Appointments Box (Transferred)

Proficiency Builder 6-2: Additional Practice Completing the Patient's Medical Record

Enter the information in **Table 6-20** for each of the following patients.

    a. Craig X. Smith

    b. Ellen Ristino

    c. Edith Robinson

    d. Barbara Watson

You will complete the patient's medical record by bringing up the patient's chart (Activity 6-6); then adding medications (Activity 6-7); and adding allergies to the patient's chart (Activity 6-8).

 TIP Be sure to access each patient's chart through the *Clinical Today* module as follows:

1. Click on *Clinical Today*.

2. In the *Appointments* screen within *Clinical Today*, bring up the date of the patient's appointment. Be sure that *Resource* reflects "All." **Hint:** If you don't recall the date of the appointment, with the patient in context, click on the *History* tab in the *Scheduling* module to locate the patient's appointment. Do not create a new encounter for this activity; use only the appointment/encounter previously scheduled.

3. Click on the patient's name. The patient's *Chart Summary* will open in a new window (refer to Figure 6-15).

Table 6-20 Medications and Allergies for Craig, Ellen, Edith, and Barbara

MEDICATION/ ALLERGY	CRAIG X. SMITH	ELLEN RISTINO	EDITH ROBINSON	BARBARA WATSON
Medication (**Note**: Select "Benefit outweighs risk" in the *Interaction Screening* dialog box when entering medications.)	None currently	Atorvastatin Calcium Oral Tablet 20 mg by mouth every night	SitaGLIPtin Phosphate Oral Tablet 50 mg by mouth daily Metoprolol Succinate Extended-Release Oral Tablet 24 Hour 50 mg by mouth daily	Ibandronate Sodium Oral Tablet 150 mg by mouth monthly
Allergy	No known drug allergies	Peanuts— Anaphylaxis (Use date January 1, 2008)	No known drug allergies	No known drug allergies

(continues)

BUILD YOUR PROFICIENCY (*continued*)

Proficiency Building 6-3: Additional Practice Recording Vital Signs

Record vital signs for Craig X. Smith, Ellen Ristino, Edith Robinson, and Barbara Watson using **Table 6-21**. Refer to Activity 6-11 for help.

 TIP Be sure to access each patient's chart through the *Clinical Today* module as follows:

1. Click on *Clinical Today*.

2. In the *Appointments* screen within *Clinical Today*, bring up the date of the patient's appointment. Be sure that *Resource* reflects "All." **Hint:** If you don't recall the date of the appointment, with the patient in context, click on the *History* tab in the *Scheduling* module to locate the patient's appointment. Do not create a new encounter for this activity; use only the appointment/encounter previously scheduled.

3. Click on the patient's name. The patient's *Chart Summary* will open in a new window (refer to Figure 6-15). Enter the information in Table 6-21 for each of the following patients.

Table 6-21 Vital Signs for Craig, Ellen, Edith, and Barbara

VITAL SIGNS	CRAIG X. SMITH	ELLEN RISTINO	EDITH ROBINSON	BARBARA WATSON
Height	N/A	5'9"	5'7"	5'10"
Weight	26 lb	165 lb	132 lb	135 lb
BMI	(automatically calculates)	(automatically calculates)	(automatically calculates)	(automatically calculates)
Blood Pressure	92/62	130/75	148/92	122/78
Pulse Rate	110 bpm	84 bpm	92 bpm	66 bpm
Temperature	100.6°	100.8°	98.4°	101°
Respiratory Rate	40	16	18	16
Pulse Oximetry	93%	96%	98%	98%
Pain Level (0–10)	(wheezing) N/A	(sore throat) 0/10	(back pain) 9/10	(Fever 101°F) 0/10
Head Circumference (Pediatric Patients only)	N/A	N/A	N/A	N/A
Length (Pediatric Patients only)	32.8" or 88.3 cm	N/A	N/A	N/A

Completing the Visit

Key Terms

accession
adjudication
advance beneficiary notice (ABN)
Ask at Order Entry (AOE)
beers
compendium
contraindication
dispensable (drug)

formulary
order
Real Time Adjudication (RTA)
routed (drug)
Rx Norm
SIG
stat
"Tall Man" lettering

Learning Objectives

1. Complete requisitions for diagnostic orders: specialists, labs, and radiology.
2. Search for pharmacies, manage a list of favorites, and create and print prescriptions.
3. View, add, and create immunization records.
4. Search for, customize, and provide patient education materials for patients.
5. Access the Correspondence application to add, filter, customize, and print patient correspondence.
6. Create outgoing and incoming patient referrals.
7. View and resolve open encounters and unsigned notes by completing the visit and signing the Progress Note.

Real-World Connection

In this chapter, you will learn additional EMR functions, such as how to enter orders in the electronic medical record. You may be tempted to enter orders at the time you create a patient prevention or maintenance plan, but you should never enter any orders until the provider has reviewed and approved each order. Entering orders without the provider's approval is equivalent to practicing medicine without a license. You will also learn to capture a visit (selecting procedure and diagnosis codes for the patient's visit). The electronic health record makes orders and visit capture a seamless process. Your challenge is to learn the proper steps for entering orders into the patient's EMR, to avoid the temptation of entering orders without the provider's approval, and to select the proper codes for the patient's visit.

INTRODUCTION

Now that you have completed the EMR activities in Chapter 6, you will move forward and complete tasks from the *Assessment* and *Plan* (A&P) tabs located in the patient's progress note. These activities are often referred to as "completing the visit." To generate claims, charges must be captured for the patient's visit. The *Visit* application allows you to capture charges and enter CPT®, NDC, and ICD codes for a patient's visit. The *Visit Summary* application enables you to define patient, provider, visit, and chart information to include in the *Visit Summary* reports generated by your group.

You will place orders and prescriptions, provide educational material for patients, create referrals, document immunizations you administer, sign the progress note, and schedule follow-up appointments as indicated. To complete activities in this chapter, you will refer back to the patient's progress note *Assessment* and *Plan* (**Figure 7-1**). Many of the advanced features of Harris CareTracker EMR's applications are introduced in this chapter, but you will also be directed to the *Help* section where appropriate for more details.

> **ASSESSMENT:**
> (N39.0) - Urinary tract infection
> (R30.0) - Dysuria
> (I10) - Essential (primary) hypertension
> (N02.9) - Recurrent and persistent hematuria
> **PLAN:**
> a. Stat lab test - "Urinalysis dipstick panel by Automated test strip
> b. Send urine out for lab test "Urinalysis microscopic panel [#volume] in urine by automated count
> c. Give patient educational handouts (1) Urinary Tract Infections in Women, and (2) What is Hematuria?
> d. Bactrim DS Oral Tabs (80-160 mg), Sig 1 tab bid for 5 days, No refills
> e. Enter Order for 3-phase CT cysturethrogram
> f. Patient to return in 10 days for a Follow-Up UA
> g. Set patient up for a referral with a urologist
> **PREVENTION GOALS**
> a. Patient to have her first Hepatitis B shot today
> b. Set patient up for a mammogram

Courtesy of Harris CareTracker PM and EMR

Figure 7-1   Assessment and Plan for Jane Morgan

Before you begin the activities in this chapter, refresh your memory on working with Harris CareTracker by referring back to the Best Practices list on page xxiii of this textbook. This list is also posted to the student companion website. Following best practices will help you complete work quickly and accurately.

COMPLETING REQUISITIONS FOR DIAGNOSTIC ORDERS

Learning Objective 1: Complete requisitions for diagnostic orders: specialists, labs, and radiology.

The *Orders* application in Harris CareTracker EMR enables you to manage and track orders such as laboratory, radiology, pathology, and physical therapy directly from the patient's medical record. This ensures that all orders placed are followed up on by the clinic for patient compliancy. The *Orders* application works simultaneously with the *Results* application by providing quick access to test results of completed orders and enables entering manual results and linking to results received electronically.

> **TIP** If you find that when you access a patient's medical record you receive a pop-up alert indicating some missing information (e.g., consent, PCP, NPP, etc.), it is best practice to update the patient's record in the demographics screen before moving forward.

Activity 7-1
Access the *Orders* Application

1. Access patient Jane Morgan's *Medical Record* module using one of the following methods:

    a. Pull patient Jane Morgan into context and click the *Medical Record* module.

    b. If the patient has an appointment, click the patient's name in the *Appointments* application of the *Clinical Today* module. (To find an appointment date, with the patient in context, click on the *History* tab of the *Scheduling* module. It displays the most current appointment for the patient in context in either the *Pending Appointments* or *Rescheduled Appointments* sections in the center of the screen.)

2. In the *Patient Health History* pane of the *Medical Record* module, click *Orders/Referrals* (**Figure 7-2**). The *Orders* window displays with outstanding orders for the patient. You will see that there are no outstanding orders at this time.

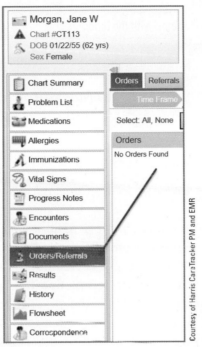

Figure 7-2   Orders/Referrals Application

 FYI If there were an open order, you would be able to see more details by clicking on the order number. You would be able to view the date and type of order, the test description, the ordering provider, encounter date, and associated diagnosis as noted in **Table 7-1**.

Table 7-1 describes the information displaying in the columns of the *Orders* window.

TABLE 7-1   Orders Columns

COLUMN	DESCRIPTION
Order #	Indicates a unique, system-assigned identifier to track the order. This identifier is often referred to as an accession.
Date	Displays the date the order must be completed. (**Note:** The *Due Date* column is updated to display "Stat" if you set the urgency to "Stat" when creating the order. **Stat** refers to "immediately" or "without delay.")
Type	Displays the type of the order. Order types include lab, diagnostic imaging, and procedure.
Test Description	Displays a description about the order.

(Continues)

TABLE 7-1 (*Continued*)

COLUMN	DESCRIPTION
Provider	Displays the provider who created the order.
Enc Date	Displays the encounter date associated with the order.
Diag	Displays the diagnoses associated with the order.

Courtesy of Harris CareTracker PM and EMR

You can view notes entered by moving the pointer over the *Note* ✍ icon. However, the *Note* ✍ icon is dimmed if notes are not available for the order.

Enter New Lab Orders

The *Orders* application, accessed by clicking *Order* 🔬 on the *Clinical Toolbar*, allows you to order tests directly from the *Medical Record* module.

An **order** consists of a list of tests to perform on one or more patient specimens; for example, blood or urine. In many cases, each order is tracked with a unique, system-assigned identifier. This identifier (which is usually a number) is often referred to as an **accession**. When an order is created, the application enables you to preview, print, fax, or send electronically to the facility that will be completing the order. The order is saved as an open order in the *Orders* application and *Open* activities sections of the patient's medical record, enabling you to track outstanding orders for the patient. Additionally, the order is saved to the *Practice* tab of the *Home* module under the *Clinical* header, as well as the *Open Orders* application of the *Clinical Today* module.

The *Open Orders* application provides a quick and efficient way to track the progress of and resolve open orders to expedite patient treatment. This process replaces the manual log books that were used to keep track of labs and other diagnostic tests. In many instances, *Orders* can be sent electronically to some labs; however, this functionality is not operational in your student version of Harris CareTracker PM and EMR.

The *Orders* application enables you to answer *Ask at Order Entry (AOE)* or custom questions, provide physician instructions, produce Medicare waivers for tests that may not be covered, and more. You can also manage a list of favorite facilities, tests, and test notes. Using patient Jane Morgan, complete the *Assessment* and *Plan* (A&P) *Orders* as outlined in the progress note from her encounter that you created in Chapter 6, Activity 6-16 (see Figure 7-1). You will refer back to her A&P throughout this chapter's activities. The first activity will be to add a new lab order (Activity 7-2).

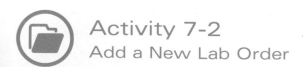

Activity 7-2
Add a New Lab Order

1. Before beginning the steps in this activity, refer back and record patient Jane Morgan's appointment you scheduled in Chapter 4. Date/Time: _____.

2. Pull patient Jane Morgan into context, and then click the *Medical Record* module.

3. In the *Clinical Toolbar*, click *Order* 🔬

4. If an encounter is in context, Harris CareTracker EMR displays the *New Order* dialog box. If an encounter is not in context, Harris CareTracker EMR displays the *Select Encounter* dialog box. Click on the encounter you created with the appointment booked in Chapter 4, Activity 4-1 and the *Order* screen (**Figure 7-3**) will appear.

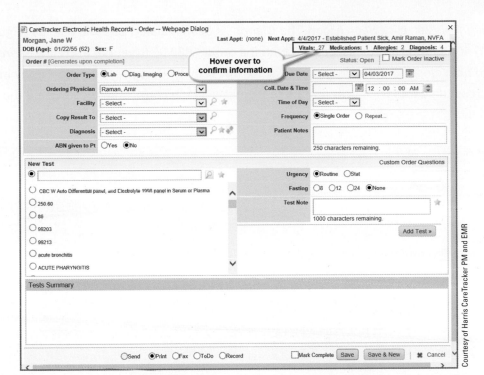

Figure 7-3 Order Screen

TIP Best practice would be to verify that patient information such as medications, allergies, and diagnoses are up-to-date in the medical record. This is done by hovering over each category in the upper-right corner of the *Order* dialog box (see Figure 7-3). This allows the opportunity for the medical assistant to add and update the information as necessary. For example, hover over the *Medications* category and the patient's medications will appear. This is informational only, and not a required step in this activity.

---

5. By default, the *Status* is set to "Open" in the *Order* dialog box (see **Figure 7-3**).

6. By default, the *Order Type* is set to "Lab." Leave this setting as is. The *Order Type* defaults to the option selected in the *Default Order Type*.

FYI The order type can be changed by selecting *Lab, Diag. Imaging,* or *Procedure.* You can only select one order type per order and you must select the correct type to view pertinent tests.

---

7. By default, the *Ordering Physician* list displays the provider associated with the encounter. Confirm that the provider listed is Dr. Raman, Ms. Morgan's, PCP.

8. The *Facility* list displays the default facility set for the order type. Click the drop-down list. A list of favorite labs will appear. Select the first lab on the list. Because this is a live educational environment, you may see multiple entries for the same facility name. Only select the first lab on the list for this activity.

FYI *If* you want to copy the result to another provider, in the *Copy Result To* list, click other providers to whom you wish to route results. If the provider is not on the list, click the *Search* 🔍 icon to search for the provider. (Skip this step.)

9. In the *Diagnosis* list, click *Search* icon. The *Diagnosis Search* dialog box will display (**Figure 7-4**). Type in the ICD-10 Diagnosis code associated with the order "R30.0" (Dysuria) and click *Search*. (**Note:** Do not select from the drop-down list for this activity. Because "favorites" may have been saved across the database it is important that you select the correct diagnosis using the *Search* feature only.)

Diagnosis Search					
R30.0 [Search]					
Diagnosis		**ICD-9**	**ICD-10**		
Dysuria		788.1	R30.0		
Burning with urination		788.1	R30.0		
Difficult or painful urination		788.1	R30.0		
Dysuria after pancreas transplant using bladder drainage technique (BDT)		788.1	R30.0 S		
Painful urging to urinate		788.1	R30.0		
Scalding pain on urination		788.1	R30.0		
Spastic dysuria		788.1	R30.0		
Stranguria		788.1	R30.0		
Strangury		788.1	R30.0		

Courtesy of Harris CareTracker PM and EMR

Figure 7-4   Diagnosis Search Dialog Box

TIP   Steps to search for a diagnosis:

*   Click the *Search* 🔍 icon next to the *Diagnosis* list. Harris CareTracker EMR displays the *Diagnosis Search* dialog box.

*   In the *Search Text* box, enter the name, partial name, or diagnosis code.

    Note: If a partial name search does not return the result expected, enter the full name of the diagnosis or the code.

*   Click *Search*. Harris CareTracker EMR displays a list of diagnoses that match the search criteria.

---

10. Click on the diagnosis you want (R30.0).

11. In the *ABN given to Pt* field, choose "Yes" or "No" to indicate if an advance beneficiary notice was given to the patient. This notifies the patient that Medicare can deny payment for that specific service and that the patient is responsible for payment if denied. Select "No" because this patient does not have Medicare as her insurance.

12. In the *Due Date* box, leave as -Select- and enter the date the order is due in MM/DD/YYYY format in the calendar field. (Select the date of the patient's encounter and collection.) If you were to select the time period from the list, Harris CareTracker EMR would automatically calculate the due date. Because you may be working in the EMR on a date other than the current date, you will need to use the MM/DD/YYYY format for consistency; however, Harris CareTracker EMR will automatically date stamp your work with the day you perform the activity.

13. In the *Coll. Date & Time* box, enter the date and time for collecting the specimen. Use the date of the encounter and a time of 30 minutes past the patient's set appointment time (e.g., if Jane Morgan's visit was on July 30, 2018, at 9:00 a.m., the UA collection time would be 9:30 a.m.).

14. In the *Time of Day* list, use the drop-down and select the time of the day for completing the order, "Morning," "Afternoon," or "Evening" indicated by the appointment time/encounter.

15. In the *Frequency* field, select "Single Order" or "Repeat" to indicate if the order is a single order or must be repeated (select "Single Order"). (**Note:** If the *Frequency* is set to "Repeat," you can click the *Repeat* link to display the *Test Frequency* dialog box (**Figure 7-5**) and select from Daily, Weekly, Monthly, or Yearly, enabling you to record additional details about the tests that must be repeated.)

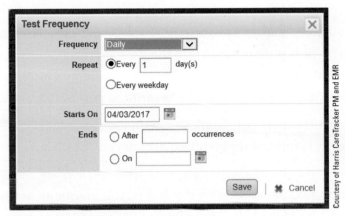

Figure 7-5   Test Frequency Dialog Box

16. *(Optional)* In the *Patient Notes* box, enter any notes about the order you want to display on the order form. Do not make any entries here.

17. The *New Test* section displays favorite tests for the order type, provider, and facility selected that had previously been entered.

18. You will search for the test by clicking on the *Search* icon. The *Search For* list defaults to the order type selected.

19. By default, the *Search Field* list displays "Description." Leave as "Description."

 TIP The options in the *Search Field* list are based on the order type you select. If you are searching for a lab-type order test, you can search by "Logical Observation Identifiers Names and Codes (LOINC) Code" and "Order Code." If you are searching for a procedure-type order test, you can search by "CPT® Code."

20. By default, the *Search Terms* list displays "Contains." However, you can change the option to "Begins with" if necessary. Leave as "Contains."

21. In the *Search Text* box, enter the keyword (enter "Urinalysis dipstick").

22. Click *Search*. Harris CareTracker EMR displays the *Orders Test Search* dialog box, which contains a list of tests that match the selected order type and the compendium associated with the facility (**Figure 7-6**).

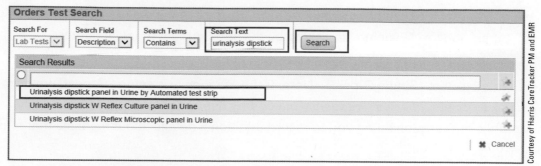

Figure 7-6　Orders Test Search Dialog Box

23. Select the tests indicated in the patient's A&P. Start by selecting "Urinalysis dipstick panel in Urine by Automated test strip" which is then pulled into the *New Test* section. (Note: You may see multiple entries in the *New Test* field. That is because each time an operator selected a test as a "favorite," it populates in the favorites field. Do NOT save as a favorite as part of this activity.)

24. In the *Urgency* field, select "Routine" or "Stat" based on the urgency level of the order. (Select "Stat" for this order.) **Note:** Select "Routine" for standard orders and "Stat" if results must be processed immediately.

25. In the *Fasting* field, select the option based on the fasting requirements for the test. (Select "None.") By default, a test that is a part of the Harris CareTracker PM and EMR compendium includes the fasting information as part of the AOE questions.

26. In the *Test Note* box, enter notes specific to the test to display on the order form. (Do not enter any additional notes in this field.)

27. Click *Add Test.* The test is added to the *Tests Summary* section. You can add multiple tests that are of the same order type, if necessary. You can also edit, view notes pertaining to the test, or remove a test from the *Test Summary* section.

28. Using the same settings (and steps 6 through 26 used to add the first test), add an additional *Stat* test named "Urinalysis microscopic panel [#/volume] in Urine by Automated count."

29. Click *Add Test.* In the *Tests Summary* section, both of the tests will now display.

30. At the bottom of the screen, select the appropriate option to process the order (select the *Print* radio dial button). Your screen of Ms. Morgan's *Order* should look like **Figure 7-7.**

31. Click *Save* to generate the order number and save the order. A copy of the order(s) is saved in the *Open Activities* section at the top of the patient's *Chart Summary*. Additionally, the open order displays in the *Today's Open Activities* dialog box when you access the patient's medical record from the *Clinical Today* module. Each option is described in the *Order Actions* listed in Table 7-2.

32. Once the order is saved, a pop-up box (**Figure 7-8**) will display the completed order. (**Note:** It may take a few moments for the completed order to display.) Print or save the order.

💾 **Print the lab order. Label it "Activity 7-2" and place it in your assignment folder.**

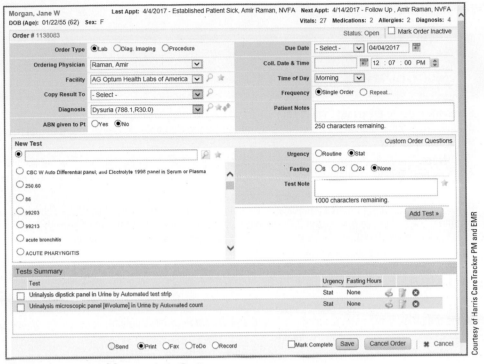

Figure 7-7   Jane Morgan Lab Order

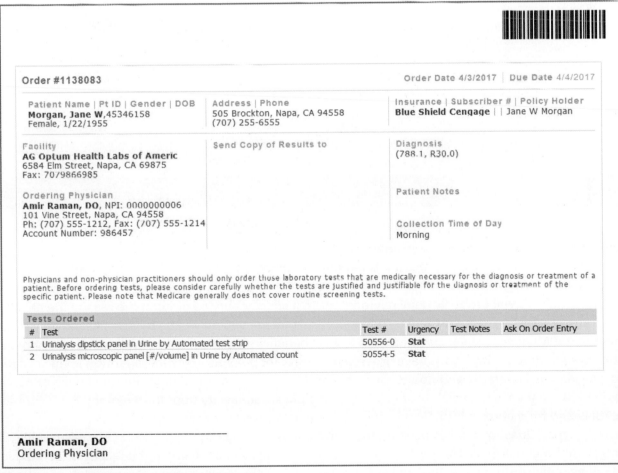

Figure 7-8   Order Completed Pop-Up Window

The possible *Order Actions* are described in **Table 7-2**.

TABLE 7-2   Order Actions

ACTION	DESCRIPTION
Send	Saves the order to the patient's medical record and the *Open Orders* application of the *Home* and *Clinical Today* modules. The order is also electronically transmitted via the Health Level Seven International (HL7) interface to the selected facility. (**Note:** The *Send* option is enabled only if an order interface is set up for the selected facility and your practice. This functionality is not available in your student version of Harris CareTracker PM and EMR.)
Print	Saves the order to the patient's medical record and the *Open Orders* application of the *Home* and *Clinical Today* modules. The order also displays in PDF format, enabling you to print. If an order has multiple tests, Harris CareTracker PM and EMR prints all tests at once. If the ABN given to Pt is set to "Yes" at the time the order is created, the ABN also displays after the order form to print. (**Note:** If your group is not activated to send orders electronically, Harris CareTracker PM and EMR defaults to the *Print* option.)
Fax	Saves the order to the patient's medical record and the *Open Orders* application of the *Home* and *Clinical Today* modules and faxes the order to the facility. (**Note:** Only the order form is sent to the facility. Additionally, a default fax number displays if the fax number is entered in the *Favorite Labs* application of the *Administration* module. If a fax number is not available for the lab, you must select the fax number from your address book.)
ToDo	Enables you to create a *ToDo*, referencing the order. For example, the provider may send a message asking the finance department to call the insurance to approve the charge for the order.
Record	Saves the order to the patient's medical record and the *Open Orders* application of the *Home* and *Clinical Today* modules to send or print at a later time.
Mark Complete	Marks the selected tests or the entire order as complete. (**Note:** By default, selecting the *Mark Complete* checkbox selects checkboxes pertaining to all tests included in the order.)

Courtesy of Harris CareTracker PM and EMR

Additional information you should know about *Orders* are described below.

The **advance beneficiary notice (ABN)** is a written notice (the standard government form CMS-R-131) that a patient receives from physicians, providers, or suppliers before they provide a service or item to the patient, notifying them that Medicare will probably deny payment for that specific service or item; the reason the physician, provider, or supplier expects Medicare to deny payment; and that the patient will be personally and fully responsible for payment if Medicare denies payment. ABNs alert beneficiaries that Medicare might not reimburse for certain services even though physicians have ordered them, ask for patients' consent regarding financial liability when Medicare denies coverage, and notify patients with Medicare insurance that either a service or services rendered will be the patient's financial responsibility to the physician/facility (lab) for payment. For information regarding ABNs and for a current form, access the CMS website (http://www.cms.gov).

The *Custom Order Questions* link is used to enter additional information for the test. Only fields with information display in the *Order* form. The *Custom Order Questions* link is unavailable if the facility selected has an associated lab-specific compendium such as LabCorp. However, if the facility does not have a lab-specific compendium associated but has additional fields defined via the *Order Questions* application, Harris CareTracker EMR activates the *Custom Order Questions* link. **Compendium** refers to a summary or abstract containing the essential information in a concise but brief form.

Ask at Order Entry (AOE) represents answers you must provide to the lab when sending an order electronically or submitting a printed order. The AOE questions are based on the compendium associated with the facility and the test selected. If you do not select a facility when you create an order, Harris CareTracker EMR displays tests and associated AOE questions from the Harris CareTracker PM and EMR master compendium.

If the practice had created *Order Sets*, when you click the OrdSet 🚿 icon, the required questions display with a red background. If the AOEs are required and you do not answer the questions, a message alerts you that the required AOEs are missing for the tests. You can choose to answer the questions in the *Order Set* window or answer the questions in the *Orders* dialog box before saving the order. You would answer the AOE questions, if required.

If creating an order that includes two or more tests with different settings, a message prompts, indicating that there is a conflict with the setting and provides you the ability to assign common settings for all tests. However, if you want each test to have different settings, you must create separate orders for each test.

The *Open Activities* section in the *Chart Summary* displays open orders that are overdue. Overdue tests display "Due" and the due date in red. An order with an urgency of "Stat" displays a bold "S" in parenthesis (**S**) in the test description. For example (see **Figure 7-9**): "Due 04/04/2017—Urinalysis microscopic panel [#volume] in Urine by Automated count; Urinalysis dipstick panel in Urine by Automated test strip."

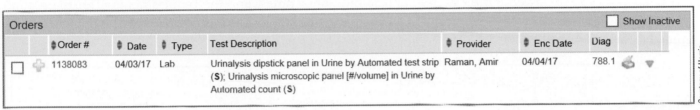

Figure 7-9   Open Orders for Jane Morgan

The *Orders* application has a number of advanced features that improve workflow in the medical practice. These include the ability to filter the list of orders on the status, the date of the order, the case associated with the order, or the tests included in the order. In addition, the *Orders* application consists of both open and complete orders for a patient. When you create an order for a patient, the order is saved in the patient's medical record, enabling you to track the progress of the order. When results are received, through mail, fax, or electronically, you can enter the results manually, or link to the electronic result, and update the status of the order in the *Open Orders* application of the *Quick Tasks* menu in *Clinical Today* and the *Practice* tab in the *Home* module. When results are entered for an outstanding order and marked as "complete," the order is removed from the *Open Activities* section of the patient's medical record. Additionally, the order is removed from the *Open Orders* application. Furthermore, you can print a copy of the order created for the patient or create a copy of the order when you want to order the same tests again. You will learn to record lab results in Chapter 8 activities.

To print patient test orders to share with other health care professionals treating the patient, click on the drop-down arrow next to the order entry and select *Print* (**Figure 7-10**). This helps to review the history of tests, enabling you to prevent unnecessary duplication of tests and increase the efficiency of patient care when ordering required tests.

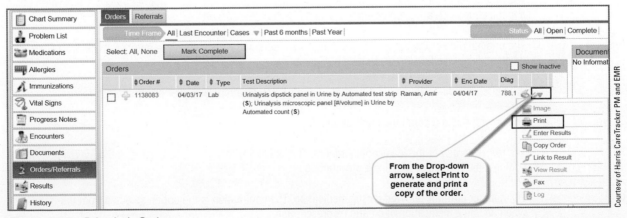

Figure 7-10   Print Lab Order

CREATING AND PRINTING PRESCRIPTIONS

Learning Objective 2: Search for pharmacies, manage a list of favorites, and create and print prescriptions.

In Chapter 6, you were introduced to the *Medications* application in Harris CareTracker EMR. This chapter focuses on managing favorite medications, searching for pharmacies, and creating and printing prescriptions.

The *Medications* application consists of the past and current medications the patient is taking. The list also includes medications prescribed, medications administered, and samples given to the patient. You can maintain the complete list of medications by manually adding, prescribing, uploading via the *Document Management* module, and importing medication information from a Continuity of Care Document (CCD).

You can manage the list by reviewing the medication history, updating medication details, flagging medications that need attention, renewing, and electronically transmitting prescribed medications, and more. All the active medications recorded for the patient display in various locations in Harris CareTracker PM and EMR.

Table 7-3 describes the columns of the *Medications* window. **Figure 7-11** allows you to review Actions regarding the medication (such as *Interactions, Print, Fax,* and more). Refer to **Table 7-3** for a further description of the columns.

In Chapter 6, you reviewed the *Rx Writer* application, Surescripts®, and the requirements prior to creating and transmitting prescriptions electronically to a pharmacy. Additional features of the *Rx Writer* application are outlined in **Table 7-4**.

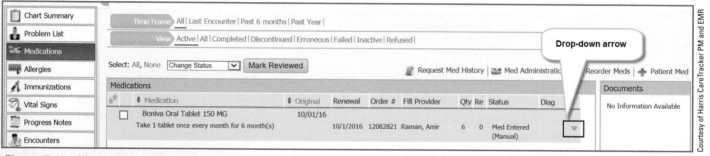

Figure 7-11   Medications Window

TABLE 7-3   Medications Columns

COLUMN	DESCRIPTION
Medication	The name of the medication dosage (SIG) information. The dosage is the information entered in the *Directions* (SIG) box when adding a medication or creating a prescription. For inactive medications, the *Medication* column displays the reason and the end date recorded in the *End Date* box when deactivating the medication. Example: Flomax Oral Capsule 0.4 MG (Inactive; Discontinued as of May 17, 2009).
Original	The original date for taking the medication. This is the date entered in the *Medication Date* box when adding a medication or creating a prescription.
Renewal	The original date or the dates the medication was reordered. This is the date entered in the *Start Date* box when adding a medication or creating a prescription.
Order #	A unique, system-assigned identification number for medications added or prescriptions ordered.
Fill Provider	The provider who ordered the medication.
Qty	The total quantity of the medication ordered. This is the quantity that is calculated in the *Fill Qty* box when adding a medication or creating a prescription.
Re	The number of refills allowed for the medication. The information is the option selected from the *Refills* list when adding a medication or creating a prescription.

COLUMN	DESCRIPTION
Status	Indicates if the medication was added manually or imported from a CCD. Additionally, the column displays the status for prescriptions based on the action option selected when creating the prescription.
Diag	The diagnoses treated with the medication. These are the diagnoses you selected from the *Diagnosis* list when adding a medication or creating a prescription.
Actions	• *Interactions*: Displays interactions that were returned when the medication was added to the patient's medical record. If no interactions were returned, the *Interactions* icon appears dimmed. • Reorder: Displays the original order for review and edit as necessary to reorder the medication. • Print: Displays the confirmation dialog box to enter information required to reprint the prescription. • Fax: Displays the *New Fax* dialog box to enter information required to fax the prescription. • Send Electronically: Displays the confirmation dialog box to enter information required to resend the prescription. • Log: Displays activity related to the medication.
Documents	Displays medications that are uploaded or scanned via the *Document Management* module. The list is sorted based on the document date entered when you upload or scan the document. You can move the pointer over the document to view a summary of the medications and click the document to open in the *Document Viewer*.

Courtesy of Harris CareTracker PM and EMR

TABLE 7-4   Rx Writer Application Features

The application is *RxHub* certified and electronically routes up-to-date patient medication history and pharmacy benefit information at every point of care. This helps improve patient safety and saves time required to create and renew prescriptions.

Allows you to verify and update information, such as the patient's last vital signs, medications, allergies, and diagnoses, to identify possible adverse effects during screening. To verify, add, or update information, hover over each category on the upper-right-hand corner of the *Rx Writer* application.

Displays easy-to-read formulary-specific messages and generic cost-effective suggestions when writing a prescription.

Calculates dosage recommendations for the medication based on weight and age.

Create provider preferences such as favorite medications, SIGs, and pharmacy notes to simplify the prescription-writing process.

Supports an extensive national drug database, interaction screening, and medication education information in different languages.

In addition to sending prescriptions electronically, allows you to print and fax prescriptions.

Courtesy of Harris CareTracker PM and EMR

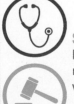

SPOTLIGHT   e-Prescribing controlled substances is now legal nationwide, a step that helps combat opioid abuse by making it harder for addicts and drug peddlers to forge prescriptions. For more information regarding Drug Schedules, visit the Drug Enforcement Agency website at www.dea.gov.

Create Prescriptions

The *Rx* application allows you to create prescriptions for both controlled (scheduled) and noncontrolled drugs. All prescriptions created through the *Rx Writer* application are recorded in the *Medications* application with the name, Rx Norm code, dosage, and other pertinent data. **Rx Norm** is a standardized nomenclature for clinical drugs and drug delivery devices produced by the National Library of Medicine (NLM). The Rx Norm code supports interoperability between EHR systems.

To check the selected medication for contraindications with the patient's active medications, problems, and allergies, set provider-level screening preferences for the provider via the *Provider Screening* application. A **contraindication** is a symptom or condition that makes a particular treatment or procedure inadvisable. For more information on the *Provider Screening* application, search for "Provider Screening" in the *Search* tab of the *Help* system.

Manage a List of Favorites

The *Rx Writer* application helps save favorite or most commonly prescribed medications, commonly used SIGs, and pharmacy notes to your list of favorites. This avoids having to search for medications, create SIGs, or enter pharmacy notes when creating future prescriptions. **SIG** is an abbreviation for the Latin word *signa* (meaning "label" or "sign"). SIG codes are specific dosage instructions that are given when prescribing medications.

Because your Harris CareTracker student version saves certain features across the database, you will <u>not</u> be saving a medication as a *Favorite*. In a live practice, the medical assistant would save medications as *Favorites* to streamline workflow. The medications saved as *Favorites* would be linked to the provider in the *Patient Medication* and *Prescription* dialog boxes.

You will now add a medication (Activity 7-3). It is important to know that you will need to click in the boxes of the dialog box vs. using the [Tab] key when adding medications/prescriptions. In addition, when you fill in the number of days in the quantity box, the SIG will populate the information into the screen.

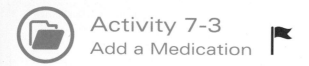

Activity 7-3
Add a Medication

1. Access the *Chart Summary* of Jane Morgan by clicking on her appointment in the *Clinical Today* module to add the medication noted in her progress note *A&P* (see Figure 7-1). If you are not in Jane Morgan's medical record, access it following the steps below:

   - Click on *Clinical Today*.

   - In the *Appointments* screen within *Clinical Today*, bring up the date of Jane Morgan's appointment. Be sure that *Resource* reflects "All." **Hint:** If you don't recall the date of the appointment, with the patient in context, click on the *History* tab in the *Scheduling* module to locate the patient's appointment. Do not create a new encounter for this activity, use only the appointment/encounter previously scheduled.

   - Click directly on the patient's name under *Appointments*, and the *Patient Health History* pane will appear (Note: Close out of the *Clinical Alerts* dialog box if displaying).

2. In the *Clinical Toolbar*, click the *Rx* icon. (This will launch the *Prescription* dialog box.)

3. Skip the *Pharmacy* field for now.

4. By default, the *Filling Provider* list displays the provider set in your batch. However, you can click another provider to add to your favorites. Confirm that the *Filling Provider* for patient Jane Morgan displays Dr. Raman.

5. Click on the *Search* 🔍 icon at the end of the *Medication* field. The *Medication Search* dialog box displays to search for a medication. By default, the *Search For* field displays "Medications." By default, the *Drug Type* list is set to "Dispensable." **Dispensable** (capable of being dispensed, administered, or distributed) includes the medication name and dosage information.

6. By default, the *Search Terms* list is set to "Contains"; however, you can change the option to "Begins with" if necessary. (Leave as "Contains.)

7. Enter a keyword in the *Search Text* box. (Enter "Bactrim.")

8. Select the *Include Generics* checkbox to include generic versions of the medication in the search results. The generic version displays in *italics* for easy identification.

9. Click *Search*. Harris CareTracker EMR displays a list of medications matching the search criteria. (**Note:** By default, the search results do not show obsolete medications. To view medications that are obsolete, select the *Show Obsolete Drugs* checkbox. The obsolete medications appear dimmed in the search results. You cannot save obsolete medications.)

 FYI In your student environment, the *Drug Type* list is grayed out and automatically set to "Dispensable." In the real-world version of Harris CareTracker EMR, you can also select "Routed Drug" to record the medication without any dosage information. **Routed** refers to the way that a drug is introduced into the body, such as oral, enteral, mucosal, parenteral, or percutaneous.

---

10. Scroll down and click on the medication noted in the *A&P*: Bactrim DS Oral Tablet 800-160 MG (**Figure 7-12**). Click on the medication selected. (**Note:** If an *Interaction Screening* dialog box appears, select "Benefit outweighs risk" as the *Override Reason* and then click *Accept*.)

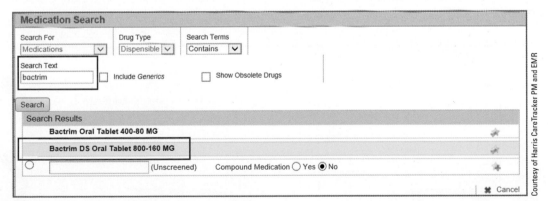

Figure 7-12   Bactrim Search Results

11. Continue completing the prescription by creating the SIG, as noted in the *Progress Note* in the *Dose* line of the *New Prescription* section ("SIG: 1 tab [tablet] bid [twice a day] for 5 days"). You can also click the *Dosing Calculator* 📱 icon, and the calculator will display the advised SIG. If the *Dosing Calculator* returned the SIG noted in the A&P, click on the radio dial, then scroll down and click *Select*. The SIG will populate in the *Prescription* dialog box. If the SIG returned by the *Dosing Calculator* is not the

same as noted in the *Progress Note*, enter the SIG manually. In this case, the SIG will need to be entered manually.

a. For *Amount*, enter "1."

b. For *Unit,* select "Tablet."

c. For *Frequency*, select "Twice a day."

d. Enter a *Duration* of "5 Days."

FYI The *Rx Writer* application includes the dosing calculator that provides dosing recommendations for the medication the provider is prescribing based on the weight and age of the patient. You must enter the patient's weight to provide weight-based decision support. Additionally, the calculator takes into consideration other factors, such as the reason for prescribing the medication, type of the dose, route, and other special conditions, enabling you to customize recommendations to suit your preference. However, the ability and the options available to customize dosage recommendations are based on the medication the provider is prescribing.

12. In your student environment, you will need to change the *Start Date* and *Original Date* to reflect the date of the patient's encounter. However, the date stamp for audit purposes will reflect the actual date and time you recorded the information.

FYI When you click the *More Information* link next to the *Med Formulary* field, Harris CareTracker EMR displays the *Formulary-Additional Information* dialog box (**Figure 7-13**) with formulary, copay, coverage, and alternatives. **Formulary** is defined by the Centers for Medicare & Medicaid Services (CMS) as a list of prescription drugs covered by a prescription drug plan or another insurance plan offering prescription drug benefits (also called a drug list) (see Table 7-5).

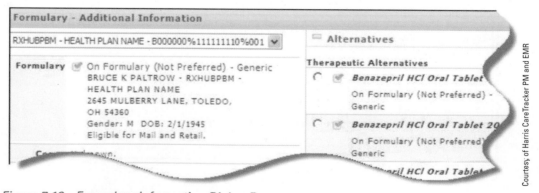

Figure 7-13   Formulary Information Dialog Box

You can select the original or an alternative medication and click *Select*. (**Note:** The selected medication is screened against the patient's active diagnoses, medications, and allergies. If the screening triggers an interaction that is higher than the severity settings set for the provider in the batch, the *Interaction Screening* dialog box displays for you to acknowledge the screening.)

13. Click *Add Rx* (**Figure 7-14**) and the prescription summary will display the newly added medication (**Figure 7-15**).

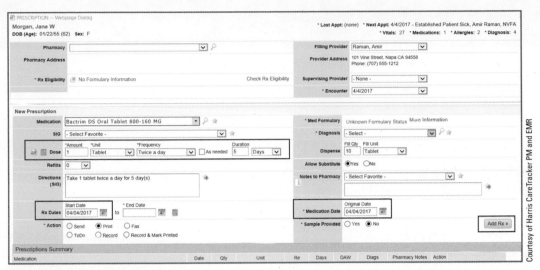

Figure 7-14   Add Rx

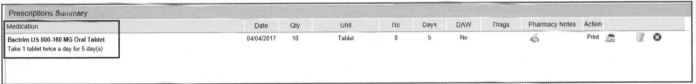

Figure 7-15   Rx Added to Prescription Summary

14. Click *Complete* to finish the prescription. The prescription will open in a new window (**Figure 7-16**). If you receive a prompt for a PIN to sign electronically, close out of the pop-up.

15. If your prescription did not print, follow the instructions in Activity 7-4 to reprint the prescription. Use reprint reason of "Printer Out Of Paper."

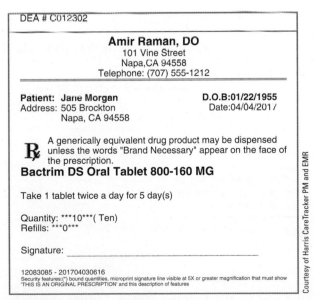

Figure 7-16   Printed Bactrim Rx

▣ **Print the Bactrim prescription ordered for Jane Morgan. Label it "Activity 7-3" and place it in your assignment folder.**

The tiered formularies are displayed with color-coded symbols, as described in **Table 7-5**.

TABLE 7-5 Formulary Symbols

SYMBOL	DESCRIPTION
☆	The medication is formulary compliant and is preferred.
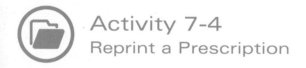	The medication is formulary compliant but not preferred.
✖	The medication is not formulary compliant and the payment is the patient's responsibility if prescribed.

Courtesy of Harris CareTracker PM and EMR

Print Prescriptions

The *Medications* application helps review and print prescription information to give to a patient or fax to a pharmacy.

Activity 7-4
Reprint a Prescription

1. With patient Jane Morgan in context, click the *Medical Record* module.

2. In the *Patient Health History* pane, click *Medications*. Harris CareTracker EMR displays the *Medications* window.

3. Click on the checkbox next to the prescription you want to reprint. (Select *Bactrim*.)

4. In the *Actions* menu, click the *Arrow* icon for the prescription and click *Print* (**Figure 7-17**).

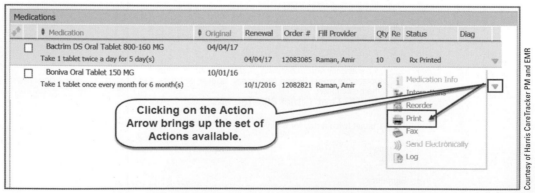

Figure 7-17   Actions Menu—Print

5. A *Reprint Prescription* dialog box will pop up. Select "Printer Out of Paper" as your *Reprint Reason* and click *Print*. The prescription displays in PDF format, enabling you to print. **Note:** If the prescription does not print, then print a screenshot of the *Reprint Prescription* dialog box with "Printer Out of Paper" selected instead. You can check your student companion website for more information.

FYI If you had uploaded a digital signature, Harris CareTracker EMR would display the *Provider Signature* dialog box. Because no digital signature has been uploaded, print the prescription as is. In the *Medication* window, the *Status* of the medication changes to "Rx Printed."

Print a copy of the prescription. Label it "Activity 7-4" and place it in your assignment folder.

TIP By default, the prescription is set up to print on 4" × 6" paper. If you want to print a prescription in one-quarter of the page, click to clear the *Auto-Rotate and Center* checkbox in the *Page* handling section of the *Print* dialog box (**Figure 7-18**).

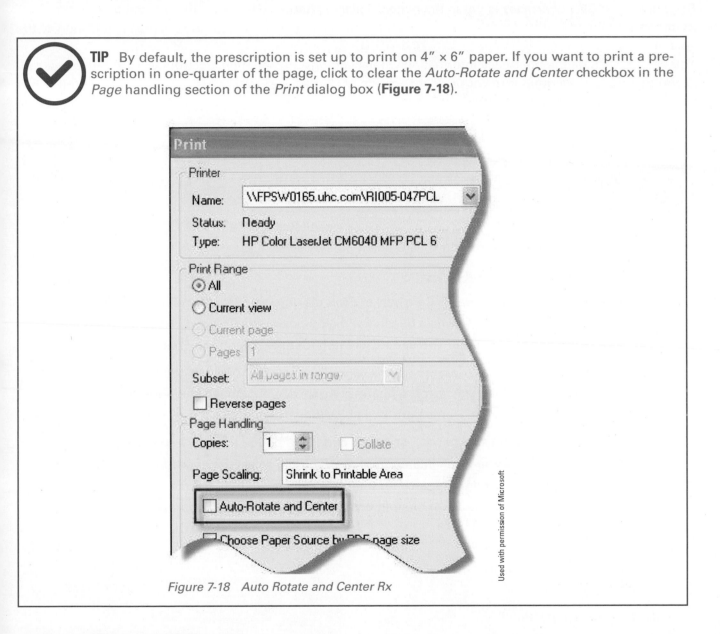

Figure 7-18   Auto Rotate and Center Rx

Search for a Pharmacy

The *Rx Writer* application includes a *Pharmacy* list that includes the following two categories:

- Patient Pharmacies: Displays patient pharmacies listed under the *Relationships* application in the *Patient* module. By default, the *Pharmacy* list displays the patient's preferred pharmacy recorded for the patient in the *Relationships* application of the *Patient* module.

- Favorite Pharmacies: Displays pharmacies your practice most frequently uses. The favorite pharmacy list is set via the *Quick Picks* application of the *Administration* module. To access the application, click the

Administration module, *Setup* tab, and then click the *Quick Picks* link under the *Financial* section. Click *Pharmacies* from the list to search and add favorite pharmacies for your practice. For more information on the *Quick Pick Setup* application, see *Administration Module > Setup > Financial > Quick Pick Setup* in the *Help* system.

Additionally, the *Rx Writer* application includes a pharmacy search feature, enabling you to search for pharmacies that are not in the patient's active pharmacy list or the practice's favorite pharmacy list. When you write a prescription for a pharmacy that is not in the list, Harris CareTracker EMR adds the pharmacy to the *Relationships* application in the *Patient* module.

For example, if CVS pharmacy is not in the patient's active pharmacy list, writing a prescription to the pharmacy automatically adds it under the *Active Patient Pharmacies* section in the *Relationships* application of the *Patient* module.

You need to include the pharmacy information when sending a prescription electronically. Because you cannot send electronic prescriptions in your student version of Harris CareTracker EMR, you can only complete this function up to the point of searching for a pharmacy. Follow the instructions in Activity 7-5 to familiarize yourself with this task.

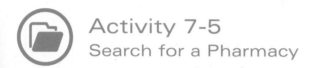

Activity 7-5
Search for a Pharmacy

1. With patient Jane Morgan in context, click the *Medical Record* module.

2. In the *Clinical Toolbar*, click the *Rx* icon.

3. If an encounter is in context, Harris CareTracker EMR displays the *Prescription* dialog box. (Note: If an encounter is not in context, the *Select Encounter* dialog box displays for you to select or create a new encounter. Click on the encounter you already created for this patient. The *Prescription* dialog box will display.)

4. If Ms. Morgan does not have any favorite pharmacies saved yet, you will need to click the *Search* icon next to the *Pharmacy* list. Harris CareTracker EMR displays the *Search Pharmacies* dialog box.

5. Enter search criteria such as name, city, state, zip code, and phone number in the specific boxes to search for the pharmacy you want. In the *Pharmacy Type* list, select the appropriate type of pharmacy. For example, if you want to search for pharmacies that can mail the medication to the patient, you would select "Mail Order." Enter the following criteria in the *Search Pharmacies* dialog box:

    a. *Name:* CVS

    b. *City:* Napa

    c. *State:* CA

    d. *Pharmacy Type:* Retail

    Note: The *State* list defaults to the patient's home address state and is a required field. In the *Name* box, enter the first few characters of the pharmacy name to display more results and prevent from eliminating results based on the way the name is spelled.
    Example: Entering *wal* will display all results with "wal" such as walmart, wal mart, and wal-mart, etc.

6. Click *Search*. Harris CareTracker EMR will return all pharmacies matching your criteria (**Figure 7-19**).

Print a copy of the Search Pharmacy dialog box. Label it "Activity 7-5" and place it in your assignment folder.

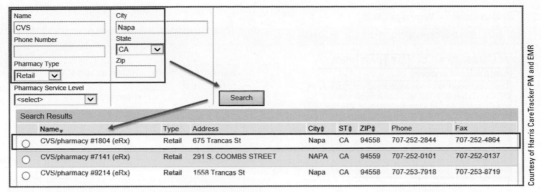

Figure 7-19   Search Pharmacy Criteria Results

7. Select CVS # 1804. (Note: If you get an error message, close the dialog box and begin the search over.)

8. Do not add in the medication name or SIG at this time because this activity is only to learn to use the *Search* feature for pharmacies.

9. Click *Cancel* in the bottom right corner of the *Prescription* dialog box.

10. Click *OK* in the *Cancel Prescription* box.

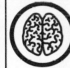

CRITICAL THINKING   State requirements for prescriptions may vary, and it is your responsibility to be sure your practice is in compliance. Because you are a medical assistant at Napa Valley Family Health Associates in Napa, California, log in to the *Help* system and click on *State Print Instructions* located under *Medical Records > Prescriptions > Printing Prescriptions*. Scroll down to locate the *State Print Instructions*. Print each of the *State Print Instructions* sheets at the bottom of the screen (California, New Jersey, and New York). Compare and contrast the differences of each state. Write a one-page paper on why you think individual states would have different requirements. Submit the forms and your paper to your instructor for class discussion.

Other Prescription Highlights

Some medication names may have mixed case lettering in the description name. This is known as **"Tall Man" lettering**; for example, NexIUM. This is a standard used to comply with the patient safety initiative endorsed by the Food and Drug Administration (FDA) and Institute for Safe Medication Practices (ISMP). This helps reduce errors between medication names that either look or sound alike.

Interaction Screenings

The *Rx Writer* application checks for interactions when prescribing a medication to a patient. The screening checks for possible contraindications with the patient's active medications, allergies, and problems and alerts you if the interaction is higher than the severity level you set.

If an interaction exists for a medication added or prescribed, you can click *Cancel* or "X" in the *Interactions Screening* dialog box and take necessary action to avoid adverse reactions. You can also choose to acknowledge the screening by selecting one or more override reasons and entering notes before clicking *Accept*. The *Interactions Screening* dialog box is color and numerically coded to highlight the severity levels of an interaction (**Figure 7-20**). It also summarizes the effects and the level of risk of the prescribed medication.

If a medication, a diagnosis, or an allergy triggered an interaction, you can click the *Interaction* icon for the item in the associated application to display a read-only dialog box with the interactions and override reasons available. The *Interaction* icon appears dimmed if interactions are unavailable.

The *Levels of Severity* (Numeric and Color Codes) listed in **Table 7-6** are the numeric severity indications. The *Levels of Interaction* are described in **Table 7-7**.

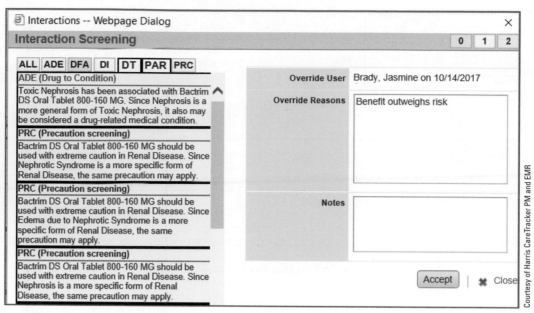

Figure 7-20   Interactions Screening

TABLE 7-6   Levels of Severity

LEVEL OF SEVERITY	DESCRIPTION
Gray (0)	Indicates minor severity (bothersome or little effect)
Yellow (1)	Indicates moderate severity (deterioration for patient's status)
Green (2)	Indicates major severity (life-threatening or permanent damage)

Courtesy of Harris CareTracker PM and EMR

TABLE 7-7   Levels of Interaction (Tab View)

LEVEL OF INTERACTION	DESCRIPTION	EXAMPLE
ADE (Drug-to-Condition Interaction)	The prescribed medication has a negative interaction with the patient's existing diagnosis.	The patient suffers from high blood pressure and the prescribed medication has an effect on blood pressure; for example, Sudafed effects on Hypertension.
DFA (Drug-to-Food Interaction)	The prescribed medication taken with certain food interacts in ways that diminish the effectiveness of the ingested medication or reduce the absorption of food nutrients.	Vitamin and herbal supplements taken with prescribed medications can result in adverse reactions; for example, latex allergy and avocados.
DI (Drug-to-Drug Interaction)	The prescribed medication has an effect with the patient's active medications that may cause new and dangerous reactions or may reduce or increase the effects of the prescribed medication.	Mixing antidiabetic medication (e.g., oral hypoglycemics) and beta blockers (e.g., Inderal) can result in decreased response of the antidiabetic drug and increase the frequency and severity of low blood sugar episodes.

LEVEL OF INTERACTION	DESCRIPTION	EXAMPLE
DT (Duplicate Therapy)	The prescribed medication is the same as a medication the patient is currently on and is treating the same diagnosis. If a provider prescribes a brand name medication and allows substitution, a duplicate medication message displays when approving a refill request for the generic version of the medication. If the refill request is approved for the generic version, the previously prescribed brand name medication is made inactive on the same date the refill request is received. Additionally, a record is also saved for the generic medication in the patient's active medication list. You can view the brand name medication that was originally ordered by hovering over the generic medication name.	Two sleep medication types are prescribed for the patient.
PAR (Drug to Allergy)	The prescribed medication has allergic reactions and cross sensitivities with the patient allergies.	For example: Patient with a sulfa allergy who is being prescribed Hydrochlorothiazide.
PRC (Precaution Screening)	The prescribed medication has precautionary warnings based on factors such as age (pediatric and geriatric) and medical conditions.	For example: Ibuprofen in patients less than 6 months; Benadryl in children less than 2 years; Beers list for geriatric patients.

Courtesy of Harris CareTracker PM and EMR

Beers is the criteria for safe medication use in older adults—for people over 65 years of age.

The *Complete Screening* icon in the *Patient Detail* bar enables you to check for interactions in real time for the patient in context. This complete screening is for informational purposes only and includes interactions based on active diagnoses, medications and allergies, patient's age and weight, duplicate therapy, food interactions, and precaution screening.

Fax Prescriptions

The *Medications* application enables you to fax prescriptions to a pharmacy using the *Message Center* application. You must have an account with *MyFax®* to use the faxing features in Harris CareTracker PM and EMR and have a *Fax* queue set up to send the prescription as a fax. Your student version of Harris CareTracker EMR does not have the *MyFax®* feature. For information and instructions on faxing prescriptions, log in to the *Help* system *Contents* tab and select *Faxing Prescriptions* (*Medical Records* module > *Prescriptions* > *Faxing Prescriptions*).

Submit Prescriptions Electronically

The *Medications* application helps transmit a saved prescription electronically to a selected pharmacy. This feature is useful to transmit a prescription that failed electronic transmission or is saved to send later. Because your student environment will not electronically transmit prescriptions, the option to send electronically is grayed out in your *Actions* drop-down list.

In a live environment, the steps to send an electronic prescription are noted in the following FYI box.

FYI Submit a Saved Prescription Electronically

1. Access the patient's *Medical Record* module.
2. In the *Patient Health History* pane, click *Medications*. The *Medications* window displays.

(*Continues*)

(*Continued*)

TIP If the prescription was previously sent, faxed, or printed, the *Transmit Rx* dialog box displays.

- In the *Resend Reason* list, click a reason for sending the prescription again. If the reason is not in the list, click "Other (See Comments)." You must select a reason for tracking purposes. The reason and comments are saved in the activity log of the prescription.

  - In the *Comments* box, enter the reason or additional comments if necessary.

3. In the *Actions* menu, click the *Arrow* ▼ icon for the prescription you want and click *Send Electronically* to electronically send the prescription to the pharmacy.

4. Click *Send.* In the *Medication* window, the *Status* of the medication changes to "Rx Queued" (for Electronic Transmit) or "Rx Sent" (Electronically).

ACCESSING THE IMMUNIZATION APPLICATION

Learning Objective 3: View, add, and create immunization records.

In Chapter 5, you learned how to manage immunization lots in Harris CareTracker EMR. In this chapter, you will view, add, and create immunization records. In Chapter 8, you will perform advanced features such as running an immunization lot number report.

The *Immunizations* application consists of a list of newly administered immunizations, immunizations administered in the past, and immunizations that the patient refused to have administered. You can maintain the complete list of immunizations by manually recording immunizations, uploading via the *Document Management* module, or importing immunization information from a CCD. You can manage the list of immunizations by reviewing the immunization history, updating, sorting, and printing. All active immunizations recorded for the patient display in various locations in Harris CareTracker PM and EMR.

Additionally, the *Immunizations* application provides access to the Centers for Disease Control and Prevention (CDC) website. The website provides quick reference for recommended child and adolescent immunization schedules and a catch-up schedule for children who missed a scheduled immunization. You can review and print the immunization schedules from the CDC site.

Activity 7-6
Access the Immunizations Application

1. Pull patient Jane Morgan into context and click the *Medical Record* module.

2. In the *Patient Health History* pane, click *Immunizations.* Harris CareTracker EMR displays the *Immunizations* window with a list of patient immunizations (**Figure 7-21**).

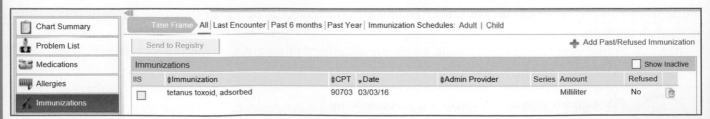

Figure 7-21 Immunizations Window

Courtesy of Harris CareTracker PM and EMR

💾 **Print a screen shot of the Immunizations window. Label it "Activity 7-6" and place it in your assignment folder.**

Table 7-8 describes the columns in the *Immunizations* window, as displayed in Figure 7-21.

TABLE 7-8 Immunizations Columns

COLUMN	DESCRIPTION
IIS	Allows you to select the immunization to send to the Immunization registry.
Immunization	The name of the immunization.
CPT®	The CPT® code associated with the immunization.
Date	The date the immunization was administered. By default, the immunization list is sorted by the immunization administered date.
Admin Provider	The provider who administered the immunization.
Series	The series associated with the immunization.
Amount	The dosage amount of the administered immunization.
Refused	Displays if the immunization was refused by the patient. If the immunization was refused, you can move the pointer over *Yes* to view the reason for refusing the immunization.
Log	Displays all activities pertaining to the immunization.
Documents	Displays immunizations that are uploaded or scanned via the *Document Management* module. The list is sorted based on the document date entered when you upload or scan the document.

Courtesy of Harris CareTracker PM and EMR

Add Immunizations

The *Immunizations* application helps maintain a complete record of a patient's immunizations by adding past immunizations administered and immunizations that the patient refused to have administered in addition to new immunizations recorded. This helps store an up-to-date record of a patient's immunization history in one location and provides the ability to track immunizations that are due.

The *Immunization Writer* application, accessed by clicking the *Immunizations* icon on the *Clinical Toolbar*, allows you to maintain an up-to-date record of immunizations by recording information about immunizations administered. This helps your practice report accurate and complete patient immunization records to other entities, track inventory of immunizations, improve patient safety, and more.

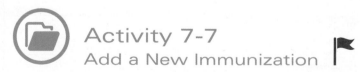

Activity 7-7
Add a New Immunization

Prior to adding a new immunization, you must set your *Administered By* list, which is defined through the *Immunization Administrator Maintenance* application accessed via the *Administration* module **(Figure 7-22).**

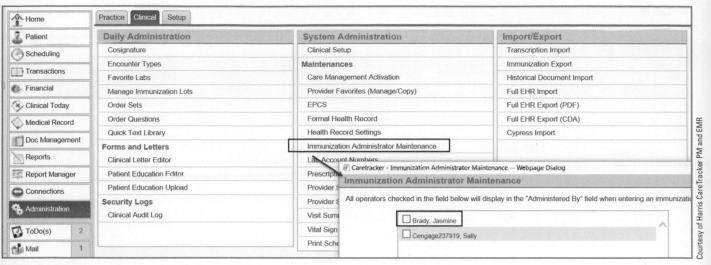

Figure 7-22 Immunization Administrator Maintenance

1. Go to the *Administration* module > *Clinical* tab and select the *Immunization Administrator Mainte-nance* link. Place a check mark next to your name (or if you didn't change your operator name in Activ-ity 2-8, select your "Training Operator" number), then click *Save*, and then click on the red "X" (Close). You are now ready to add immunizations. (Note: You may receive an error message that the web page is trying to close; if so, click *Yes*. You can close out of the *Immunization Administrator Maintenance* dialog box by clicking the "X" in the upper-right corner. You have been added as an administrator to *Immunization Maintenance*.)

2. Pull patient Jane Morgan into context, and then click the *Medical Record* module.

3. In the *Clinical Toolbar*, click the *Immunizations* 📌 icon.

4. If an encounter is in context, Harris CareTracker EMR displays the *Immunization Writer* dialog box. If there was no encounter in context, the *Select Encounter* dialog box would display for you to select an encounter. Select the appointment date/encounter you created for this patient in Chapter 4, which will launch the *Immunization Writer* dialog box.

> **TIP** As Best Practice at this step, the medical assistant would want to verify that patient information such as diagnoses, medications, and allergies are up-to-date in the medical record by hovering over each category in the upper-right corner of the *Immunization Writer* application and clicking on the number next to it (**Figure 7-23**).

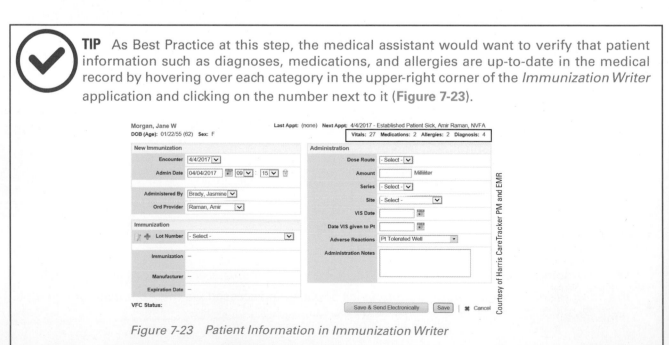

Figure 7-23 Patient Information in Immunization Writer

5. The *Encounter* list defaults to the encounter date selected or created. (Leave as is.) If the encounter date is different, select the date of the encounter using the calendar icon.

6. The *Admin Date* defaults to today's date. To change the date of administration, enter the date or click the *Calendar* icon to select the date. (Change the *Admin Date* so that it matches the encounter date.) Select the time the immunization is administered. (Enter a time that is 15 minutes past the patient's appointment time.)

 TIP You can also click the *Reset* icon to reset to the current date and time.

7. In the *Administered By* list, click the provider who administered the immunization. The screen should populate with your name or operator number. (Leave as is.)

8. In the *Ord Provider* list, click the provider who ordered the immunization. (Select "Dr. Raman.")

9. Click on the *Add Lot* ✚ icon in the *Immunization* section. Referring to the details in **Figure 7-24**, add immunization lot information and enter the following information in the *Lot Management* dialog box.

    a. Enter the *Lot Number* (enter "Hep" followed by your operator number as the lot number).

    b. Click the *Search* icon next to *Immunization*.

        i.   Enter "Hep B" in the *Search Text* field. Click *Search*.

        ii. Select "Hep B, adult" from the *Search Results* list.

    c. Click the *Search* icon next to *Manufacturer*.

        i.   Enter "me" in the *Search Text* field. Click *Search*.

        ii. Select the radio dial button next to "Merck & Co." under *Search Results*.

    d. Enter *Received Date* of January 1, 20XX (current year).

        (**Note:** Adjust the years in the *Received Date* and *Expiration Date* fields depending on the date of the encounter. For example, if your encounter takes place in 2018, the *Received Date* should occur in 2018, and the *Expiration Date* should be on the same month/day in 2019.)

    e. Enter *Expiration Date* of January 1, 20XX (following year). (See prior note on the *Expiration Date*.)

    f. Enter "20" in the *# Doses in Lot* field.

    g. Enter *Standard Dose* of "1.0" mL (note: the screen may reflect ml vs. mL).

    h. Select *Standard Route* of "IM."

    i. *State Supplied* defaults to "No. "

    j. *Active* defaults to "Yes."

    k. Click *Save*.

10. Select the lot you just created from the *Lot Number* drop-down list.

Napa Valley Family Health Associates-cengage237919 -

Add Immunization Lot: Napa Valley Family Health Associates 2

Lot Number	Hep228134
Immunization	Hep B, adult
Manufacturer	Merck & Co.
Received Date	01/01/2017
Expiration Date	01/01/2018
# Doses in Lot	20
Standard Dose	1.0 ml
Standard Route	IM
State Supplied	○Yes ●No
Active	●Yes ○No

Save | ✖ Cancel

Courtesy of Harris CareTracker PM and EMR

Figure 7-24   Add Immunization Lot

SPOTLIGHT   Important!!

- If the lot number is not selected, a warning message displays, prompting you to select a lot number.
- All state departments of health require reporting the amount of an immunization administered in milliliters (mL).

11. By default, the *Dose Route* list displays the standard route information selected in the *Lot Management* dialog box. However, you can change the method by which the immunization is administered by making another selection from the *Dose Route* list. (Leave the *Dose Route* as "IM.")

12. By default, the *Amount* field displays the amount entered in the *Lot Management* dialog box. You can change this by manually entering another amount. (Leave the *Amount* as "1" Milliliter.)

13. In the *Series* list, select the appropriate sequence when the immunization administered is from a series of several shots (i.e., initial challenge and boosters). For example, if administering the patient with a series of hepatitis immunizations and it is the first immunization in the series, select "1" in the *Series* list. (Select "1.")

SPOTLIGHT   Three doses are generally required to complete the hepatitis B vaccine series for adults.

- First injection—given at any time
- Second injection—at least one month after the first dose
- Third injection—six months after the first dose

When documenting a patient encounter, the series information displays in the narrative.

14. In the *Site* list, click the area of the patient's body where the immunization or drug is administered. (Select "Left Deltoid.")

15. In the *VIS Date* box, Harris CareTracker EMR automatically fills in the date from the *Support* database (leave as is). **Note:** If the date does not display, enter the date on the *Vaccine Information Statements* (VIS) handed out to the patient when the immunization was administered. (Enter date of the first day of the current year you are working in. For instance, if you are working in 2018, you would enter "01/01/2018.") **(FYI)** This feature only works on immunizations given via the *Immunization Writer*, and will not display for the information entered via the *Add Past/Refused Immunization* historical data.

16. In the *Date VIS given to Pt* box, enter the date the VIS was given to the patient. (Enter the date of the patient encounter.)

17. By default, the *Adverse Reactions* list is set to "Pt Tolerated Well." However, you can select one or more other reactions the patient had as a result of the immunization administered. (Leave the selection as is.)

18. In the *Administration Notes* box, enter additional comments about the immunization if necessary. (Enter: "Patient to return in 4–5 weeks for second injection, and return 6 months after the 1st dose for 3rd injection.") Your screen should look like **Figure 7-25**.

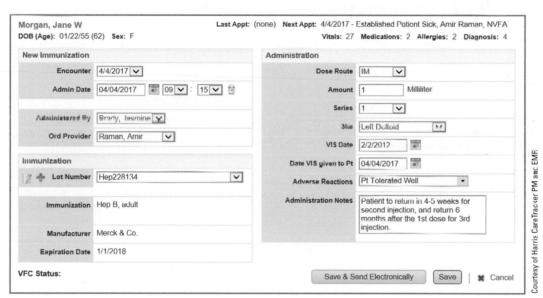

Figure 7-25   Immunization Writer

19. Click *Save* to save the administered immunization to the patient's medical record, *Chart Viewer*, and the narrative of the *Progress Note* template. (**Note:** To save and send the immunization information to the Department of Health in your state, you would click *Save & Send Electronically*.)

20. Refresh your *Immunizations* screen by clicking on the *Immunizations* application, and you will see the newly added Hep B immunization (**Figure 7-26**).

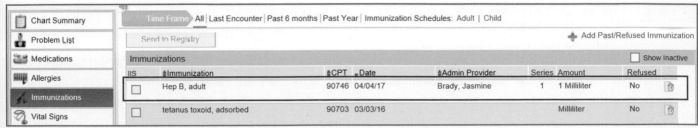

Figure 7-26   Refreshed Immunization Screen

Courtesy of Harris CareTracker PM and EMR

💾 **Print the updated Immunizations window. Label it "Activity 7-7" and place it in your assignment folder.**

Print Immunization Records

The *Immunizations* application allows you to print immunization records to give to patients. This printed record helps to review the immunization history, provides the ability to know when an immunization is due, and prevents over-immunization. It also shares the patient immunization history with other entities such as clinics, schools, and camps, enabling compliance with safety and health regulations.

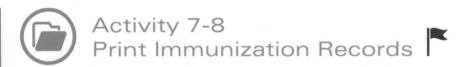

Activity 7-8
Print Immunization Records

1. Pull patient Jane Morgan into context, and then click the *Medical Record* module.

2. In the *Patient Health History* pane, click *Immunizations*. Harris CareTracker EMR displays the *Immunizations* window with a list of immunizations administered to the patient.

3. Click on your name or operator number in the *Admin Provider* column. The information regarding the immunization displays.

4. After viewing the dialog box, close out by clicking on the "X" in the upper-right-hand corner of the dialog box.

5. Click the drop-down arrow next to *Print* 🖨 on the *Patient Detail* bar, and click *Print Immunization*.

6. The patient immunization record opens in a new window (**Figure 7-27**).

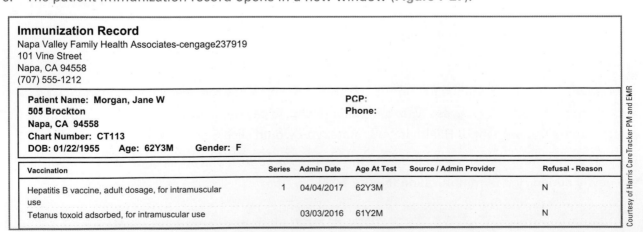

Figure 7-27   Print Immunization Record

Print the Immunization Record. Label it "Activity 7-8" and place it in your assignment folder.

7. Close out of the *Immunization Record* tab.

> **TIP** The *Immunization Record* displays a detailed list of active immunizations for the patient. Immunizations marked as inactive do not display in the report.

View the Activity Log of an Immunization

The *Activity Log* tracks all activity related to immunizations recorded in the patient's medical record. It is a helpful reference for audit purposes and displays information such as date, user responsible for the action, the action performed, and comments associated with an action. The log provides protection to patients, and helps providers demonstrate compliance with privacy laws and regulations such as HIPAA.

Activity 7-9
View the Activity Log of an Immunization

1. With patient Jane Morgan in context, click the *Medical Record* module.

2. In the *Patient Health History* pane, click on the *Immunizations* application. Harris CareTracker EMR displays the *Immunizations* window with a list of immunizations administered to the patient.

3. Now click the *Log* icon for the immunization you entered in Activity 7-8 and the *View Clinical Logs* dialog box displays each event as listed in **Table 7-9**, based on the type of action performed. (**Note:** If the log is not displaying, you may need to adjust the date in the *From Date* [e.g., select "01/01/2018"] and *To Date* [use current date] boxes to include previously administered immunizations [**Figure 7-28**].)

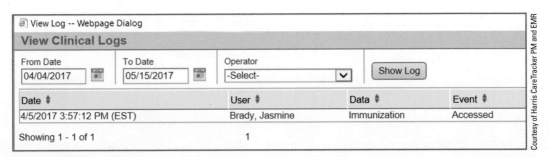

Figure 7-28   View Clinical Logs

 Print a screen shot of the Immunization Log. Label it "Activity 7-9" and place it in your assignment folder.

4. Close out of the *Log* by clicking the "X."

TABLE 7-9 Immunizations Activity Log

ENTRY	DESCRIPTION
Immunization Added	Displays when the immunization is added to the patient's medical record.
Immunization Accessed	Displays when immunization information is viewed.
Immunization Modified	Displays when information about the immunization is updated. However, this does not include updates to the status of the immunization.
Immunization Removed	Displays when the immunization is changed to an inactive status.

Courtesy of Harris CareTracker PM and EMR

PULLING UP AND RECORDING PATIENT EDUCATION

Learning Objective 4: Search for, customize, and provide patient education materials for patients.

The *Patient Education* application provides a comprehensive library of patient education material available through Krames StayWell that covers the most common conditions. You can search for education material using keywords, ICD or CPT® codes, or search for material by navigating the tree structure. The content in this site is updated quarterly based on material received from Krames StayWell. You can also browse a list of favorite education materials via the *Favorites* tab. The material includes access to a database of health care advisories and clinical education handouts in different languages. You can give these materials to the patient based on the patient's condition and treatment options. The application enables searching through hundreds of education material, saving common material given out to patients as favorites, or linking to other online sites with professionally written material. Education handouts given to a patient are recorded in the *Correspondence* and the *Progress Notes* sections of the patient's medical record.

Activity 7-10
Access and Search for Patient Education

1. With patient Jane Morgan in context, click on the *Medical Record* module.

2. In the *Clinical Toolbar*, click the *Patient Education* (Edu) ![icon] icon.

3. If an encounter is in context, the *Patient Education* dialog box displays and defaults to the tab set in the *Patient Education Default* list in the *Set Chart Summary Defaults* dialog box. If an encounter is not in context, Harris CareTracker EMR displays the *Select Encounter* dialog box. Select the appointment date/encounter you created for the patient in Chapter 4. This will launch the *Patient Education* dialog box.

4. By default, the *Search By* option is set to "Keywords." However, you can change the search option to CPT®, ICD-9, or ICD-10 code if necessary. (Leave as is.)

5. By default, the age and gender criteria default to the information saved for the patient in context. However, you can change the age and gender selections if necessary. (Change the *Age* selection to "All.")

6. In the *Language* list, click the language of the education material you want. (Select "English.")

7. In the blank box above *Language* type in the keywords "Urinary Tract Infection."

8. Click *Search*.

9. Under *Search Results* scroll down and select "Urinary Tract Infections in Women." Click on the *Favorite* ⭐ icon in the *Search Results* bar to save in your list of *Favorites*.

10. Now enter "Hematuria" in the text box above *Language*.

11. Click *Search*.

12. Scroll down and select "What Is Hematuria?" under the *Urinary Tract Problems* header. Click on the *Favorite* ⭐ icon to save in your list of *Favorites*.

13. To print the handouts for "Urinary Tract Infections in Women" and "What Is Hematuria":

    a. Click on the *Favorites* tab at the top of the *Patient Education* dialog box (**Figure 7-29**).

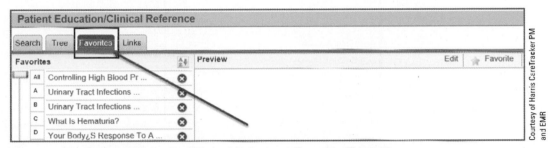

Figure 7-29   Patient Education/Clinical Reference Favorites Tab 7.32

    b. Select the required handout(s) from the *Favorites* list. The handout displays in the *Preview* section of the window.

    c. Click *Print* on the top right of the window to print the handout. **Hint:** You must actually print (or print to PDF) the handout for it to appear in the *Correspondence* section.

🖫 **Label the printed Patient Education Sheet(s) "Activity 7-10a and 7-10b" and place them in your assignment folder.**

14. Close out of the *Patient Education/Clinical Reference* tab.

You can also search for handouts via the *Tree* tab and via the *Favorites* tab (**Figure 7-30**). For more information on these alternative search methods, log in to *Help*, click on the *Contents* tab, and select *Searching for Handouts* (Go to *Medical Records > Patient Education > Searching for Handouts*).

Advanced Features for Patient Education

The *Patient Education* application enables you to customize the content of patient education material based on your requirements. However, the changes you make are only valid for the current encounter and the customized handout cannot be saved as a favorite. If you print the customized handout, the *Patient Education Printed* entry, and a copy of the customized handout are recorded in the *Correspondence* application of the patient's medical record.

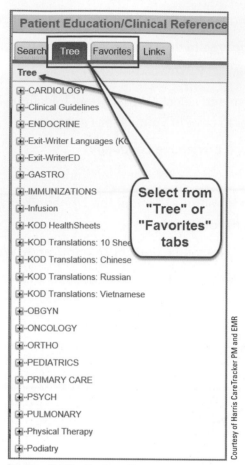

Figure 7-30   Patient Education/Clinical
Reference Search Tab 7.33

The *Patient Education* application enables you to search other online sites for professionally written material as well. Refer to instructions in *Help* for accessing websites for handouts.

CREATING CLINICAL LETTERS

Learning Objective 5: Access the Correspondence application to add, filter, customize, and print patient correspondence.

The *Letters* application provides the ability to use letter templates to create letters for patients. You can include the company logo; patient information, such as progress note data; lab reports; and more, in the letter. You can utilize the editor that is similar to other desktop editors like MS Word® to format and edit each letter. After creating the letter, you can save, print, or attach the letter to a *ToDo*, mail, or fax.

FYI If a live practice would like to include a company-specific logo on any letters printed from the *Clinical Letter Editor*, you would complete the following steps to define and set up letter templates via the *Clinical Letter Editor* application:

- To access the *Clinical Letter Editor* application, click on the *Administration* module, select the *Clinical* tab, and then click on the *Clinical Letter Editor* link under the *Forms and Letters* heading.

- You can include the company logo in a letter by uploading the logo via the *Company Logo* application. To access the *Company Logo* application, click on the *Administration* module, and then select the *Setup* tab and *Company Logo* link.

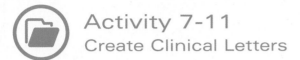

Activity 7-11
Create Clinical Letters

1. Pull patient Jane Morgan into context, and then click the *Medical Record* module.

2. In the *Clinical Toolbar*, click the *Letters* icon.

3. If an encounter is in context, Harris CareTracker EMR displays the *Letter Manager* dialog box. (**Note:** If an encounter is not in context, Harris CareTracker EMR displays the *Select Encounter* dialog box. Select the appointment date/encounter you created for the patient in Chapter 4. This will launch the *Letter Manager* dialog box.)

4. To select the *Letter Template* you want to use ("NVFHA Consult Letter COPY"):

    a. Click the *Manage Favorites* ☆ icon to search for the required letter.

    b. In the *Manage Letter Favorites* dialog box, select "NVFHA Consult Letter COPY" under *Clinical Note* (**Figure 7-31**). The selected letter template will now appear in the *Letter Manager* dialog box.

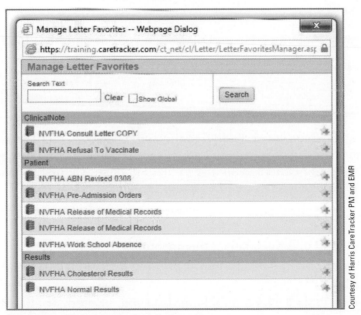

Figure 7-31   Manage Letter Favorites

5. The Harris CareTracker EMR *Letters* application pulls in the referring provider (Dr. Richard Shinaman) and information from the patient encounter, creating the *Consult Letter* to send to Dr. Shinaman (**Figure 7-32**). **Note:** There must be a *Progress Note* associated with the encounter for the *Letter*(s) to pull in.

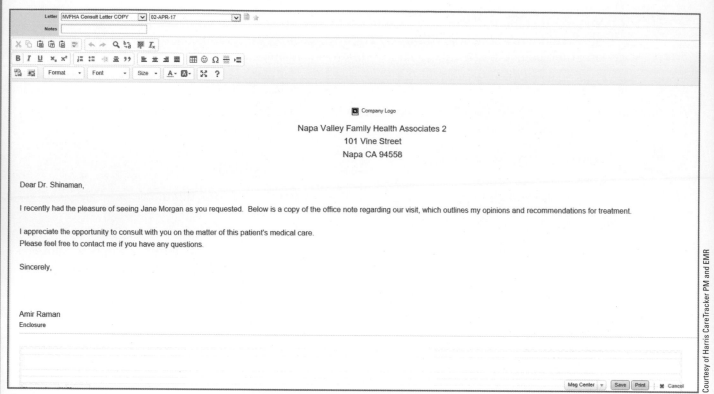

Figure 7-32   NVFHA Consult Letter

6. In the bottom right corner of the screen, select *Print* to print a copy of the consult letter. (All letter actions are described in Table 7-10.)

 Label the printed consult letter "Activity 7-11" and place it in your assignment folder.

7. Close out of the *Letter* screen.

> **TIP** To save a letter as a favorite and add it to the *Letter* list, click the *Add as Favorite* ✚ icon to the right of the letter name in the *Manage Letter Favorites* dialog box. You can check the box next to "Show Global" and the *Letters* available in the database will display. Any *Letter* previously added as a *Favorite* will have the *Saved as Favorite* ✚ icon displayed.

If printing a *Clinical Note* type letter, you must select the encounter. This allows you to generate a letter with information and progress note data from the encounter. If printing a *Results* letter type, you must select the specific result to include in the letter.

All letter actions are described in **Table 7-10**. When a letter is saved, printed, or attached to a *ToDo*, an entry is recorded in the clinical log.

TABLE 7-10 Letter Actions	
ACTION	**DESCRIPTION**
Save	Click to save and print the letter at a later date. The letter is saved in the *Correspondence* application and displays the *Letter Generated* entry. The name of the letter displays under the *Name* column and notes display under the *Document* column of the *Correspondence* application.

ACTION	DESCRIPTION
Print	Click to print the letter. When a letter is printed, an entry is recorded with the date and time in the *Correspondence* application.
Msg Center	Point to the *Arrow* ▼ icon next to *Msg Center*, and click the required option to attach the letter as a PDF to a *ToDo* or fax or mail the letter.

Courtesy of Harris CareTracker PM and EMR

Access the Correspondence Application

The *Correspondence* application displays any correspondence your practice has had with the patient in context and with another provider regarding the patient. This includes items such as *ToDo*(s), emails, phone calls, letters pertaining to the patient, patient education material given to the patient, and more. This helps keep track of all communications associated with the patient in a central location. The *Correspondence* application is accessible from the following locations:

- *Name Bar > Corr* icon 👤
- *Patient Info* 👤 icon on the *Name Bar > Documents* tab > *Correspondence* tab (**Figure 7-33**)
- *Home* module > *Practice* tab > *Unprinted Correspondence* link (*Front Office* section)
- *Financial* module > *Correspondence* tab
- *Medical Record* module > *Correspondence* pane

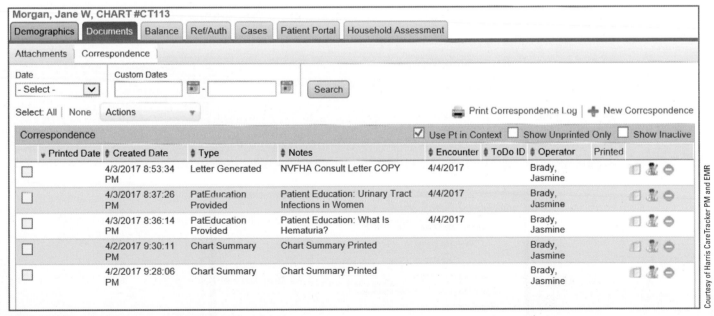

Figure 7-33   Patient Info—Correspondence Tab

Add Patient Correspondence

The *Correspondence* application allows you to add any correspondence, including medical record disclosures associated with a patient. When recording a medical record disclosure, a dialog box displays to enter additional details such as date and information disclosed. Additionally, you can link a correspondence to a specific encounter or to a document uploaded to the patient's medical record.

Activity 7-12
Add a Patient Correspondence

Patient Jane Morgan requested that a copy of her medical records be mailed to her home address because she is considering relocating to Colorado and wants to have all her records in her possession. She has completed the required authorization form.

1. Pull patient Jane Morgan into context, and then click the *Medical Record* module.

2. In the *Patient Health History* pane, click *Correspondence*. Harris CareTracker EMR displays the *Correspondence* window.

3. Click *+ New Correspondence* (**Figure 7-34**). Harris CareTracker EMR displays the *Add Correspondence* dialog box. The *Printed Date* box is grayed out, so no dates can be entered here.

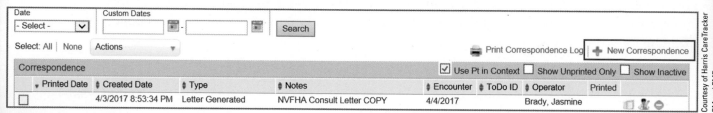

Figure 7-34   Add New Correspondence

4. In the *Type* field, scroll down to "Medical Record Disclosure" and select it.

5. In the pop-up *Correspondence Type: Medical Records* dialog box, enter the following details (**Figure 7-35**):

   a. *Date of Disclosure*: Enter today's date

   b. *Operator Name*: Enter your name or operator number

   c. *Reported to*: Enter "Patient, Jane Morgan"

   d. *Recipient's Address*: Leave blank

   e. *Information Disclosed*: Enter "Medical Record"

   f. *Purpose of Disclosure*: Enter "Pt requested copy of medical record"

   g. Click *Save*.

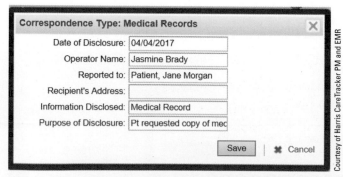

Figure 7-35   Correspondence Type: Medical Records

6. You will be taken back to the *Add Correspondence* dialog box. In the *Encounter ID* list, select the encounter to link to the correspondence. Use the last encounter you created for the patient.

7. In the *Document* list, you would click the attachment given to the patient. No document appears in the list.

8. By default, *Active* is set to "Yes." (Leave as is.)

9. In the *Notes* box, you can enter additional comments about the patient correspondence. Enter "Mailed copy to patient's home address on (use today's date)." Verify that the information entered in the *Correspondence Type* dialog box appears here (**Figure 7-36**).

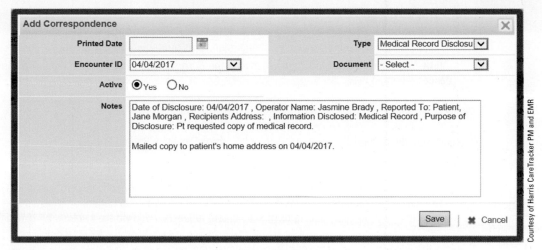

Figure 7-36   Review Patient Correspondence Notes

10. Click *Save* (**Figure 7-37**).

11. You will receive a *Success!* box. Close out of the *Success!* box. Close the *Add Correspondence* window if still displaying.

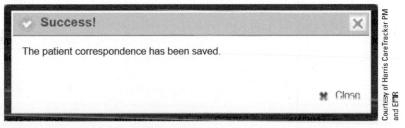

Figure 7-37   Correspondence Saved

The correspondence is saved in the *Correspondence* window of the *Correspondence* module (**Figure 7-38**).

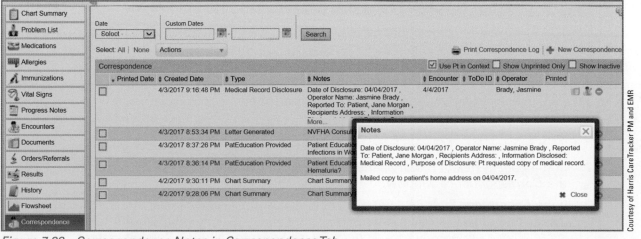

Figure 7-38   Correspondence Notes in Correspondence Tab

📧 **Print a screenshot of the Patient Correspondence window. Label it "Activity 7-12" and place it in your assignment folder.**

Table 7-11 describes the information that displays in the columns of the *Correspondence* window. You can click a column heading to sort the items on the window.

TABLE 7-11   Correspondence Columns

COLUMN	DESCRIPTION
Printed Date	The original date the correspondence is printed or marked as printed. (**Note**: You can click the *Mark Printed* action in the *Correspondence* application to mark a correspondence as printed.)
Created Date	Displays the date the correspondence is created in MM/DD/YY, HH:MM:SS format.
Type	The correspondence type. For example, Patient Education Provided, Patient Portal, and Patient Visit Summary.
Notes	Displays notes entered in the *Note* field when manually entering the correspondence or creating a *ToDo* or *Fax*. Additionally, the columns display titles of patient education given to a patient or attached to a *ToDo*, names of letters created, approval status of amendment requests made via the *Patient Portal*, and more.
Encounter	Displays the encounter date associated with the correspondence.
ToDo ID	Displays the *ToDo* number associated with *ToDo*-type correspondence.
Operator	Displays the operator who created the correspondence.
Printed	Indicates if practice management letters are generated.
Documents	Allows viewing documents attached to the correspondence.
Letters	Allows viewing letters attached to the correspondence.
Activate/Deactivate	Allows activating and deactivating a correspondence.

Courtesy of Harris CareTracker PM and EMR

Work with Patient Correspondence

The *Correspondence* application allows you to view correspondences and any attachments. You can view any documents or letters attached to patient correspondences in the *Correspondence* window.

FYI In a live environment, to view and print correspondence attachments, follow the instructions below:

1. With patient Jane Morgan in context, click the *Medical Record* module.

2. In the *Patient Health History* pane, click *Correspondence*. Harris CareTracker EMR displays the *Correspondence* window.

3. If the *Letters* icon is grayed out, you cannot view the actual correspondence in this tab. To view a letter in a live environment, click the *Letters* icon on the right-hand side of your screen. For example, click the *Letters* icon next to "NVFHA Consult Letter COPY" to open the letter in a new window. It may take a few moments for the *Letter* to pull up.

4. Click *Print* to print the selected letter(s).

Activate and Deactivate Correspondence

You can set items as inactive in the *Correspondence* window. Inactive items display the *Set Active* ⓘ icon. You can also change the status of an inactive item to active.

ACTIVITY 7-13
Set an Item as Inactive or Active

1. With patient Jane Morgan in context, click the *Medical Record* module.

2. In the *Patient Health History* pane, click *Correspondence*. Harris CareTracker EMR displays the *Correspondence* window.

3. First, mark the "Patient Education: What Is Hematuria?" document as inactive. Click the *Set Inactive* ◇ icon pertaining to this correspondence and then click *OK* to confirm the change (**Figure 7-39**).

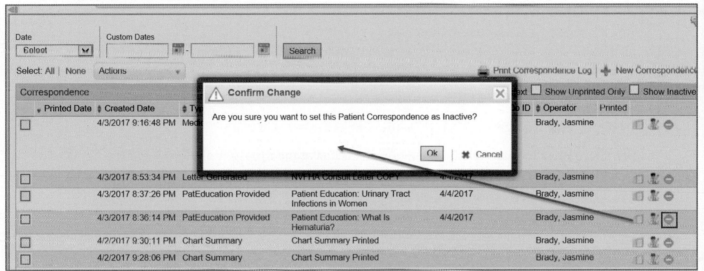

Figure 7-39   Set as Inactive Confirmation Box

Courtesy of Harris CareTracker PM and EMR

4. Check the box in the upper-right-hand corner of your screen to "show inactive" (**Figure 7-40**).

	Printed Date	Created Date	Type	Notes	Encounter	ToDo ID	Operator	Printed	
☐		4/3/2017 9:16:48 PM	Medical Record Disclosure	Date of Disclosure: 04/04/2017 , Operator Name: Jasmine Brady , Reported To: Patient, Jane Morgan , Recipients Address: , Information More...	4/4/2017		Brady, Jasmine		🗐 🛉 ⊖
☐	4/3/2017 8:53:34 PM		Letter Generated	NVFHA Consult Letter COPY	4/4/2017		Brady, Jasmine		🗐 🛉 ⊖
☐	4/3/2017 8:48:51 PM		Letter Generated	NVFHA Consult Letter COPY	4/4/2017		Brady, Jasmine		🗐 🛉 ⓘ
☐	4/3/2017 8:37:26 PM		PatEducation Provided	Patient Education: Urinary Tract Infections in Women	4/4/2017		Brady, Jasmine		🗐 🛉 ⊖
☐	4/3/2017 8:36:30 PM		PatEducation Provided	Patient Education: What Is Hematuria?	4/4/2017		Brady, Jasmine		🗐 🛉 ⓘ

Figure 7-40   Show Inactive Box

Courtesy of Harris CareTracker PM and EMR

💾 **Print the screen of the Inactive Patient Correspondence, label it "Activity 7-13a," and place it in your assignment folder.**

5. Now, mark the inactive document "Patient Education: What is Hematuria?" as active by clicking the *Set Active* ⏻ icon pertaining to the inactive correspondence.

6. Click *OK* to confirm the change.

🖨 **Print the screen of the Activated Patient Correspondence, label it "Activity 7-13b," and place it in your assignment folder.**

Print the Correspondence Log

The *Correspondence Log* is a summary of all patient correspondences.

Activity 7-14
Print the Correspondence Log

1. Pull patient Jane Morgan into context, and then click the *Medical Record* module.

2. In the *Patient Health History* pane, click *Correspondence*. Harris CareTracker EMR displays the *Correspondence* window.

3. Uncheck *Show Inactive*.

4. Click the *Print Correspondence Log* (**Figure 7-41**) link at the top right of the screen. The application displays the log in a new window (**Figure 7-42**). (**Note:** If the log does not appear within a few seconds, go on to step 5.)

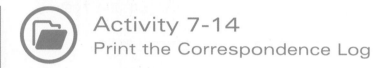

	Printed Date ⬍	Created Date	⬍ Type	⬍ Notes	⬍ Encounter	⬍ ToDo ID	⬍ Operator	Printed	
☐		4/3/2017 9:16:48 PM	Medical Record Disclosure	Date of Disclosure: 04/04/2017 , Operator Name: Jasmine Brady , Reported To: Patient, Jane Morgan , Recipients Address: , Information More...	4/4/2017		Brady, Jasmine		📄 🧍 ⊖
☐		4/3/2017 8:53:34 PM	Letter Generated	NVFHA Consult Letter COPY	4/4/2017		Brady, Jasmine		📄 🧍 ⊖
☐		4/3/2017 8:37:26 PM	PatEducation Provided	Patient Education: Urinary Tract Infections in Women	4/4/2017		Brady, Jasmine		📄 🧍 ⊖
☐		4/3/2017 8:36:30 PM	PatEducation Provided	Patient Education: What Is Hematuria?	4/4/2017		Brady, Jasmine		📄 🧍 ⊖
☐		4/2/2017 9:30:11 PM	Chart Summary	Chart Summary Printed			Brady, Jasmine		📄 🧍 ⊖

Select: All | None   Actions ▾   🖨 Print Correspondence Log | ➕ New Correspondence

Correspondence   ☑ Use Pt in Context ☐ Show Unprinted Only ☐ Show Inactive

Figure 7-41   *Print Correspondence Log*

5. Click back on the home screen (first tab in your browser), where you will see the PDF report on the lower part of your screen (**Figure 7-43**). You will be asked if you want to *Open* or *Save* the PDF. Click *Open* and then *Print* by right-clicking your mouse in the screen and selecting *Print* from the *Menu*. **Note:** If you still don't see the report, follow the steps in the Tip Box at the end of this activity.

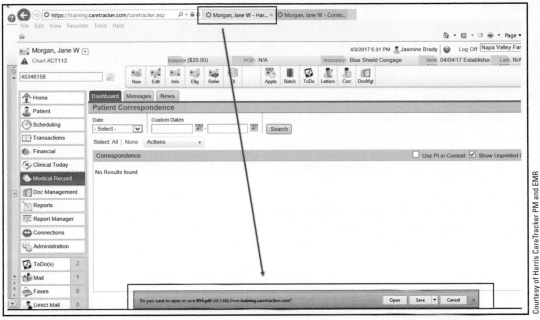

Figure 7-42   Correspondence Log

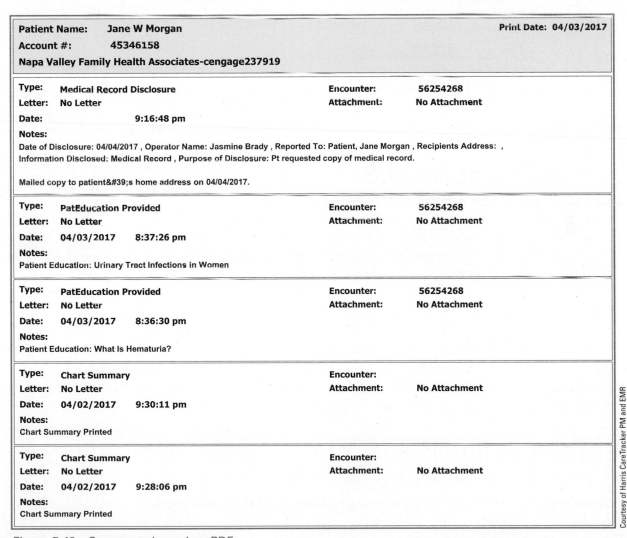

Figure 7-43   Correspondence Log PDF

TIP Depending on the version of Internet Explorer you are working in, you may have some difficulty loading the *Correspondence Log*. If you are experiencing difficulty, you can try to troubleshoot as follows:

1. Click back on the home screen, where you will see a message at the top of the screen indicating that Internet Explorer has blocked the correspondence file from downloading. Click on the message and select "Download file" from the drop-down menu (see **Figure 7-44**). The home page will reload.

   a. Go back into the patient's medical record, and in the *Correspondence* module click on the *Print Correspondence Log* link.

   b. A *Generating Report* window will pop up, telling you that the log is processing. (Note: If the correspondence log is taking too long to load, you can close out of the *Generating Report* window and the patient's medical record. Go back to the home screen and click the *Medical Record* module. Click the *Correspondence* tab and select the *Print Correspondence Log* link again. The correspondence log PDF should now load quickly.)

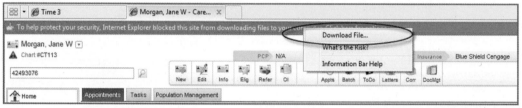

Figure 7-44   Select Download File

Courtesy of Harris CareTracker PM and EMR

📧 Print the Correspondence Log. Label it "Activity 7-14" and place it in your assignment folder.

CREATING REFERRALS

Learning Objective 6: Create outgoing and incoming patient referrals.

The *Referrals and Authorizations* application enables providers to create inbound and outbound referrals and associated authorizations directly via the patient's medical record. You can provide data about the patient's condition and needs, referring and referred-to provider details, treatment authorization data, and referral dates and ranges. Referrals enable you to track patient compliance with the referral instructions, eliminating the need for paperwork.

You can set the *Referrals and Authorizations* application to default to a referral type in the *Referral Default* field (Referral-Incoming, Referral-Outgoing, or Referral-Outgoing New) when creating a batch. Referrals and authorizations in "pending" status do not display in the *Authorization* list of the *Additional Claim Information* dialog box. This prevents you from linking an incomplete referral or authorization to a claim.

All referrals added via the *Referrals and Authorizations* application display in the patient medical record as well as the *Ref/Auth* application of the *Patient* module, and vice versa.

Access the Referrals and Authorizations Application

There are several ways to access the *Referrals and Authorizations* application:

- Click the *Patient* module and then click the *Referrals & Authorizations* tab.
- Click the *Refer* icon on the *Name Bar*.
- Click the *Medical Record* module and then click the *Refer* icon on the *Clinical Toolbar*.

Create Outgoing Referrals

Outgoing referrals are requests made by the physician to specialists, ancillary providers, or clinics. Most primary care physicians (PCPs) create outgoing referrals; however, many specialists refer out for ancillary services and/ or for consults with other specialties.

If a PCP sends a patient to a dermatologist to treat a psoriasis condition, the PCP gives the patient a referral, which is referred to as an outgoing referral. (**Note:** The authorization number, provider information, from and to dates, and number of authorized visits are mandatory information required to link a referral to a charge.)

The *Referral To* list displays the providers in your *Refer Provider To* quick picks list. The *Referral From* list displays the providers in your *Refer Provider From* quick picks list. The quick picks list is set up via the *Quick Picks* application. The *Quick Picks* application is accessible by clicking the *Administration* module, *Setup* tab, and then clicking the *Quick Picks* link under the *Financial* section.

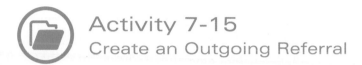

Activity 7-15
Create an Outgoing Referral

1. Pull patient Harriet Oshea into context.

2. With the patient in context, click on the *Medical Record* module. Harriet had been seen by Dr. Brockton on March 20, 2017, and complained of hip and back pain. She was to follow up with Dr. Brockton in one month. However, Harriet called the office on today (use today's date) complaining that the pain had increased and requested a referral to an orthopedic specialist.

3. In the *Clinical Toolbar*, click the *Refer* ![icon] icon. A *Select Encounter* dialog box will pop up. Select the encounter dated March 20, 2017. Harris CareTracker EMR displays the *Referrals and Authorizations* dialog box (**Figure 7-45**).

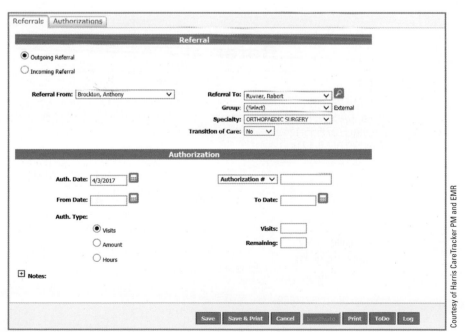

Figure 7-45   Referral to Dr. Rovner

4. If the default selection is set to *Outgoing Referral* in your batch, leave as is. If not, change the field to *Outgoing Referral* for this activity.

5. If the *Default Referral to Billing Provider* list is set to "Yes" in your batch, then the *Referral From* list defaults to the billing provider set in the batch. However, you can select a different provider if needed. Confirm that Dr. Brockton is listed as the referring provider. If not, use the drop down and select Dr. Brockton.

6. From the *Referral To* list, select the provider to whom you want to refer the patient. Click the *Search* 🔍 icon to search for a provider.

    a. In the *Provider Search* dialog box, enter the *Name* and *State* information for Dr. Robert Rovner in San Ramon, California. Click *Search*.

    b. Click on Robert Rovner's name under the *Provider Name* heading and Harris CareTracker EMR will pull his information into the referral dialog box.

7. If the provider is outside the practice (external), you must select the provider's group and specialty. (Select "Orthopaedic Surgery" in the *Specialty* field.)

 FYI If the provider you are referring to is within the same practice as the referring from provider (internal), Harris CareTracker EMR automatically populates the information in the *Group* and *Specialty* lists.

---

8. By default, the *Transition of Care* list is set to "Yes" to indicate that the outgoing referral is a transition of care to another provider. However, you can change the option if necessary. (Select "No.")

9. Change the *Auth. Date* to today (use today's date/the date Harriet called, requesting a referral).

10. (*Optional—Authorization*) Harriet's insurance does not require an authorization. Leave blank.

11. Click *Save & Print* (see **Figure 7-45**) at the bottom of the screen. Harris CareTracker EMR saves the referral (**Figure 7-46**). (**Note:** Once you have saved the referral, you may have to close out of the *Referral* and *Authorization* dialog box to see the *Referral Print* screen.)

Referral

Referred From:	Anthony Brockton	Referred To:	Robert Rovner
	101 Vine Street Napa, CA 94558 (Phone):(707)555-1212 (Fax):(707)555-1214		ORTHOPAEDIC SURGERY 5801 Norris Canyon Rd Ste 210 San Ramon, CA 945835440 (Phone):(925)355-7350 (Fax):(925)244-1457

Chart #:	CT151	**DOB:** 11/22/1972 **Age:** 45	
Patient Name:	HARRIET OSHEA	**Sex:** F	
Address:	5545 Wilson Way Sonoma, CA 95476		
Phone:	(Home): (707)222-5707 (Work): (800)967-4663		
PCP:	No Provider Found		

Primary Insurance Plan:	Proplan	**Subscriber #:**	
Auth Date:	4/3/2017	**Authorization:**	PENDING
From Date:	1/1/1900	**To Date:**	1/1/1900
Notes:			

Figure 7-46   *Referral Form for Harriet Oshea*

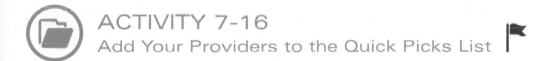 **Print the Outgoing Referral by clicking on the Print button, or by right-clicking your mouse and selecting Print from the menu. Label it "Activity 7-15" and place it in your assignment folder.**

12.   Close out of the *Referral* print dialog box.

Create Incoming Referrals

Incoming referrals are generally received by specialty physicians and must be processed during check-in or on a pre-visit basis. The referral is necessary for the specialty provider to receive appropriate payment. For example, if a women's health care specialist receives a referral from an outside practice to treat a patient for polycystic ovarian syndrome, this is referred to as an incoming referral.

Prior to creating incoming *Referrals*, you must set up your providers in the "Refer Provider To" list via the *Quick Picks* link. In previous chapters, you learned how to create *Quick Picks*. Follow the steps in Activity 7-16 to add your providers to the *Quick Picks* list.

ACTIVITY 7-16
Add Your Providers to the Quick Picks List

1.   Click on the *Administration* module > *Setup* tab > *Financial* header > *Quick Picks* link.

2.   In the *Screen Type* drop-down, scroll down and select *Refer Provider To*.

3.   Your screen will display either (a) "Paul T Endo" in the *Refer To Providers* box (if you completed Case Study 2-1) who is not a NVFHA provider, or (b) "There are no quick picks" (if you did not complete Case Study 2-1).

4.   Click the *Search* 🔍 icon and enter the providers of NVFHA (Rebecca Ayerick, Anthony Brockton, Gabriella Torres, and Amir Raman).

   a.   In the *Provider Search* dialog box, enter the provider's last name (Ayerick) and state (California) to narrow your search (**Figure 7-47**). Click *Search*.

   b.   Click on Rebecca Ayerick's name.

   c.   You will receive a *Success* box stating "Quick Pick information has been updated."

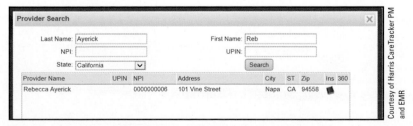

Figure 7-47   *Quick Pick—Refer Providers To*

5.   Repeat step 4 for each of the remaining providers in the NVFHA group (Anthony Brockton, Amir Raman, and Gabriella Torres).

6.   Click *Close* to exit out of the *Success* box after each provider has been added. When you have completed each entry, your screen should look like **Figure 7-48**.

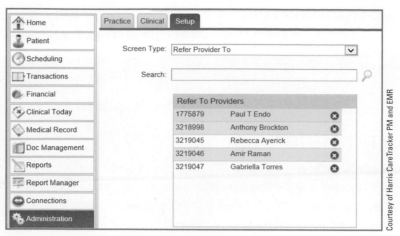

Figure 7-48 Refer Provider To Quick Pick List

 Print the Refer Provider To Quick Picks screen, label it "Activity 7-16" and place it in your assignment folder.

Now that your referring provider *Quick Picks* have been set up, you will be able to create an incoming referral (Activity 7-17).

Activity 7-17
Create an Incoming Referral

1. Pull patient Edith Robinson into context and then click on the *Medical Record* module. Ms. Robinson was referred to Dr. Raman of NVFHA as her new PCP by orthopedic specialist Dr. David Dodgin.

2. In the *Clinical Toolbar*, click the *Refer* 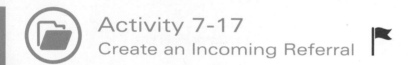 icon.

   a. If you are taken to a *Select an Encounter* dialog box, select the most recent encounter for the patient. If no encounter is available to select, then follow the Tip box steps below.

   b. If the *Referral and Authorization* dialog box displays, you can proceed with Step 3.

TIP Only if the patient does not have a previous encounter listed, select the *Create a New Encounter* link and enter the following information in the *Create a New Encounter* dialog box:

a. *Type*: Select "Other"

b. *Service Date*: Enter the date of the appointment you scheduled for Ms. Robinson in Chapter 4.

c. *Responsible Provider*: Select "Dr. Raman"

d. *Patient Case*: Leave as "Default"

e. *Location*: Leave as "NVFA"

f. *Transition of Care*: Leave as "No"

g. Click *Ok*.

---

3. In the *Referrals* dialog box, select *Incoming Referral* if not already selected (**Figure 7-49**). (The default selection for this field is set in your batch.)

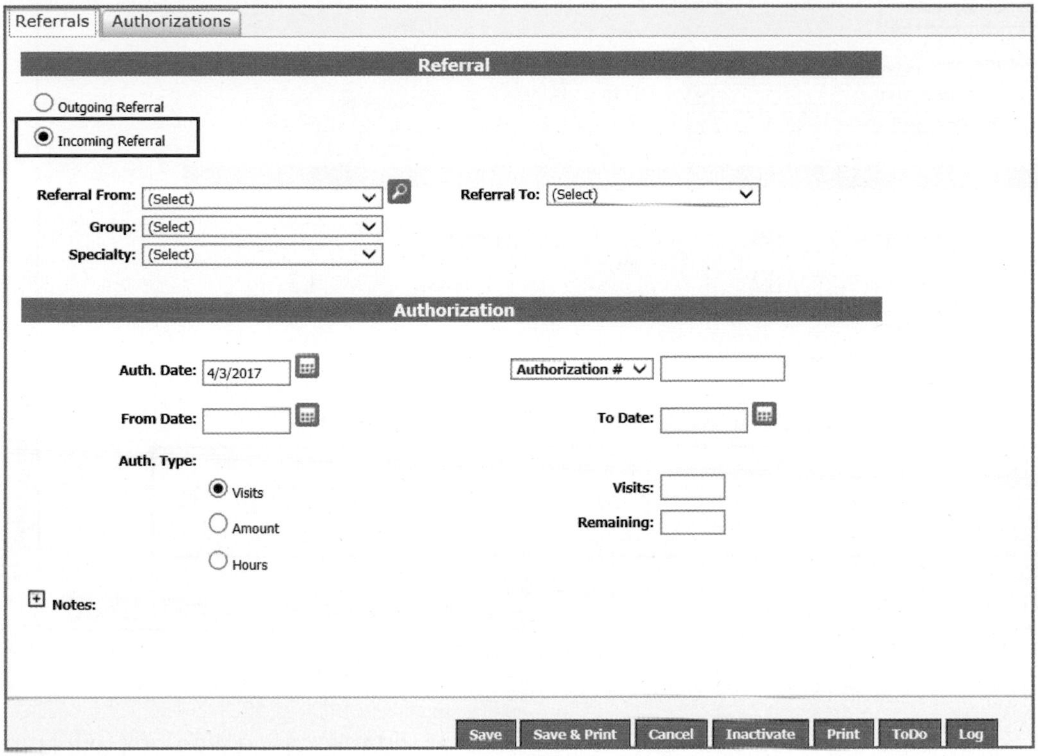

Courtesy of Harris CareTracker PM and EMR

Figure 7-49 Incoming Referral

4. Click *New*. Harris CareTracker PM and EMR displays the incoming referral fields. (**Note:** If the patient did not have a previous encounter, the *New* button will not display until you save this incoming referral, allowing you to create another. Skip this instruction and continue with the rest of the activity if the *New* button is not displayed.)
5. In the *Referral From* list, select the provider referring the patient. (Select "David Dodgin.")

   Alternatively, click the *Search* icon to search for a provider. If you use the search feature to select a provider, Harris CareTracker EMR automatically adds the provider to the *Providers* (tab) application of the *Patient* module.
6. Leave the *Group* field as "(Select)."
7. In the *Specialty* field, select "Orthopaedic Surgery" from the drop-down list.
8. The *Referral To* list defaults to the billing provider set in your batch (if the batch setting of *Default Referral* to Billing provider is listed as "Yes"), but you can select a different provider if needed using the drop-down arrow. Select "Dr. Raman."
9. No authorization is required; however, change the *Auth. Date* to your encounter date (the first appointment date that the patient has/had with Dr. Raman).
10. Click + *Notes* to enter comments related to the authorization. Enter notes: "Edith Robinson is a patient of Dr. Dodgin and has recently moved to Napa and would like to establish with Dr. Raman as her PCP" (**Figure 7-50**).

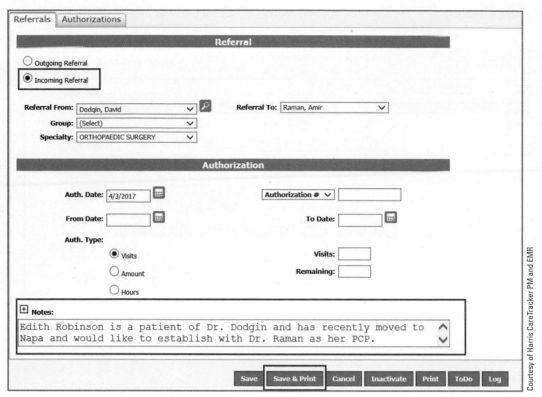

Figure 7-50   Incoming Referral for Edith Robinson

11. Click *Save & Print.* Harris CareTracker EMR saves the referral and the *Print* dialog box will appear (**Figure 7-51**). (**Note:** You may need to close out of the *Referral and Authorization* dialog box to see the *Referral Print* box.)

Print

Referral

Referred From:	David Dodgin 5201 Norris Canyon Rd Ste 300 San Ramon, CA 945835405 (Phone):(925)820-6720	Referred To:	Amir Raman 101 Vine Street Napa, CA 94558 (Phone):(707)555-1212 (Fax):(707)555-1214

Chart #:	CT143		
Patient Name:	EDITH ROBINSON		
Address:	3072 Sacramento St Sonoma, CA 95476	DOB: 1/1/1948 Sex: F	Age: 69
Phone:	(Home): (707)245-9898 (Work): (800)941-7044		
PCP:	No Provider Found		

Primary Insurance Plan:	Medicare Cengage	Subscriber #:	
Auth Date:	4/3/2017	Authorization:	PENDING
From Date:	1/1/1900	To Date:	1/1/1900

Notes:	Edith Robinson is a patient of Dr. Dodgin and has recently moved to Napa and would like to establish with Dr. Raman as her PCP.

Figure 7-51   Incoming Referral Print Box

Print the Incoming Referral by clicking the Print button in the Referral Print dialog box, or by right-clicking your mouse and selecting Print from the menu. Label it "Activity 7-17" and place it in your assignment folder.

12.   Close out of the *Referral* print screen.

You can generate a report in Harris CareTracker PM and EMR to help manage patient referrals and authorizations. For more information on generating referral authorization reports, see *Reports* module > *Patient Reports* > *Referral Authorizations Report* in the *Help* system.

COMPLETING A VISIT FOR BILLING PURPOSES

Learning Objective 7: View and resolve open encounters and unsigned notes by completing the visit and signing the Progress Note.

In Chapter 6, you completed much of the patient work-up to the point of completing and printing the progress note. In order for a patient visit to be billable, any open encounters must be resolved and the visit must be completed and the note signed. The provider is the person who is responsible for signing the progress note; however, to enhance your understanding of workflows in the EMR, you will be completing the visit, resolving open encounters, and electronically signing the note.

Completing a Visit

To generate claims, charges must be captured for the patient's appointment. The *Visit* application allows you to capture charges and enter procedure, NDC, and diagnosis codes for a patient's appointment.

Visits can be entered into Harris CareTracker PM and EMR via several applications. Access the *Visits* application by one of the following methods:

- Left-click on a patient's appointment in the *Book* application and select *Visit* from the pop-up mini-menu.

- Pull a patient into context, click the *Appts* button in the *Name Bar,* pull the appointment into context, and select *Visit* from the *Actions* menu.

- Click the *Appointments* link under the *Appointments* section of the *Dashboard* tab in the *Home* module, pull the patient appointment into context, and then select *Visit* from the *Actions* menu.

- Click the *Visits* link from the *Actions* drop-down list for a patient listed in the *Appointments* application of the *Clinical Today* module.

- Click the *Visit* icon on the *Clinical Toolbar* within the *Medical Record* module.

> **TIP**   If a patient is flagged as VIP in the *Demographic* application of the *Patient* module, the patient name displays as **VIP** in the appointment list unless you have the VIP overrides assigned to your profile. The overrides include *VIP Patient Access Break Glass* or *VIP Patient Access.* The VIP status is set in the *Demographic* application of the *Patient* module and overrides in the *Operators & Roles* application of the *Administration* module.

The *Visit* window contains a number of applications, but to save a visit you only need to enter the procedure and diagnosis code(s). Please note that a visit can only be edited prior to becoming a charge. For our first *Visit* activity, refer to patient Harriet Oshea's appointment on March 20, 2017, with Dr. Brockton. Best practice would be to access the *Assessment* tab in the *Progress Note* (**Figure 7-52**) and review the problem list to determine which diagnoses were selected for this visit. You would then capture the *Visit* following the instructions in Activity 7-18.

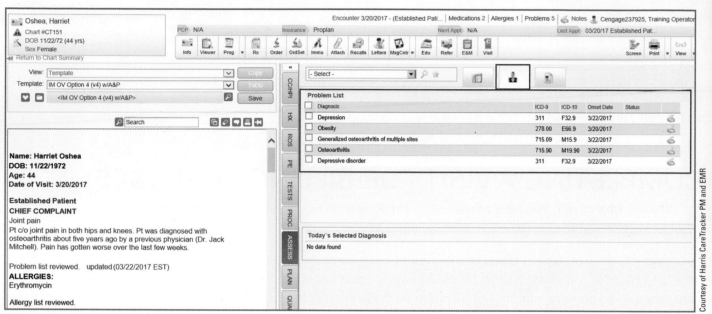

Figure 7-52   Harriet Oshea A&P

Courtesy of Harris CareTracker PM and EMR

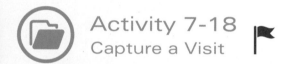

Activity 7-18
Capture a Visit

1. Click the *Scheduling* module. Harris CareTracker PM and EMR opens the *Book* application by default.

2. Move the schedule to display the date of service for which you want to confirm an appointment. This can be done by manually entering in the date in the *Date* box, by clicking the *Calendar* icon, or by selecting a time period from the *Move* list. (Enter "March 20, 2017" in the *Date* box.)

3. You will need to set the *Resources* field (just to the right of the calendar) to "All Resources" using the drop-down to select "All Resources" in order for the full schedule and all providers to display.

4. Click *Go*.

5. Left-click the appointment for which you want to enter visit information and select *Visit* from the mini-menu (select Harriet Oshea's appointment). The application displays the *Visit* window (**Figure 7-53**). When you first bring up the *Visit* window, it automatically displays the procedures section (*Procedures* tab located at the top left of the window).

6. The *Procedures* screen contains a list of procedure codes that mirror the CPT® codes on the encounter form. Place and verify that the checkboxes next to each code associated with the patient's appointment are selected. Select CPT® codes 99213, 73565, 73520, and 36415 for this visit. (**Note:** If no *Visit* had yet been entered for the patient, the encounter form would display with no checkboxes next to procedure or diagnosis codes. If you see the code you want to select for the *Visit*, you can select the checkbox next to the code. Alternatively, you could enter either a code or key term in the *Procedure Search* box and click *Search* to locate the desired code.)

Procedures	Diagnosis	Visit Summary						EncoderPro.com

Pt Name Oshea, Harriet (F)   **PCP**   **Admit Date** N/A   **Notes**

DOB 11/22/1972 (44 yrs)   **Ref Provider** Brockton, Anthony   **Last Surgery Date** N/A

Primary Ins Proplan   **Case Ins** Proplan   **Next Appointment** None   **Complaint** Joint Pain

Procedure Search: [   ] 🔍

OFFICE VISIT EST PTS	Mod	Units	OFFICE PROCEDURES	Mod	Units	PREVENTIVE MEDICINE EST	Mod	Units
☐ 99212 Office Outpatient Visit 10 Min		1	☐ 93000 Ecg Routine Ecg W/Least 12 Lds		1	☐ 99395 Periodic Preventive Med Est Pa		1
☐ 99213 Office Outpatient Visit 15 Min		1	☐ G0102 Pros Cancer Screening; Digtl R		1	☐ 99396 Periodic Preventive Med Est Pa		1
☐ 99214 Office Outpatient Visit 25 Min		1	☐ 94760 Noninvasive Ear/Pulse Oximetry		1	☐ 99397 Periodic Preventive Med Est Pa		1
☐ 99215 Office Outpatient Visit 40 Min		1	☐ J7650 Isoetharine Hci Inhal Thru Dme		0	**PREVENTIVE MEDICINE NEW**	**Mod**	**Units**
OFFICE VISIT NEW PTS	**Mod**	**Units**	☐ 94620 Pulmonary Stress Testing Simpl		1	☐ 99384 Initial Preventive Medicine Ne		1
☐ 99201 Office Outpatient New 10 Minut		1	☐ D7911 Complicated Suture-Up To 5 Cm		1	☐ 99385 Initial Preventive Medicine Ne		1
☐ 99202 Office Outpatient New 20 Minut		1	☐ 93225 Xtrnl Ecg < 48 Hr Recording		1	☐ 99386 Initial Preventive Medicine Ne		1
☐ 99203 Office Outpatient New 30 Minut		1	☐ V5008 Hearing Screening		1	☐ 99387 Initial Preventive Medicine Ne		1
☐ 99204 Office Outpatient New 45 Minut		1	☐ 3210F Group A Strep Test Performed		1	**INJECTIONS**	**Mod**	**Units**
RADIOLOGY	**Mod**	**Units**	**OTHER SERVICES**	**Mod**	**Units**	☐ 90471 Imadm Prq Id Subq/Im Njxs 1 Va		1
☐ 71020 Radiologic Exam Chest 2 Views		1	☐ Q0091 Screen Pap Smear; Obtain Prep		1	☐ 90658 Influenza Virus Vaccine Split		1
☐ 72100 Radex Spine Lumbosacral 2/3 Vi		1	☐ 88143 Cytp C/V Flu Auto Thin Mnl Scr		1	☐ G0008 Administration Of Influenza Vi		1
☐ 73100 Radex Wrist 2 Views		1	☐ 99051 Svc Prv Office Reg Schedd Evn		1	☐ G0009 Administration Of Pneumococcal		1
☐ 73500 Radex Hip Unilateral			☐					

Figure 7-53   Harriet Oshea Visit Window

TIP   If you need to search for a CPT® code:

- Enter a partial code, complete code, or a keyword in the *Procedure Search* field, and then click the *Search* icon. The application opens the *Procedure Search* window.

- (*Optional*) To search for an NDC Code, select *NDC Code* from the *Search Type* list and then click *Search*.

- Click on the desired procedure to select it. The codes selected from the search are added to the patient's *Visit* window, and there is no limit to the number of codes you can select.

7. Enter any modifiers in the *Mod* field next to each selected procedure code, if applicable. (No modifier is required.)

8. If needed, enter the number of units in the *Units* field for each selected procedure code. (Number of units is "1" per CPT® code for this activity [as noted in **Figure 7-53**].)

9. Click the *Diagnosis* tab in the *Visit* window. The application displays the *Diagnosis* application.

10. The *Diagnosis* screen displays a list of codes that mirror the ICD codes on the encounter form. Select the checkbox next to each code associated with the patient's appointment. (Select ICD-10 code M15.0 as in **Figure 7-54**.)

TIP   If you need to search for a diagnosis code:

- Enter a partial code, a complete code, or a keyword in the *Diagnosis Search* field, and then click the *Search* icon. The application opens the *Diagnosis Search* window.

- Click on the desired ICD-10 code to select it. The codes selected from the search are added to the patient's *Visit* window.

| Procedures | Diagnosis | Visit Summary | | | EncoderPro.com |

☐ F32.9 Major Depressive Disorder Single Episode Uns   ☐ M15.9 Polyosteoarthritis Unspecified

GASTROENTEROLOGY

☐ R10.84 Generalized Abdominal Pain

☐ K76.9 Liver Disease Unspecified

☐ K59.00 Constipation Unspecified

☐ K57.30 Diverticulosis Lg Intest W/O Perf/Absc W/O Bleed

☐ K21.9 Gastro-Esoph Reflux Disease Without Esophagitis

☐ K58.9 Irritable Bowel Syndrome Without Diarrhea

☐ R11.2 Nausea With Vomiting Unspecified

CARDIAC / HYPERTENSION

☐ I48.91 Unspecified Atrial Fibrillation

☐ I25.10 Ashd Native Coronary Artery W/O Angina Pectoris

☐ I65.29 Occlusion & Stenosis Unspecified Carotid Artery

☐ R07.9 Chest Pain Unspecified

☐ I50.20 Unspecified Systolic Congestive Heart Failure

☐ I10   Essential Primary Hypertension

☐ E78.5 Hyperlipidemia Unspecified

☐ I10   Essential Primary Hypertension

GYNECOLOGIC

☐ N94.6 Dysmenorrhea Unspecified

☐ N95.1 Menopausal And Female Climacteric States

☐ N94.9 Uns Cond Assoc W/Fe Genit Orgn & Menstrual Cycl

☐ N76.0 Acute Vaginitis

SKIN / SUBCUTANEOUS TISSUE

☐ L03.90 Cellulitis Unspecified

☐ L03.119 Cellulitis Of Unspecified Part Of Limb

☐ L25.9 Unspecified Contact Dermatitis Unspecified Cause

☐ R60.9 Edema Unspecified

MISC.

☐ B19.20 Uns Viral Hepatitis C Without Hepatic Coma

☐ B02.9 Zoster Without Complications

☐ A69.20 Lyme Disease Unspecified

☐ J02.9 Acute Pharyngitis Unspecified

☐ H61.20 Impacted Cerumen Unspecified Ear

V-CODES

☐ Z00.00 Encounter Gen Adult Med Exam W/O Abnormal

PSYCHIATRY

☐ G30.9 Alzheimers Disease Unspecified

☐ F41.9 Anxiety Disorder Unspecified

☐ F32.9 Major Depressive Disorder Single Episode Uns

HEMATOLOGY

☐ D64.9 Anemia Unspecified

☐ D50.9 Iron Deficiency Anemia Unspecified

MUSCULOSKELETAL

☐ M79.1 Myalgia

☐ M54.5 Low Back Pain

☐ M62.838 Other Muscle Spasm

☐ M19.90 Unspecified Osteoarthritis Unspecified Site

☐ M81.0 Age-Related Osteoporosis W/O Currnt Path Fx

☐ M79.2 Neuralgia And Neuritis Unspecified

☑ M15.0 Primary Generalized Osteoarthritis

☐ Z51.89 Encounter For Other Specified Aftercare

☐ M54.30 Sciatica Unspecified Side

NEUROLOGY

Figure 7-54   Harriet Oshea Diagnosis Codes

11. Click the *Visit Summary* tab in the top-left corner of the *Visit* window. Harris CareTracker PM displays a summary of the visit information.

12. To check out the patient directly from the *Visit* application, select the *Check out Patient?* checkbox (**Figure 7-55**) at the bottom of the screen.

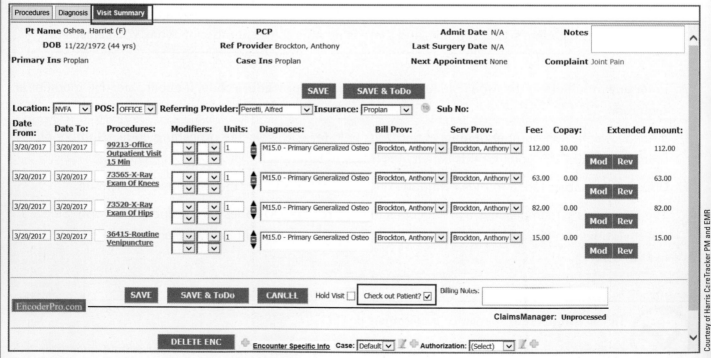

Figure 7-55   Harriet Oshea Visit—Summary Window

13. Review the screen (see **Figure 7-55**) and verify the accuracy of the information including the *Location, Place of Service (POS), Referring Provider, Insurance, Billing,* and *Servicing Provider.*

14. (If applicable) To link the visit to a case, you would select a case from the *Case* list. (No *Case* number is associated with this visit.)

15. Select an authorization number from the *Authorization* list, if applicable (not applicable in this activity).

16. From the *Billing Type* list, select the billing type "Professional" at the bottom of the *Visit* screen (**Figure 7-56**).

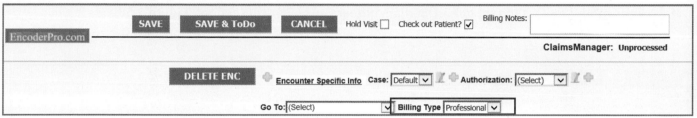

Figure 7-56   Billing Type—Professional

Courtesy of Harris CareTracker PM and EMR

17. (*Optional*) Click *EncoderPro.com* to obtain coding information from *EncoderPro*. This information can be used as a guide to correct the visit information.

 Print the Visit Summary screen. Label it "Activity 7-18," and place it in your assignment folder.

18. Click *Save* at the top or bottom of the screen. Once you hit *Save*, you will receive a pop-up message (**Figure 7-57**) stating "An error occurred connecting to Claims manager. Transaction saved." You must *wait* for this error message before continuing with the activity. Once you receive the error message, click *OK* on the pop-up. When the visit is saved, the coding information is sent to *ClaimsManager* for screening. In addition, Harris CareTracker PM and EMR automatically checks out the patient on the schedule and a check mark appears next to the patient's name confirming that the visit has been captured. Your *ClaimsManager* feature is not active in your student version of Harris CareTracker which is why you receive the error message, but the visit is saved for this activity and future billing activities.

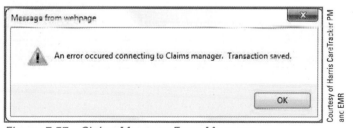

Figure 7-57   ClaimsManager Error Message

Courtesy of Harris CareTracker PM and EMR

CRITICAL THINKING **Real Time Adjudication (RTA)** refers to the immediate and complete adjudication of a health care claim upon receipt by the payer from a provider. If RTA is available in a live practice for the payer, you would click *RTA* to receive preliminary payment information. **Adjudication** is the final determination of the issues involving settlement of an insurance claim, also known as a claim settlement. The payment from the insurer then occurs the next day in an electronic funds transfer (EFT) payment deposited to the provider's bank account.

After Harriet Oshea has been examined by her PCP for back and hip pain, she proceeds to check out. The medical assistant realizes that Ms. Oshea is a member of a health insurance plan operated by a payer that supports RTA. What should the medical assistant do?

Open Encounters

An encounter is an interaction with a patient on a specific date and time. Encounter types include visits, phone calls, referrals, results of a test, and more. The *Open Encounters* application displays a list of appointment-based "visit" type of encounters that do not have a corresponding clinical note and also identifies patients who have a clinical note for a specific date of service but no encounter billed for that same date. Additionally, the *Open Encounters* application displays customized encounters that require billing or a signed note. The *Open Encounters* application is accessible from the following locations:

- *Home* module > *Dashboard* tab > *Open Encounters* link (*Clinical* section) (**Figure 7-58**)

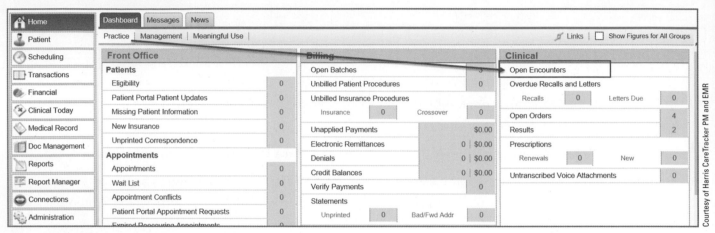

Figure 7-58   Open Encounters Link on Dashboard Tab

- *Clinical Today* module > *Tasks* tab > *Open Encounters* (from the *Tasks* menu on the right side of the window) (**Figure 7-59**)

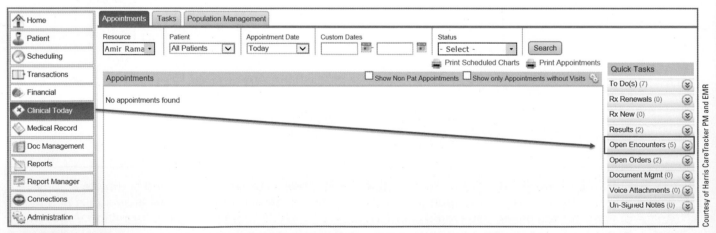

Figure 7-59   Open Encounters from the Clinical Today module

Table 7-12 describes the information displaying in the columns of the *Open Encounters* window. Refer to Figure 7-58 while reviewing Table 7-12.

Table 7-12   Open Encounters Columns

COLUMN	DESCRIPTION
Date	The date of the encounter.
Type	The type of encounter.
Patient	The name of the patient with an open encounter.
Complaint	The complaint recorded on the appointment associated with the encounter.
Provider	The name of the billing provider associated with the encounter.
Description	The diagnoses associated with the encounter. You can point to the diagnoses codes to view the associated descriptions. • Visit Diags: Displays diagnosis codes selected in the *Visit* application in the order of priority. • Associated Diags: Displays diagnosis codes selected from the progress note template.
Note	A note can have four different statuses that include *Not Signed, Missing (Required), Missing (Not Required)*, or *Complete.* It is important to focus on notes that are in the *Not Signed* or *Missing (Required)* statuses and complete the note (by clicking the *Progress Notes* 📇 icon on the *Clinical Toolbar* of the *Medical Record* module). Additionally, if a note consists of an untranscribed file, you must first transcribe the note prior to signing. When the note is signed the *Note* column displays the *Show Note* icon.
Visit	This column displays a *Visit* icon if visit information is required. When the appropriate CPT and ICD codes are saved and the visit is complete, the *Visit* icon displays a check mark on the visit. If an encounter does not require visit information, the *Visit* icon appears dimmed.

Courtesy of Harris CareTracker PM and EMR

Viewing a List of Open Encounters

Access the list of *Open Encounters* by going to your *Home* module > *Dashboard* tab > *Open Encounters* link (*Clinical* section). You may need to change the *Provider* to "All" using the drop-down arrow; otherwise the encounters might not display (**Figure 7-60**).

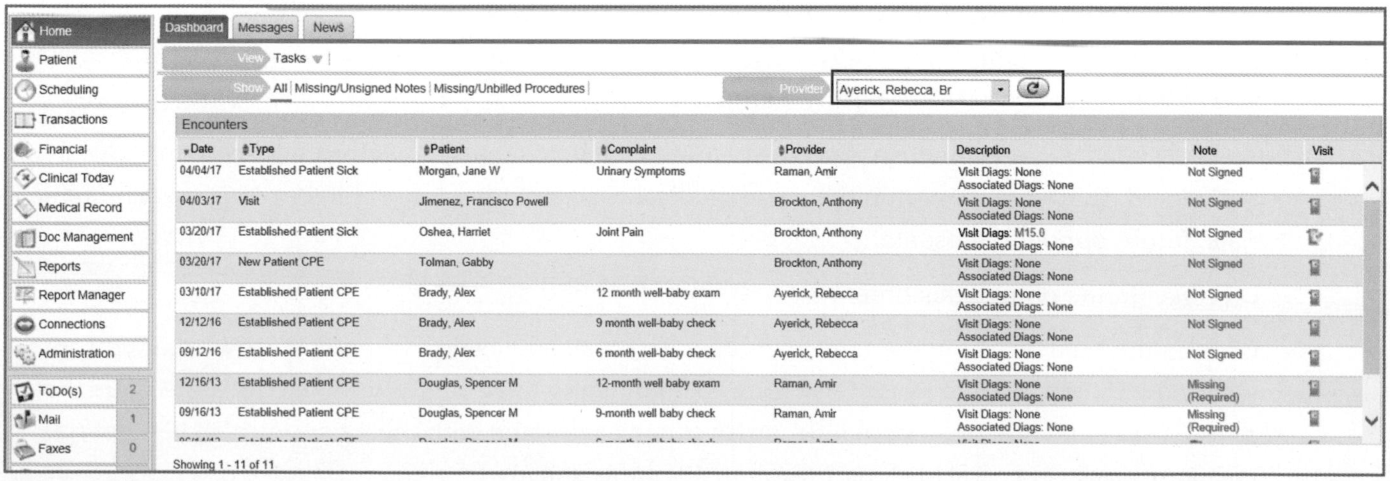

Figure 7-60   Open Encounters—Select All Providers

Courtesy of Harris CareTracker PM and EMR

There are advanced features available in the *Open Encounters* application, such as the ability to filter the list of open encounters by clicking on the column header (e.g., Provider, Appointment Type/Complaint, etc.).

Resolve Open Encounters

The *Open Encounters* application helps resolve appointment-based "visit" type of encounters by entering the visit information, reviewing, transcribing (if the note contains an untranscribed file), signing the note, and then billing. All tasks related to the note can be completed via the *Progress Note* application in the *Medical Record* module. *Visit* information is captured by entering the appropriate CPT® and ICD codes using the *Visit* application. For this activity, you will want to view the *Progress Note* and confirm (resolve) that all items in the A&P for the encounter have been completed. If there are any outstanding items, complete them before you sign the note.

An open encounter with an unsigned note, untranscribed file, is billable if visit information is captured; however, it is recommended and best practice to enter, transcribe, and sign the note, and then complete the billing.

It is important to complete transcription on a note before signing. The application prevents you from signing notes with untranscribed files. When the note is signed, the *Note* column status changes to *Complete*.

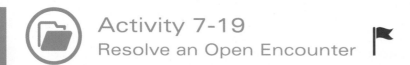

Activity 7-19
Resolve an Open Encounter

1. Access the *Open Encounters* application from the *Home* module > *Dashboard* tab > *Open Encounters* link (*Clinical* section). If the encounter you are looking for does not display, use the drop-down feature next to *Provider*, select *All*, and then click the *Change Resource* ⟳ icon.

2. Find the encounter you want to resolve (**Figure 7-61**). (Locate the encounter you created for Jane Morgan.)

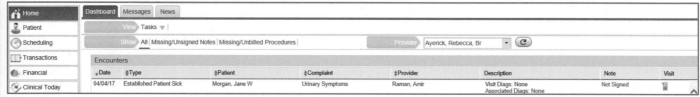

Figure 7-61   Jane Morgan Open Encounter   Courtesy of Harris CareTracker PM and EMR

3. Under the *Note* column, click the *Not Signed* link. The *Progress Note* application displays, enabling you to complete and sign the note if instructed.

4. As Best Practice, you would confirm (resolve) that all items in the *A&P* for the encounter have been completed. This is the opportunity for the medical assistant to complete any orders, education materials, future appointments, etc.

5. Do *not* sign the note at this time.

6. Click on the *Visit* 🗋 icon in the *Clinical Toolbar*. The *Visit* application will display. (**Note:** If you completed the Billing Module Quick Start prior to completing this activity, you will get a message that says, "There are already Financial Records written associated with this Encounter." If you get this message, click *OK* and skip steps 7 through 13 of this activity.)

7. Enter/select the appropriate CPT® (99213 and 90746) in the *Procedures* tab.

Source: Current Procedural Terminology © 2017 American Medical Association.

8. Click on the *Diagnosis* tab and enter ICD-10 codes (N39.0, R30.0, and I10). Be sure a check mark is placed next to each ICD-10 code you selected, and de-select any codes not listed in this activity that may have been previously entered.

9. Click on the *Visit Summary* tab. Review the information on the *Visit Summary* tab to confirm that the correct codes are displaying.

10. Once the information is confirmed in the *Visit Summary* screen (**Figure 7-62**), click *Save.*

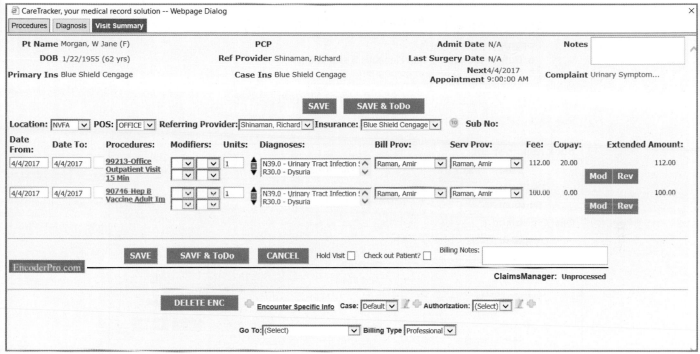

Figure 7-62   Jane Morgan Visit Summary Screen

Courtesy of Harris CareTracker PM and EMR

11. You must wait for the message "An error occurred connecting to Claims manager. Transaction saved" before moving on.

12. Click on the "OK" button.

13. When the visit information is saved, the icon in the *Visit* column changes to "Visit Complete." (**Note:** If you don't see the change, "Refresh" the *Open Encounters* screen to see the updated *Visit* column entry. You can refresh clicking on the *Refresh* ⟳ icon located next to the Provider name field.)

💾 **Print a screenshot of the updated Open Encounters window, label it "Activity 7-19," and place it in your assignment folder.**

14. Now that you have completed the tasks assigned, click back on Ms. Morgan's medical record, and review the *Progress Note* for the appointment date/encounter you scheduled for her in Chapter 4. Scroll down to the bottom and confirm that all orders, immunizations, referrals, and educational materials ordered in the A&P have been completed (**Figure 7-63**).

15. You note that the patient is to return in 10 days for a follow-up UA. Schedule a Follow-Up Appointment for Jane Morgan with Dr. Raman for 10 days from her original encounter (**Figure 7-64**). Write "10-day follow up for UA" in the chief complaint. (Refer to Chapter 4, Activity 4-1, if you need to review the instructions for making an appointment.)

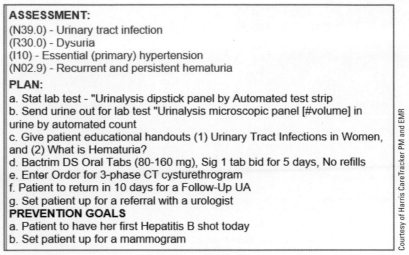

ASSESSMENT:
(N39.0) - Urinary tract infection
(R30.0) - Dysuria
(I10) - Essential (primary) hypertension
(N02.9) - Recurrent and persistent hematuria

PLAN:
a. Stat lab test - "Urinalysis dipstick panel by Automated test strip
b. Send urine out for lab test "Urinalysis microscopic panel [#volume] in urine by automated count
c. Give patient educational handouts (1) Urinary Tract Infections in Women, and (2) What is Hematuria?
d. Bactrim DS Oral Tabs (80-160 mg), Sig 1 tab bid for 5 days, No refills
e. Enter Order for 3-phase CT cysturethrogram
f. Patient to return in 10 days for a Follow-Up UA
g. Set patient up for a referral with a urologist

PREVENTION GOALS
a. Patient to have her first Hepatitis B shot today
b. Set patient up for a mammogram

Figure 7-63   Completed A&P for Jane Morgan

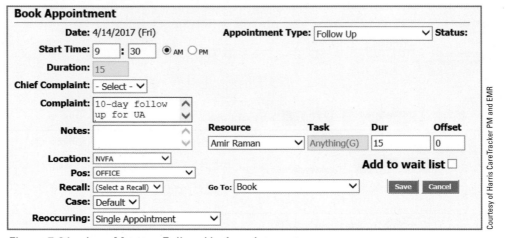

Figure 7-64   Jane Morgan Follow-Up Appointment

16. You will sign the note in Activity 7-20. After both the progress note and billing process are complete, the encounter is deleted from the *Open Encounters* application and is saved under the *Encounter* section of the patient's medical record for reference. Harris CareTracker PM and EMR updates the status of the *Note* and *Visit* columns to "Complete," and "Visit Complete."

TIP Copies of billable open encounters are saved with other unbillable encounters in the *Encounters* section of the *Medical Record* module. Therefore, you can also resolve an open encounter for a patient using the *Encounter* application in the *Medical Record* module.

Unsigned Notes

The *Unsigned Notes* application displays a list of progress notes that are not signed or require a co-signature by the provider set in the batch. A co-signature is required when a progress note is documented by a nonphysician provider such as a physician assistant (PA) or a nurse practitioner (NP). Co-signing for activities performed by others helps determine who is responsible for the supervision and quality of care.

CRITICAL THINKING   To determine the scope of practice and legal requirements regarding nurse practitioners that would apply to the NVFHA practice, log on to the website of the State of California Department of Consumer Affairs and select the "General Information: Nurse Practitioner Practice" document at *http://www.rn.ca.gov/pdfs/regulations/npr-b-23.pdf*. Determine if Gabriella Torres, the NP at NVFHA, requires supervision and a co-signature on the *Progress Note*. What actions would you need to take in Harris CareTracker PM and EMR? Write a summary of the actions required in Harris CareTracker and a one-page paper on NP status in the state of California. Submit to your instructor for class discussion.

Additionally, the *Unsigned Notes* application works the same as the *Progress Note* application and allows you to edit, preview, sign, attach the note to a *ToDo*, print, and view the activity log. The *Unsigned Notes* application (**Figure 7-65**) is accessible from the following locations:

- *Clinical Today* module > *Tasks* tab > *Unsigned Notes* (from the *Tasks* menu on the right side of the window) or click an unsigned notes task in the *All Tasks* window. You can sort on the *Tasks* column to easily identify unsigned note tasks. (**Note:** If the *Unsigned Note* is not displaying, change the provider to "All" and click the refresh icon.)

- An alternative method is to click the *Clinical Today* module, and then click *UnSigned Notes* from the *Quick Tasks* menu (on the right side of the window).

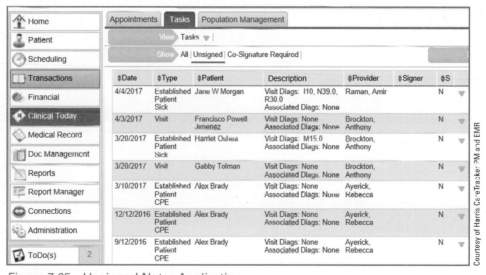

Figure 7-65   Unsigned Notes Application

Table 7-13 describes the columns of the *Unsigned Notes* window. Refer to Figure 7-65 as you review Table 7-13.

View and Filter the List of Unsigned Notes

The *Unsigned Notes* application enables you to filter the list of progress notes by provider and the signed status. You can sort on the *Tasks* column to easily identify unsigned notes tasks and filter the list of unsigned notes based on your requirements. The notes that display under each tab are based on the provider selected in your list and the setup for your company.

Table 7-13   Unsigned Notes Columns

COLUMN	DESCRIPTION
Date	The date of the encounter associated with the note.
Type	The type of encounter or the short name for the appointment type. If the encounter type is linked to an appointment, the column displays the appointment short name only. If the encounter type is not linked to an appointment, the column displays the encounter type.
Patient	The patient name associated with the note.
Description	The diagnoses associated with the encounter. You can point to the diagnoses codes to view the associated descriptions. • Visit Diags: Displays diagnosis codes selected in the *Visit* application in the order of priority. • Associated Diags: Displays diagnosis codes selected from the progress note template.
Provider	The author of the note.
Signer	Both the provider signature and the co-signature. The co-signature is indicated with "(CS)" next to the name.
Signed(S)	Indicates that the document requires a signature. The *Signed* column displays one of two statuses that include "N" or "CS." "N" indicates that the note is not signed and "CS" indicates that the note requires a co-signature.
Action	The *Action* menu allows you to do the following: • *Edit Note*: Allows you to edit the note. • *ToDo*: Allows you to attach the note to a *ToDo*. • *Print*: Allows you to print the note. • *Log*: Allows you to view activity related to the note.

Courtesy of Harris CareTracker PM and EMR

Signed Notes

The *Unsigned Notes* application lists notes that the treating and supervising provider must review and sign. The note can be signed directly from the following locations:

- *Unsigned Notes* application
- *Progress Note* application

It is important to know that once a *Progress Note* is signed, you can no longer make changes to it, and any open items/orders that were not completed prior to signing the note will not display within the A&P. When a note is signed, the provider's name displays at the bottom of the progress note as the treating provider with a signature and date stamp. If the note requires a co-signature, the *Signed* column displays "CS" until signed off by the supervising provider. In addition, the provider can make changes to the signed note until it is signed by the supervising provider.

The *Co-signature* maintenance application allows practices to set up providers requiring a co-signature on progress notes. You can assign one or more supervising providers who are authorized to provide a co-signature.

When the supervising provider signs the note, the signature is appended to the end of the note. In addition, the *Signed* column changes to "Y" and the supervising provider name displays under the *Signer* column with "CS" in parentheses. This locks the note by making *Edit* unavailable to prevent changes being made. However, either provider can add an addendum to the locked note if necessary. **Table 7-14** indicates the information that must display in the *Signed* and *Signer* columns during the signing process.

Table 7-14   Progress Note Signing Workflow

SIGN REQUIREMENT	SIGNED COLUMN	SIGNER COLUMN
(For Single Provider Signing) Note Created and Saved	N (Not Signed)	—
(For Single Provider Signing) Note Signed	Y (Signed)	Treating provider name
(For Notes Requiring Co-Signature) Note Created and Saved	N (Not Signed)	—
Treating Provider Signs the Note	CS (Indicates that a co-signature is required	Treating provider name
Supervising Provider Signs the Note	Y (signed and co-signed)	Treating provider name; Supervising provider name (CS)

Courtesy of Harris CareTracker PM and EMR

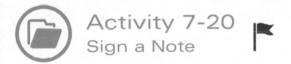

Activity 7-20
Sign a Note

Once you have confirmed that all tasks outlined in the *A&P* are completed:

1. Access the *Unsigned Notes* application by clicking on the *Home* module, *Open Encounters* under the *Clinical* column.

2. In the *Encounters* screen, *Note* column you will find Ms. Morgan's note, stating "Not Signed."

3. Click on "Not Signed" in the *Note* column and the progress note launches. **Hint**: If you do not see the note, remember to change the "Resource" (Provider) to *All* and then search.

4. Review the progress note for accuracy then click the *Sign* 🖉 icon.

5. A message prompts to confirm the action (**Figure 7-66**). Click *OK.* (Note: Alternatively, you could point to the *Arrow* icon in the *Action* menu and click *Edit Note* to open the note in a new window, review, make changes, and sign or co-sign the note.)

6. Once the *Progress Note* is signed, it will disappear from the *Unsigned Notes* application. **Note:** You may need to click the *Refresh* icon first.

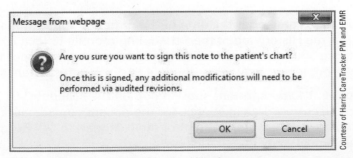

Figure 7-66   Sign Note Pop-Up Window

7. With patient Jane Morgan in context, click on the *Medical Record* module.

8. Click on *Progress Notes* from the *Patient Health History* pane, and select the progress note you created for Jane Morgan. The note launches on the right side of the pane.

9. Click the *Print* 🖫 icon on the *Progress Note* (**Figure 7-67**) tab that you just signed. A dialog box will display where you can select *Print* or *PDF*. Select *Print*.

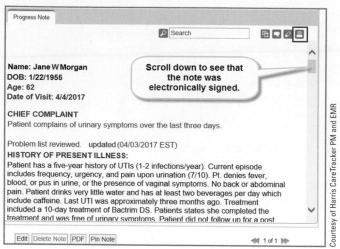

Figure 7-67   *Progress Note with Print Icon*

🖫 **Print the signed Progress Note. Label it "Activity 7-20," and place it in your assignment folder.**

10. Close the dialog box when you have finished printing.

11. Now access the *Open Encounters* application again from the *Home* module > *Dashboard* tab > *Open Encounters* link (*Clinical* section). Using the drop-down feature next to *Provider*, select *All*, and then click the *Change Resource* icon to refresh the screen. You will note that Jane Morgan's encounter is no longer listed in the *Open Encounters* link.

Activity 7-21
Capture a Visit 🚩

Using what you learned in Activity 7-18, capture the visit for the following patients. This activity is required in order to create the data needed to complete billing and collections activities in Chapters 9 and 10.

TIP   Before you begin work, review these helpful hints for capturing visits.

- **What do I do if I can't remember the date of the patient's appointment?** With the patient in context, look in the History tab of the Scheduling module to locate the patient's appointment. Once you have the patient's appointment date, go back to the Book tab of the Scheduling module and move the schedule to display the patient's date of service.

- **Why isn't the patient's appointment showing up on the schedule?** Be sure you moved the schedule to the correct date of service for the patient you are working with. Be sure to set the Resources field (just to the right of the calendar) to "All Resources" in order for the full schedule and all providers to display.

A—Ellen Ristino

1. Using steps you learned throughout this chapter (refer to Activity 7-18), and using the information below, capture the visit for Ellen Ristino for the appointment/encounter you created in Chapter 4.
   - *CPT® Codes: 99213; 3210F; 36415; 94760; 86308*
   - *ICD-10 Codes: J06.9; J20.9*
   Source: Current Procedural Terminology © 2017 American Medical Association.

2. Remember to wait for the pop-up error message to appear before moving on.

Print a screenshot of the completed visit and label it "Activity 7-21A." Place the document in your assignment folder.

B—Craig X. Smith

3. Referring to Activity 7-18, and using the information that follows, capture the visit for patient Craig X. Smith. Refer to the appointment/encounter you created for Mr. Smith in Chapter 4.
   - *CPT® Codes: 99213; J7650; 71020 (Note: for CPT® code J7650 you will need to enter "1" in the Units field of the Visit Summary screen.)*
   - *ICD-10 Code: R06.2*
   Source: Current Procedural Terminology © 2017 American Medical Association.

4. Remember to wait for the pop-up error message to appear before moving on.

Print a screenshot of the completed visit and label it "Activity 7-21B" and place in your assignment folder.

C—Barbara Watson

5. Referring to Activity 7-18, and using the information that follows, capture the visit for patient Barbara Watson. Refer to the appointment/encounter you created for Ms. Watson in Chapter 4.
   - *CPT® Codes: 99213; 94760*
   - *ICD-10 Code: R50.9*
   Source: Current Procedural Terminology © 2017 American Medical Association.

6. Remember to wait for the pop-up error message to appear before moving on.

Print a screenshot of the completed visit and label it "Activity 7-21C." Place the document in your assignment folder.

D—Edith Robinson

7. Referring to Activity 7-18, and using the information that follows, capture the visit for patient Edith Robinson. Refer to the appointment/encounter you created for Ms. Robinson in Chapter 4.
   - *CPT® Code: 99203*
   - *ICD-10 Codes: M54.5; M99.03; M99.05; I10; E11.9*
   Source: Current Procedural Terminology © 2017 American Medical Association.

8. Remember to wait for the pop-up error message to appear before moving on.

Print a screenshot of the completed visit and label it "Case Study 7-21D." Place the document in your assignment folder.

E—Alex Brady

9. Referring to Activity 7-18 and using the information that follows, capture the three visits for patient Alex Brady's encounters. Refer to the *History* tab in the *Scheduling* module to obtain the date/time/provider for Alex's appointments. Use the CPT and ICD-10 codes noted below for the visit dated 09/12/2016:
   - *CPT® Code: 99391*
   - *ICD-10 Code: Z00.129*
   Source: Current Procedural Terminology © 2017 American Medical Association.

10. Remember to wait for the pop-up error message to appear before moving on.

11. Once the visit has been captured, sign the *Progress Note* for Alex Brady's 09/12/2016, encounter. Refer to Activity 7-20 if you need a refresher of the instructions.

Print screenshots of the completed visits and label them "Activity 7-21E1." Print the signed *Progress Note* **and label it "Activity 7-21E2." Place all the documents in your assignment folder.**

12. Now capture the visit for Alex Brady for his encounter dated 12/12/2016. (Note: Do *not* sign the Progress Note for this encounter at this time.)
    - *CPT® Code: 99391*
    - *ICD-10 Code: Z00.121*
    Source: Current Procedural Terminology © 2017 American Medical Association.

13. Remember to wait for the pop-up error message to appear before moving on.

Print a screenshot of the completed visits and label it "Activity 7-21E3." Place the document in your assignment folder.

14. Now capture the visit for Alex Brady for his encounter dated 03/10/2017. (Note: Do *not* sign the *Progress Note* for this encounter at this time.)
    - *CPT® Code: 99391*
    - *ICD-9 Code: Z00.121*
    Source: Current Procedural Terminology © 2017 American Medical Association.

15. Remember to wait for the pop-up error message to appear before moving on.

Print screenshots of the completed visits and label them "Activity 7-21E4." Place the document in your assignment folder.

F—Francisco Powell Jimenez

16. Referring to Activity 7-18, and using the information that follows, capture the visit for patient Francisco Powell Jimenez. Refer to the appointment/encounter you created for Francisco in Chapter 4.
    - *CPT® Code: 99214*
    - *ICD-10 Code: Z00.129*
    Source: Current Procedural Terminology © 2017 American Medical Association.

17. Remember to wait for the pop-up error message to appear before moving on.

Print screenshots of the completed visit and label it "Activity 7-21F." Place the document in your assignment folder.

G—Gabby Tolman

You can also capture a visit through the *Clinical Today* module. For Gabby's visit, you will need to access her appointment through the *Clinical Today* module/*Appointments* application.

18. Pull Gabby Tolman into context. Click on the *Clinical Today* module (on the left side of your screen) and set the following search criteria;

    a. Change *Resource* to "All."

    b. Change *Patient* to "All Patients."

    c. Enter "03/20/17" in the *Custom Dates* fields.

    Then click *Search*.

19. In the row for Gabby Tolman, click on the drop-down arrow next to *Actions*, and select *Visit*.

   - *CPT® Codes: 99202*
   - *ICD-10 Codes: K59.00 and R39.15*

   Source: Current Procedural Terminology © 2017 American Medical Association.

20. Remember to wait for the pop-up error message to appear before moving on.

 Print a screenshot of the completed visit and label it "Activity 7-21G." Place the document in your assignment folder.

 CRITICAL THINKING Throughout this chapter, you have completed activities where you might see a *Select Encounter* dialog box and need to select the appropriate encounter. Do you now feel comfortable with your level of understanding and proficiency to select patient encounters? Having now worked in both the practice management side and the clinical side of Harris CareTracker, do you have a better understanding of the reasoning behind the settings in the *Batch*? How does having the batch redirect set to *Clinical* save you time? If you are still being redirected to *Home* or *Admin*, have you checked your *Batch* settings?

CRITICAL THINKING At the beginning of this chapter, you were challenged to learn the proper steps for entering orders into the patient's EMR, to avoid the temptation of entering orders without the provider's approval, and to select the proper codes for the patient's visit. Having completed the activities, what do you rate your level of understanding and proficiency for entering orders and capturing visits with the appropriate codes? Were there any activities that seemed difficult? If yes, what steps did you take to resolve the issue? Did you remember to read through the entire activity first before beginning to enter data? Would you have entered a lab order before the patient was seen by the provider if the reason for the visit was burning and urgent urinary symptoms? Explain your decision.

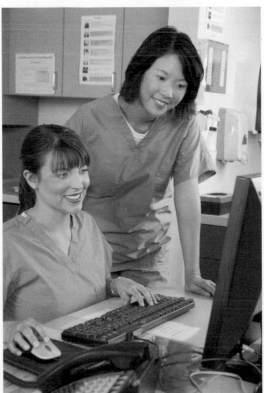

© sirtravelalot/Shutterstock.com.

SUMMARY

Congratulations on completing the patient work-up: placing *Orders, Prescriptions, Immunizations, and Referrals* and completing the *Visit* and signing the *Progress Note*. This simulates the actual EMR workflows in a medical practice combined with practice management features, enhancing the coordination and quality of patient care. This chapter provides in-depth knowledge, practice, and application of the EMR functions in Harris CareTracker PM and EMR.

In summary, the *Orders* application is where you manage and track orders such as laboratory, radiology, pathology, and physical therapy directly from the patient's medical record. This ensures that all orders placed are followed up by the office for patient compliancy. The *Medications* application consists of the past and current medications that the patient is taking. The list also includes medications prescribed, medications administered, and samples given to the patient. In addition you used the *Rx* feature to search for pharmacies, create, and print prescriptions. The list of newly administered immunizations, immunizations administered in the past, and immunizations that the patient refused to have administered, are found in the *Immunizations* application.

You learned to search for patient educational materials through the *Patient Education* application using keywords, ICD or CPT® codes, or by searching for material by navigating the tree structure. The *Letters* application was used to search for and create letters for patients.

The *Referrals and Authorizations* application enables providers to create incoming and outgoing referrals and associated authorizations directly via the patient's medical record. Use of electronic referrals provides the data about the patient's condition and needs, referred from and referred-to provider details, treatment authorization data, and referral dates and ranges. Using the *Referrals* application enables you to track patient compliance with the referral instructions and eliminates paperwork.

To wrap up the patient encounter, you learned to complete the visit, resolve open encounters, and electronically sign the note. Having signed the *Progress Note*, you will no longer be able to make changes or add orders. Chapter 8 will instruct you on how to unsign and to make addendums to the *Progress Note* when needed. In addition you will be introduced to and complete other advanced features such as recording results for open *Orders*, recording telephone calls, creating and updating patient *Recall Letters,* and using the *Clinical Export* feature to run an immunization report.

CHECK YOUR KNOWLEDGE

Select the best response.

_____1. Which is a method to access the *Medical Record* module?

a. Pull the patient into context and click the *Appointments* module

b. Click the patient's name in the *Appointments* application and select *Open*

c. Pull the patient into context, and then click the *Medical Record* module

d. Click the patient's name in the *Administration* tab, *Open Encounters*

_____2. Which icon indicates that an order includes multiple tests?

a. Orders icon

b. Expand icon

c. Results icon

d. Notes icon

_____3. Open orders in the *Open Activities* section displays a test that is overdue in:

a. Italics

b. Highlights

c. Gray

d. Red

_____ 4. If no interactions were returned in the *Medication* column *Actions,* the *Interactions* icon appears:

a. Green

b. Gray

c. Dimmed

d. Italicized

_____ 5. What method is used to process a controlled (scheduled) drug prescription?

a. Print

b. Via electronic transmission

c. Fax

d. All of the above

_____ 6. Generic versions of drugs are displayed in _____ for easy identification.

a. italics

b. green

c. gray

d. red

_____ 7. Which application provides access to the Centers for Disease Control and Prevention (CDC) website?

a. *Open Orders*

b. *Medications*

c. *Immunizations*

d. *Clinical Today*

_____ 8. A *Visit* can only be edited:

a. Prior to becoming a charge

b. Before procedure and diagnosis codes are entered

c. Before payment is received

d. None of the above

_____ 9. In *Open Encounters*, a *Note* can have four different statuses. Which of the following is not one of the four statuses?

a. Not signed

b. Missing (required)

c. Counter signature (required)

d. Complete

_____ 10. You can sign the note directly from which of the following locations?

a. *Unsigned Notes* application and *Progress Notes* application

b. *Encounter* and *Medical Records* pane

c. *Dashboard, Unsigned Notes* application

d. None of the above

CASE STUDIES

If the demographic pop-up alerts you to missing information when you pull a patient into context, it is best practice to update as necessary. Update patients' PCP, subscriber numbers, and confirm (Y) to Consent, HIE, and NPP as needed throughout the remainder of your activities and case studies.

Case Study 7-1

Complete an *Order* for a mammogram referral for patient Jane Morgan. Refer to Activity 7-2 for help.

- *Order Type:* Diag. Imaging

- *Ordering Physician*: Dr. Raman

- *Due Date*: The date of the encounter

- *Diagnosis*: Select "Encounter for screening mammogram for malignant neoplasm of breast (Z12.31)" (**Note**: Search under "Mammogram" to locate the diagnosis).

(Continues)

CASE STUDIES *(Continued)*

- *New Test*: Search for and select this test from the database "Mammography; bilateral." Do *not* free text and add your own entry. Patient information is entered into a reminder system with a target due date for the next mammogram (RAD).

- Scroll down under *New Test* and select the type of test ordered (see above "Mammography; bilateral").

- Click *"Add Test."*

- Scroll to the bottom of the *Order* screen. With "Print" selected, click "Save."

🖬 **Print the mammogram order for Ms. Morgan. Label it "Case Study 7-1" and place it in your assignment folder.**

Case Study 7-2

To complete Case Study 7-2, you must have completed the case studies from the previous chapters for patient James Smith. If you did not complete the previous case studies for James Smith, skip Case Study 7-2 and complete Case Study 7-3.

Patient James Smith was seen by Dr. Ayerick to review lab and EKG results. Based on the findings in the lab and EKG reports, Dr. Ayerick would like Mr. Smith to see a cardiologist and recommends Dr. Mark Nathan in Walnut Creek, California.

a. Refer patient to Dr. Mark Nathan in Walnut Creek, California, a well-respected Cardiologist (**Note:** you will not select a "Specialty" for this *Referral* and this is not a transition of care). Follow the steps in Activity 7-15 for help.

b. Schedule a follow up appointment (refer to Activity 4-1 for help) for repeat lab work and visit with Dr. Ayerick. Schedule the appointment four weeks from today.

c. Now that the visit is complete, capture the visit for James Smith. Use steps you learned in Activity 7-18 and the procedure and diagnosis codes that follow.

- *CPT® Codes:* 99213 and 93000

- *ICD-10 Codes:* I48.91; R00.2; and I10

  Source: Current Procedural Terminology © 2017 American Medical Association.

d. Once the visit has been captured, sign the *Progress Note* for James Smith. Refer to Activity 7-20 for help if needed.

🖬 **Print a screenshot of the Referral, Visit Capture, and signed Progress Note, and label them "Case Study 7-2." Place the documents in your assignment folder.**

Case Study 7-3

To complete Case Study 7-3 in its entirety, you must have completed Case Study 6-3 for patient Adam Thompson. If you did not complete Case Study 6-3, skip Part A and complete only Part B of Case Study 7-3 (Capture the Visit).

a. Complete the outstanding orders for patient Adam Thompson. Use the steps you learned throughout this chapter and in Activity 7-2 for help. To accurately complete the order, refer to the information contained in the A&P of the *Progress Note* you created for Mr. Thompson in Case Study 6-3 and the information that follows:

- *Order Type*: Lab

- *Due Date:* The date of the encounter

- *Ordering Physician* (select Mr. Thompson's PCP)

- *Facility*: Select the first facility noted in the drop-down list

- *Frequency:* Select "Single Order"
- *Diagnosis:* Select ICD-10 code "Z00.00"
- *ABN given to Pt:* Yes
- *Due Date:* The date of the encounter
- *New Tests:* Add the following tests:
    1. CBC W Auto Differential panel in Blood
    2. Electrolytes 1998 panel in Serum or Plasma
- *Urgency:* Routine
- *Fasting:* 12
- When the order information has been entered, select "Print" and then click *Save*.

b. Using the information that follows, capture the visit for Adam Thompson. Refer to Activity 7-18 for help if needed.

- *CPT® Codes:* 99213; 71020; 94760; 93000
- *ICD-10 Codes:* J18.9; K21.9; I10; M19.90

Source: Current Procedural Terminology © 2016 American Medical Association.

c. Once the visit has been captured, sign the *Progress Note* for Adam Thompson following the steps in Activity 7-20.

💾 **Print a copy of the order and label it "Case Study 7-3." Place the document in your assignment folder.**

BUILD YOUR PROFICIENCY

Proficiency Builder 7-1: Update Missing Demographic Information
Update the missing demographic information for patient Harriet Oshea, as indicated by the pop-up alert:

- Subscriber Number: PPHC5634
- *Consent and NPP:* Yes
- PCP: Dr. Brockton

💾 **Print a copy of the updated patient demographics and label it "BYP 7-1." Place the document in your assignment folder.**

Proficiency Builder 7-2: Search for a Provider When Adding a New Lab Order
In Activity 7-2, you added a new lab order. If the provider was not listed, you would need to search for a provider following the steps below. Complete this activity to become familiar with the process of searching for a provider when adding a new lab order.

1. Pull a patient into context, and then click the *Medical Record* module. (You may select any patient in the database that you have not yet worked on. For example, select patient Larry T. Jeorge, PCP Dr. Ayerick.)

2. In the *Clinical Toolbar*, click *Order* ⚕

3. If an encounter is in context, Harris CareTracker EMR displays the *New Order* dialog box. If an encounter is not in context, Harris CareTracker EMR displays the *Select Encounter* dialog box. You will need to click on "Create a New Encounter" and select

BUILD YOUR PROFICIENCY *(Continued)*

"Other." You can then free text in the following "BYP 7-2" in the *Description* field. Click *OK*. After entering the encounter information, the *Order* screen will appear.

4. By default, the *Status* is set to "Open" in the *Order* dialog box (see Figure 7-6).

5. By default, the *Order Type* is set to "Lab." Leave this setting as is.

6. By default, the *Ordering Physician* list displays the provider associated with the encounter. Confirm that the provider listed is the PCP for the patient you selected. If the provider listed is not the patient's PCP, use the drop-down and change to the correct provider.

7. The *Facility* list displays the default facility set for the order type. Click the drop-down list. A list of favorite labs will appear. Select the first lab that displays on the list. (**Note:** because numerous labs may have been added to the database, do not attempt to locate a specific lab, but instead select the first available that displays.)

8. You want to copy the result to another provider for this activity. The *Copy Result To* indicates providers to whom you wish to route results. You want to send these results to Dr. Vikram Talwar. Check to see if he is in the *Copy Result To* drop-down list. If he is, select him. If not, click the *Search* 🔍 icon to search for the provider.

   • To search for a provider, enter the last name, UPIN, or NPI in the specific boxes. You may select any provider not in the NVFHA group. For example, search for Dr. Vikram Talwar, located in California.

   • Click *Search*. Harris CareTracker PM and EMR displays a list of providers matching the search criteria.

   • Click the provider you want. The selected provider auto populates in the *Copy Result To* list.

      Note: The *Copy Result To* list includes all providers in the group, the patient's active providers, and providers listed in the *Refer Provider From* and *Refer Provider To* lists in the *Quick Picks* application of the *Administration* module. If you select a provider from the search results, the provider name displays under the *Current Encounter* section in the *Copy Result To* list.

9. Continue on with the test information by entering the following data:

   a. In the *Diagnosis* field, search for "CHF" and select ICD-10 code I50.9, CHF (congestive heart failure).

   b. *New Test*: Digoxin [Moles/volume] in Serum or Plasma

   c. In the *Patient Notes* field, enter "Do not take your digoxin medication within 12 hours of lab work."

4. Click *Add Test*.

5. Confirm that *Print* is checked and then click *Save*.

💾 **Print a copy of the order and label it "BYP 7-2." Place the document in your assignment folder.**

6. Click X to close out of the order screen.

7. For additional practice, you may enter orders for additional patients, using an order scenario for *Lab*, *Diagnostic Imaging*, or *Procedure* for a fictitious patient and scenario, or a patient in the database not yet having an encounter.

Proficiency Builder 7-3: Prerequisites for Creating a Prescription

As best practice, you can set up the patient's preferred pharmacy(s) prior to using the *Rx* application to create a prescription. This will also make the process for creating a prescription quick and easy. You can also add pharmacies to your *Quick Picks* as well.

1. To see a patient's frequently used pharmacies in the list, set up the patient's favorite pharmacies via the *Relationships* application in the *Patient Demographics* module.

   a. Pull patient Frank Powell into context.

   b. Click on the *Patient* module. The *Demographics* display.

   c. Click on the *Relationships* tab. You will note "There are currently no pharmacies for this patient."

   d. Click on the "Add Relationship" link and select "Pharmacy."

   e. The "Add Pharmacy" dialog box displays.

   f. Click on the *Search* icon and the "Search Pharmacies" dialog box displays.

   g. In the *Name* field enter "CVS."

   h. In the *City* field, enter "Napa."

   i. In the *State* field, select "CA."

   j. Then click *Search*. All the pharmacies matching the description entered populate.

   k. Click on the radio dial next to "CVS/pharmacy #9214."

   l. The pharmacy is now included in the "Add Pharmacy" *Relationships* field.

   m. Change *Preferred Retail* to "Yes."

   n. Leave *Preferred Mail Order* as "No."

   o. Leave *Active* as "Yes."

   p. Then click *Save*.

   q. You have now successfully added the patient's preferred retail pharmacy in the patient's *Demographics* application.

   For more information on adding patient pharmacies, see *Patient* module > *Relationships* > *Adding a Patient Pharmacy* in the *Help* system.

2. To see pharmacies frequently used by the practice, set the list of practice pharmacies via the *Quick Picks* application in the *Administration* module, *Setup* tab.

   a. Click on the *Administration* module.

   b. Click on the *Setup* tab.

   c. Click on the *Quick Picks* link under the *Financial* header.

   d. Using the drop-down next to *Screen Type*, select "Pharmacies."

   e. Click on the *Search* icon and the "Search Pharmacies" dialog box opens.

   f. In the *Name* field, enter "Safeway."

   g. In the *City* field, enter "Napa."

(Continues)

BUILD YOUR PROFICIENCY *(Continued)*

  h. In the *State* field, enter "California."

  i. Click on the *Search* button.

  j. All the Safeway pharmacies matching the parameters enter display.

  k. Select "SAFEWAY #25-0911."

  l. The "Success" box displays, and now the Safeway Pharmacy has been added to your *Quick Picks.*

  m. Click the red "X" to close the *Success* box.

  n. You will now see the pharmacy in your *Quick Picks* list.

For more information on the *Quick Picks* application, see *Administration Module > Setup > Financial > Quick Pick Setup* in the *Help* system.

Print a copy of the pharmacy added to Quick Picks and label it "BYP 7-3." Place the document in your assignment folder.

Proficiency Builder 7-4: Add a New Lab Order

Complete the outstanding order for patient Ellen Ristino with information noted below. Follow the steps you learned throughout this chapter and refer to Activity 7-2 for help.

- *Facility:* Select the first lab on the facility drop-down list
- *Diagnosis:* ICD-10 code J06.9
- *Due Date:* The date of the encounter
- *Urgency:* Routine
- *Fasting:* 12
- *Tests:* 1) CBC W Auto Differential panel in Blood; 2) Heterophile Ab [Titer] in Serum by Agglutination

Print a copy of the order and label it "BYP 7-4." Place the document in your assignment folder.

Close out of the *Order* by clicking on the *X.*

Other Clinical Documentation

8

Key Terms

addendum
progress note
titer

Learning Objectives

1. Edit, add an addendum to, sign, and print a *Progress Note*.
2. Manually enter *Results* into the patient's medical record to view, customize, graph, and print those results.
3. Record messages in Harris CareTracker PM and EMR.
4. Create and update patient *Recall Letters*.
5. Run an immunization report using the *Clinical Export* feature.

Real-World Connection

In the past, medical assistants have often had the responsibility of retrieving faxed or printed lab results for the provider to review; however, with electronic connectivity, this task will diminish over time. Whether lab results are automatically uploaded to the provider's portal or scanned into the EMR, the medical assistant should always consider the patient's peace of mind. Unfortunately, health care workers often view the retrieval of lab results as secondary to other tasks, but to an anxious patient, the wait can be agonizing. When you have a patient who is anxious about a result, watch for the result and alert the provider once it is available. This will reduce the patient's wait time. You will learn how to enter lab results into the patient's EMR in this chapter, but I urge you to think about the flip side of the result—the patient's peace of mind. Another very important consideration is that as you input data into the *Results* application, think about the integrity of the data entered. Imagine what would happen if you made an entry error that would adversely affect the results and the effect it would have on the patient and patient care.

INTRODUCTION

This chapter expands on other clinical documentation in the EMR. Moving forward, you will perform advanced features in an EMR that streamline workflows and promote continuity of patient care. You will complete activities that simulate real-world office workflows of a medical assistant, which include navigating the *Progress Notes*, *Results*, and *Messages* applications and creating *Recall Letters* and using the *Export* tool.

Your activities will include viewing and entering patient's lab results via the *Results* application. In addition, you will customize, graph, and print patient results. You will expand on the *ToDos* activities that were reviewed in earlier chapters, now focusing on the clinical side of Harris CareTracker PM and EMR. In the *Messages* application, you will record messages; create new mail messages; access and view mail messages; reply to, move, and manage your inbox.

The final features introduced are the *Recalls* application and the *Clinical Export* feature. *Recalls* are reminders to patients that an appointment needs to be booked. Harris CareTracker PM and EMR tracks all recalls, enabling you to generate recall letters at the appropriate time intervals.

The *Clinical Export* feature provides the ability to export a batch of patient clinical data in PDF. You can select the time period to cover and the level of patient information to include. You will use the *Immunization Export* application to generate a record of all vaccinations given during a specified time period, monitor inventory, and provide a database of information should there be a recall of a medication.

Upon completion of this chapter's activities, you will have gained useful knowledge and application skills using Harris CareTracker EMR—transferable skill to a wide variety of EMR products available in the market.

> Before you begin the activities in this chapter, refresh your memory on working with Harris CareTracker by referring back to the Best Practices list on page xxiii of this textbook. This list is also posted to the student companion website. Following best practices will help you complete work quickly and accurately.

THE *PROGRESS NOTES* APPLICATION

Learning Objective 1: Edit, add an addendum to, sign, and print a Progress Note.

The *Progress Notes* application allows you to navigate the list of notes saved for the patient and click a note to view and manage from the right pane. A **progress note** is a document, written by the clinician or provider that describes the details of a patient's encounter and is sometimes referred to as a chart note. To navigate and view the progress notes listed in a patient's medical record:

- Click *Next* and *Previous* buttons on the bottom of the *Progress Note* window to navigate through the list of notes (**Figure 8-1**).

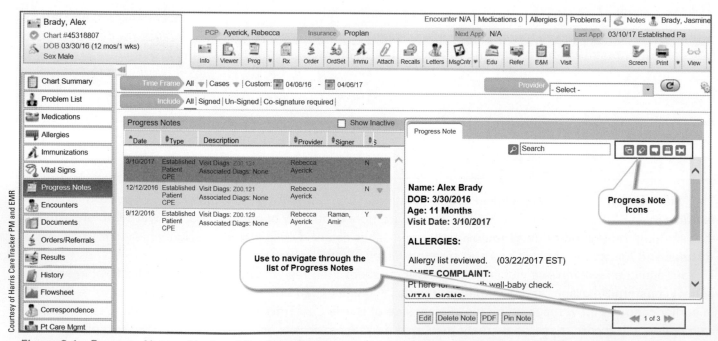

Figure 8-1   Progress Notes—Next and Previous Buttons

Courtesy of Harris CareTracker PM and EMR

- Click the *Expand/Collapse* icon in the upper-right-hand corner of your screen to maximize the view for readability.

Various ways to manage the progress note include:

- *Edit* and *Overwrite* edits of a progress note

- Sign or unsign a note

- Add an addendum to a note

- Create a PDF of the note

- Sign or print a note

- Pin /unpin a note (pinning a note will lock in a narrative to a progress note template, displaying the same narrative each time you access the template)

IMPORTANT!!   Complete and sign all progress notes before any billing information is submitted to the payers.

Access and View Progress Notes

The *Progress Notes* application displays a list of notes recorded during each patient visit and progress note–type documents that are uploaded. Progress notes include information such as the patient's history, medications, allergies, as well as a complete record of all that happened during the visit. This information is required for medical, legal, and billing purposes.

You can use the application to browse through all the patient notes, including uploaded notes, on the right pane of the window. When viewing uploaded notes, the right pane displays the document in the *Document Viewer* and fits the width of the pane. However, you can click the *Expand/Collapse* icon to control the view.

Activity 8-1
Access the *Progress Notes* Application

There are several ways to access the *Progress Notes* application. Use the following method for this activity.

1. Pull patient Alex Brady into context.

2. Click the *Medical Record* module.

3. Click on the *Progress Notes* application in the *Health History* pane. (**Note:** This patient has three visits that were scheduled on 09/12/2016, 12/12/2016, and 03/10/2017.)

4. The *Progress Notes* window displays a list of signed and unsigned notes for the patient (**Figure 8-2**).

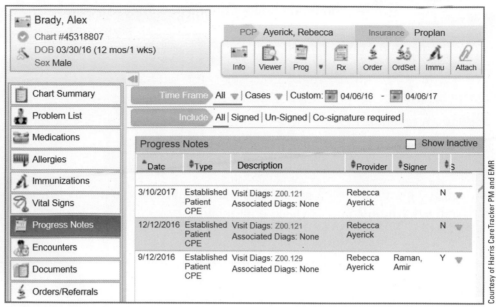

Figure 8-2   Alex Brady Progress Notes

5. On a blank sheet of paper (or new document), write down (or type) the list of the signed and unsigned progress notes for the patient. Label the page "Activity 8-1" and place it in your assignment folder.

Table 8-1 describes the columns in the *Progress Notes* window. The documents that are attached or scanned to the application only display the information in the specific columns that are marked with an asterisk (*) in the table. Refer to **Figure 8-2** while reviewing **Table 8-1**.

In addition to the *Progress Notes* application, Harris CareTracker EMR provides quick access to progress notes via two other locations:

- *Progress Note* icon on the *Clinical Toolbar*
- *Select Encounter* dialog box

TABLE 8-1	*Progress Notes* Columns
COLUMN	**DESCRIPTION**
*Date	The date of the encounter associated with the note or the document date selected when uploading the note via the *Document Management Upload* application.
*Type	The type of encounter or appointment. If the encounter type is linked to an appointment, the column displays the appointment type only. If the encounter type is not linked to an appointment, the column displays the encounter type. If the note is uploaded, the column displays the subtype selected when uploading the document.
*Description	The diagnosis associated with the encounter. You can point to the diagnosis codes to view the associated descriptions. This provides the flexibility of reviewing previous notes for a recurring problem or similar symptoms and helps reduce time to issue orders. • *Visit Diags*: Displays diagnosis codes selected in the *Visit* application • *Associated Diagnosis*: Displays diagnosis codes selected from the progress note template If the note is uploaded, the column displays the *Document* icon and the document name.
*Provider	The author of the note or the provider selected when uploading the document.
Signer	Both the provider signature and the co-signature. The co-signature is indicated with (CS) next to the name.

COLUMN	DESCRIPTION
*S	Indicates that the document requires a signature. The *Signed* column displays the following: •N: Indicates that the note is not signed and requires a signature •CS: Indicates that the note requires a co-signature by the supervising provider •Y: Indicates that the note is signed
*Action	The *Action* drop-down menu allows you to do the following: • *Edit Note*: Allows you to edit the note • *ToDo*: Allows you to attach the note to a *ToDo* • *Print*: Allows you to print the note • *Log*: Allows you to view activity related to the note The *Action* drop-down menu for uploaded documents displays the following options. • *View Document*: Allows you to view the document attached • *ToDo*: Allows you to attach the document to a *ToDo* • *Print*: Allows you to print the document • *Delete*: Allows you to delete the document

Courtesy of Harris CareTracker PM and EMR

TIP You can also access the *Progress Note* application by clicking the *Encounters & Progress Notes* section (**Figure 8-3**) title in the *Chart Summary*.

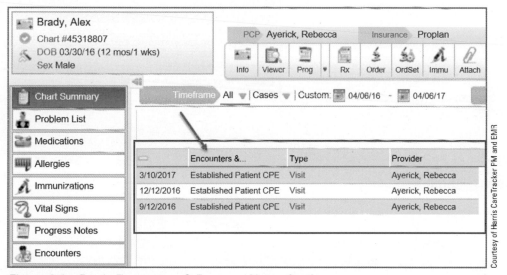

Figure 8-3   Brady Encounters & Progress Notes Section

Activity 8-2
Access *Progress Notes* from the *Clinical Toolbar*

1. Pull patient Alex Brady into context and click the *Medical Record* module.

2. In the *Clinical Toolbar*, click the *Arrow* ▼ icon next to the *Progress Notes* 📄 icon. Harris CareTracker EMR displays the *Note* 📑 icon next to the encounters that have a progress note. A pop-up with the *Progress Note* summary will appear.

3. Click the *Note* icon next to the encounter dated September 12, 2016. Harris CareTracker EMR displays the *Viewing Clinical Note* dialog box with the selected progress note to the right of the date (see **Figure 8-4**).

 ALERT! You must actually click on the *Note* icon, not just on the encounter date (**Figure 8-4**) to receive the pop-up summary. If you click on the encounter date, the entire progress note application will pull in to context.

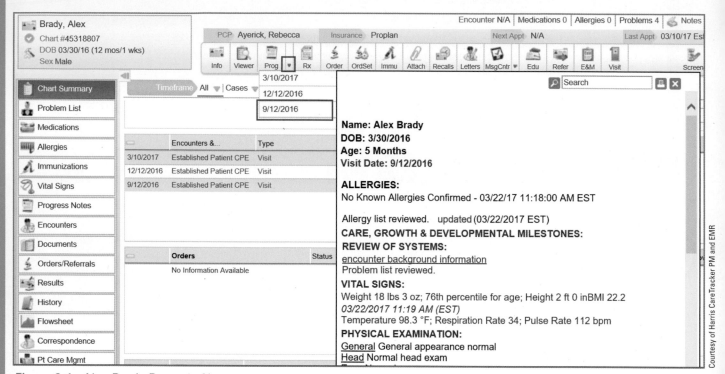

Figure 8-4   *Alex Brady Progress Note*

🖫 **Print a screenshot of the *Viewing Clinical Note* dialog box for the patient. Label it "Activity 8-2" and place it in your assignment folder.**

4. Click on the "X" to close out of the *Viewing Clinical Note* dialog box.

Activity 8-3 instructs you to use the alternative method of accessing the *Progress Note* from the *Encounter dialog* box.

Activity 8-3
Access the *Progress Note* from the *Encounter* Dialog Box

1. Pull patient Jane Morgan into context and click the *Medical Record* module.

2. In the *Patient Detail* bar, click the *Encounter* link (**Figure 8-5**).

3. Harris CareTracker EMR displays the *Select Encounter* dialog box (**Figure 8-6**). Encounters with progress notes display the *Note* 📓 icon next to the encounter.

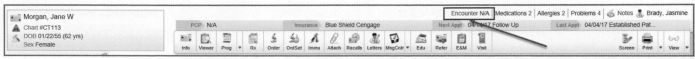

Figure 8-5   Encounter Link

Courtesy of Harris CareTracker PM and EMR

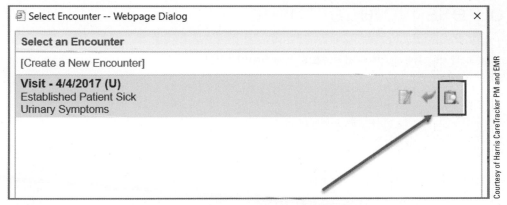

Figure 8-6   Select Encounter Dialog Box

4. Click the *Note* 📄 icon next to the encounter you created for the patient in Chapter 6. Harris CareTracker EMR displays the *View Clinical Note* dialog box with the selected progress note (**Figure 8-7**).

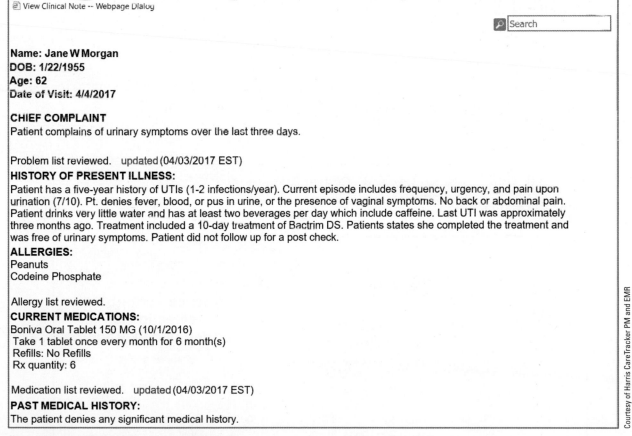

Figure 8-7   View Clinical Note Dialog Box

🖨 Print a screenshot of the *View Clinical Note* dialog box for the patient. Label it "Activity 8-3" and place it in your assignment folder.

5. Click on the "X" to close the *View Clinical Note* dialog box.

6. Click on the "X" to close the *Select Encounter* dialog box.

Filter Progress Note Templates

The *Progress Notes* application can filter a list of notes documented during a patient encounter. You can filter the list of notes based on the approval status, document date, or the diagnoses associated with the note.

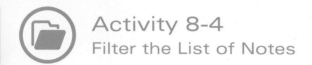

Activity 8-4
Filter the List of Notes

1. Pull patient Alex Brady into context.

2. Click on the *Medical Record* module.

3. In the *Patient Health History* pane, click *Progress Notes*. The *Progress Notes* window displays with a list of signed and unsigned notes for the patient.

4. Practice filtering by doing each of the following (**Figure 8-8**), and then take a screenshot of each for your Activities folder:

   a. To filter the list of notes by approval status, click the *Signed, Un-Signed*, or *Co-signature required* in the *Include* tab just below the *Time Frame* tab

   b. To filter the list of notes by documented date, select *Last Encounter, Past 6 months*, or *Past Year* from the *All* drop-down menu directly to the right of the *Time Frame* tab.

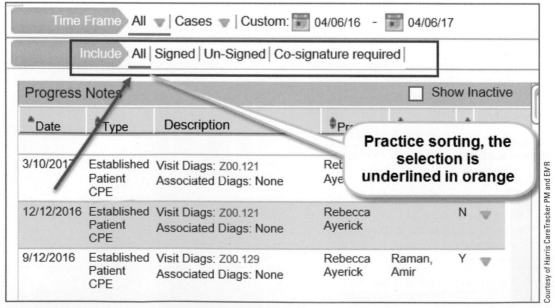

Figure 8-8   Filter the List of Progress Notes

FYI To filter the list of notes by case:
- Click the *second drop-down menu to the right of the Time Frame tab.*
- Select *Cases*, *All Cases*, or *Default*.

c. To filter the list of notes by diagnoses selected in the *A&P* (*Assessment*) tab of a progress note:

   i. Select *Diag. Filter* from the *All* drop-down menu to the right of the *Time Frame* tab. Harris Care-Tracker EMR displays the *Select Diagnosis* dialog box (**Figure 8-9**). (**Note:** If no diagnoses have been entered in the *A&P* (*Assessment* tab) of the *Progress Note*, the dialog box will be blank. If a diagnosis appears, you would select the checkbox pertaining to the diagnosis you want.)

   ii. Click *Select*. Harris CareTracker EMR displays the notes associated with the selected diagnoses.

Figure 8-9   Select Diagnosis Dialog Box

 SPOTLIGHT The *Diag. Filter* tab displays all diagnoses selected in the *A&P* (*Assessment*) tab of a progress note when documenting a patient encounter. It does not display the primary diagnosis selected via the *Visit* application.

📰 **Print a screenshot of the filtering methods that displays the Time Frame of "All" and includes "Un-Signed" only. Label it "Activity 8-4" and place it in your assignment folder.**

Manage Progress Note Templates

You will now perform various activities related to managing progress notes such as:

- *Edit* and *Overwrite* edits of a progress note

- Unsign a signed note

- Add an addendum to a note

- Send a *ToDo*

- Create a PDF of the note

- Sign or print a note

Edit a Progress Note. Edits can be made to a progress note until it is signed by the provider. If the note requires a co-signature, it can be edited until the supervising provider signs the note. If a note is signed, the template is unavailable to prevent changes being made to the note. However, the signing provider (you, in this case of student training) can unsign a note to make changes if necessary.

Harris CareTracker EMR provides a notification if the content of the note changes before the operator has a chance to save his or her edits. You can overwrite the edits by reviewing the options in the *Override Edits* box, selecting the edit you want, and clicking *Apply* (**Figure 8-10**).

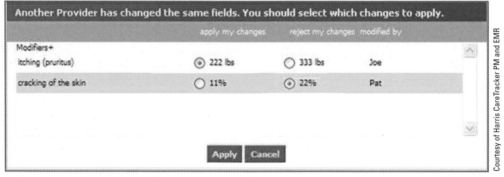

Figure 8-10   Override Edits Box

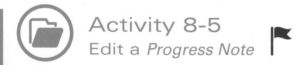

Activity 8-5
Edit a *Progress Note*

1. In the *Clinical Today* module, set the calendar to December 12, 2016, and click on Alex Brady's name in the *Appointments* window. This will launch his medical record. **Hint:** If you do not see the appointment, you will need to set the *Resources* field (just to the right of the calendar) to "All Resources" using the drop-down to select "All Resources" in order for the full schedule and all providers to display, then click *Search*, and then click on Alex Brady's name in the *Appointments* window.

2. In the *Patient Health History* pane, click *Progress Notes*. Harris CareTracker EMR displays the *Progress Notes* window.

TIP If you had previously signed the progress note, unsign it so that you can make edits (see Activity 8-9).

3. To edit from the *Actions* menu:

   a. Click the *Arrow* ▼ icon next to the note dated December 12, 2016, and then click *Edit Note*. If the *Copy prior note* dialog box appears, click *Cancel*. Harris CareTracker EMR displays the *Progress Note Template* window (**Figure 8-11**). In the *Template* field, select "9 Month Well Child Visit" if not already displaying.

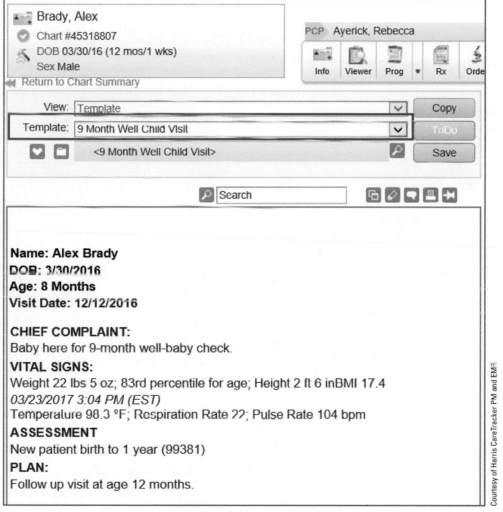

Figure 8-11   *Progress Note Template Window*

   b. Notice that there is only a small amount of information recorded in the *Progress Note*. Refer back to Chapter 6 and, using the steps outlined in Activity 6-17, edit and update the progress note using the information packet for Alex Brady's 9-month exam (see Source Document 8-1, found at the end of this activity).

c. When you have finished entering the data from Source Document 8-1 into the progress note, click *Save*. **Note:** If your screen turns gray, close out of the *Progress Note* window, click back on the patient's medical record and open the *Progress Note*. You will see the information entered has been saved.

d. Sign the note (refer to Activity 7-20 if you need to review the steps). Recall that although your name/operator will display as the signer on the note, in the *Progress Notes* module, the signer will be noted as the provider set in your batch.

4. Using an alternate method (steps a–f following), edit the progress note dated March 10, 2017 from the preview in the *Progress Notes* screen. Repeat Steps 1 and 2 of this activity but set the calendar to March 10, 2017 if needed.

a. Click on the progress note (not the *Actions Arrow* icon) you want to edit. Select the progress note dated March 10, 2017. The progress note displays on the right pane of the window.

b. Click *Edit* at the bottom of the screen (**Figure 8-12**).

c. If the *Copy prior note* dialog box displays, click *Cancel*. The *Progress Note* window launches, enabling you to edit the unsigned note. **Note:** If this *Progress Note* has already been signed, first *Unsign* it and then make your edits.

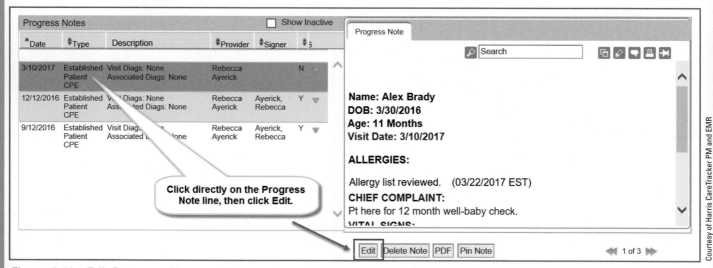

Figure 8-12   Edit Button on Progress Note

d. Using the steps outlined in Activity 6-15, edit and update the note using the information packet for Alex Brady's 12-month exam (see Source Document 8-2, found at the end of this activity).

e. When you have finished entering the data from Source Document 8-2, click *Save*.

f. Now sign the note.

Print the edited progress notes. Label the December 12, 2016 progress note "Activity 8-5a" and the March 10, 2017 progress note "Activity 8-5b," and then place them in your assignment folder.

Source Document 8-1

PATIENT'S NAME: Alex Brady

DATE OF BIRTH: 03/30/2016 (**Note:** Since patient Alex Brady's date of birth is fixed in the database, his age may show as older than 9 months when you are completing this activity. However, he was 9 months old at the time of his December 2016 appointment.)

PROVIDER: Dr. Ayerick

PROGRESS NOTE

Template: Pediatric: 9-month well-child visit (You may need to search for this template)

Tab	Entry
Interval History	*Accompanied by:* Mother *Concerns and Questions:* Mother has no questions or concerns at this time. *Interval History:* Pt. is here a bit early for 9-month visit. Family will be out of the country for the next two months so mother wanted to bring Alex in before leaving for their trip.
ROS	**Nutrition** Select "Y" for *breast fed* *Times per day:* 3 *Minutes per side:* 10 Check the following boxes: *Drinks from cup, source of water, solid foods, juice* Add comment to the *solid foods* note box: "Eats approximately 3 jars of baby food/day. Solid foods include cereal with applesauce, peas, squash, and bananas." **Elimination** *Wet diapers per day:* 6 *Bowel movements per day:* 1 **Sleep** Select "Y" for *sleeping through the night* **Development** *Gross Motor:* Select "Y" for *sits well,* and *crawls;* Select "N" for *pulls to feet with support* *Fine motor:* Select "Y" for *Feeds self, bangs objects together,* and *pincer grasp* *Communication:* Select "Y" for *Responds to name, waves bye-bye,* and *imitates sound* *Social:* Select "Y" for *Peekaboo, Patty-cake,* and *Stranger anxiety*
PE	**Vital Signs** *Weight:* 22 lbs 05 oz *Height:* 30 in 76.2 cm *Temperature:* 98.3 F *Heart Rate:* 104 bpm *Respiration Rate:* 22 **Physical Examination** Select "N" for normal for all categories except female genitalia (leave that blank)
Anticipatory Guidance	*Nutrition:* Select "avoid choke foods" *Injury Prevention:* Select "crib safety," "choking hazards," "First Aid, CPR," and "sun exposure"
Assess & Plan	Assessment: Click on the box beside "established patient birth to 1 year (99391)" Immunizations: Click on the box beside "DTap-HepB-IPV (90723)" *Plan:* Click on the drop-down box beside *Follow-up/Next Visit* and select "3 months"

Source Document 8-2

PATIENT'S NAME: Alex Brady

DATE OF BIRTH: 03/30/2016 (**Note:** Since patient Alex Brady's date of birth is fixed in the database, his age may show as older than 12 months when you are completing this activity. However, he was 12 months old at the time of his March 2017 appointment.)

PROVIDER: Dr. Ayerick

PROGRESS NOTE

Template: Pediatric: 12-month well-child visit (You will need to search for this template.)

Tab	Entry
Interval History	*Accompanied by:* Father *Concerns and Questions:* Father has no questions or concerns at this time.
ROS	**Nutrition** Select "N" for *breast fed.* Add comment to the *breast fed* note box: "Mom stopped breast feeding last month. Patient has adjusted well according to dad." Select "Y" for the following: *Drinks from cup, table foods, finger foods* **Elimination** *Wet diapers per day:* 6 *Bowel movements per day:* 2 **Sleep** Select "Y" for *sleeping through the night* **Development** *Gross Motor:* Select "Y" for *walks without assistance,* and *stands well alone* *Fine motor:* Select "Y" for *has a pincer grasp, bangs objects together, scribbles spontaneously* *Communication:* Select "Y" for *says mama/dada specifically, imitates simple daily tasks, language at 12 months* *Social:* Select "Y" for *plays pat-a-cake, waves bye-bye*
PE	**Vital Signs** *Weight:* 21 lbs *Length 33 in / 83.8 cm* *Temperature:* 98.2 F *Heart Rate:* 100 bpm *Respiration Rate:* 22 **Physical Examination** Select "N" for normal for all categories except female genitalia (leave that blank)
Anticipatory Guidance	*Nutrition:* Select "whole milk," "healthy food choices," and "nutritious snacks, limit sweets" *Social competence:* Select "toilet training" *Injury Prevention:* Select "electrical outlets"
Assess & Plan	Click on the box beside "established patient birth to 1 year (99391)" *Immunizations:* Select "DTAP/HIB/IPV (90698)," "Polio Virus Vaccine (90713)," and "Measles, Mumps, Rubella Vaccine (90707)." Click on the drop-down box beside *Follow-up/Next Visit* and select "1 Month." *Plan:* Enter "Will bring patient back in for a weight check in 30 days."

Delete a Progress Note.

You can only delete unsigned notes. When a note is signed, *Delete Notes* appears dimmed.

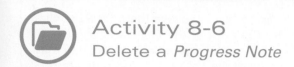

Activity 8-6
Delete a *Progress Note*

In a recent audit, you discovered a progress note from the year 2013 that was entered in error. To correct the error, you will delete the progress note.

1. Pull patient Donald Schwartz into context.

2. Click on the *Medical Record* module.

3. In the *Patient Health History* pane, click *Progress Notes*. Harris CareTracker EMR displays the *Progress Notes* window.

4. Click the progress note you want to delete. Select the note dated May 14, 2013. The progress note displays on the right pane of the window.

5. Click *Delete Note* (**Figure 8-13**). Harris CareTracker EMR displays the *Void* dialog box.

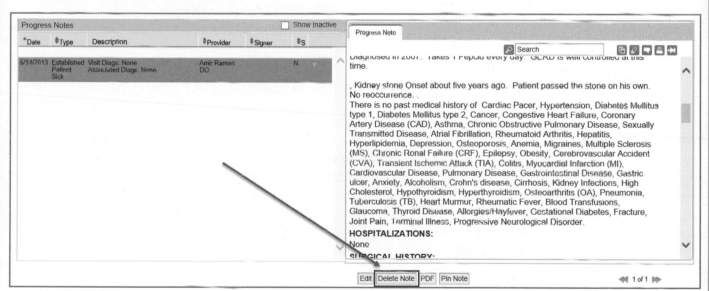

Figure 8-13   Delete Note Tab

Courtesy of Harris CareTracker PM and EMR

6. Select *Delete Reason*: "Other" (**Figure 8-14**).

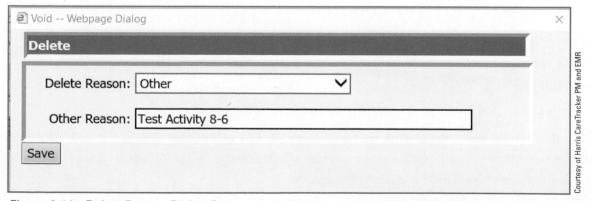

Figure 8-14   Delete Reason Dialog Box

7. You will be prompted to enter a reason. Enter "Test Activity 8-6."

8. Click *Save*. (**Note:** It may take a few moments for the note to be deleted.)

> **TIP** A record of the deleted note is maintained in the *Clinical Log.* To access the *Clinical Log,* click the drop-down arrow next to the *View* 👓 icon at the top right of the *Chart Summary* screen, and then select *View Clinical Log.* The *View Log* dialog box will display (**Figure 8-15**). **Note:** You may need to adjust the *Time Frame* parameters to include the date of the *Progress Note* you deleted.

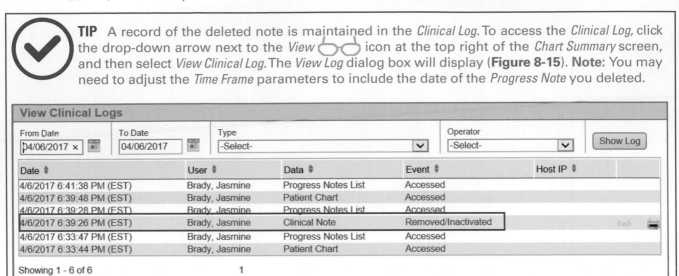

View Clinical Logs

From Date	To Date	Type		Operator	
04/06/2017 ×	04/06/2017	-Select- ▾		-Select- ▾	Show Log

Date ⬍	User ⬍	Data ⬍	Event ⬍	Host IP ⬍	
4/6/2017 6:41:38 PM (EST)	Brady, Jasmine	Progress Notes List	Accessed		
4/6/2017 6:39:48 PM (EST)	Brady, Jasmine	Patient Chart	Accessed		
4/6/2017 6:39:28 PM (EST)	Brady, Jasmine	Progress Notes List	Accessed		
4/6/2017 6:39:26 PM (EST)	Brady, Jasmine	Clinical Note	Removed/Inactivated		
4/6/2017 6:33:47 PM (EST)	Brady, Jasmine	Progress Notes List	Accessed		
4/6/2017 6:33:44 PM (EST)	Brady, Jasmine	Patient Chart	Accessed		

Showing 1 - 6 of 6   1

Figure 8-15 View Clinical Logs   Courtesy of Harris CareTracker PM and EMR

🖥 **Print a screenshot of the *Clinical Log*, which shows the deleted progress note (see Tip box above). Label it "Activity 8-6" and place it in your assignment folder.**

9. Close out of the *View Clinical Logs* dialog box by clicking on the "X" in the upper-right-hand corner.

Add an Addendum to a Progress Note.

You can add an addendum to both a signed and an unsigned note to accommodate any clinical workflow your practice follows. An **addendum** is text that is added to a progress note after it is signed. The addendum displays at the end of the original progress note and helps track updates made to the note. Additionally, the "Addended By" label displays with the operator's name and the date and time of the addendum. This tracks changes made to the note and the person responsible for the change.

Activity 8-7
Add an Addendum to a *Progress Note*

1. Pull patient Harriet Oshea into context.

2. Click on the *Medical Record* module.

3. In the *Patient Health History* pane, click *Progress Notes*. Harris CareTracker EMR displays the *Progress Notes* window.

4. Click the progress note to which you want to add an addendum. Select the note dated March 20, 2017. The progress note displays on the right pane of the window.

5. Click the *Add Addendum* 🖳 icon. Harris CareTracker EMR displays the *Add Clinical Note Addendum* dialog box. (**Note:** If you receive an error message, close the dialog box and click on the *Add Addendum* icon again until the prompt displays.)

6. Enter additional note: "Pt requests referral to Dr. Robert Rovner for Orthopedic evaluation" (**Figure 8-16**).

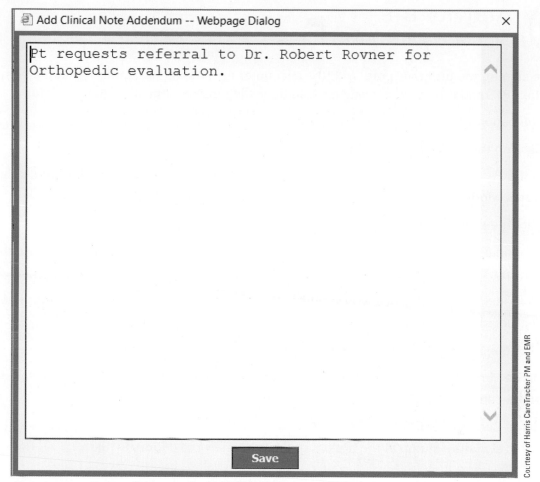

Figure 8-16   Harriet Oshea Addendum Text

7. Click *Save*.

 SPOTLIGHT You can also choose to dictate the addendum or use the quick text feature to enter additional notes.

8. In the right pane, scroll to the bottom of the progress note where the *Addendum* has been added (**Figure 8-17**).

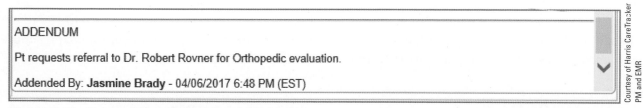

Figure 8-17   Harriet Oshea Addendum Added to Note

💾 **Print the progress note that now reflects the Addendum. Label it "Activity 8-7" and place it in your assignment folder.**

Sign the Progress Note.

Having previously learned to sign the progress note in Chapter 7 (Activity 7-20), you will now sign the progress note(s) you have worked on in this chapter. (**Note:** Before you sign a progress note, be sure the visit has been captured with CPT® and ICD codes entered. Refer to Activity 7-18 if you need to review these steps.)

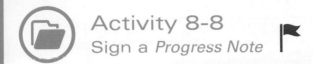

Activity 8-8
Sign a *Progress Note*

Before signing the progress note, with the encounter in context, first confirm that there is a captured *Visit* with the CPT® and ICD codes already entered (following instructions from Activity 7-18).

1. Pull patient Harriet Oshea into context.

2. Click on the *Medical Record* module.

3. In the *Patient Health History* pane, click *Progress Notes*. Harris CareTracker EMR displays the *Progress Notes* window.

4. Click the progress note you want to sign. Select the note dated March 20, 2017.

5. (Optional) Click on the *Expand* 🔳 icon to maximize the readability of the progress note you are viewing. You can click the icon again to collapse the narrative.

6. (Optional) As Best Practice, you would confirm that the addendum to the note has been added as instructed in Activity 8-7.

7. Click the *Sign* 🖊 icon on the right pane of the window to sign the note.

8. Harris CareTracker EMR will display a pop-up window asking "Are you sure you want to sign this note to the patient's chart?" Click *OK*.

9. Harris CareTracker EMR will update the status of the note. When complete, you will note the electronic signature stamp at the bottom of the progress note (**Figure 8-18**).

Electronically Signed By: Jasmine Brady
Electronically signed: 4/6/2017 6:55:44 PM

Courtesy of Harris CareTracker PM and EMR

Figure 8-18   *Electronically Signed Progress Note*

💾 **Print the signed progress note. Label it "Activity 8-8" and place it in your assignment folder.**

Unsign the Progress Note.

You can unsign a signed note, if necessary. However, only the operator who signed the note is allowed to unsign a note based on the operator's role. Enter a reason for unsigning the note if required to complete the action. For audit purposes, a copy of the original note is maintained in the patient's clinical log.

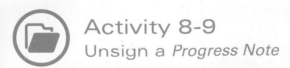

Activity 8-9
Unsign a *Progress Note*

1. After signing Ms. Oshea's progress note in the previous activity, you realize that Dr. Brockton is the provider who needs to sign the note, not you.

2. To unsign the note, with patient Harriet Oshea in context, click the *Medical Record* module.

3. In the *Patient Health History* pane, click *Progress Notes*. Harris CareTracker EMR displays the *Progress Notes* window.

4. Click the progress note you want to unsign. Select the note dated March 20, 2017. The progress note displays on the right pane of the window.

5. Click the *Unsign* ✐ icon. Harris CareTracker EMR displays a confirmation message.

6. Click *OK* to unsign the note.

7. In the *Progress Notes* window, the note will now be listed as unsigned (**Figure 8-19**).

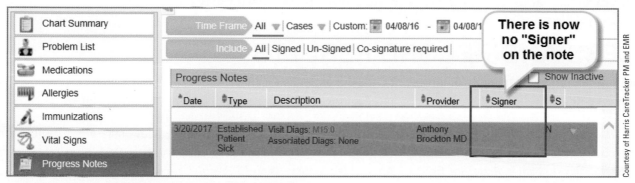

Figure 8-19   *Progress Note Window—Unsigned Note*

🖶 **Print a screenshot of the unsigned progress note. Label it "Activity 8-9" and place it in your assignment folder.**

8. Now sign the progress note once again and save it so you can use this encounter in later activities.

Print the Progress Note.

To print the progress note, follow the instructions in Activity 8-10.

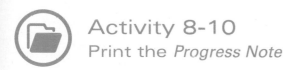

Activity 8-10
Print the *Progress Note*

1. With patient Harriet Oshea in context, click the *Medical Record* module.

2. In the *Patient Health History* pane, click *Progress Notes*. Harris CareTracker EMR displays the *Progress Notes* window.

3. With the March 20, 2017 progress note in context, use each of the following three print functions:

   a. Print from the *Actions* menu:
      • Click the *Arrow* ▼ icon and click *Print*. Harris CareTracker EMR displays the *Clinical Note* dialog box.
      • Click *Print*. A copy of the notes prints to the printer attached to your computer.
      • Close out of the print dialog box when finished.

   b. Print from the preview in the right pane:
      • Click the progress note you want to print. The progress note displays on the right pane of the window.
      • Click the *Print* 🖶 icon. Harris CareTracker EMR displays the *Clinical Note* dialog box.
      • Click *Print*. A copy of the note prints to the printer attached to your computer.
      • Close out of the print dialog box when finished.

c. Create a PDF of the progress note:
- Click the progress note you want to convert to PDF. The progress note displays on the right pane of the window.
- Click *PDF* at the bottom of the screen. Harris CareTracker EMR creates a PDF version of the documented progress note. You can print or save a copy.
- Close out of the print dialog box when finished.

💾 **Print the progress note using each of the methods in the activity. Label the pages "Activity 8-10a," "Activity 8-10b," and "Activity 8-10c" and place them in your assignment folder.**

ACCESS AND RECORD RESULTS

Learning Objective 2: Manually enter Results into the patient's medical record to view, customize, graph, and print those results.

The *Results* application is where lab and radiology results are displayed. The medical assistant should monitor results on a continuous basis, determining that results are received, reviewed, and handled in an efficient manner. Be certain to reset the *Provider* field to *All* and then click *Search*. Results received electronically are saved in the following locations:

- *Home* module > *Dashboard* tab > *Clinical* section > *Results* link
- *Clinical Today* module > *Tasks* tab > *Results* (from the *Tasks* menu on the right side of the window) (**Figure 8-20**)

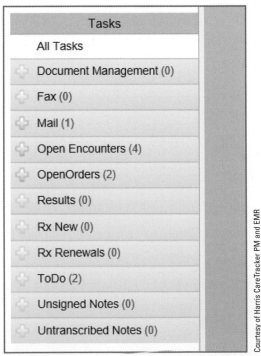

Tasks
All Tasks
✛ Document Management (0)
✛ Fax (0)
✛ Mail (1)
✛ Open Encounters (4)
✛ OpenOrders (2)
✛ Results (0)
✛ Rx New (0)
✛ Rx Renewals (0)
✛ ToDo (2)
✛ Unsigned Notes (0)
✛ Untranscribed Notes (0)

Courtesy of Harris CareTracker PM and EMR

Figure 8-20 Results in Tasks Pane

- *Open Activities* section of the *Chart Summary*
- *Results* section of the *Chart Summary*.

The results displaying in the *Medical Record* module are color coded based on the status of the results, as shown in **Table 8-2**.

Table 8-2   *Results* Statuses

RESULT COLOR	STATUS
Black	Final result
Gray	Preliminary result
Bright Red	Abnormal result **Note:** If any component within a result is returned with an abnormal value, the entire result is considered as an abnormal result.
Light Red	Preliminary Abnormal result

Courtesy of Harris CareTracker PM and EMR

Results received into Harris CareTracker EMR are automatically linked to the corresponding patient based on the demographic information and the order. If a result has an "Unmatched" status, the result is saved only in the *Results* application of the following locations:

- *Home* module
- *Clinical Today* module

Your student version of Harris CareTracker will not receive results electronically. However, you are able to manually enter lab results into the patient's medical record.

Manual results can be entered, scanned, or attached to the patient's medical record. If a result has an *Unmatched Patient* icon, it indicates that the computer was unable to find any patients with the same exact demographics, thus the result is saved only in the *Results* application.

> **FYI** Electronic results received into Harris CareTracker EMR automatically link to the corresponding patient based on the demographic information.

The result is not saved in the *Results* application in the *Medical Record* module unless it is manually matched. If a matching patient is not found, Harris CareTracker EMR displays the *Match* icon, enabling you to manually link the results to the corresponding patient. Additionally, any test result that falls outside of normal parameters displays the observation in red to alert you and get your immediate attention (**Figure 8-21**).

	↓Reported	⬍Collected	⬍Patient	⬍Sex	⬍DOB (Age)	⬍Type	⬍Facility	⬍Provider	⬍Status	⬍S			
☐	04/07/17		Morgan, JaneW	F	01/22/1955 (62)	LAB	EastSide	Raman, Amir	Final	N			
	Urinalysis microscopic panel [#/volume] in Urine by Automated count, Urinalysis dipstick panel in Urine by Automated test strip												
☐	04/07/17		Morgan, JaneW	F	01/22/1955 (62)	LAB	EastSide	Raman, Amir	Final	N			

Results — ☐ Show Abnormal Only   ☐ Show Unsigned Only

Figure 8-21   Abnormal Result Displayed in Red

Courtesy of Harris CareTracker PM and EMR

> **FYI**
> - There are several ways to browse through results that continue on additional pages:
>   - By clicking the specific page number or
>   - By clicking the *Previous Page* icon or *Next Page* icon.
> - From the *Results* application, you can also link results to orders, send a *ToDo* regarding the result, enter recalls for required tests, print results, and more.

Entering Results Manually

The *Open Orders* application enables you to manually enter the results of lab tests into the system or automatically download them from the facility. If the delivery method of results includes fax, phone, paper, or download, you must manually enter the results for the specific order. This automatically updates the order status and the results in the patient's medical record. When the result is entered, both the order and the result are removed from the *Open Orders* application under *Quick Tasks* and the *Open Activities* section of the *Chart Summary* in the *Medical Record* module.

In the Build Your Proficiency activities at the end of this chapter, you will manually record *Results* for patient Jane Morgan's urinalysis lab order you created in Chapter 7, Activity 7-2 and perform more advanced features, such as creating customized result views, filtering the patient's result list, graphing patient results, and printing a single result.

For Activity 8-11, you will perform only an abbreviated results entry in the *Office Tests* section of the *Tests* tab in the *Progress Note*.

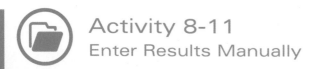

Activity 8-11
Enter Results Manually

1. Pull patient Jane Morgan into context.

2. Click on the *Medical Record* module.

3. Access the *Progress Note* for the appointment/encounter you created for Ms. Morgan in Chapter 4.

4. If you had previously signed Ms. Morgan's *Progress Note*, unsign the note, following the steps in Activity 8-9, then click *Edit*.

5. Select the *TESTS* tab of the *Progress Note*.

6. In the *Office Tests* field, enter "Negative" into the *Rapid Streptococcus Group Identification (Kit)* field drop-down at the top of the *Tests* tab of the *Progress Note*.

7. Click on *Save*.

8. Sign the *Progress Note*.

🖫 **Print the Progress Note that displays the Rapid Strep Test result, label it "Activity 8-11", and place it in your assignment folder.**

Viewing Results

The *Results* application accessed via the *Medical Records* module consists of two tabs:

- *List View* tab
- *Chart Results* tab

Table 8-3 describes the information displaying in the columns of the *Results* window (*List View* tab). However, manual results (attached or scanned) only display information in specific columns marked with an (*) in **Table 8-3**. Refer to **Figure 8-22** while reviewing this table.

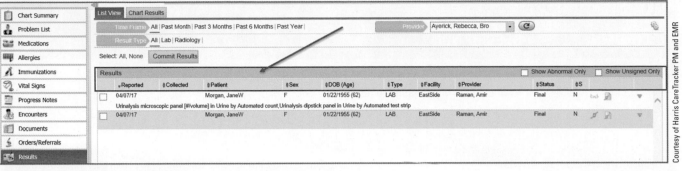

Figure 8-22   Results Columns

Courtesy of Harris CareTracker PM and EMR

Table 8-3   *Results* Columns

COLUMN	DESCRIPTION
*Reported	The date and time the results were transmitted into Harris CareTracker EMR or selected when uploading the result via the *Document Management Upload* application. Additionally, the column displays the name of the result below the reported date. Manual results displays the *Document* icon to the left of the document name, the subtype in parentheses, and notes entered when uploading the document.
Collected	The date and time the specimen is collected.
Patient	The name of the patient.
Sex	The sex of the patient.
DOB (Age)	The patient's date of birth in mm/dd/yyyy format and the age of the patient.
Type	The type of the result.
Facility	The name of the facility.
*Provider	The name of the ordering provider or the provider selected when uploading the result document. Additionally, if a provider was copied on the result, the name displays below the ordering provider's name and is indicated with "CC." **Note:** The provider who was copied on the result can see the result only if the *Include Copy To* checkbox is selected.
*Status	The status of the result.
*S	"S" represents whether or not the result has been reviewed and signed and can have one of two values. Results reviewed and committed to the patient's medical record are indicated with a "Y." Results that are not reviewed by the ordering provider are indicated with an "N."
*Linked to Order	Allows you to link the result to an order. When a result is linked to a document, the *Link to Order* icon is replaced by the *View* icon. You can click the *View Linked Order* icon to view the order linked to the result.
Link to Document	Allows you to link the result to a document associated with the patient. When a result is linked to the document, the *View Linked Order* icon displays, allowing you to view the document linked to the result. **Note:** The *Link to Document* icon appears dimmed if the result is an attached or a scanned document.

(continues)

Table 8-3 *(continued)*

COLUMN	DESCRIPTION
Action ▼	The *Action* menu allows you to do the following: • *Print.* Allows you to print the result. • *ToDo.* Allows you to attach the result to a *ToDo.* • *Log.* Allows you to view the *Result Activity Log.*
Observation (below the result row)	Comments about the result. *Abnormal* results display the specific test values in red in the observation row.
Notes (below the observation row)	Displays any comments you entered when signing the result.

Courtesy of Harris CareTracker PM and EMR

Customize Patient Results View.

The *Results* application enables you to create an operator-specific default view for both the *List View* and *Chart Results* tabs. You can select the time frame, result type, and the providers for the list view. You can select the default chart type and the reported date for the chart view.

Filter Patient Results.

The list of results pertaining to the patient can be filtered on the result type, date, or provider.

 SPOTLIGHT It is important that all results are signed and committed to the patient's chart in a timely manner.

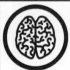 **CRITICAL THINKING** A patient calls to inquire about some tests she had performed three days ago. She states that she checked the patient portal but no results are showing up. She is quite nervous about the testing. You check the patient's EMR but the results have not been uploaded. Where else in the EMR might you look for these results? What can be done if you are unable to locate the results?

Graph Patient Results.

The *Chart Results* tab in the *Results* application allows you to plot all or specific lab test values that pertain to a specific time period in three different views. The views include *Vertical Chart*, *Horizontal Chart*, and *Graph*. Results in chart or graph views are color coded based on the status of the result and display the measurements associated with each result as shown in **Table 8-2**. You can only graph results that were entered, not results that were scanned into the chart.

Print Patient Results.

The *Results* application helps print test result records to give to the patient and other entities such as specialists and hospitals that are treating the patient. Fewer laboratory tests will be ordered because health practitioners across the provider network will have the results of earlier tests, eliminating the need to reorder tests that were previously completed. The *Results* application provides two methods to print a specific result: You can use the *Action* menu in the *Result* application or open the result to print.

RECORDING MESSAGES

Learning Objective 3: Record messages in Harris CareTracker PM and EMR.

In Chapter 2, you were introduced to the *Message Center* where you created *ToDos* and *Mail* messages and viewed *Queues* and *Fax* options. In this chapter, we expand on your previous activities: simulate the office environment and workflows, and record patient messages in Harris CareTracker PM and EMR.

Message Center Templates

The *Messages* application is a communication tool accessed via the patient's medical record that allows you to manage customer, staff, and patient communications. The application supports the clinical workflow by providing the ability to create a *ToDo* by attaching PDF documents or image files (jpg, gif, tif, etc.) and links with patient information. This helps the provider coordinate patient care activities during a patient visit and electronically communicate that information in real time to front office and clinical staff in your practice. This also helps the clinical staff monitor and complete tasks efficiently as a patient goes through the visit and ensures that no important tasks are left undone.

When a patient checks out from an appointment, the patient is automatically pulled into context, and all *ToDos* for orders, prescriptions, referrals, educational handouts, and the chart summary display as patient *ToDos*, enabling the person responsible to manage and complete the tasks efficiently. Patient-related *ToDos* also display in the *Correspondence* and *Open Activities* sections of the patient's medical record. The *Messages* application is a combination of *ToDos*, *Mail*, *Queues*, and *Fax*.

Use the steps outlined in Activity 8-12 to access the *Messages* application each time you are instructed to create a *ToDo* or *Mail* message. The *ToDo* application is also accessible by clicking the *ToDo* 🗹 icon or the *ToDo* button in other applications accessed via the patient's medical record.

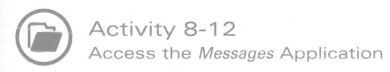

Activity 8-12
Access the *Messages* Application

1. Pull patient Jane Morgan into context and click the *Medical Record* module.

2. In the *Clinical Toolbar*, click the drop-down arrow next to *Msg Cntr* 🗹 and select *New ToDo*. Harris CareTracker EMR displays the *New ToDo* dialog box.

🖬 **Print a screenshot of the *ToDos* screen, label it "Activity 8-12", and place it in your assignment folder.**

3. Click "X" in the top right corner of the window to close it.

You can use templates to create preformatted content for *ToDos*, faxes, and mail messages. For example, you can create a standard mail message used for outgoing referrals. Anytime that template is selected, the mail message is automatically populated with the text in the template. Templates help improve workflow, and are discussed in detail in Chapter 2.

ToDos

ToDos are Harris CareTracker PM and EMR's internal messaging system that serves two primary functions: assigning a co-worker a task and communicating with the Harris CareTracker PM and EMR support team. You can also view *ToDos* for a patient if the *Messages* application is accessed when a patient is in context.

If the *ToDo* is for a patient, it is saved under the *Correspondence* application of the *Financial* module when the patient is in context, and the *Correspondence* and *Open Activities* section of the patient's medical record. In addition, all *ToDos* are also saved in the *ToDo* list of the people involved in the *ToDo*, the owner of the *ToDo*, and the person who was assigned the *ToDo*.

Create a ToDo.

In Chapter 2, you created a "test" *ToDo* (see Activity 2-14). Now you will create a clinical *ToDo* related to EMR.

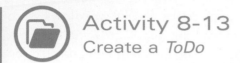

Activity 8-13
Create a *ToDo*

1. Pull patient Harriet Oshea into context.

2. Click on the *Medical Record* module.

3. Click on the *Msg Center* ☑ icon in the *Clinical Toolbar*. This will launch the *New ToDo* window.

4. By default, the *From* list displays your operator name/number.

5. Of the options available in the *To* list, select "Operator."

6. If a patient is in context when sending a *ToDo*, the patient's name displays in the *Patient* box. If no patient is in context, click the *Search* 🔍 icon next to the *Patient* list. The *Patient Search* dialog box displays, enabling you to enter the required parameters to search for the patient. Patient Harriet Oshea should be in context.

7. By default, the *Subject* box displays information based on the selection in the *Type* and *Reason* lists. However, you can change the subject if necessary. Leave as is.

8. In the *Due Date* and *Due Time* boxes, enter the date and time by which the *ToDo* must be completed. This is important to track overdue items. Change to the date Ms. Oshea called the office requesting the referral (use today's date). Leave *Due Time* box blank.

9. From the *Template* list, select the template you want to use. Leave this blank.

10. From the *Category* list, select the appropriate *ToDo* category. (For example, if the *ToDo* created is for the Harris CareTracker PM and EMR *Support* entity, select "Support Center" from the *Category* list.) Select "Interoffice" for this activity.

11. By default, the *Type* list displays "EHR." Leave as is.

12. In the *Reason* field, use the drop-down and select "Phone Call (Patient)."

13. In the *Severity* list, click the priority of the *ToDo*. Select "Medium." Click the *Info* i icon to view a description of each severity level.

14. By default, the *Status* list is set to "Open." Leave as is.

15. Leave the *Duration* box blank.

16. In the *Notes* box, enter additional notes pertaining to the *ToDo*. You can format the note and spell-check the note entered. This is similar to the formatting toolbar in MS Word®. Enter the following text regarding referral to Dr. Rovner. "Patient called saying that her hip and back pain has increased and

is requesting referral to Orthopedic Specialist. She has a friend that sees Dr. Robert Rovner in San Ramon and is very happy with him. Can you arrange a referral to Dr. Rovner? Her insurance does not require authorization." (**Figure 8-23**)

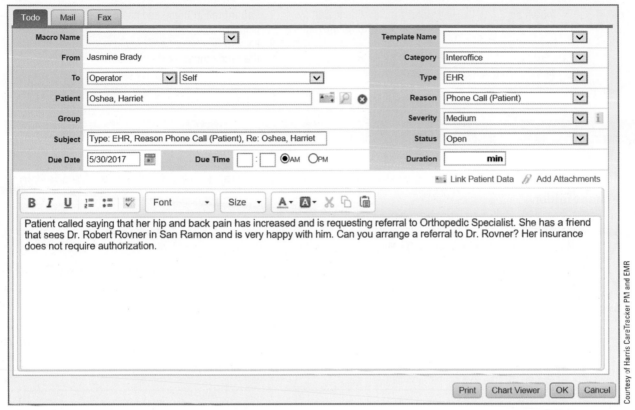

Figure 8-23   *Harriet Oshea ToDo Requesting Referral*

17. Click *OK*.

18. Refresh your *Home* module screen. The *ToDo* will be listed in the bottom left corner of the screen. Click on the *ToDo* link to view the *ToDo List* window (**Figure 8-24**).

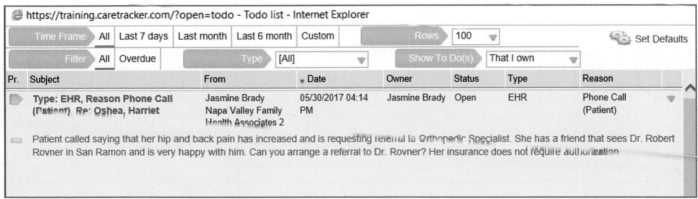

Figure 8-24   *ToDo on Home Module Screen*

Courtesy of Harris CareTracker PM and EMR

19. Now repeat the activity and create *ToDo* as listed in **Table 8-4**. For the *ToDo* in **Table 8-4** use the *Category* "Interoffice," *Type* "EHR," and *Reason* "Phone Call (Patient)."

Table 8-4   New *ToDo* Messages

FROM	TO	SUBJECT	REASON/ SEVERITY	NOTES (MESSAGE)	PATIENT
You	You *(in an actual practice, you would send this message to the provider)*	Fall/Refer to X-ray	Phone Call (Patient/High	Patient fell at home and hand is in extreme pain. He wants to know if he can get an X-ray in the office today, or if he should go to Urgent Care. Please call on cell phone ASAP. OK to leave message.	Domenic Scott

Courtesy of Harris CareTracker PM and EMR

 Print a screenshot of the contents of the *ToDo* you created. Label it "Activity 8-13" and place it in your assignment folder.

TIP Additional/Optional *ToDo* Features:

- You can click *Chart Viewer* to access clinical information for the patient in context. The *Chart Viewer* button displays only if you have the EHR-Mid and EHR-Provider roles or have the *ToDo – Chart Viewer* override included in your operator profile. The *Chart Viewer* button is active only if a patient is attached to the *ToDo*.

- If a patient is in context, Harris CareTracker PM and EMR displays the *Link Patient Data* link. You can click the link to attach other documents for the patient using the *ToDo Attachments/Links* dialog box.

FYI Additional/Optional *ToDo* Features:

- Click the *Add Attachments* link to attach a document to the *ToDo*. The *Document Management Upload* dialog box displays, enabling you to attach or scan a document or link a voice attachment to the *ToDo*. (This feature is not available in your student environment.)

- You can click the attachment name to view the document in the document viewer. All markups made to a document attached to a *ToDo* can be saved by clicking *Save*. However, if you edit the document information, you must click *Upload* to save the changes made.

CRITICAL THINKING What would happen if you closed a *ToDo* that had not been resolved? For example, MA Sally closed a *ToDo* sent to her by Dr. Raman regarding patient Mr. Scott before she had called him back with instructions to go immediately to the hospital (call 911), to follow up regarding his status, and to make a follow-up office visit. Where does the original message go? Who would know it was not completed or that MA Sally had not followed Dr. Raman's instructions? What are the ramifications of closing *ToDo* messages? Write a one-page paper answering these questions, and then prepare another document creating what you consider to be "Best Practice" instructions for closing *ToDos*. Submit to your instructor for class discussion.

Mail

The *Mail* application is similar to any standard email application and allows you to send, receive, organize, and reply to mail messages. In Chapter 2, Activity 2-15, you created a "Test Mail Message." This chapter expands by creating new *Mail* messages that mimic clinical workflows.

Create a New Mail Message.

The *Mail* application allows you to communicate electronically with staff members, providers in your *Provider Portal*, and patients activated in the *Patient Portal*. The mail feature works similarly to other email applications, enabling you to open, view, create, send and receive, and delete messages. In Harris CareTracker PM and EMR, the mail application is a secure messaging system that users can participate in by invitation only and allows a user to send secure messages outside of the Harris CareTracker system to patients through the patient portal or to referring doctors who are part of the referral network. This is different from email because it is on a secure server, but the use and functions within the mail system are similar to standard email. In addition, you can link attachments such as patient encounter notes, documents, results, referrals, and authorization forms and set priorities and more. As a general rule, the *Mail* feature should only be used when sending a message to someone outside the practice, for example, to refer to providers (outside the practice), or to patients active in the *Patient Portal*. **Figure 8-25** lists the tabs available to use when selecting a mail recipient (*My Company*, *Provider Portal*, or *Patients*). (**Note:** For your training environment, you will use only the *My Company* tab.)

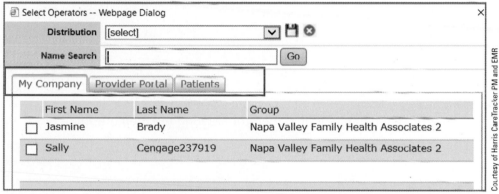

Figure 8-25   Select Mail Recipients

 TIP Important !! If you want a task to be completed by a specific person within the practice, send a *ToDo* and not a *Mail* message.

 SPOTLIGHT If sending *Mail* messages to a patient, be sure to follow HIPAA policy and protocol.

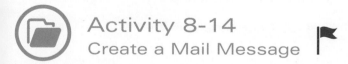

Activity 8-14
Create a Mail Message

This will be a simulated activity because your student version of Harris CareTracker does not include an active *Patient Portal* or *Provider Portal*. For this activity, you will remain in the *My Company* tab.

1. With no patient in context, click the *Home* module.

2. Click on the *Messages* tab. The *Messages Center* opens and displays all of your open *ToDos*.

3. Click *Send Mail* in the bottom right corner of the screen (**Figure 8-26**), which opens the *New Mail* dialog box.

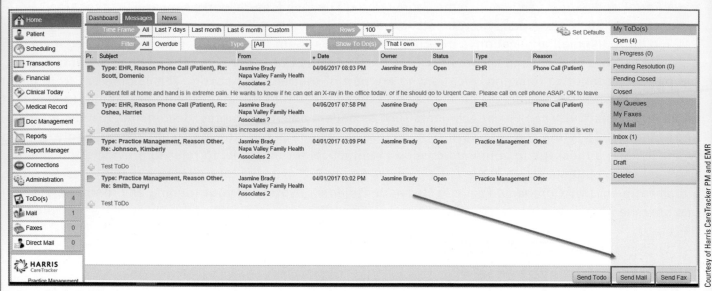

Figure 8-26   Send Mail Button

> **FYI** The *From* list defaults to the operator creating the mail message (you) and cannot be edited.

4. In the *To* field, click the *Search* 🔍 icon. Harris CareTracker PM and EMR opens the *Select Operators* dialog box. You will be the only operator available to select (along with any operators you have created). In a live environment, you would select the most appropriate person (this could also be a provider or a patient). Check the box next to your operator name or number, and click *Select* at the bottom of the screen.

5. If a patient is in context, the patient's name displays in the *Patient* box. However, you can also send a mail message about a different patient by clicking on the *Search* 🔍 icon. You can delete a patient from the list by clicking the *Remove Patient* ❌ icon. There should be no patient in context, so leave the *Patient* field blank.

6. In the *Subject* box, enter "Cardiology Group Presentation." If the subject is patient related, be sure the correct patient's name displays in the *Subject* box. If the message does not relate to a patient, be sure to remove the patient's name. Remove any patient from the *Subject* box.

7. By default, the *Severity* list displays "Medium." However, you can change the priority of the mail message if necessary. Leave as is.

8. In the *Notes* box, enter the message and format the information as directed in **Figure 8-27**. "Hello Dr. Raman, the Napa Valley Cardiology Group would like to make a presentation at your next providers meeting. Would you like me to arrange it? Thanks." (Sign the note with your operator name/number.)

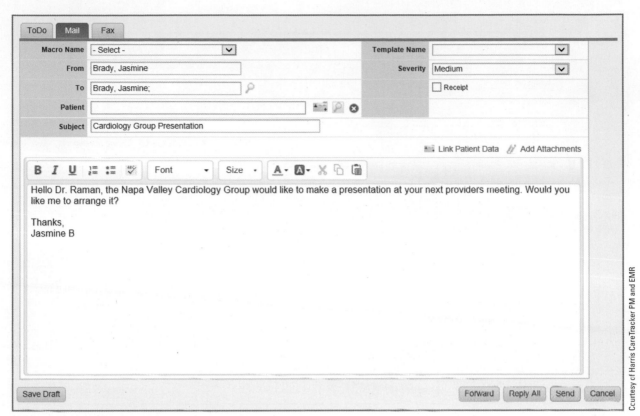

Figure 8-27   Mail Message—Cardiology Group

9. Click *Send* to send the mail message to the selected operators. The message(s) you created will now appear in your *Inbox* (see **Figure 8-30**) listed under *My ToDo(s)* on the right-hand side of the screen.

10. Repeat these steps to create the "Patient Portal" and "Office Holiday Party" messages in **Figures 8-28** and **8-29**. **Figure 8-30** shows your *Inbox* with all these messages. You would click the + sign to expand the message and the – sign to collapse the message.

    a. Patient Portal message (with patient Jane Morgan in the *Patient* field): ***This is a simulated mail message as Patient Portal is not active in the student version of Harris CareTracker***

        Subject: Medical Records

        Message Text: "Hello Ms. Morgan, your medical records have been copied and mailed per your request. If there is anything else I can do for you, please let me know. Sincerely, (your operator name/number)"

    b. Office Holiday Party message (with no patient in context):

        Subject: Office Holiday Party

        Message Text: "Hello all Providers and Staff. We are planning an Office Holiday Party on December 15th. Reservations have been made at Vic Stuart's Restaurant for 6:30 pm. You may invite a guest as well. Please respond no later than December 1st if you are planning to attend and if you will be bringing a guest or not. Should be lots of fun!! Hope you can attend. Best, (your operator name/number)"

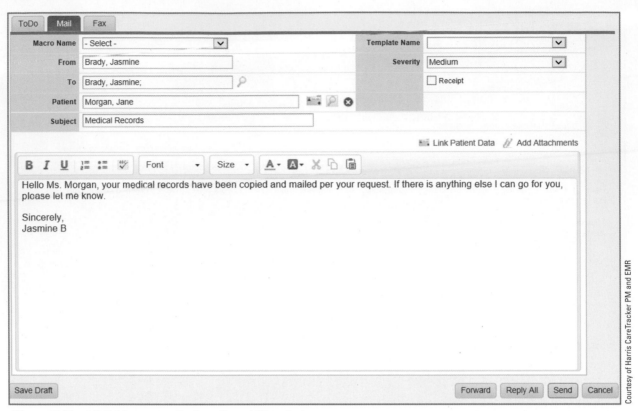

Figure 8-28   Mail Message—Patient Portal Simulation

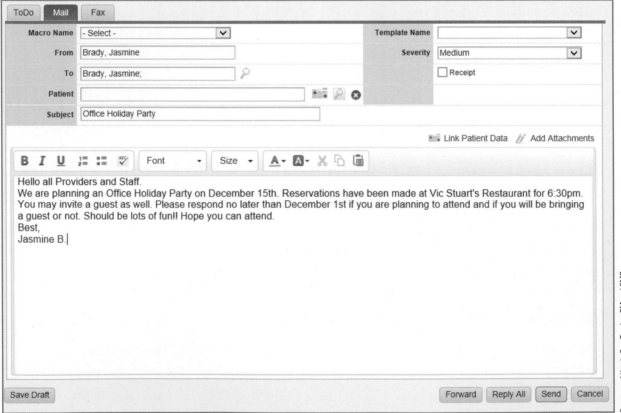

Figure 8-29   Mail Message—Office Holiday Party

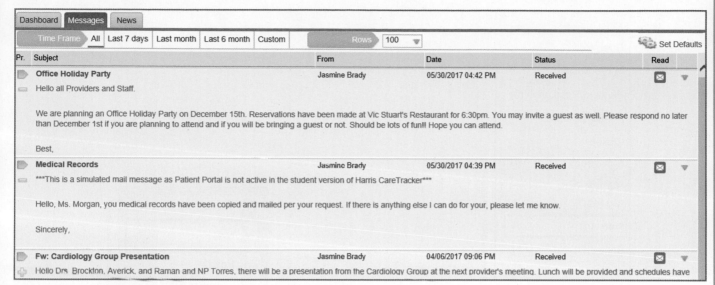

Figure 8-30   *Mail Messages in Inbox*

📇 **Print the screen that displays the contents of each mail message by clicking on the *Inbox* under *My ToDo(s)* on the right-hand side of the screen. Label it "Activity 8-14" and place it in your assignment folder.**

Manage Mail.

Similar to any standard email application, the *Mail* application allows you to send, receive, organize, and reply to mail messages. *Managing Mail* consists of:

- Accessing *Mail* Messages
- Viewing *Mail* Messages
- Moving *Mail* Messages
- Replying to a *Mail* Message
- Forwarding a *Mail* Message
- Deleting a *Mail* Message
- Working with Attachments

Accessing Mail Messages.   There are two ways to access your mail:

- In the *Home* module, click the *Messages* tab and then click the *Inbox* link below the *My Mail* section on the right side of the window. The number next to the *Inbox* indicates the total number of unread mail messages (**Figure 8-31**).
- Click the *Mail* link at the bottom of the left navigation pane. The number displayed indicates the number of unread messages in your inbox (**Figure 8-32**).

View Mail Messages.   The *Mail* application displays all mail messages sent to you. A mail message is used as a method of sharing information and may or may not require a return action. The functionality is similar to any other email application such as *Outlook®*, *Outlook Express®*, *Yahoo!*, and *Gmail*. The inbox is easy to customize (**Figure 8-33**):

- Click any of the column headings to sort the messages in the inbox by *Priority, Subject, From, Date, Status,* and so on.

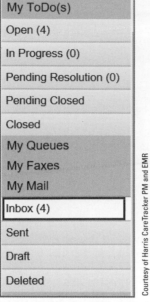

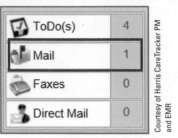

Figure 8-31   Access Mail Messages from the Inbox Link

Figure 8-32   Access Mail Messages from the Mail Link

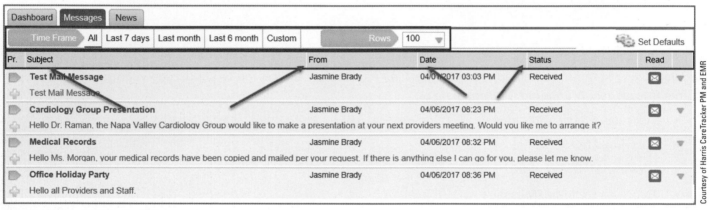

Figure 8-33   Customize Inbox

- Click the filters at the top of the page to view mail messages based on the time period (*Last 7 days*, *Last month*, etc.), or click the *Custom* tab to enter a specific date range.

- Click the *Rows* list to select the number of messages to display.

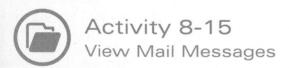

Activity 8-15
View Mail Messages

1. Access your mail messages from the *Home* module.

2. Click the *Messages* tab.

3. Click on the *Inbox* link below the *My Mail* section on the right side of the window. (**Note:** You may have to refresh your screen for the recent activity to display.)

4. Click on the plus sign [+] next to the messages to quickly review the message thread without opening the message.

5. Now click the minus sign [−] to close the thread (**Figure 8-34**).

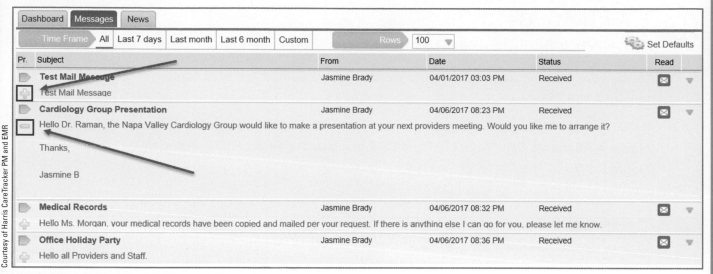

Figure 8-34   Review Mail Message Thread

6. To open the mail message, either click on the *Subject* line or point to the *Arrow* ▼ icon at the far right end of the row, and then select "Open." Harris CareTracker PM and EMR opens the message.

7. From the *Actions* column, you can choose to move to folder, open, delete, reply, reply all, or forward (**Figure 8-35**). (You will move, reply, forward, and delete messages in later activities.)

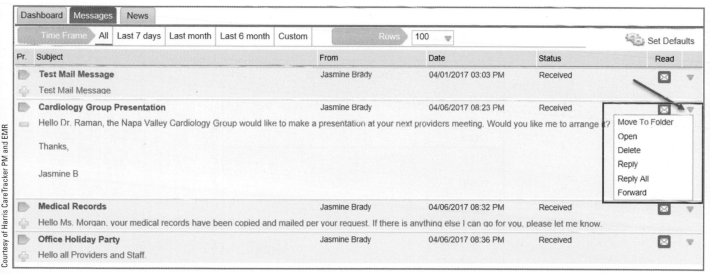

Figure 8-35   Action Column Options

⊞ **Print the screen that displays the contents of the Mail Messages Inbox. Label it "Activity 8-15" and place it in your assignment folder.**

Moving Mail Messages. You have the option to move mail messages to the *Inbox*, *Sent*, *Draft*, and *Deleted* folders.

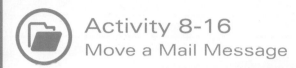

Activity 8-16
Move a Mail Message

1. Access your mail messages. You will be moving the message "Test Mail Message" (created in Activity 2-15).

2. In the "Test Mail Message" row, point to the *Arrow* ▼ icon and then select "Move To Folder" (**Figure 8-36**). Harris CareTracker PM and EMR displays the *Select Folder* dialog box (**Figure 8-37**).

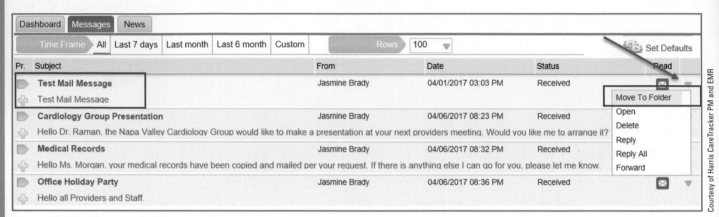

Figure 8-36   Move to Folder

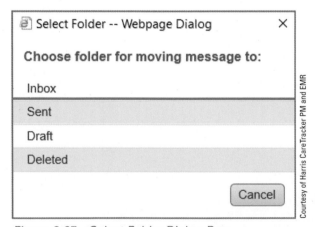

Figure 8-37   Select Folder Dialog Box

3. Click on the folder you want to move the mail message to: Move to "Deleted." The mail is moved to the selected folder.

4. Under *My Mail,* click the *Deleted* link (**Figure 8-38**). The message you deleted will display (**Figure 8-39**). **Note:** You may need to click "Last 6 months" or "Custom" in the *Time Frame* section in order for the message to appear.

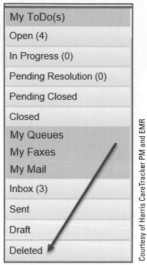

Figure 8-38   Deleted Link

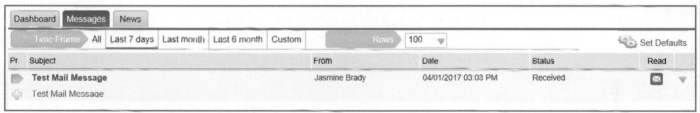

Figure 8-39   Deleted Test Mail Message

Courtesy of Harris CareTracker PM and EMR

🖨 **Print the Deleted message screen. Label it "Activity 8-16" and place it in your assignment folder.**

Replying to a Mail Message.

To reply to a *mail message*, follow the instructions in Activity 8-17.

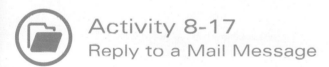

Activity 8-17
Reply to a Mail Message

1. Access the mail messages in your *Inbox.* You will reply to the mail message "Office Holiday Party."

2. To reply to only the sender, point to the *Arrow* ▼ icon in the *Actions* column and then click "Reply."
    Note: If there were multiple recipients on a mail message, you could reply to all of the recipients by pointing the *Arrow* ▼ icon in the *Actions* column and clicking *Reply All.*

3. Type the reply message as noted in **Figure 8-40**: "Count me in for 2 !! Thank you."

4. Click *Send.* You may need to refresh your screen before the message appears in your *Inbox.*

5. Repeat the activity and reply to the "Cardiology Group Presentation." Type the reply message as noted in **Figure 8-41**: "Yes, please arrange the presentation and advise other providers in the group and block off schedules. Please order lunch from Tulio's for the presentation. Thanks, Dr. R."

6. Click *Send.*

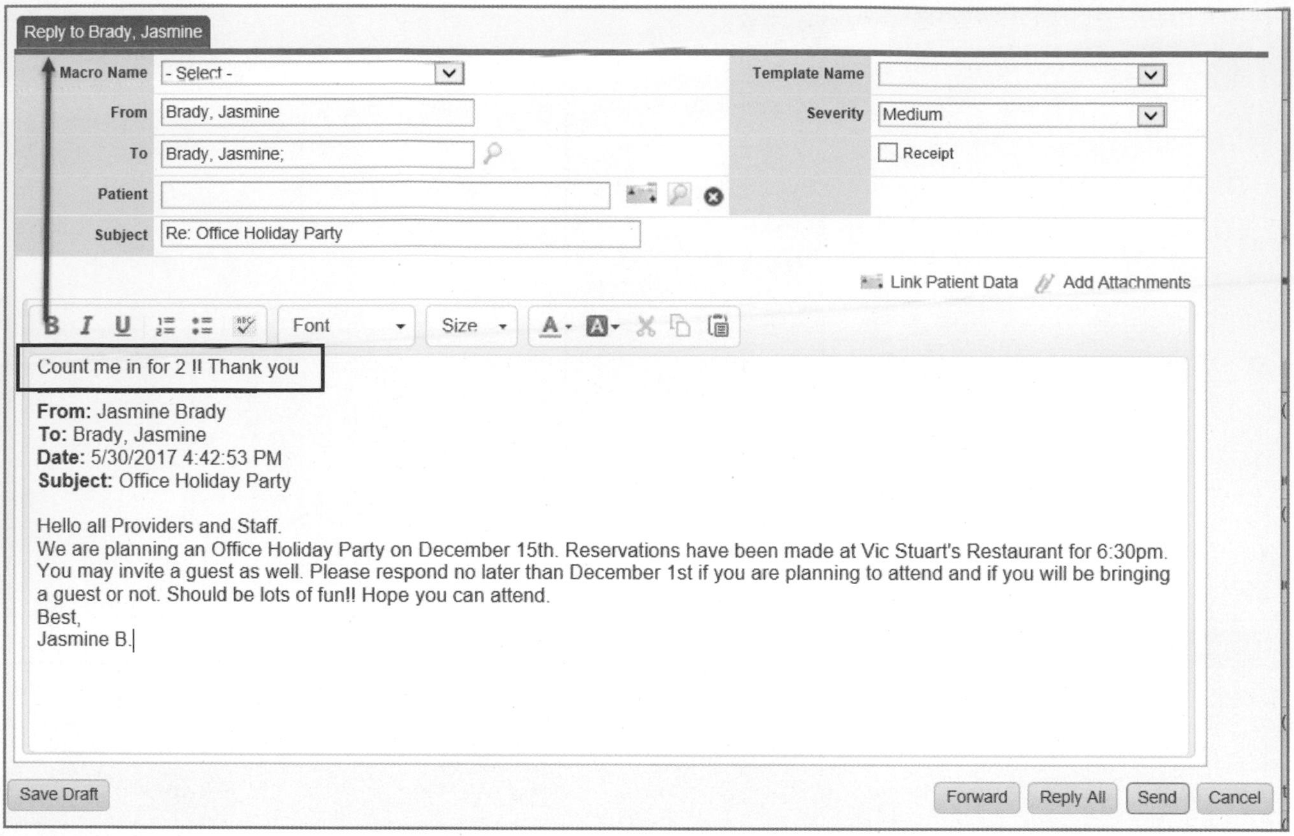

Figure 8-40   Holiday Party Reply Mail Message

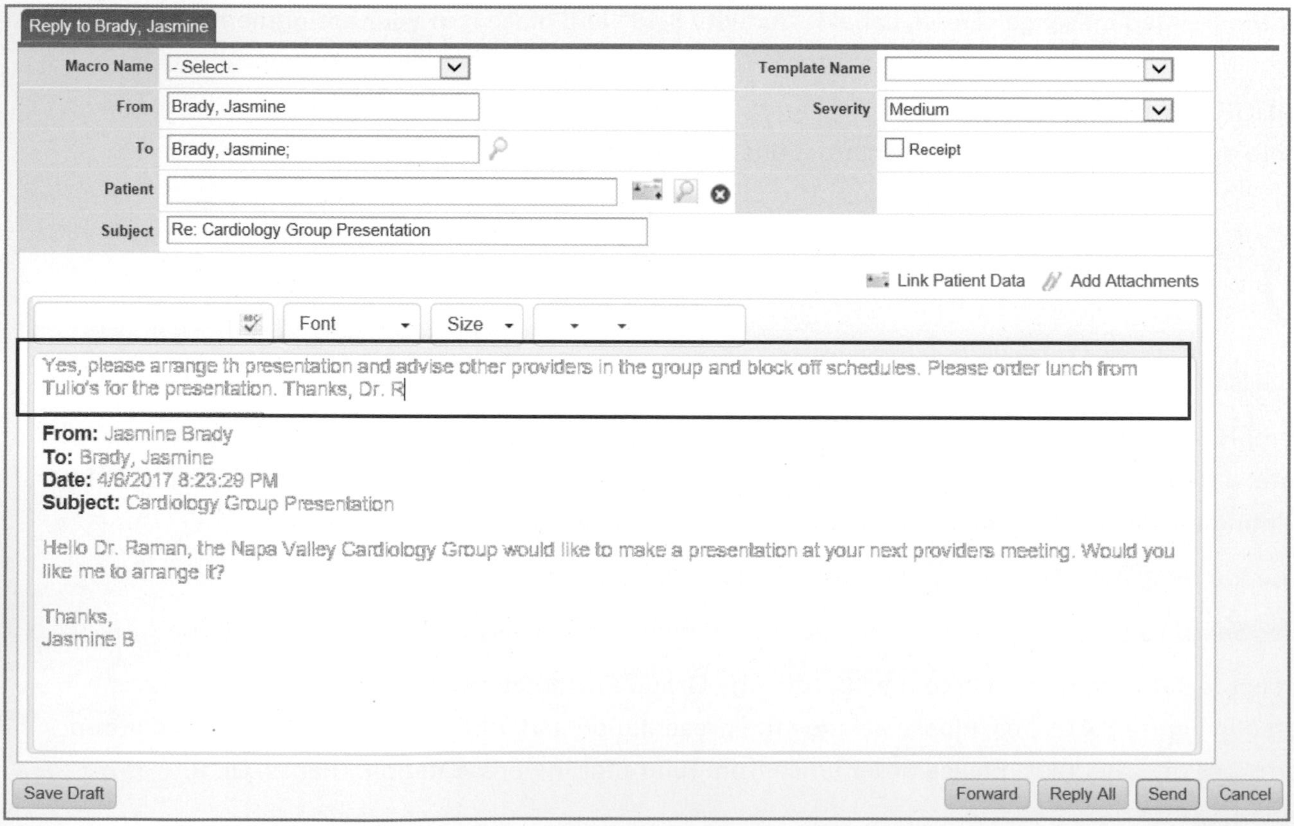

Figure 8-41   Cardiology Reply Mail Message

🖥 **Print the screen that displays the mail message replies. Label it "Activity 8-17" and place it in your assignment folder.**

Forwarding a Mail Message.

Forwarding allows you to send the original mail message to a new recipient.

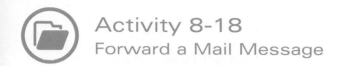

Activity 8-18
Forward a Mail Message

1. Access your *Inbox*. You will forward the mail message "Cardiology Group Presentation" (forward the message reply, not the original message).

2. In the *Actions* column, point to the *Arrow* ▼ icon and then select "Forward." Harris CareTracker PM and EMR displays the *Forward Message* window.

3. In the *To* field, click the *Search* 🔍 icon. The *Select Operators* dialog box displays. In this training environment, you will be the only operator listed (along with any operators you have created).

4. Select the checkbox next to the person (you) to whom you want to forward the message.

5. Click *Select*. Harris CareTracker PM and EMR closes the *Select Operators* dialog box. Free text the following message to forward: "Hello Drs. Brockton, Ayerick, and Raman and NP Torres, there will be a presentation from the Cardiology Group at the next provider's meeting. Lunch will be provided and schedules have been blocked. Thank you, (your name/operator number)" (**Figure 8-42**).

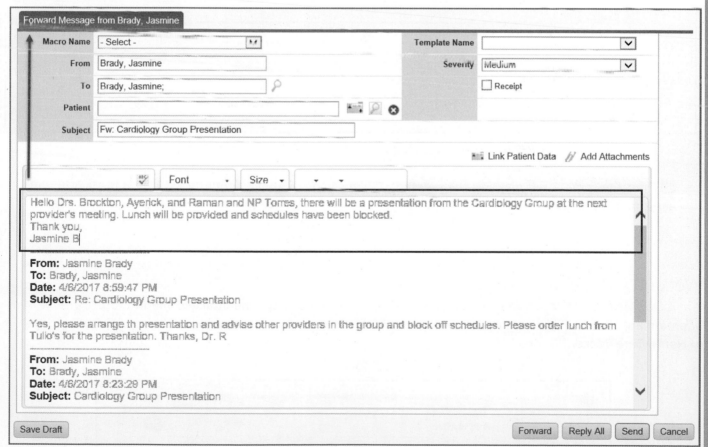

Figure 8-42 Cardiology Forwarded Mail Message

Courtesy of Harris CareTracker PM and EMR

6. Click *Send*. The message is forwarded to the selected recipients.

🖳 **Print the screen that displays the forwarded mail message. Label it "Activity 8-18" and place it in your assignment folder.**

Deleting a Mail Message.

Once you finish with a mail message, it is best practice to clean up your mail box. This means you should delete messages that no longer require attention or a response.

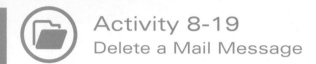

Activity 8-19
Delete a Mail Message

1. Access your *Inbox*. You will delete the original "Office Holiday Party" and "Cardiology Group Presentation" messages.

2. In the *Actions* column for each message, point to the *Arrow* ▼ icon and then select "Delete." Harris CareTracker PM and EMR deletes the message from the list.

3. Click the *Deleted* link under *My Mail* to view your deleted message. **Figure 8-43** represents the *Deleted Mail Messages* in your *My Mail* tab.

	Dashboard	Messages	News						

Time Frame	All	Last 7 days	Last month	Last 6 month	Custom	Rows	100 ▼		Set Defaults

Pr.	Subject	From	Date	Status	Read	
▶	**Test Mail Message**	Jasmine Brady	04/01/2017 03:03 PM	Received	✉	▼
✚	Test Mail Message					
▶	**Office Holiday Party**	Jasmine Brady	04/06/2017 08:36 PM	Received	✉	▼
✚	Hello all Providers and Staff.					

Figure 8-43   Deleted Messages

🖳 **Print the screen that displays the deleted mail messages. Label it "Activity 8-19" and place it in your assignment folder.**

Working with Attachments.

If a *ToDo, Mail* message, or *Fax* contains an attachment, you can save the attached file in the *Document Management* application (**Figure 8-44**). The *Document Management* feature is not available in your student version of Harris CareTracker PM and EMR.

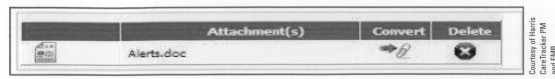

	Attachment(s)	Convert	Delete
🖼	Alerts.doc	➜🖉	✖

Figure 8-44   Working with Attachments

FYI In a live practice, the steps to work with attachments are:

1. Click the attachment name to view a preview of the file.
2. Click the *Upload Document* 📋 icon to upload the attachment to the *Document Management* application.
3. Click the attachment name to view a preview of the file.
4. Click the *Convert* ➥🖉 icon to convert a file or link into a PDF. This is important if you are sending the attachment to someone who cannot access Harris CareTracker PM and EMR.
5. Click the *Delete* ✖ icon to remove the attachment.

RECALL LETTERS

Learning Objective 4: Create and update patient Recall Letters.

Recalls are reminders to patients that an appointment needs to be booked. Rather than scheduling a future appointment, a recall date is set for the appointment in the *Scheduling* module. Harris CareTracker PM and EMR tracks all recalls, enabling you to generate recall letters at the appropriate time intervals. The *Recalls/Letters Due* application allows you to generate and print letters and labels for the following:

*   Appointment recalls
*   Appointment reminders
*   Missed/cancelled appointments

Recalls are categorized by recall type and age. A recall is considered overdue if the recall has not been linked to a patient appointment prior to the date of the recall. When a patient calls to schedule an appointment, his or her recall will be linked to the appointment and will be removed from the *Recall* application.

Harris CareTracker PM and EMR automatically generates an appointment reminder for any patient entered into the *Recall* application and generates letters and envelope labels for printing. This application helps keep track of patient visits and provide proper medical care.

For example, when a patient schedules an appointment, you can manually link the recall to the appointment if necessary. If the appointment type scheduled is the same as the existing recall, Harris CareTracker PM and EMR links the appointment to the recall, making it inactive. If the patient cancels an appointment linked to a recall, the recall changes to an active recall and displays on the *Overdue Recalls and Letters* link on the *Dashboard* (**Figure 8-45**). The *Recall* application helps review, add, and update recalls saved for the patient.

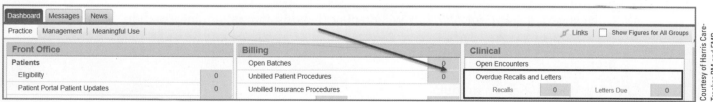

Figure 8-45   *Overdue Recalls and Letters Link*

Add Recalls

The *Recall* application is where you add reminders about follow-up treatments and appointments that patients need. This enables the staff to generate reports about patients who need follow-up appointments and additional testing. Adding recalls helps develop robust and responsive disease management and health maintenance programs for improved patient care outcomes. It also helps the practice generate revenue that might be lost when follow-up care is neglected or appointments are missed.

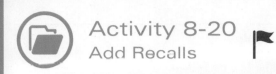

Activity 8-20
Add Recalls

1. Pull patient Gabby Tolman into context.

2. The *Patient Alerts* pop-up alert will note any missing information (**Figure 8-46**).

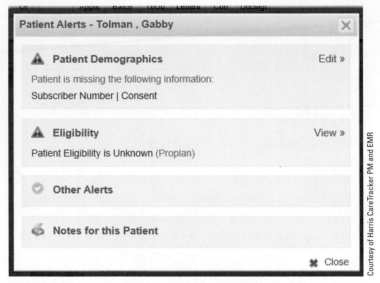

Figure 8-46   Pop-up Alert—Edit/Update Missing Information

3. As best practice, update Ms. Tolman's demographics screen as noted below.

   a. Click on the *Patient* module

   b. Click on *Edit*

   c. Change her *Group Provider*, *Referred By*, and her *PCP* all to Dr. Brockton

   d. Change *Consent* to *Yes*

   e. Click on *Yes* in the *NPP* field

   f. In the *Subscriber #*, enter the same information contained in the *Group #* in the *Insurance Plan(s)* section

   g. Click *Save*

   h. Once saved, the *Patient Alert* box will display "No missing patient information" in the *Patient Demographics* section. It is best practice to always update a patient's chart when needed and prompted.

4. Click the *Medical Record* module.

5. You see that Ms. Tolman's *Last Appt* displays as "03/20/17 New Patient CPE" (**Figure 8-47**).

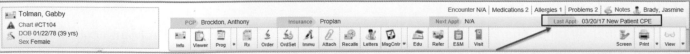

Figure 8-47   Last Appointment Displayed for Gabby Tolman

Courtesy of Harris CareTracker PM and EMR

6. In the *Clinical Toolbar*, click the *Recalls* icon.

7. If an encounter is in context, Harris CareTracker EMR displays the *Recalls* dialog box. If an encounter is not in context, Harris CareTracker EMR displays the *Select Encounter* dialog box. Select the encounter dated March 20, 2017.

8. Click + *New Recall* (**Figure 8-48**). Harris CareTracker EMR displays the *Add Patient Recall* dialog box.

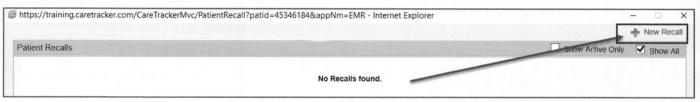

Figure 8-48   *Add New Recall*   Courtesy of Harris CareTracker PM and EMR

9. In the *Time Frame* list, click the time interval when the patient is expected to return to the office for a comprehensive physical exam (CPE). Select "2 Years."

10. In the *Appointment Type* list, click the reason for the patient recall. Select "Established Patient CPE."

11. In the *Resource* list, click the provider assigned to the recall (Dr. Brockton). This is the preferred provider the patient wants to see during the appointment. (**Note:** If there is no preference, select "Any Resource" from the list.)

12. In the *Location* list, click the preferred location for the appointment. If there is no preference, click "Any Location" from the list. Select "Napa Valley Family Associates."

FYI In the *Case* list, click the case associated with the recall. If no case is associated with a recall, click "Default." A case list would apply in the case of workers' compensation. No case list applies. **Note:** If a recall is associated with a case, it is linked to the appointment when scheduled. For example, you can link workers' compensation and auto accident cases to an appointment.

13. By default, the *EMR Alert Status* is set to "No Alert." If required, add an alert to the recall by clicking either "Soft Alert" or "Pop-Up Alert." Select "Soft Alert."

14. In the *Recall Notes* box, enter additional comments for the recall. Enter "Schedule CPE and send Lab Order 30 days prior to appointment for complete panel." (**Figure 8-49**).

TIP The *pop-up alert* ⚠ displays when the patient's medical record is launched. The alert displays each time the patient's medical record is accessed and stops displaying when the alert is closed. You can also click the *Alert* icon next to the patient's chart number on the *Patient Detail* bar to view both soft and pop-up alerts.

15. In the *Active* field, select "Yes."

16. Click *Save* to save the recall to the patient's record. (You could also click *Save and ToDo* to send a *ToDo* for the recall saved.) The *Recalls* dialog box displays with the recall just created (**Figure 8-50**).

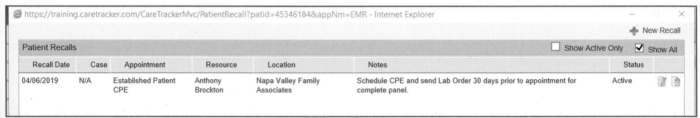

Figure 8-49   Add Recall for Gabby Tolman

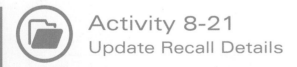

Figure 8-50   Patient Recalls Dialog Box

Courtesy of Harris CareTracker PM and EMR

Print a copy of the patient's recall. Label the recall summary "Activity 8-20," and place it in your assignment folder.

17. Close out of the *Patient Recalls* dialog box by clicking the "X" in the upper right-hand corner.

Update Recall Details

The *Recall* application updates recall details recorded for the patient.

Activity 8-21
Update Recall Details

1. Pull patient Gabby Tolman into context.

2. Click on the *Medical Record* module.

3. In the *Clinical Toolbar*, click the *Recalls* icon.

4. If an encounter is in context, Harris CareTracker PM and EMR displays the *Recalls* dialog box. If an encounter is not in context, Harris CareTracker PM and EMR displays the *Select Encounter* dialog box. Select the encounter dated March 20, 2017.

5. Find the recall you want to update ("Established Patient CPE" you created in Activity 8-20).

6. Click on the *Edit* icon next to the recall and make the necessary changes to the available information. Dr. Brockton is having his non-Medicare patients see NP Torres for CPEs. Change the provider (*Resource*) to NP Torres.

7. Click *Save.* The existing recall for the patient is updated.

 Print a copy of the updated recall, label it "Activity 8-21," and place it in your assignment folder.

8. Close out of the *Patient Recalls* dialog box by clicking the "X" in the upper right-hand corner.

> ✔ **TIP** To deactivate an open recall, click the *Edit* ✎ icon and change the *Active* field to "No." To activate a recall, click the *Edit* ✎ icon and change the *Active* field to "Yes."

RUNNING AN IMMUNIZATION LOT NUMBER REPORT

Learning Objective 5: Run an immunization report using the Clinical Export feature.

There are many reasons to run immunization lot number reports. For example, occasionally you will receive a notice that certain lot numbers of a product have been recalled by the Food and Drug Administration (FDA). Lot numbers provide a source of comfort during a recall because each immunization is recorded in the EMR and various reports can be run to track that patients received the immunization. In addition, a practice can monitor inventory and expiration of immunizations on hand and also use the report for internal audit purposes.

Immunization Export

The *Immunization Export* application allows a practice to generate a record of all vaccinations given during a specified time period. This application pulls the Harris CareTracker PM and EMR data into a state-specific format that can be downloaded and then sent to the state's department of health.

In Activity 8-22, you will take the appropriate steps after your practice has received a letter from a drug company recalling a specific lot number. The *Immunization* records will be generated on the report so that you can contact any patient who received the immunization. You would then relay to the patient that the drug may not be effective and that it is recommended that the patient come in to have a **titer** (labs drawn). A titer determines how much antibody is present in the patient's blood to fight a specific antigen (disease-causing agent). If the levels are at an acceptable level to protect the patient, the test results will indicate that the patient has reached full immunity against the disease. In this case, it would mean that the immunization given reached its desired effect. However, if the test results indicate that the patient is not immune, the patient will need to return for another immunization to reach full immunity.

Immunization Lot Number Report

Now that you have learned the steps to run the *Immunization Export* report, you will run an *Immunization Lot Number* report.

Activity 8-22
Run an Immunization Lot Number Report

1. With no patient in context, click on the *Reports* module and then click the *Reports* tab.

2. Under *Medical Reports*, click on the *Other Reports* link.

3. Click the *Report* drop-down menu and select "Global – Immunization by Lot Number" (**Figure 8-51**).

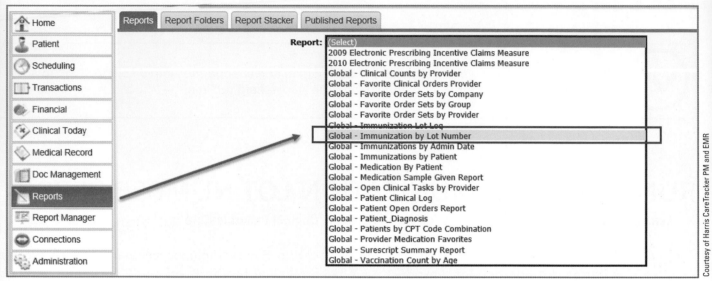

Figure 8-51   Select Global – Immunization by Lot Number

4. Enter the lot number you created in Activity 7-7 in the *Enter the Lot Number* box and also in the *Saved Report Name* box (see **Figure 8-52**). **Hint**: The lot number should be "Hep" followed by your operator number.

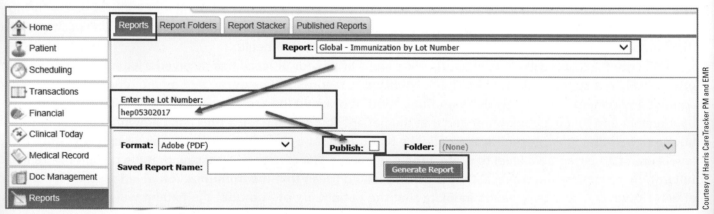

Figure 8-52   Enter the Hep vs hep

5. Uncheck "Publish."

6. Click *Generate Report*.

7. In the lower portion of your screen, you will see the report generated (**Figure 8-53**).

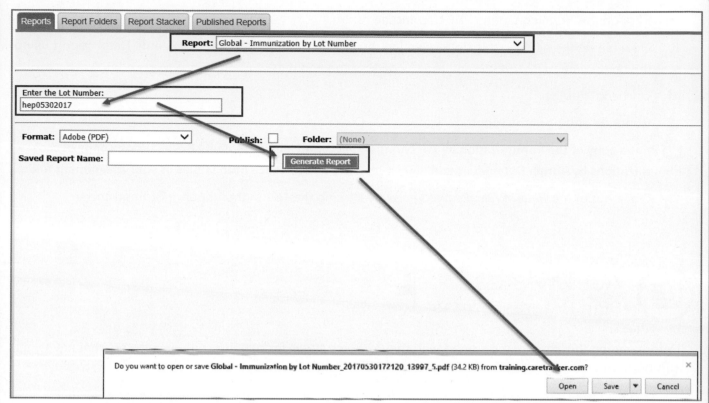

Figure 8-53   Generate Report

Courtesy of Harris CareTracker PM and EMR

8. Click *Open* on the *PDF generated report* to view the report (**Figure 8-54**). **Note:** You also have the option to "Save," "Save as," or "Save and open" so you can store the file on your computer to print later (**Figure 8-55**). **Hint:** You might get a pop-up window asking if you want to Open or Save the PDF report. Select Open and the report will display.

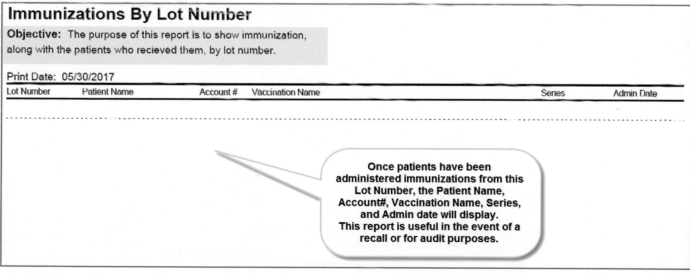

Figure 8-54   PDF Format of Published Reports

Courtesy of Harris CareTracker PM and EMR

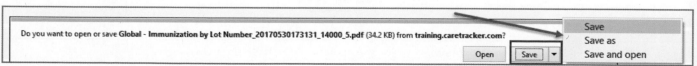

Figure 8-55   Alternative Methods to Save PDF Format of Published Reports

Courtesy of Harris CareTracker PM and EMR

9. Click on the *Print* icon in the PDF to print the report.

10. Now repeat the activity, this time selecting the "Global – Immunizations by Admin Date" report using the begin date of 01/01/2013 and today's date as the end date.

11. Uncheck "Publish."

12. Generate and print the report.

💾 **Print a copy of the Immunization by Lot Number report and label it "Activity 8-22a." Print a copy of the Immunizations by Admin Date report and label it "Activity 8-22b." Place both copies in your assignment folder.**

13. Close out of the *Patient Recalls* dialog box by clicking the "X" in the upper-right-hand corner.

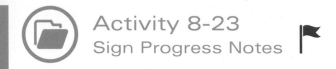

Activity 8-23
Sign Progress Notes 🚩

Before ending this chapter, be sure to sign the *Progress Notes* for patients with encounters that have visits captured. You may refer to the instructions in Activity 7-20 to complete this activity.

1. Click on the *Home* module > *Dashboard* tab > *Practice* tab > *Clinical* heading > *Open Encounters* link.

2. Select *All* providers and click on the refresh icon to the right of the *Provider* dropdown.

3. The screen will display any unsigned notes and whether or not the visit has been captured.

4. To determine if a visit has been captured, look at the *Description* column. A saved visit will display the *Visit Diags* codes. A visit that has not been captured will say "None" after "*Visit Diags*" as illustrated in **Figure 8-56**. In addition, a *Visit* that has not been captured displays the *Visit* icon 🖥. A *Visit* that has been captured will display the *Visit* icon with a checkmark 🖥✓.

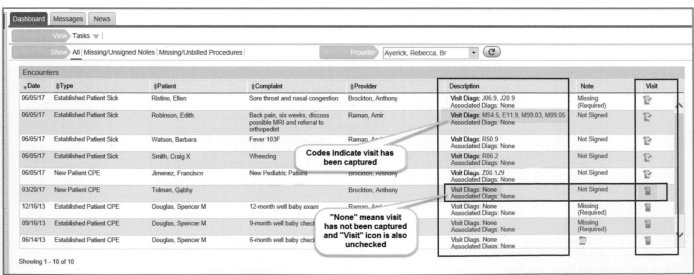

Figure 8-56   Description Column in Encounters

5. Sign <u>all</u> of the progress notes for the patients with captured visits () by clicking on "Not Signed" in the *Note* column. Do <u>not</u> sign any *Notes* that are noted *as Missing (Required)*.

6. The progress note will display.

7. Change the *Template* to "IM OV Option 4 (v4) w/A&P" (except for patient Francisco Jimenez, leave the *Template* as "Pediatric OV Option 4 (v1)").

8. Click on the *Sign* icon in the *Progress Note*.

9. Click back on the *Open Encounters* link on the *Dashboard*, change *Provider* to *All*, and click the *Refresh* icon. The *Note*(s) with the captured visit that has been signed will disappear from the screen.

10. Continue steps 5 through 9 for the remaining patients with a completed *Visit* and a *Note* that is "Not Signed."

11. If there are any *Encounters* displaying at this time without *Visits*, do <u>not</u> sign the *Note*(s). Do <u>not</u> sign any *Note* noted *as Missing (Required)*.

12. You will now be able to complete the *Billing* and *Collection* activities in Chapters 9 and 10.

Print a screenshot of the *Open Encounters* screen after signing any unsigned notes with *Visits* captured. Label it "Activity 8-23" and place it in your assignment folder.

CRITICAL THINKING   Having completed the activities in this chapter, reflect on your ability to integrate the patient relationship aspect and the clinical side of your duties. At the beginning of the chapter, you were encouraged to think about the patient's peace of mind as you receive and enter lab results, and the process of promptly notifying the provider. The other very important piece of processing and recording lab results is the integrity of the data entered. When you complete the Build Your Proficiency *Results* activities, keep in mind the following: What steps did you take to enter lab data? What measures were taken to ensure data accuracy? Although the majority of lab results are sent electronically to the patient's EMR in a live practice, there are still some instances where the practice will receive lab result by paper and/or fax. Some practices scan the results to the patient's chart; some enter the data into the patient's electronic chart; some do both. After completing the activities and Build Your Proficiency activities in this chapter, what conclusions have you reached about lab results? Would you advocate one method over another? Why or why not? Describe the "best practice" for entering lab results.

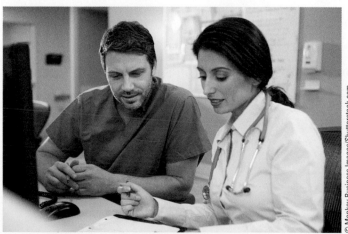

© Monkey Business Images/Shutterstock.com

SUMMARY

This chapter has focused on other clinical documentation and advanced features in Harris CareTracker EMR. You learned to navigate the *Progress Notes* application, which allows you to view and manage the list of notes saved for the patient, and complete advanced activities.

The *Results* application was also introduced. Although results are not received electronically in your student version of Harris CareTracker EMR, you will learn to manually enter lab results and to customize, graph, and print patient results in the Build Your Proficiency activities.

We expanded on the knowledge you learned from earlier chapters and completed activities related to the *ToDo* application, focusing now on the clinical side of Harris CareTracker. Activities performed that mimic a medical assistant's clinical responsibilities included creating new *ToDos* and *Mail* messages, accessing and viewing mail messages, as well as replying to, moving, and managing your inbox. We also reviewed advanced features of Harris CareTracker EMR such as generating *Recall Letters* and running *Immunization Lot* reports.

Congratulations on completing Practice Management and EMR components, functions, and activities in your student version of Harris CareTracker PM and EMR ! You will now advance to the *Billing* and *Collections* features in Chapters 9 and 10.

CHECK YOUR KNOWLEDGE

Select the best response.

_____ 1. The *Progress Notes* application displays a list of notes recorded during each patient appointment. *Progress Notes* include information such as:

      a. Patient's history   c. Allergies

      b. Medications   d. All of the above

_____ 2. In addition to the *Progress Notes* application, you have quick access to progress notes via other locations. Which is not one of the alternate ways to access progress notes?

      a. *Quick Picks*   c. *Progress Notes* icon in the *Clinical Toolbar*

      b. *Select Encounter* dialog box   d. *Progress Notes* application

_____ 3. When can you make edits to a progress note after it has been signed by the provider and supervising provider?

      a. Never   c. If the signing provider unsigns the note first

      b. At any time   d. When there is no addendum on the progress note

_____ 4. Which statement is true regarding deleted progress notes?

      a. Progress notes can never be deleted.   c. You can only delete a signed note.

      b. You can only delete an unsigned note.   d. None of the above.

_____ 5. Who can "unsign" a progress note?

      a. An operator with "Break the Glass" privileges   c. The supervising physician

                                   d. Any operator with access to the progress note

      b. The operator who signed the note

_____ 6. If a progress note requires a co-signature, the *Signed* column displays:

      a. "Y"   c. *Edit* icon

      b. "CS"   d. *Pencil* icon

_____ 7. If a *Result* has an "unmatched status," the result is saved only in the *Results* application of which of the following locations?

    a. Patient alerts   c. *Clinical Today* module

    b. *Home* module   d. Both b and c.

_____ 8. The *Action* menu in the *Results* column allows you to do the following:

    a. Print the result   c. Delete the result

    b. Attach the result to a *ToDo*   d. All of the above

_____ 9. Which of the following is not a type of *Recall Letter* available when using the *Recalls/Letters Due* application?

    a. Appointment recalls   c. Appointment reminders

    b. Outstanding orders   d. Missed/cancelled appointments

_____ 10. Which of the following is a reason to run an *Immunization Lot* report?

    a. Product recall   c. Monitor expiration dates

    b. Monitory inventory   d. All of the above

CASE STUDIES

Case Study 8-1

Patient: Adam Thompson

(**Note**: You must have completed Case Study 7-3 in order to complete Case Study 8-1.) Add an *Addendum* to Adam Thompson's progress note as follows: "Patient went to ED and was admitted to NVGH for treatment." Refer to Activity 8-7 for guidance if needed.

🖳 **Print a screenshot of the screens that illustrate you entered the addendum. Label them "Case Study 8-1" and place it in your assignment folder.**

Case Study 8-2

Patient: Alex Brady

    a. Create an addendum for Alex Brady's encounter dated December 12, 2016 as follows: "Mother called on 12/18/2016 to inquire if any vaccinations are required for overseas travel. Sent the CDC recommendations for traveling to South America." Refer to Activity 8-7 for guidance if needed.

🖳 **Print a screenshot that illustrates you entered the addendum. Label it "Case Study 8-2a" and place it in your assignment folder.**

    b. Create an addendum for the patient's encounter dated March 10, 2017 as follows: "Mother called on 03/12/2017 at 4:50 pm to say Alex is refusing to eat solid foods; asked her to bring him into office for immediate follow-up. She will go to Urgent Care for after-hours visit." Refer to Activity 8-7 for guidance if needed.

🖳 **Print a screenshot that illustrates you entered the addendum. Label it "Case Study 8-2b" and place it in your assignment folder.**

(*Continues*)

(Continued)

Case Study 8-3

Create *ToDos* as listed in **Table 8-5**. For each *ToDo* in **Table 8-5** use the *Category* "Interoffice," *Type* "EHR," and *Reason* "Phone Call (Patient)." Refer to Activity 8-13 for guidance if needed.

Table 8-5   New *ToDo* Messages

FROM	TO	SUBJECT	SEVERITY	NOTES (MESSAGE)	PATIENT
You	You *Though you have selected You for the To field, in the real world, you would be sending this to Dr. Raman.*	Medication Question	Medium	Patient wants to know if he can take a multivitamin while he is taking Coumadin. Please advise and I will return call to patient. Thank you.	Bradley Torez
You	You (see above comment)	Referral/ Authorization Status	Medium	Patient called and wants to know if her request for referral and authorization for MRI has been ordered. Please call patient at home phone between 3:00 p.m. and 5:00 p.m. OK to leave message on voicemail.	Kimberly Johnson

Courtesy of Harris CareTracker PM and EMR

🖥 **Print a screenshot from the Messages tab that reflects the *ToDo*s you created. Label it "Case Study 8-3" and place it in your assignment folder.**

Case Study 8-4

Create *Recalls* for the following patients, using each patient's PCP as provider. Refer to Activity 8-20 for guidance if needed.

   a. Jane Morgan (recall for CPE due two years from today). Include a note to send lab (complete panel) and mammogram orders one month prior to CPE.

   b. Harriet Oshea (recall for CPE due two years from today). Include a note to send lab (complete panel) and mammogram orders one month prior to CPE.

🖥 **Print a screenshot that illustrates you entered the recalls. Label it "Case Study 8-4" and place it in your assignment folder.**

BUILD YOUR PROFICIENCY

Proficiency Builder 8-1: Enter Results Manually

Note: This activity is required in order to complete Proficiency Builders 8-2, 8-3, 8-4 and 8-5. Although not typical, there are times when results may be manually recorded in the patient's electronic health record. With today's technology and integrated electronic medical records, most lab results come across electronically, into the provider's inbox and to the patient's EMR. In the case where results are received from a lab or facility that is not electronically integrated with your practice's EHR, the results would normally be first reviewed and signed off (validated) by the provider, and then either scanned into the patient's electronic health record, or entered into the EHR manually, depending on the provider's/practice's preference and protocol. There are two schools of thought on this. Entering laboratory results into the EMR allows for tracking results electronically and enabling historical data to compare and graph; however, there is also the increased chance for data-entry error. Given the sensitive nature of the lab values, any data-entry error could have a detrimental effect to the patient's care. In order to understand the steps to manually enter results, you will now manually record *Results* for patient Jane Morgan's urinalysis lab order you created in Activity 7-2. Enter the *results* found in Source Document 8-3, found at the end of this activity.

Prior to beginning this activity, make a note of the encounter date and collected time (if recorded) for which the lab order was created. You will need this information when you enter results manually. If the collected time is not recorded on the *Order*, refer back to the *Scheduling* module and *History* tab to identify the date and time of the patient's appointment.
Date/Time: _____

This activity requires in-depth review and careful data entry. Read through the entire activity before beginning to enter data. Have your source document available, and review the figures provided to help guide your entries.

1. With patient Jane Morgan in context, click on the *Medical Record* module.

2. In the *Patient Health History* pane, click on *Orders/Referrals*. This will launch the *Orders* window.

3. Click the *Arrow* ▼ icon next to the order for which you want to enter results (urinalysis) and select "Enter Results" (**Figure 8-57**). Harris CareTracker EMR displays the *Manual Lab Results* dialog box. In the *Manual Lab Results* dialog box, scroll down and you will see that both of the Lab Orders previously entered are located on the same page.

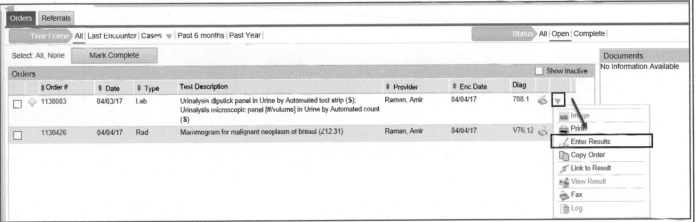

Figure 8-57   Enter Results Link

Courtesy of Harris CareTracker PM and EMR

4. Review the order information. The information is based on the entries made at the time of creating the order.

5. In the top part of the *Manual Lab Results* box, enter the selections at the time of the order (as listed in Source Document 8-3, located at the end of this activity):

   a. *Laboratory*: Select the first lab that displays in the drop-down (or leave as is if a *Laboratory* is already displaying).

   b. *Ordering Provider*: Amir Raman

   c. *Result Type*: Lab

(*Continues*)

(*Continued*)

    d.   *Filler Order #*: Leave blank

    e.   *Fasting or Non-Fasting*: Non-Fasting

    f.   *Collected Date*: Enter the date of the appointment you created for Jane Morgan in Activity 4-1.

    g.   *Collected Time*: Enter the time that was recorded in the original order, or if no time was recorded, enter a time that is 15 minutes after the start of Jane Morgan's appointment.

6. In the *Manual Lab Results* screen, be sure to scroll down to locate the "Urinalysis dipstick panel in Urine by Automated test strip" fields. Because both urinalysis orders were entered at the same time they both appear on the *Manual Lab Results* screen, but not necessarily in the same order.

7. Enter the results in the *Value, Units* (if applicable), *Abnormal,* and *Reference Range* fields for the codes selected, as noted in Jane Morgan's lab result form (Source Document 8-3), using **Figure 8-58** as a reference. When you have finished entering the results for this test, your screen should match **Figure 8-58**. (**Note:** You will notice that both tests and results are on one lab order. Scroll up/down the Order to locate.)

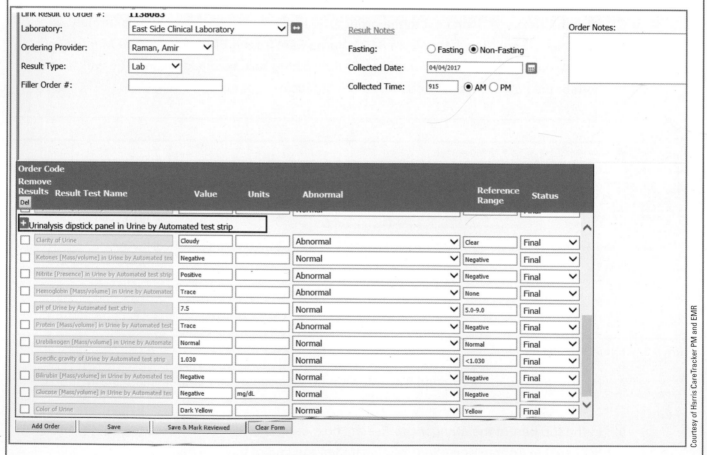

Figure 8-58   *Manual Lab Results Screen (Urinalysis dipstick)*

Courtesy of Harris CareTracker PM and EMR

    a.   In the *Value* box, enter the "Results" or "Abnormal Results" entry as indicated on the lab result form.

    b.   In the *Units* box, enter the units if indicated on the lab result form.

c.   In the *Abnormal* box, indicate whether the results were "Normal" or "Abnormal."

d.   In the *Reference Range* box, enter the normal range for the test.

e.   In the *Status* list, click the status of the result code. For example, if the result received states "incomplete," click *Incomplete* in the *Status* list; otherwise select *Final.* For Jane Morgan's results, select *Final.*

 TIP You can enter partial results on panels by entering a value for the result under the *Value* column and selecting the correct option under the *Abnormal* column. **Example**: If the order is for a CBC (panel) and there are multiple individual tests that are part of that panel, you do not have to enter values for all tests to save the result.

8.   Now scroll up using the inner scroll line just to the right of the *Status* column (not the outer left scroll line) and enter the results for the remaining test: "Urinalysis microscopic panel [#/volume] in Urine by Automated count." Refer to the lab results form (refer to Source Document 8-3, located at the end of this activity). Your entries should mirror **Figure 8-59**.

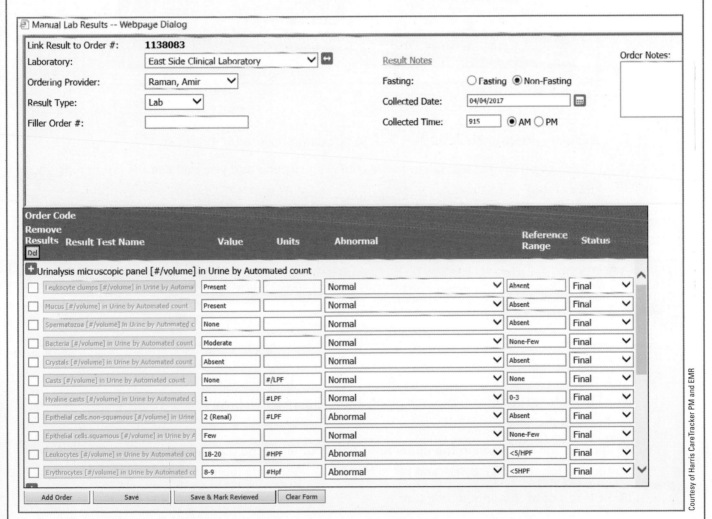

Figure 8-59   Manual Lab Results Screen (Urinalysis microscopic panel)

💾 **Print the Manual Lab Results screen for the Urinalysis Lab Order. Label it "BYP 8-1A" and place it in your assignment folder.**

(Continues)

(Continued)

9. Based on your requirements, click one of the following action buttons: *Add Order, Save, Save & Mark Reviewed,* or *Clear Form* (**Figure 8-60**). Select *Save.*

Add Order
Save
Save & Mark Reviewed
Clear Form

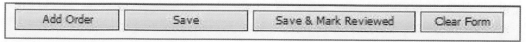

Figure 8-60 Results Action Buttons

Courtesy of Harris CareTracker PM and EMR

10. Once you click *Save,* you will receive a pop-up asking if you want to mark the order as complete (**Figure 8-61**). Select *No.*

Do you want to mark this order complete?
Yes
No

Courtesy of Harris CareTracker PM and EMR

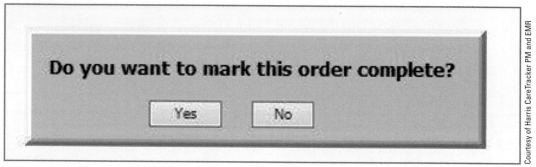

Figure 8-61 Mark Order Complete

11. You will receive another pop-up stating "Update Successful." Click *OK.*
12. Now click on the *Results* tab in the *Health History* pane and you will see the lab results you just entered.
13. Click directly on the lab result you entered (**Figure 8-62**).

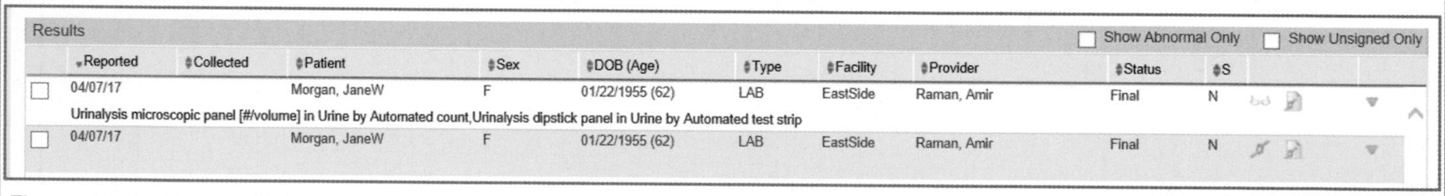

Results
Show Abnormal Only
Show Unsigned Only
Reported
Collected
Patient
Sex
DOB (Age)
Type
Facility
Provider
Status
S
04/07/17 Morgan, JaneW F 01/22/1955 (62) LAB EastSide Raman, Amir Final N
Urinalysis microscopic panel [#/volume] in Urine by Automated count,Urinalysis dipstick panel in Urine by Automated test strip
04/07/17 Morgan, JaneW F 01/22/1955 (62) LAB EastSide Raman, Amir Final N

Figure 8-62 Results Columns

Courtesy of Harris CareTracker PM and EMR

14. The *Lab Results* dialog box will display (see **Figure 8-63**). Note that "Abnormal" results display in red.

Click on the *Print* icon in the upper-right-hand corner of the dialog box to print a copy of the lab results, label it "BYP 8-1B," and place in your assignments folder.

15. Close out of the print dialog box.
16. Close out of the Lab Results Report dialog box.

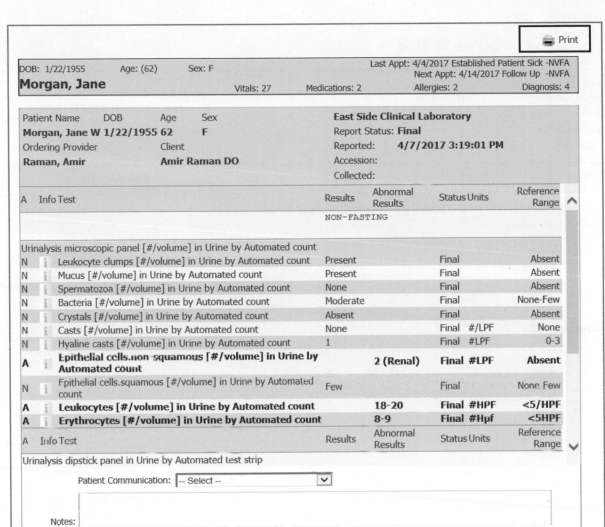

DOB: 1/22/1955	Age: (62)	Sex: F		Last Appt: 4/4/2017 Established Patient Sick -NVFA
Morgan, Jane				Next Appt: 4/14/2017 Follow Up -NVFA
		Vitals: 27	Medications: 2	Allergies: 2 Diagnosis: 4

Patient Name	DOB	Age	Sex	**East Side Clinical Laboratory**
Morgan, Jane W 1/22/1955 62			**F**	Report Status: **Final**
Ordering Provider		Client		Reported: **4/7/2017 3:19:01 PM**
Raman, Amir		**Amir Raman DO**		Accession:
				Collected:

A	Info Test	Results	Abnormal Results	Status Units	Reference Range
			NON-FASTING		
	Urinalysis microscopic panel [#/volume] in Urine by Automated count				
N	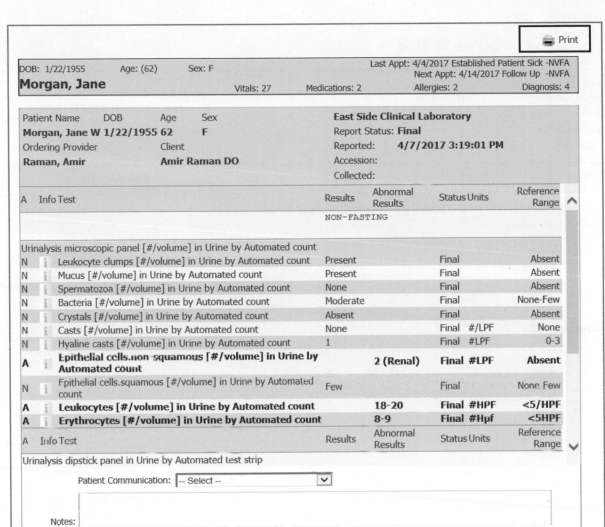 Leukocyte clumps [#/volume] in Urine by Automated count	Present		Final	Absent
N	Mucus [#/volume] in Urine by Automated count	Present		Final	Absent
N	Spermatozoa [#/volume] in Urine by Automated count	None		Final	Absent
N	Bacteria [#/volume] in Urine by Automated count	Moderate		Final	None-Few
N	Crystals [#/volume] in Urine by Automated count	Absent		Final	Absent
N	Casts [#/volume] in Urine by Automated count	None		Final #/LPF	None
N	Hyaline casts [#/volume] in Urine by Automated count	1		Final #LPF	0-3
A	**Epithelial cells.non-squamous [#/volume] in Urine by Automated count**		**2 (Renal)**	**Final #LPF**	**Absent**
N	Epithelial cells.squamous [#/volume] in Urine by Automated count	Few		Final	None-Few
A	**Leukocytes [#/volume] in Urine by Automated count**		**18-20**	**Final #HPF**	**<5/HPF**
A	**Erythrocytes [#/volume] in Urine by Automated count**		**8-9**	**Final #Hpf**	**<5HPF**
A	Info Test	Results	Abnormal Results	Status Units	Reference Range

Urinalysis dipstick panel in Urine by Automated test strip

Patient Communication: [-- Select -- ▼]

Notes:

Figure 8-63   Jane Morgan—Lab Results Form

(Continues)

(*Continued*)

Source Document 8-3

Patient Name	DOB	Age	Sex		
Morgan, Jane W	**1/22/1955**	**62**	**F**	Report Status:	**Final**
Ordering Provider				Reported:	**08/01/20XX (2 days after the Collected date) 10:07:05 PM**
Amir Raman DO				Accession:	
A = Abnormal N = Normal				Collected:	**7/30/2017 (use actual Order date)**

A	Test	Results (Value)	Abnormal Results	Units	Reference Range
URINALYSIS DIPSTICK PANEL IN URINE BY AUTOMATED TEST STRIP					
A	**Clarity of Urine**		**Cloudy**		**Clear**
N	Ketones [Mass/volume] in Urine by Automated test strip	Negative			Negative
A	**Nitrite [Presence] in Urine by Automated test strip**		**Positive**		**Negative**
A	**Hemoglobin [Mass/volume] in Urine by Automated test strip**		**Trace**		**None**
N	pH of Urine by Automated test strip	7.5			5.0-9.0
A	**Protein [Mass/volume] in Urine by Automated test strip**		**Trace**		**Negative**
N	Urobilinogen [Mass/volume] in Urine by Automated test strip	Normal			Normal
N	Specific gravity of Urine by Automated test strip	1.030			< 1.030
N	Bilirubin [Mass/volume] in Urine by Automated test strip	Negative			Negative
N	Glucose [Mass/volume] in Urine by Automated test strip	Negative		mg/dL	Negative
A	**Color of Urine**	**Dark Yellow**			**Yellow**
URINALYSIS MICROSCOPIC PANEL [#/VOLUME] IN URINE BY AUTOMATED COUNT					
A	**Leukocyte clumps [#/volume] in Urine by Automated count**		**Present**		**Absent**
A	**Mucus [#/volume] in Urine by Automated count**		**Present**		**Absent**
N	Spermatozoa [#/volume] in Urine by Automated count	None			Absent
A	**Bacteria [#/volume] in Urine by Automated count**		**Moderate**		**None-Few**
N	Crystals [#/volume] in Urine by Automated count	Absent			Absent
N	Casts [#/volume] in Urine by Automated count	None		#/LPF	None

Patient Name	DOB	Age		Sex
Morgan, Jane W	**1/22/1955**	**62**		**F**
Ordering Provider				
Amir Raman DO				
A = Abnormal N = Normal				

Report Status: **Final**
Reported: **08/01/20XX (2 days after the Collected date) 10:07:05 PM**
Accession:
Collected: **7/30/2017 (use actual Order date)**

A	Test	Results	Abnormal Results	Units	Reference Range
N	Hyaline casts [#/volume] in Urine by Automated count	1		#/LPF	0-3
A	**Epithelial cells.non-squamous [#/volume] in Urine by Automated count**		**2 (Renal)**	**#/LPF**	**Absent**
N	Epithelial cells.squamous [#/volume] in Urine by Automated count	Few			None-Few
A	**Leukocytes [#/volume] in Urine by Automated count**		**18-20**	**#/HPF**	**<5/HPF**
A	**Erythrocytes [#/volume] in Urine by Automated count**		**8-9**	**#/HPF**	**<5/HPF**

Proficiency Builder 8-2: Create Customized *Result* Views

Depending on provider preferences, you can customize the view in the *Results* tab. You can select one or more providers and set the defaults for the customized view.

1. With patient Jane Morgan in context, click the *Medical Record* module.

2. In the *Patient Health History* pane, click *Results*. Harris CareTracker EMR displays the *Results* window with a list of patient results.

3. Click the *Settings* ⚙ icon in the top right corner of the screen, which will open the *Set Results Default* window.

4. Select the options you want to set as the default in both the *List View Operator Defaults* and *Chart View Operator Defaults* sections (**Figure 8-64**).

    a. Set *Time Frame*, *Result Type*, and *Provider* to "All."

    b. Set *View* to "Graph" and *Reported Date* to "All."

(Continues)

(*Continued*)

Set Results Default   ✕

List View Operator Defaults

Time Frame   All | Past Month | Past 3 Months | Past 6 Months | Past Year

Result Type   All | Lab | Radiology |

Provider   - Select -   ▾

Chart View Operator Defaults

View   ○ Vertical Chart ○ Horizontal Chart ● Graph

Reported Date   All | Past Month | Past 3 Months | Past 6 Months | Past Year

Save | ✖ Cancel

Courtesy of Harris CareTracker PM and EMR

Figure 8-64   Set Results Default Dialog Box

Print a screenshot of the Set Results Default box. Label it "BYP 8-2" and place it in your assignment folder.

5. Click *Save*. A "Success" message displays to confirm the action.

6. Click *Close*.

Proficiency Builder 8-3: Filter the Patient's *Result* List

To further customize provider preferences, you can also filter the view in the *Results* tab to include only abnormal results, show only unsigned results, and more. This activity is designed to familiarize you with the various settings you can select for sorting multiple labs only.

1. With patient Jane Morgan in context, click the *Medical Record* module.

2. In the *Patient Health History* pane, click *Results*. Harris CareTracker EMR displays the *Results* window with a list of patient results.

3. Complete each the following:

   a. You have the option to change the display of results based on the *Time Frame* of the result by selecting the *All*, *Past Month*, *Past 3 Months*, *Past 6 Months*, or *Past Year* tabs. Select *All* (**Figure 8-65**).

   b. You can filter the results based on the *Result Type* by selecting the *All*, *Lab*, or *Radiology* tab. Select *All*.

   c. You can view results pertaining to one or more providers by selecting the checkboxes in the *Provider* list. Click *All* so that you will view results pertaining to all providers and click the *Refresh* icon.

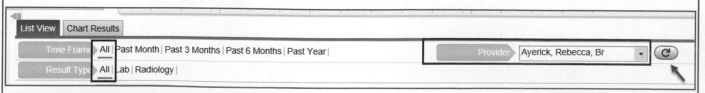

Figure 8-65   Select Option "All" for Viewing Results

Courtesy of Harris CareTracker PM and EMR

d. View abnormal results by selecting the *Show Abnormal Only* checkbox. An abnormal result displays the specific test values in red in the observation row.

e. Now uncheck the box.

f. View the unsigned results by selecting the *Show Unsigned Only* checkbox. You can also sort signed and unsigned results by clicking on the *Signed* column.

g. Now uncheck the box.

Print a screenshot of the window after you have filtered the patient results as directed. Label it "BYP 8-3" and place it in your assignment folder.

Proficiency Builder 8-4: Graph Patient Results

Depending again on provider preferences, you can customize the view in the *Results* tab by creating graphs and more.

1. With patient Jane Morgan in context, click the *Medical Record* module.

2. In the *Patient Health History* pane, click *Results*. The *List View* tab opens by default.

3. Click on the *Chart Results* tab.

4. In the *Lab Test Values* list, you have the option of selecting *All* or selecting the checkbox of the results you want to include in the chart. Select *All*.

5. In the *Reported Date* list, click the time period you want. Select *Past Year*.

6. In *View*, you have the option to select *Vertical Chart*, *Horizontal Chart*, or *Graph* (**Figure 8-66**). Select *Vertical Chart*.

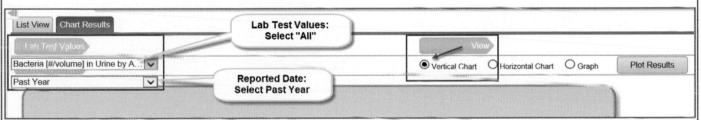

Figure 8-66   *Select Vertical Chart Results View*   Courtesy of Harris CareTracker PM and EMR

7. Click *Plot Results*. Your screen will look like **Figure 8-67**.

8. Repeat steps 6 and 7, and select and plot the results in *Horizontal Chart* and *Graph* view as well. **Hint:** If you receive an error when you click *Graph* view, then proceed without printing the *Graph* view. See your student companion website for more information.

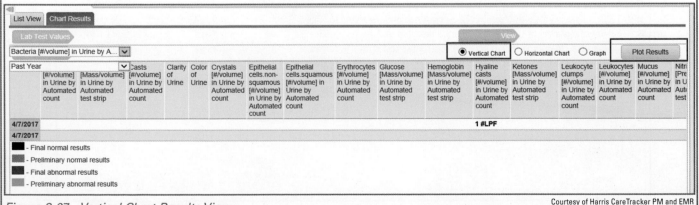

Figure 8-67   *Vertical Chart Results View*   Courtesy of Harris CareTracker PM and EMR

(*Continues*)

(*Continued*)

Print a screenshot of each of the final chart views selected and plotted. Label it "BYP 8-4" and place It in your assignment folder.

Proficiency Builder 8-5: Print a Single Result

The *Results* application prints test result records to give to the patient and other entities such as specialists and hospitals that are treating the patient. Fewer laboratory tests will be ordered because health practitioners across the provider network will have the results of earlier tests, eliminating the need to reorder tests that were previously completed. The *Results* application provides two methods to print a specific result: you can use the *Action* menu in the *Result* application or open the result to print.

1. With patient Jane Morgan in context, click the *Medical Record* module.

2. In the *Patient Health History* pane, click *Results*. Harris CareTracker EMR displays the *Results* window with a list of patient results.

3. For each printing option, clicking *Print* will open a new screen with the printable results. Click *Print* on the shortcut menu to print the result. Do one of the following:

   a. Click the result (urinalysis lab order) to open it (**Figure 3-68**) and then click *Print* in the *Lab Results Report* dialog box.

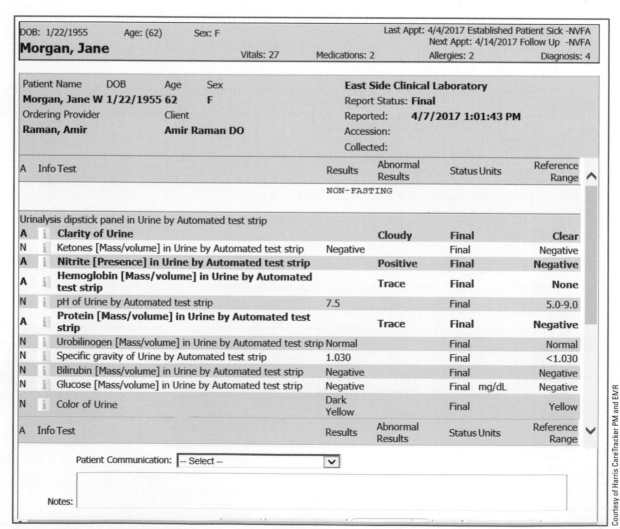

Figure 8-68   Lab Results Screen

b. In the *Results* window, click the *Arrow* ▼ icon (**Figure 8-69**) beside the urinalysis order and click *Print*.

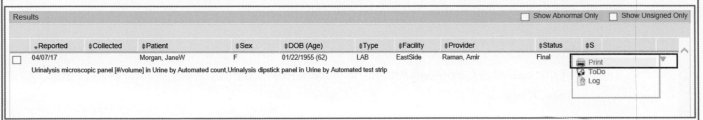

Figure 8-69   *Print from the Actions Menu*

c. Go to the *Clinical Today* module > *Quick Tasks* pane. Click the arrow next to the *Results* link (**Figure 8-70**). (**Note**: If there are no *Results* showing, check your *Batch* and make sure the ordering provider is displaying.) Click on the result, which opens a new screen. Click the *Print* 🖫 icon at the top right of the screen.

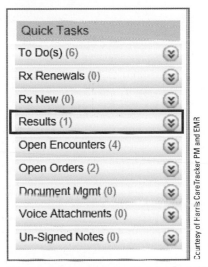

Figure 8-70   *Results Link in Quick Tasks Pane*

d. Go to the *Home* module > *Dashboard* tab > *Clinical* section > *Results* link (**Figure 8-71**), and then click the *Print* 🖫 icon next to the urinalysis results.

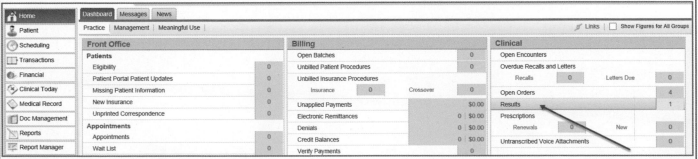

Figure 8-71   *Results Link from Home Dashboard*

🖫 **Print the patient's result, label it "BYP 8-5" and place it in your assignment folder.**

(*Continues*)

(Continued)

Proficiency Builder 8-6: Enter Results Manually

Note: For patient Adam Thompson, you must have completed Case Study 7-3 to complete this activity. For patient Ellen Ristino, you must have completed Proficiency Builder 7-4 in order to complete this activity.

a.   Enter *results* for the *Open Lab Orders* found in Source Document 8-4 (located at the end of this activity) for patient Adam Thompson. Refer to Proficiency Builder 8-1 for guidance, if needed.

b.   Enter *results* for the *Open Lab Orders* found in Source Document 8-5 (located at the end of this activity) for patient Ellen Ristino. Refer to Proficiency Builder 8-1 for guidance, if needed.

💾 **Print the patients' results, label them "BYP 8-6a and 8-6b," and place them in your assignment folder.**

Source Document 8-4

Patient Name	DOB	Age	Gender		
Thompson, Adam	**1/1/1942**	**75**	**M**	Report Status:	**Final**
Ordering Provider				Reported:	**08/01/20XX (2 days after the Collected date) 7:17:14 PM**
Anthony Brockton MD				Accession:	
N = Normal H = Above High Normal L = Below Low Normal				Collected:	**8/12/2017 (use actual Order date)**

A	Test	Results (Value)	Abnormal Results	Units	Reference Range
	CBC W AUTO DIFFERENTIAL PANEL IN BLOOD				
N	Granulocytes %				
N	Erythrocyte distribution width				
N	Neutrophils.band form #				
N	Platelet distribution width				
N	Platelet mean volume				
N	Neutrophils.band form %				
N	Lymphocytes Variant %				
N	Lymphocytes Variant #				
N	Hematocrit %	41.2		%	39.0-50.0
N	Leukocytes other #				
N	Auto Differential panel in Blood				
N	Other cells %				
N	Complete blood count (hemogram) panel in Blood by Automated count				
N	Other cells #				
N	Monocytes %	12.9		%	0.0-13.0
N	Leukocytes #	5.2		Thous/cu. mm	3.9-11.1
N	Basophils #				
H	**Basophils %**		**3.0**	**%**	**0.0-2.0**
N	Eosinophils #				
N	Eosinophils %	0.6		%	0.0-8.0
N	Hemoglobin	14.5		g/dL	13.2-16.9
N	Lymphocytes #				
N	Lymphocytes %	46.1		%	15.0-48.0
N	Monocytes #				
N	Neutrophils #				
N	Neutrophils %	40.1		%	38.0-80.0
N	Platelets #	172		Thous/cu. mm	140-390
H	**Erythrocyte mean corpuscular hemoglobin**		**41.4**	**pg**	**27.0-34.0 pg**
N	Erythrocyte mean corpuscular hemoglobin concentration	35.3		%	32.0-35.5 g/dL
H	**Erythrocyte mean corpuscular volume**		**117**	**fL**	**78.0-100.0 fL**

(Continues)

(*Continued*)

Patient Name	DOB	Age	Gender		
Thompson, Adam	**1/1/1942**	**75**	**M**	Report Status:	**Final**
Ordering Provider				Reported:	**08/01/20XX (2 days after the Collected date) 7:17:14 PM**
Anthony Brockton MD				Accession:	
N = Normal H = Above High Normal L = Below Low Normal				Collected:	**8/12/2017 (use actual Order date)**

A	Test	Results	Abnormal Results	Units	Reference Range
N	Erythrocyte distribution width %				
L	**Erythrocytes #**		**3.51**	**Mil/cu.mm**	**4.2-5.7 Mil/cu.mm**
	ELECTROLYTES 1998 PANEL IN SERUM OR PLASMA				
N	Carbon dioxide, total [Moles/volume] in Serum or Plasma	31		mEq/L	22-32
N	Chloride [Moles/volume] in Serum or Plasma	122		mEq/L	118-132
N	Potassium [Moles/volume] in Serum or Plasma	4.2		mEq/L	3.5-5.0
N	Sodium [Moles/volume] in Serum or Plasma	140		mEq/L	135-145
H	**Anion gap in Serum or Plasma**		**18**	**mEq/L**	**7-16**

Source Document 8-5

Patient Name	DOB	Age	Gender	
Ristino, Ellen	**11/1/1956**	**61**	**F**	Report Status: **Final**
Ordering Provider				Reported: **08/01/20XX (2 days after the Collected date) 8:12:58 AM**
Anthony Brockton MD				Accession:
A = Abnormal N = Normal				Collected: **7/29/2017 (use actual Order date)**

A	Test	Results	Abnormal Results	Units	Reference Range
		FASTING			
HETEROPHILE AB [TITER] IN SERUM BY AGGLUTINATION					
N	Heterophile Ab [Titer] in Serum by Agglutination	Negative			Negative
CBC W AUTO DIFFERENTIAL PANEL IN BLOOD					
N	Granulocytes %				
N	Erythrocyte distribution width				
N	Neutrophils.band form #				
N	Platelet distribution width				
N	Platelet mean volume				
N	Neutrophils.band form %				
N	Lymphocytes Variant %				
N	Lymphocytes Variant #				
N	Hematocrit %	42		%	39.0-50.0
N	Leukocytes other #				
N	Auto Differential panel in Blood				
N	Other cells %				
N	Complete blood count (hemogram) panel in Blood by Automated count				
N	Other cells #				
N	Monocytes %	3		%	0.0-13.0
N	Leukocytes #	4.2		Thous/cu. mm	3.9-11.1
N	Basophils #				
N	Basophils %	0		%	0.0-2.0
N	Eosinophils #				
N	Eosinophils %	1		%	0.0-8.0
N	Hemoglobin	14		g/dL	13.2-16.9
N	Lymphocytes #				
H	**Lymphocytes %**		**52**	**%**	**15.0-48.0**
N	Monocytes #				
N	Neutrophils #				
N	Neutrophils %	44		%	38.0-80.0
N	Platelets #	320		Thous/cu. mm	140-390

(Continues)

(Continued)

Patient Name	DOB	Age	Gender		
Ristino, Ellen	**11/1/1956**	**61**	**F**	Report Status:	**Final**
Ordering Provider				Reported:	**08/01/20XX (2 days after the Collected date) 8:12:58 AM**
Anthony Brockton MD				Accession:	
A = Abnormal N = Normal				Collected:	**7/29/2017 (use actual Order date)**

A	Test	Results	Abnormal Results	Units	Reference Range
N	Erythrocyte mean corpuscular hemoglobin	31.8		pg	27.0-34.0
N	Erythrocyte mean corpuscular hemoglobin concentration	33.3		%	32.0-35.5
N	Erythrocyte mean corpuscular volume	95.5		fl	78.0-100.0
N	Erythrocyte distribution width %				
N	Erythrocytes #	4.4		Mil/cu.mm	4.2-5.7

MODULE 4
Billing Skills

This module includes:

- Chapter 9: Billing

- Chapter 10: ClaimsManager and Collections

As a health care professional, you may use Harris CareTracker PM and EMR to manually enter and edit charges, and generate claims. Once claims are generated, you will perform the steps to work claims, print patient statements, review overdue accounts, and perform collection actions. All the activities you will complete in this module mimic a real-world setting using the administrative and financial features of electronic health records.

QUICK START

In the patient workflow, billing tasks are performed after the patient has been seen by the provider. Because Harris CareTracker is a live EMR, you will need to complete several tasks to simulate a live clinic where patient accounts are ready for billing. The following activities are required in order to complete the activities in this module. **If you have been following along in this book from the beginning and have completed all Required** ▶ **activities as you've moved sequentially through the text, then you have already completed the activities below and can move forward. If you are beginning with this module, then you will need to complete the activities below *before* you can complete any other activities in this module.**

Be sure you are working in a supported browser (Internet Explorer 11 or Safari for iPad) before you begin. Other browsers (such as Chrome and Firefox) are not supported. Review Best Practices.

- ❑ Activity 1-1: Disable Toolbars
- ❑ Activity 1-2: Set Up Tabbed Browsing
- ❑ Activity 1-3: Turn Off Pop-Up Blocker
- ❑ Activity 1-4: Change Page Setup
- ❑ Activity 1-5: Add Harris CareTracker to Trusted Sites
- ❑ Activity 1-6: Clear Your Cache
  - *Note: Remember that you should clear your cache each time before you begin working in CareTracker.*
- ❑ Activity 1-8: Disable Download Blocking
  - *Note: Once you have completed the system set-up requirements (Activities 1-1, 1-2, 1-3, 1-4, 1-5, and 1-8), you will not need to repeat these activities unless you change the device you are using or the settings automatically default back to prior settings.*
- ❑ Activity 1-9: Register Your Credentials and Create Your Harris CareTracker PM and EMR Training Company
  - *Note: It will take up to 24 hours for your CareTracker "Student Company" to be created. Plan accordingly.*
- ❑ Activity 2-1: Log in to Harris CareTracker PM and EMR
  - *Note: Be sure to write down your new password inside the front cover of your book for easy reference.*

- ❑ Activity 2-5: Open a New Fiscal Year
  - *Note: Every January 1, you will need to open a new fiscal year.*
- ❑ Activity 2-6: Open a Fiscal Period
  - *Note: Every first of the month, you will need to open a new fiscal period.*
- ❑ Activity 3-1: Searching for a Patient by Name
  - *Complete steps 1 and 2 only.*
  - *Note: You will search for patients throughout the text using the steps in Activity 3-1.*
- ❑ Activity 4-1: Book an Appointment
  - *Book an appointment for Jane Morgan, Ellen Ristino, Craig X. Smith, Adam Thompson, and Edith Robinson, but do **NOT** book an appointment for Francisco Powell Jimenez at this time.*
  - *The directions for this activity state to book the appointment for one week from today. Instead, book the appointment for today (the day you are working). If no appointments are available today, then book the appointment for a day within the past week.*
  - *Also book an "Established Patient Sick" appointment for today for Barbara Watson with Amir Raman. Her chief complaint is "Fever—103F."*
- ❑ Activity 4-14: Create a Batch
  - *Note: At various times throughout the activities, you will be directed to create batches.*
- ❑ Activity 4-15: Accept/Enter a Payment
- ❑ Activity 4-17: Accept/Enter a Payment
  - *Complete steps 1 through 12 only. You do not need to print receipts for this activity at this time.*
- ❑ Activity 4-19: Post a Batch
  - *Note: At various times throughout the activities, you will be directed to post batches.*
- ❑ Activity 7-18: Capture a Visit
  - *Also capture the visit for Jane Morgan. Enter the CPT codes 99213 and 90746 in the Procedures tab. Enter the ICD-10 codes N39.0, R30.0, and I10 in the Diagnosis tab. View the Visit Summary tab and save the information, making sure to receive the message "An error occurred connecting to Claims manager. Transaction saved" before moving on.*
- ❑ Activity 7-21(a-d): Capture a Visit
  - *Complete only parts A-D for Ellen Ristino, Craig X. Smith, Barbara Watson, and Edith Robinson at this time. Do **NOT** complete parts E, F, or G.*

Once you have completed these activities as part of this Quick Start, you will not need to complete them again if you come across the activities while working in Chapters 1–7.

PREREQUISITES FOR CASE STUDIES

In addition to the activities listed in the Quick Start, you will need to complete the following case study if you plan to complete case studies in this module:

- ❑ Case Study 7-3
  - *Complete part B only.*

Billing

Key Terms

batch
clearinghouse
explanation of benefits
  (EOB)
explosion code

mnemonics
remittance advice (RA)
scrub
variance

Learning Objectives

1. Create a batch for financial transactions.
2. Manually enter a charge.
3. Edit an unposted charge.
4. Generate electronic and paper claims.
5. Perform activities related to electronic remittance including: posting payments and adjustments, and reconciling insurance payments.

Real-World Connection

Your challenge is to become familiar with the many different types of insurance plans and the effects on the practice when there is an issue regarding noncovered services. In order for the medical practice to be profitable, fees must be collected from patients for services rendered. The fees and copay can be collected at the time of the visit, or you can bill the patient after a claim has been submitted to the insurance company, depending on the type of insurance and the policy of the practice. It is NVFHA policy that copays must be collected from the patient at the office for each encounter. We only bill the copay when the patient does not have any form of payment available at the time of service. Upon receipt of payment from the insurance company and after any adjustment to the contracted rate is applied, the balance due will be billed to the patient.

Although it may be a delicate issue, you will be responsible for communicating the fees for services to patients. This discussion should take place prior to the patient's appointment with the physician to avoid an awkward situation, and again at any time there is a test ordered that will also include separate fees. With the ever-changing insurance environment and mandates from the Affordable Care Act (ACA), and the possible repeal and replacement of the ACA, you must verify the patient's insurance plan, deductibles, out-of-pocket amounts, and confirm that NVFHA is in fact contracted with the patient's insurance company before providing services. The deductibles with insurance plans available through the ACA and exchanges are extremely high (average for individuals is $6,500 per year or more and $10,000 or more per family). Consider how such a high deductible and out-of-pocket expenses will affect the patient's ability to pay and also the possibility that the patient may delay seeking health care due to the high insurance deductible.

If the patient's insurance is not contracted with NVFHA, the patient will be responsible for the entire fee. In some cases, patients will be forced to change providers to one that is contracted with their insurance; otherwise the costs would be unaffordable to the patient. Changing doctors is very stressful to many patients. Often they have developed relationships that span many years or decades. Therefore, it is important that you have an understanding of the various types of insurance and how to communicate effectively with patients in an articulate and compassionate manner. Even within the many types of insurance, copays and deductibles can vary widely. Some health plans have large deductibles and large copays. Other plans may require no copay at the time of visit, but the patient will pay a percentage of the contracted rate for the service.

(Continues)

Real-World Connection (*Continued*)

When you register a new patient and collect patient demographic information over the phone, you will gather insurance information as well. This will help determine what type of fee or payment will be required of the patient, and confirm that our practice is contracted with the patient's insurance carrier. The office policy must be clearly stated to the patients on the telephone, by written communication (on forms the patient must complete and sign), and by way of posted notices in the waiting room. Patients should be gently reminded in a very professional manner that payment will be expected at the time of service. Our automated answering system also conveys fee and payment options available.

INTRODUCTION

Harris CareTracker PM and EMR provides a secure environment to ensure that the billing process goes smoothly and the quality of the information sent to insurance carriers is clean. The *Billing* feature crosses many modules, applications, and functions. The normal flow for a claim in Harris CareTracker PM and EMR starts with a patient appointment, followed by checking in the patient where patient information is confirmed and updated. At the end of the patient visit, the services are recorded and reviewed before the claims are sent out.

Harris CareTracker PM and EMR will **scrub** the claim before it is sent to payers. Claim scrubbing ensures that claims are correctly coded before being sent to the insurance company, which reduces denials and increase payments to the practice. *ClaimsManager,* the claim scrubber in Harris CareTracker PM, provides a comprehensive set of coding and technical edits. Each individual edit may be enabled or disabled completely for a specific claim type or for an individual payer. Most claims are sent electronically in Harris CareTracker PM and any claims that have been identified as having a problem that would prevent them from being paid will show up on a *Worklist* list to be resolved.

This chapter introduces you to billing activities in Harris CareTracker PM and EMR. Having learned the concept and created a batch in Chapter 4, you will build upon activities previously completed. The **batch** is the essential component required before entering and posting any financial transaction such as charges, payments, adjustments, and refunds. In this chapter, you will perform billing functions, enter and edit charges and remittances, run a journal to verify your batch and entry information, view all open batches, and then post your batch into the system.

Once charges are entered, you will learn how to generate an insurance claim by using (by simulating) the electronic remittance features of Harris CareTracker PM. Activities include posting payments and adjustments, reconciliation, matching unmatched transactions, and working denials and credit balances. An **explanation of benefits (EOB)** (**Figure 9-1**) is the insurance company's written explanation to a claim provided to the patient, showing the amount paid by the insurance company, any contractual write-off amounts, and any balance that the patient must pay. The **remittance advice (RA)** is the notice of payment that explains and itemizes the payment and any adjustment(s) made by a payer during the adjudication of claims process and sent to the provider. Often times the terms EOB and RA are used interchangeably.

Before you begin the activities in this chapter, refresh your memory on working with Harris CareTracker by referring back to the Best Practices list on page xxiii of this textbook. This list is also posted to the student companion website. Following best practices will help you complete work quickly and accurately.

CREATE A BATCH

Learning Objective 1: Create a batch for financial transactions.

As discussed in Chapter 4, you must create a batch to enter any financial information into Harris CareTracker PM and EMR, for example, charges, payments, and adjustments. For this learning objective, you will create a new batch for billing activities.

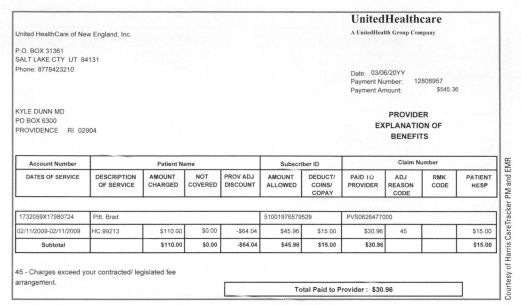

Figure 9-1   Example of an EOB (RA)

Setting Operator Preferences

In order to perform any financial transactions, you must create a batch or have a batch open. Harris CareTracker PM will prompt you to create a batch unless you have already created a batch that has not yet been posted. You can view open batch(es) by clicking on the *Home* module > *Dashboard* tab > *Billing* header > *Open Batches* link (**Figure 9-2**). Activities related to searching for a patient or scheduling a patient do not require that a batch be created. You begin by setting the operator preferences as completed in Chapter 4, Activity 4-13. Following the instructions in Activity 9-1, create a *Batch* as instructed to begin your activities in this chapter.

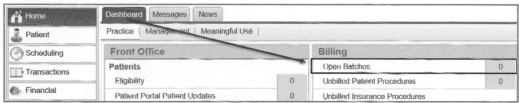

Figure 9-2   Open Batches Link   Courtesy of Harris CareTracker PM and FMR

Because you will have been working in various activities in more than one fiscal period, always work in the "current" fiscal period unless otherwise instructed (e.g., if you begin an activity in September, complete all the related activities in that period. If you start a new activity unrelated to a previous period [e.g., in December], you would then use the new period [December]). Although you will be instructed to complete activities and post batches, *never* close a period.

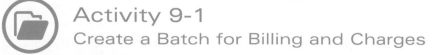 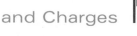

Activity 9-1
Create a Batch for Billing and Charges

1. Prior to creating a batch, you will need to open the fiscal period for which you will be entering activities. Go to the *Administration* module > *Practice* tab > *System Administration, Financial* headers > *Open/Close Period* link (**Figure 9-3**).

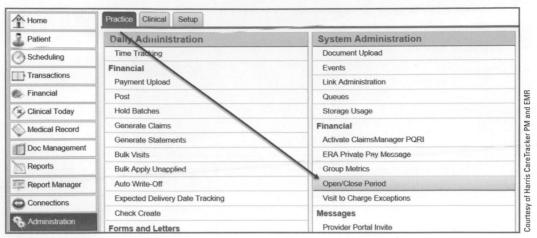

Figure 9-3   Open/Close Period Link

2. Open the fiscal period for the activities you are posting. Since you will be posting financial information for patient Alex Brady whose visit was in September 2016, open the fiscal period (2016) and month (September). **Note:** You will first need to change the current *Fiscal Year* box field to 2016.

3. Click *Save* (**Figure 9-4**).

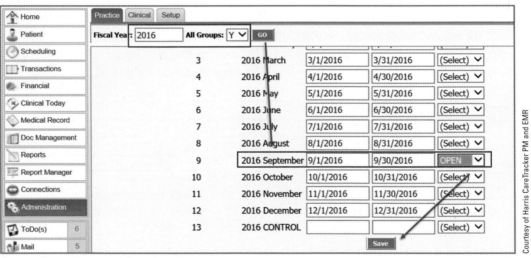

Figure 9-4   Open Fiscal Period for June 2016

4. Click the *Batch* ▌ icon on the *Name Bar* and the *Operator Encounter Batch Control* dialog box will display.

5. Then click *Edit*. (**Figure 9-5**).

6. Click *Create Batch*. The *Batch Master* dialog box displays (**Figure 9-6**).

7. Name the batch "Ch9Charges" (**Figure 9-7**). Do not use symbols when editing the name. By default, the *Batch Name* box displays a batch identification name. The name consists of your user name followed by the current date. However, you can edit the batch name if necessary to identify the types of financial transactions associated with the batch.

8. By default, the *Group Id* displays the name of your group.

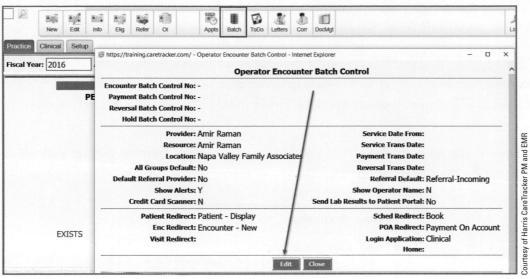

Figure 9-5   Operator Encounter Batch Control Dialog Box—Edit

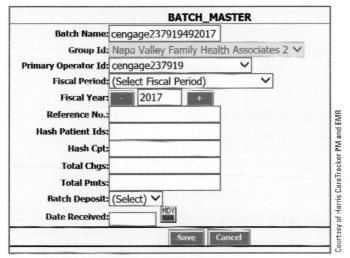

Figure 9-6   Batch Master Dialog Box

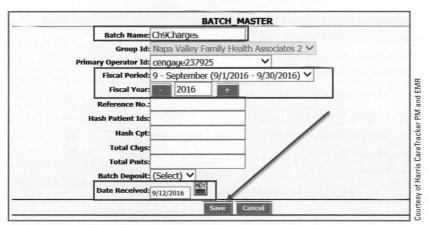

Figure 9-7   Change Batch Name

9.   By default, the *Primary Operator Id* displays your user name. This cannot be changed.

10.   By default, the *Fiscal Year* displays the current financial year set up for your company. Change the year to "2016."

11. In the *Fiscal Period* list, click the period to post financial transactions. The list only displays fiscal periods that are currently open. Select "September 2016" as the *Fiscal Period*.

12. Leave the *Reference No*; *Hash Patient Ids*; *Hash Cpt*; *Total Chgs*; *Total Pmts*; and *Batch Deposit* fields blank.

13. In the *Date Received* box, enter the date the encounter was created in MM/DD/YYYY format or click the *calendar* 🔲 icon and select the date. Select the date of Alex Brady's first appointment (September 12, 2016).

14. Click *Save*. If you have more than one period open, a pop-up warning (**Figure 9-8**) will appear asking you to confirm the fiscal period. Click *OK*.

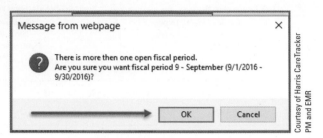

Figure 9-8   Fiscal Period Pop-Up Warning

15. Harris CareTracker PM and EMR displays the *Operator Encounter Batch Control* dialog box with the new batch information (**Figure 9-9**).

16. Further *Edit* your batch using the drop-down arrow next to each field and updating the provider, resource, location, and so on, if needed.

    a. If not already selected, select "Rebecca Ayerick" as the *Provider* and *Resource*.

    b. Change your *Login Application* to *Home*.

    c. Leave the *Home* field as *Practice*.

17. Click *Save*.

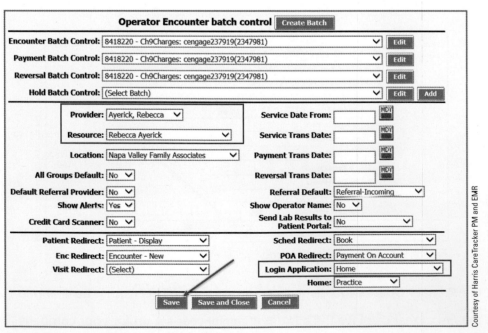

Figure 9-9   Charges Batch Information

18. Write down your "Encounter Batch Control No." for future reference (should include "Ch9Charges").

_____

📠 **Print the Operator Encounter Batch Control screen, label it "Activity 9-1," and place it in your assignment folder.**

19. Click the "X" in the upper-right corner to close the dialog box.

MANUALLY ENTER A CHARGE

Learning Objective 2: Manually enter a charge.

Charges are financial transactions that require a batch to be created before entering and saving a charge. Having created your batch in Activity 9-1, complete Activity 9-2 to post a patient payment.

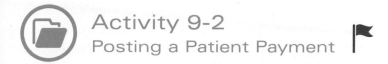

Activity 9-2
Posting a Patient Payment

1. Pull patient Alex Brady into context.

2. Open the *Transactions* module. The *Charge* application displays by default.

3. Click on the *Pmt on Acct* tab.

4. In Chapter 4, you learned how to enter and print copay receipts for patients. Following the instructions in Activity 4-17, enter the copay amount for patient Alex Brady. Because Alex is a pediatric patient, use the drop-down at the top of the screen and change from *Patient* to *Responsibly Party*.

5. Refer to the patient demographics or click on the *Info* 🪪 icon to determine the amount of copay required ($10).

6. Enter Payment Type "Payment-Patient Check."

7. In the Reference # field, enter check number "4434."

8. Enter the appointment date (*Trans. Date*) to be applied to Alex's payment (September 12, 2016). Your screen should look like **Figure 9-10**. (**Note:** Be sure to check the "Copay?" box.)

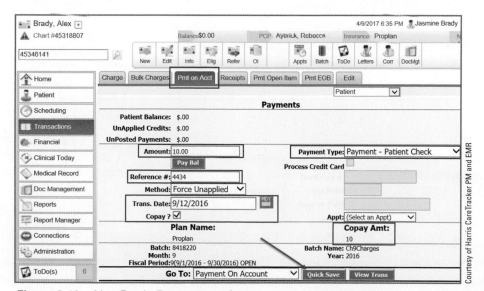

Figure 9-10   Alex Brady Payment on Account

9. Click *Quick Save.*

10. Click on the *Receipts* tab and print a receipt for Alex Brady.

💾 **Print the receipt, label it "Activity 9-2," and place it in your assignment folder.**

You will <u>not</u> post the batch at this time because you will complete additional activities before running a journal and posting a batch.

Coding Tips

ICD codes are internationally recognizable code sets, representing medical conditions or signs and symptoms. ICD-10 replaced the ICD-9 code set on October 1, 2015. To accommodate the change to ICD-10, Harris CareTracker has a *View Mappings* link (**Figure 9-11**) that will enable you to find ICD-9 and ICD-10 codes as needed. The *Visit Diagnosis, Visit Summary*, and *Claim Edit* screens for visits after October 1, 2015 display a code set ⑩ icon next to the insurance field that indicates that the insurance company or plan is configured to receive ICD-10 diagnosis codes (**Figure 9-12**) based on the encounter date. A diagnosis code in the *Diag* box can be removed by double-clicking on the code. The order of multiple codes can also be changed in the *Diag* box by highlighting the code to move up or down and then clicking on the corresponding up or down black arrow next to the *Diag* box.

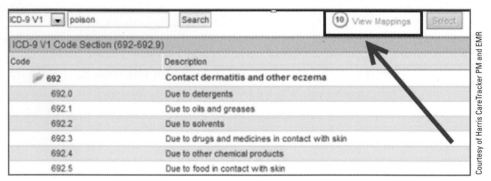

Figure 9-11   View Mappings

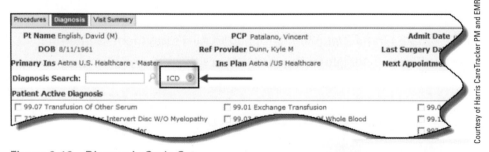

Figure 9-12   Diagnosis Code Set

Mapping Screen

The ICD mapping screen is accessed by clicking the *View Mappings* link at the top of the search results. This screen acts as a basic mapping tool, allowing the operator to see which current ICD-10 codes map to ICD-9 codes if needed (**Figure 9-13**) and vice versa. Basic mapping is available for:

- ICD-9-CM Vol. 1 to ICD-10-CM

- ICD-10-CM to ICD-9-CM Vol. 1

The mapping screen contains several columns with information about the relationship between the ICD-9 and ICD-10 codes. Because ICD-10 has been in use since October 1, 2015, it is unlikely you will encounter any ICD-9 codes.

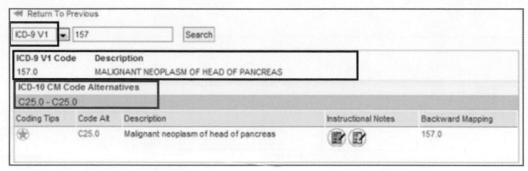

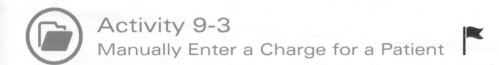

Figure 9-13   ICD-9 to ICD-10 Mapping

Having entered the copay for Alex Brady in Activity 9-2, continue your billing activities by manually entering a charge for a patient not on the schedule.

Activity 9-3
Manually Enter a Charge for a Patient

1. Because you will be manually entering a charge in a different period, follow the steps in Activity 9-1 to create a new batch using today's current month and year. (**Note:** If the fiscal period and fiscal year are not already open, you will need to open them before creating the batch.) Set the batch parameters as follows:

    a. Batch Name: RobinsonSNF

    b. Fiscal Year: Use the current year

    c. Fiscal Period: Use the current month

    d. Provider and Resource: Raman, Amir

2. After the current fiscal period is open and you have the new batch created, pull patient Edith Robinson into context.

3. Open the *Transactions* module. The *Charge* application displays by default, displaying the charge screen.

TIP You may get a pop-up stating "Please check Batch." If so, click *OK*. The *Operator Encounter Batch* screen will display. In the *Encounter Batch Control* field, you'll see that the "Robinson-SNF" batch you created is selected. Click "Save and Close."

4. Manually enter a "Skilled Nursing Facility" charge using the following charge-related information:

    a. Using the *Location* drop-down, select "NVSNF."

    b. Using the [Tab] key will automatically populate the *POS* with "SKILLED NURSING FACILITY."

    c. Enter *Ref Provider* "Dr. Raman."

FYI In the center of the screen, the *Visit* button will be grayed out (**Figure 9-14**). In a live application, clicking the *Visit* button allows you to access the *Visit* window in which CPT and ICD-10 codes can be selected for the patient.

(Continues)

(*Continued*)

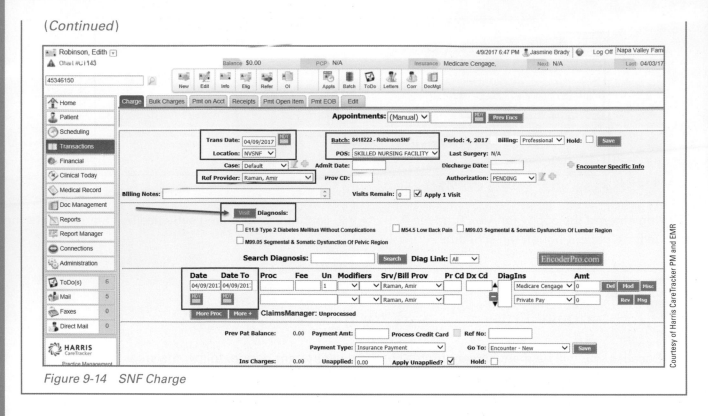

Figure 9-14   SNF Charge

5. If there have been previous ICD codes entered for this patient, you can place a check mark by the desired code to select it. Select codes E11.9, I10, M54.5, M99.03, and M99.05. If any of these codes are not listed, type the code (e.g., "I10") in the *Search Diagnosis* field and then click *Search*. Harris Care-Tracker PM will pull in the diagnosis code of I10 in the *Diag* field (**Figure 9-15**). Repeat code searches as necessary until you have all the five codes listed.

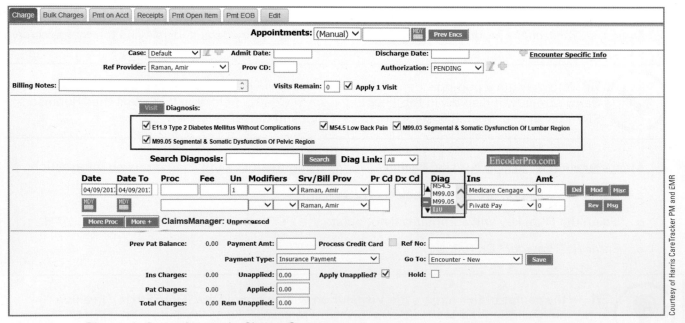

Figure 9-15   Diagnosis Codes Selected—Charge Screen

6. Click on *EncoderPro.com* to review the codes selected and determine if they are appropriate for the visit/charge. Click "X" to close the *EncoderPro* window.

7. Enter today's date in the *Date* and *Date To* fields. A date can either be entered manually in MM/DD/YYYY format or can be selected from the *Calendar* ![MDY] function. The date must be within the open period in your current batch.

8. Enter the code "99212" in the *Proc* field, and hit the [Tab] key. The procedure description, fee, and the amount to be charged to the patient's insurance and to the patient will be populated, and the *Modifiers* will become the active field.

9. Click on the *More Proc* button, which brings up another billing line. Enter CPT® code "G0180" in the *Proc* field. Hit the [Tab] key and the *Procedure Search* pop-up box will appear (**Figure 9-16**). Click on the code or description and the procedure will be pulled in to the charge box.

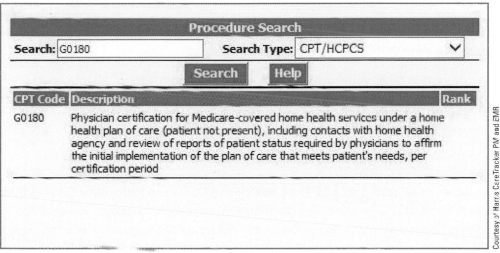

Figure 9-16   G0180 Procedure Search Window

10. Enter $100 in the *Fee* field because this CPT® code is not on the NVFHA fee schedule.

11. Select "Raman, Amir" from the *Srv/Bill Prov* drop-down list, if not already selected (**Figure 9-17**).

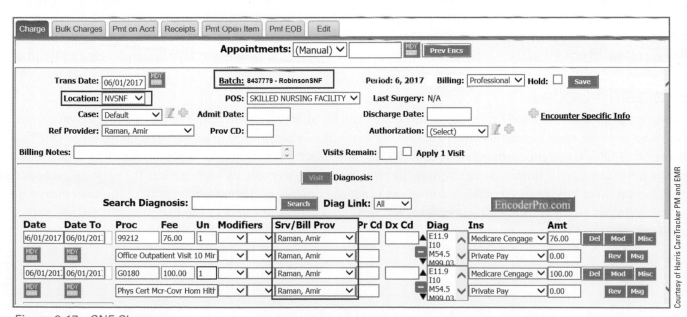

Figure 9-17   SNF Charge

💾 **Print the Charge Screen, label it "Activity 9-3," and place it in your assignment folder.**

12. Click *Save*. You will receive an error message (**Figure 9-18**) because your student version is not connected to *ClaimsManager*. However, the transaction will be saved, and the patient is taken out of context. (**Note:** It may take a few moments for this task to save. You <u>must</u> wait until you receive the "error" message "Transaction Saved" before moving on.)

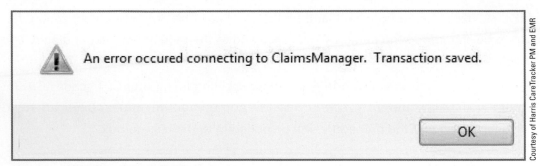

Figure 9-18   Error Message When Saving a Charge

13. Click *OK* and the patient is removed from context and "Encounter Added" displays on your screen.

14. Your manually entered charge is now saved.

Modifiers

A **modifier** is a two-character code added to a CPT® or **Healthcare Common Procedure Coding System (HCPCS)** (pronounced "hick picks") code that is used to help in the reimbursement process. For example, a modifier is used to explain that a procedure is not normally covered when billed on the same day as another, but is actually a separate and significant process, or that it is a rural health procedure that gets higher reimbursement. Up to four modifiers can be attached to each CPT® code, although in most cases only one or two are used. HCPCS (level II) is managed by the Center for Medicare and Medicaid Services (CMS) and classifies durable medical equipment (DME), injectable drugs, transportation services, and other services not classified in CPT®.

A common modifier in an outpatient setting is Modifier 25, which is defined as a significant, separately identifiable evaluation and management service by the same physician on the same day of the procedure or other service (e.g., an office visit for a facial lesion and a separate charge for destroying the lesion, vaccination(s) given at time of office visit, etc.). Refer to **Figure 9-19** for modifier selections in Harris CareTracker PM and EMR.

Explosion Codes

In Harris CareTracker PM and EMR, **explosion codes** can be built to include multiple CPT codes, which eliminates the need to enter each procedure individually. For example, in cardiology practices, the same three CPT® codes are used to bill every echocardiogram (93307, 93320, and 93325). Creating one explosion code for this procedure reduces the amount of time it takes to enter the charge into the system. Valid modifiers for each procedure code can also be linked to them. Explosion codes are practice specific, and you can determine the descriptive name of the code set along with the CPT® codes it will include. There is no limit to the number of different explosion code sets you can build for your practice.

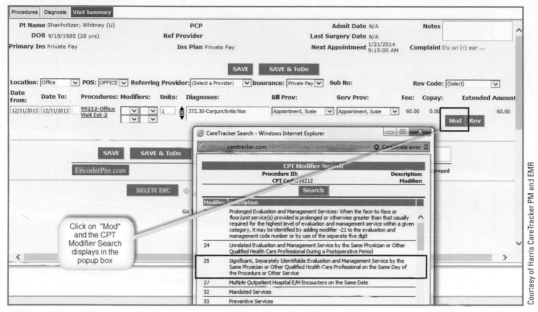

Figure 9-19   *Modifier Search*

HCPCS Codes

When a patient has both Medicare and a commercial insurance, always use the HCPCS code when billing inject-ables, DME, and others. If the HCPCS code is linked via a **crosswalk** code set to the CPT® code, the application will automatically pull the corresponding CPT® code onto the claim when the claim goes to the commercial insurance. Crosswalk (sometimes referred to as a "link") refers to a relationship between a medical procedure (CPT®/HCPCS code) and a diagnosis (ICD code). Not all HCPCS codes are linked via a crosswalk code set to CPT® codes.

FYI **Checking Procedure and Diagnosis Codes**

• When all procedure and diagnosis codes have been entered, click on the *EncoderPro.com* button at the top of the screen to verify that all the codes you have entered will be paid. Clicking the *EncoderPro.com* button displays basic information on all procedure codes that pertain to the charge. *EncoderPro* is Harris CareTracker's partner for online code verification, which can be run to verify all the procedures, diagnoses, and modifiers entered for a patient. Running *EncoderPro* helps to ensure that correct coding information is entered and that claims are processed and paid quickly.

• When *EncoderPro* has finished code verification, click *Save* at the bottom of the *Charge* screen. When the *Save* button is clicked, the associated procedures, diagnoses, and mod-ifiers are sent to *ClaimsManager* instantly for screening. (If you click *Save* in your stu-dent environment you will receive an error message because the *ClaimsManager* feature is not active in your student version.) The screening can result in one of three statuses that include "Passed," "Failed," or "Warning" (**Figure 9-20**). If the screening results in the "Passed" status, the patient's charge is saved in Harris CareTracker PM and EMR.

(Continues)

(Continued)

CLAIMSMANAGER SCREENING STATUS		
Color	**Status**	**Description**
☐	**Not Processed**	Not processed status indicates that the item has not been screened by the ClaimsManager.
▨	**Passed**	Passed status indicates that the item has passed the ClaimsManager screening.
☐	**Warning**	Warning status indicates that the item may fail or the ClaimsManager has suggested edits.
▪	**Failed**	Failed status indicates that the item does not meet the rules set by ClaimsManager and further edits are required.
▨	**CMS Edits**	This status indicates that the claim was flagged for CMS edits. **Note:** The CMS Edits status is deactivated by default. You must send a ToDo to CareTracker Support to request this feature.

Courtesy of Harris CareTracker PM and EMR

Figure 9-20   Claims Manager Screening Status

 TIP When the *Save* button is clicked, an *alert* will display if a charge for the same procedure codes on the same date of service for the same provider has already been entered into Harris CareTracker PM and EMR, preventing the creation of duplicate charges.

- If the *ClaimsManager* screening triggers an edit, Harris CareTracker PM and EMR opens the *ClaimsManager Edit* window. (See *ClaimsManager Edits for Charges* for a detailed description of each status and edit option in the *Help* section.) All edits are categorized into mnemonics for easy identification and each edit is color coded to indicate its severity (**Figure 9-21**). **Mnemonics**, defined as assisting memory, are added in the *Administration* module > *Setup* tab > *Financial* section > *Provider Mnemonics* link.

- If an action option is not clicked when a *ClaimsManager Edit* is triggered, the *Hold* checkbox is automatically selected and the charge is held until further action is taken. If waiting for reports or additional information, you can select the *Hold* checkbox manually to hold the charge and avoid further processing.

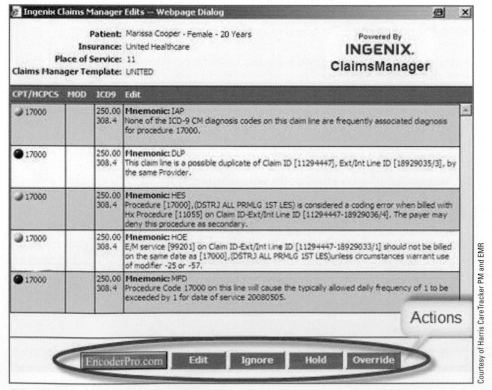

Courtesy of Harris CareTracker PM and EMR

Figure 9-21   Claims Manager Edits

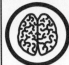

CRITICAL THINKING   Coding is quite detailed, and improper coding can be considered "fraudulent billing," subjecting you, the practice, and providers to monetary and criminal penalties. In addition, "under-coding," which is often the result of coders using a "cheat-sheet" of common codes, leaves substantial reimbursement to the provider/practice on the table.

Pull patient Edith Robinson into context. Click on the *Open Items* (*OI*) icon in the Name Bar. Without making any changes, examine the *Procedure* (CPT®) codes selected for the patient. If you are familiar with coding, identify and justify the proper codes, analyze, and question the code(s) entered on the encounter form to ensure that the most appropriate and accurate code(s) have been selected. If you are not familiar with CPT codes, do an Internet search to see if the CPT codes selected (G0180 and 99212) for the Skilled Nursing Facility (SNF) visit are appropriate. Explain how you reached your conclusion. Did you consider other code(s) that would also be appropriate? Would any of the selected codes not be appropriate for a SNF encounter?

Close out of the *Open Items* dialog box by clicking on the "X" in the upper-right-hand corner.

EDIT AN UNPOSTED CHARGE

Learning Objective 3: Edit an unposted charge.

Although it is not required to edit charges, there will be times when you will find it necessary to edit an unposted charge (e.g., a biller is reviewing a charge and sees that an incorrect CPT® code was assigned to the claim). Using the charge entered in Activity 9-3, edit the unposted charge.

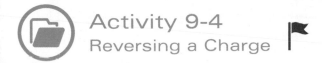

Activity 9-4
Reversing a Charge

1. Review the batch screen to confirm you are still working in the "RobinsonSNF" batch.

2. Pull patient Edith Robinson into context.

3. Click the *Transactions* module. Harris CareTracker PM and EMR opens the *Charge* application.

4. Click on the *Edit* tab. When *Edit* is clicked, all of the procedures entered in the patient's account along with each financial transaction linked to it will display (**Figure 9-22**) beginning with the most recent date of service. Locate the procedure that needs to be entirely reversed on the patient's account. (**Note:** You may need to scroll down the screen to locate the charge in question.) As a biller, you have noticed that CPT® code 99212 is incorrect, and want to change it to CPT® code 99214.

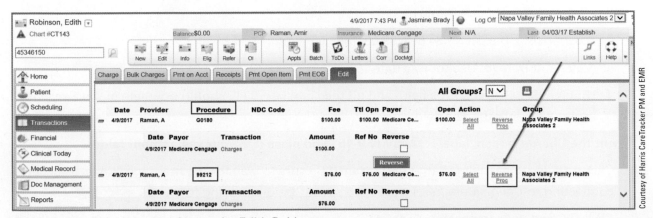

Figure 9-22   Edit Unposted Charge for Edith Robinson

5. Select the *Reverse Proc* link on the 99212 charge only (see **Figure 9-22**). (**Note:** If you click on the *Reverse* button, all of the selected transactions are reversed. Do <u>not</u> click on *Reverse*.)

6. You will receive a pop-up warning message (**Figure 9-23**) asking "Are you sure you want to reverse the selected Financial Transactions?" Click *OK*. The transaction will be reversed (see **Figure 9-24**). (**Note:** If you receive the error message "The Reversal Date must be within Period Start and End Dates: xx/xx/20xx and: xx/xx/20xx," it may be due to a "compatibility" issue with your browser. Refer to Best Practices regarding compatibility.)

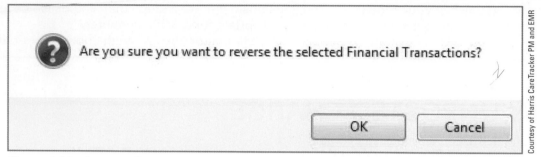

Figure 9-23   *Reverse Financial Transaction Warning*

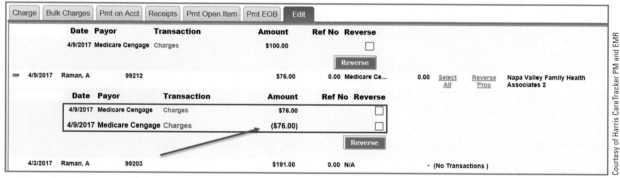

Figure 9-24   *Reversed Charge*

💾 **Print the Edit Unposted Charge screen, label it "Activity 9-4a," and place it in your assignment folder.**

7. Click back on the *Charge* tab in the *Transactions* module and complete the charge screen:

   a. *Location*: NVSNF

   b. *POS*: SKILLED NURSING FACILITY

   c. *Ref Provider*: Raman, Amir

   d. *Diagnosis*: E11.9, I10, M54.5, M99.03, M99.05

   e. *Date* and *Date To*: Use today's date

   f. Enter "99214" in the *Proc* field, and hit the [Tab] key. $245 should populate in the *Fee* field. If not, enter $245 into the *Fee* field.

💾 **Print the Charge screen, label it "Activity 9-4b" and place it in your assignment folder.**

8. Click on *Save* to save the charge. *Important!!* Be sure to wait for the message "An error occurred connecting to *ClaimsManager*. Transaction saved" before moving forward.

9. Click *OK*, and your transaction is saved.

Now that you have manually entered and edited unposted charges, the common workflow would be to complete the process by running a journal and posting your batch. Once having verified the balance with the journal (by completing Activity 9-5), you will the post a batch in Activity 9-6.

Journals

When you have finished entering data into your batch, you will run a journal to verify your batch and entry information. It is best practice to run a journal (as in Activity 4-18) prior to posting your batch to verify that you have entered all the financial transactions correctly in Harris CareTracker PM.

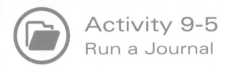

Activity 9-5
Run a Journal

1. Go to the *Reports* module > *Reports* tab > *Financial Reports* header > *Todays Journals* link (**Figure 9-25**).

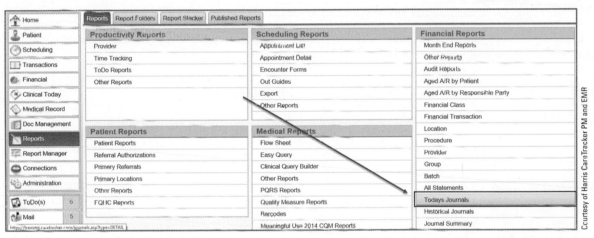

Figure 9-25   *Today's Journals Link*

2. Harris CareTracker PM displays the *Todays Journal Options* screen. All of your group's open batches are listed in the *Todays Batches* box. You may need to click on the [+] sign to expand the *Batches* field (see **Figure 9-26**).

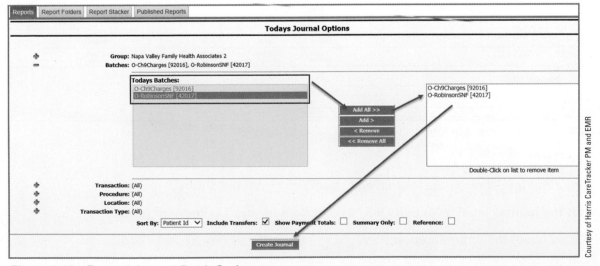

Figure 9-26   *Expand Journal Batch Options*

3. Select a batch to include in the journal either by double-clicking on the batch name or by clicking on the batch and then clicking *Add >*. Harris CareTracker PM adds the selected batches to the box on the right. Select batches "Ch9Charges" and "RobinsonSNF."

4. Scroll down to the bottom of the screen. From the *Sort By* drop-down list, select *Entry Date* (**Figure 9-27**).

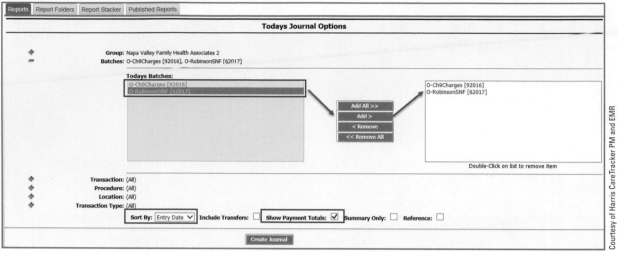

Figure 9-27   *Create Journal—Sort By Entry Date*

5. Select the *Show Payment Totals* checkbox (see Figure 9-27).

6. Click *Create Journal*. Harris CareTracker PM generates the journal (**Figure 9-28**).

| Reports | Report Folders | Report Stacker | Published Reports | |

Financial Report
Journal
Print Date: Saturday, October 28, 2017 (10:58:49 AM)
Run By: Training Operator Cengage238039
Napa Valley Family Associates

	Procedure:	(All)
Location:	(All)
Group:	Napa Valley Family Health Associates 2
Transaction Type:	(All)
Transaction Class:	(All)

Patient	Serv Dt	Trans Dt	Transaction	Charges	Payments	Adjustments	Provider	Payer	CPT	MOD	Diag
Batch: Ch9Charges-8488221											
(45757117) Brady, Alex		9/12/2016	Payment - Patient C...		($10.00)			Unapplied			
Batch Totals:				**Batch Chg** $0.00	**Batch Pmts** ($10.00)	**Batch Adj** $0.00		**Batch Net** ($10.00)			
Batch: RobinsonSNF-8488222											
(45757126) Robinson, Edith	10/28/2017	10/28/2017	Charges	$76.00			Raman, Amir	Medicare Cengage	99212		(E11.9, M99.03, M99.05, I10)
(45757126) Robinson, Edith	10/28/2017	10/28/2017	Charges	$100.00			Raman, Amir	Medicare Cengage	G0180		(E11.9, M99.03, M99.05, I10)
(45757126) Robinson, Edith	10/28/2017	10/28/2017	Charges	-$76.00			Raman, Amir	Medicare Cengage	99212		(E11.9, M99.03, M99.05, I10)
(45757126) Robinson, Edith	10/28/2017	10/28/2017	Charges	$245.00			Raman, Amir	Medicare Cengage	99214		(E11.9, M99.03, I10, M99.05)
Batch Totals:				**Batch Chg** $345.00	**Batch Pmts** $0.00	**Batch Adj** $0.00		**Batch Net** $345.00			
Grand Totals:				**Tot Chg** $345.00	**Tot Pmts** ($10.00)	**Total Adj** $0.00		**Net Total** $335.00			

Payment Totals

Payment Description.	Payment Amount
Payment - Patient Check	($10.00)
Payment Grand Total	($10.00)

Figure 9-28   *Journal—Financial Report*

7. To print, right-click on the journal and select *Print* from the shortcut menu.

💾 **Print the journal, label it "Activity 9-5," and place it in your assignment folder.**

8. Close out of the *Journal* report.

Having generated a journal for the batch(es) you would like to post, review and identify any transactions errors that may have been made, and correct them prior to posting (using the steps in Activity 9-4, *Reversing a Charge*). We will assume that there are no errors in the *Journal Report* created in Activity 9-5.

Having balanced the money in your journal, post an open batch as directed in Activity 9-6 following the alternate method of posting outlined in the steps.

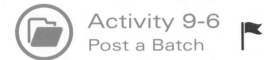

Activity 9-6
Post a Batch

1. Go to the *Administration* module > *Practice* tab > *Daily Administration* section > *Financial* header > *Post* link (**Figure 9-29**). Harris CareTracker PM displays a list of all open batches for the group.

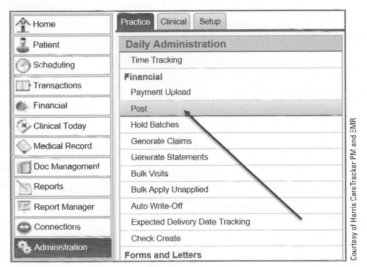

Figure 9-29   Post Link from Practice Tab

2. Check the box next to the batch(es) you want to post. Select <u>only</u> the batch "Ch9Charges" (**Figure 9-30**). Do <u>not</u> select or post the "RobinsonSNF" batch at this time.

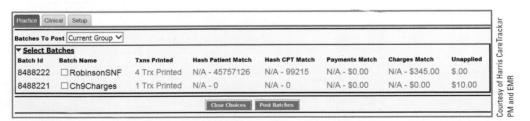

Figure 9-30   Post Batches

💾 **Print the Post Batches screen, label it "Activity 9-6," and place it in your assignment folder**

3. Then click *Post Batches*.

BUILD AND GENERATE CLAIMS

Learning Objective 4: Generate electronic and paper claims.

Harris CareTracker PM transmits electronic claims directly to insurance companies and to **clearinghouses**. After an electronic claim batch has been received by either an insurance company or a clearinghouse, Harris CareTracker PM will receive an electronic acknowledgment indicating that the file has been accepted. After the insurance company or clearinghouse has reviewed the electronic claims batch, Harris CareTracker PM will then receive a report indicating whether the claims have been accepted or rejected. Any claims that have been rejected must be corrected and rebilled. After you have received and reviewed the report from the insurance company or clearinghouse, the electronic claim batch should then be closed and removed from your *Dashboard*. In the medical field, a clearinghouse is a private or public company that provides connectivity and often serves as a "middleman" between physicians and billing entities, payers, and other health care partners for transmission and translation of claims information (primarily electronic) into the specific format required by payers.

Claims can only be generated after your batch has been posted. Most claims in a medical practice are transmitted electronically to a clearinghouse or directly to an insurance company; however, some claims will need to be printed out and mailed. To manually print out paper claims in Harris CareTracker PM, you would go to the *Home* module > *Dashboard* tab > *Billing* header > *Unprinted Paper Claim Batches* link. Because *ClaimsManager* is not active in your student version, you will not be able to perform this function.

Electronic Submission of Claims

In a live environment, after completing the activities of posting payments, charges, running the journal, and posting the batch, Harris CareTracker PM will electronically submit the claims through *ClaimsManager*. You will simulate generating claims by following the steps in Activity 9-7. Because the *ClaimsManager* feature is not active in your student version of Harris CareTracker PM, the claim will not actually generate, but you will be able to complete the steps.

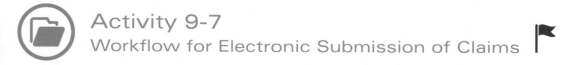

Activity 9-7
Workflow for Electronic Submission of Claims

1. Go to the *Administration* module > *Practice* tab > *Daily Administration* section > *Financial* header > *Generate Claims* link (**Figure 9-31**). Harris CareTracker PM launches the *Generate Claims* application.

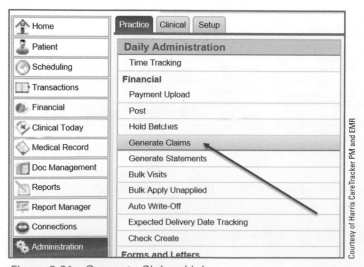

Figure 9-31 Generate Claims Link

2. Click *Generate Claims For This Group* (**Figure 9-32**). You may receive an error message stating "Error Queuing Claims" (**Figure 9-33**) or a message saying "Claims are being Generated..." because the *Claims-Manager* feature of your student version is not active. In a live environment, your screen would look like **Figure 9-34**, which states "Claims are Queued for all Groups under this Parent Company."

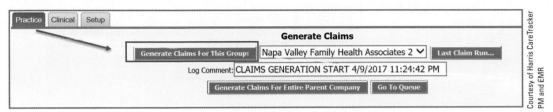

Figure 9-32   *Generate Claims for This Group*

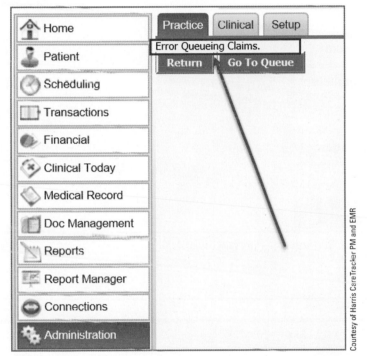

Figure 9-33   *Error Queuing Claims (Your message might say "Claims are being Generated for Group [#]" instead.)*

3. Whether or not you have received an error message, click on *Go to Queue* and a report will generate (**Figure 9-35**). **Figure 9-36** represents an example of the *Claims Queue* in a live environment, which displays the *Claims Worklist*. Since you are working in a student environment, all of your queues will be empty.

📧 **Print the Claims Queue window, label it "Activity 9-7," and place it in your assignment folder.**

4. Click back on the *Administration* module to exit the claims queue. (**Note:** Claims wait in *Queue* to be processed at 5 p.m.)

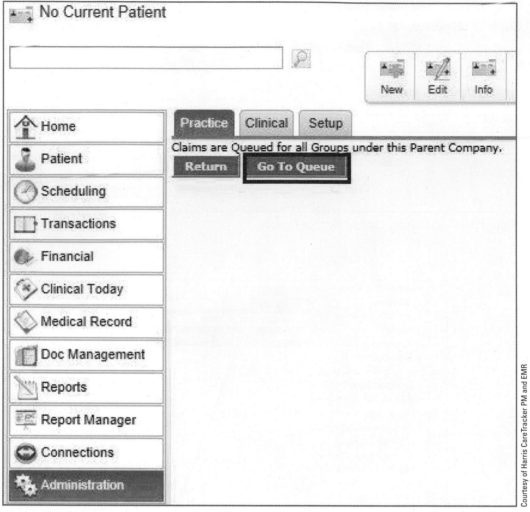

Figure 9-34   *Claims Generated*

Courtesy of Harris CareTracker PM and EMR

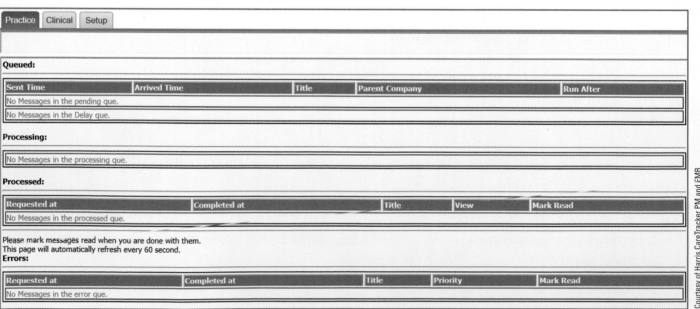

Figure 9-35   *Claims Queue (The messages on your screen may differ.)*

Courtesy of Harris CareTracker PM and EMR

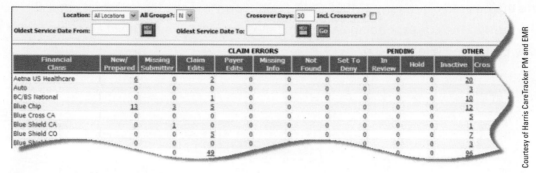

Location: All Locations	All Groups?: N				Crossover Days: 30	Incl. Crossovers? ☐					
Oldest Service Date From:				Oldest Service Date To:		Go					

				CLAIM ERRORS					PENDING		OTHER	
Financial Class	New/ Prepared	Missing Submitter	Claim Edits	Payer Edits	Missing Info	Not Found	Set To Deny	In Review	Hold	Inactive	Cros
Aetna US Healthcare	6	0	2	0	0	0	0	0	0	20	
Auto	0	0	0	0	0	0	0	0	0	3	
BC/BS National	0	0	1	0	0	0	0	0	0	10	
Blue Chip	13	3	5	0	0	0	0	0	0	12	
Blue Cross CA	0	0	0	0	0	0	0	0	0	5	
Blue Shield CA	0	1	0	0	0	0	0	0	0	1	
Blue Shield CO	0	0	5	0	0	0	0	0	0	7	
Blue Shield	0	0	0	0			0	0	0	3	
		0	49					0	0	96	

Figure 9-36   Claims Worklist

Courtesy of Harris CareTracker PM and EMR

FYI In a live environment, claims would be electronically transmitted to their intended payer/insurance company. A typical workflow would be:

- For claims transmitted electronically, you would receive a *Report* response back from the insurance company that needs to be reviewed. This can be done by clicking on the *Open Electronic Claim Batches* link on the *Dashboard* tab in the *Home* module.
- Your *Dashboard* should be reviewed daily; however, your student version of Harris CareTracker PM will not show a *Report* back.
- On the day after you have generated your claims, you would check to see if any claims that were supposed to be transmitted or dropped to paper were unable to be billed out by Harris CareTracker PM. You would do this by clicking on the *Claims Worklist* link under the *Billing* section of the *Dashboard* tab in the *Home* module.
- The system would separate electronic vs. paper claims with *ClaimsManager*.
- As a biller, you would see what dropped to paper and then generate a paper claim.

Paper Claim Batches

Although paper claims are rare, there are occasions when you will need to submit one. In Harris CareTracker PM, paper claims are generated by way of the method outlined in Activity 9-9. To print paper claims, you must first apply print settings, as in Activity 9-8.

Activity 9-8
Apply Settings to Print Paper Claims

There are two ways to apply print settings in Harris CareTracker. For this activity, use the Harris CareTracker *Dashboard*.

1. Go to the *Home* module > *Dashboard* tab > *Billing* section > *Unprinted Paper Claim Batches* link. The application displays the *Print Options* window.

2. Click the *Print Options* button in the upper-right corner of the screen.

3. Locate the desired claim form ("1500 CMS Paper Form") in the list and then enter the margin size for the form in the corresponding *Offset Top* field (enter "10") and *Offset Left* field (enter "10") if not already populated (**Figure 9-37**).

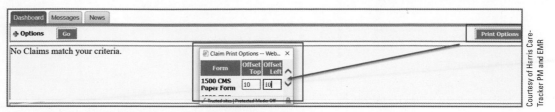

Figure 9-37   *Apply Settings to Print Paper Claims*

💾 **Print the Claim Print Options window, label it "Activity 9-8," and place it in your assignment folder.**

4. Scroll to the bottom of the dialog box and click *Update*. You must log out and then log back in to Harris CareTracker PM and EMR before the setting takes effect.

Now that you have entered your print settings, you will be set to generate paper claims. Harris CareTracker PM sends all electronic claims to the appropriate insurance company clearinghouse and captures all paper claims that cannot be transmitted electronically in the *Unprinted Paper Claim Batches* application. The paper claim batches should be printed and marked as printed in a timely fashion, per practice protocol.

Live practices have the option to automatically update the status of batch paper claims when the *Print Forms* button is used. This eliminates the need to manually mark each claim as printed. For this feature to be activated, the live practice would send a *ToDo* to its support entity.

In a live practice, Harris CareTracker PM is able to do real-time claim status checks from any application in Harris CareTracker PM and EMR where the *Claim Summary* screen displays. If the practice does not use the *Claims Status* application, the billing staff should call the insurance companies two weeks after claims are mailed to verify that the claims have been received, are on file, and are set to pay.

📁 **Activity 9-9**
Build and Generate a Paper Claim 🚩

1. Pull patient Edith Robinson into context.

2. Click the *Ol▢* tab in the *Name* bar.

3. Click on *Instant Claim* in the *First Clm* column (**Figure 9-38**) for Procedure code 99214. Harris CareTracker PM displays the *Claims Summary* in the lower frame of the screen.

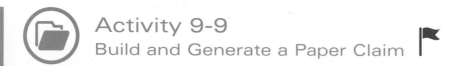

Figure 9-38   *First Clm Column—Edith Robinson*

4. Place a check mark in the rows for Procedure codes 99214 and G0180. Do **not** place a check mark in the row for Procedure code 99212.

5. Then click *Build Claim.* You will then note that the date you performed the activity is listed in the *First Clm* column.

6. Click on the date in the *First Clm* column for Procedure 99214 (**Figure 9-39**). Harris CareTracker PM displays the *Claims Summary* in the lower frame of the screen.

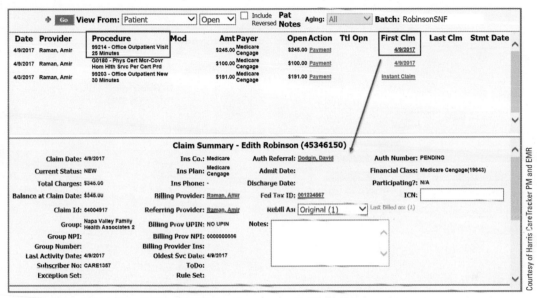

Figure 9-39   First Clm Column—Claim Summary; Edith Robinson

🖶 **Print the Claims Summary window, label it "Activity 9-9," and place it in your assignment folder.**

7. Scroll down and click the *Rebill To= = >* drop-down list at the bottom of the screen and select *Paper 1500.* Click *Rebuild Paper* (**Figure 9-40**). Because this is a simulated activity you will receive an error message (see **Figure 9-40**).

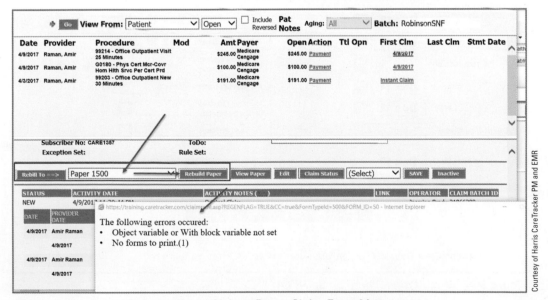

Figure 9-40   Select Rebuild Paper Claim—Paper Claim Error Message

8. Close out of the *Open Items* screen by clicking on "X."

 FYI In a live environment, Harris CareTracker PM would have generated the HCFA 1500 CMS Paper Form (**Figure 9-41**). To print this form, you would right-click on the form and select *Print* from the shortcut menu. **Figures 9-42** and **9-43** provide examples of the HCFA and Workers Comp HCFA forms.

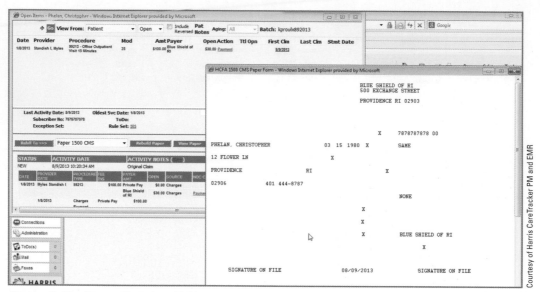

Figure 9-41 Paper Claim to 1500

Courtesy of Harris CareTracker PM and EMR

What Prints Where on a HCFA

Patient Case Detail

Claim Information | Workers Comp\ Auto | Ancillary | UB-04

Admission: **Box 18**
Discharge: **Box 18**
Consultation:
Illness: **Box 14**
LMP: **Box 14**
Local Use Code: (Select)
Local Use: **Box 19**

Onset Date: **Box 15**
Date Last Seen: **Box 19**
Supervising Prov: (Select) **Box 19**
Authorization: (Select) **Box 23**
Initial Treatment:
Last X-Ray:

Save Detail Template | **Cancel**

Figure: Patient Case Detail: Claim Information tab HCFA form mapping

Figure 9-42 What Prints Where on an HCFA

Courtesy of Harris CareTracker PM and EMR

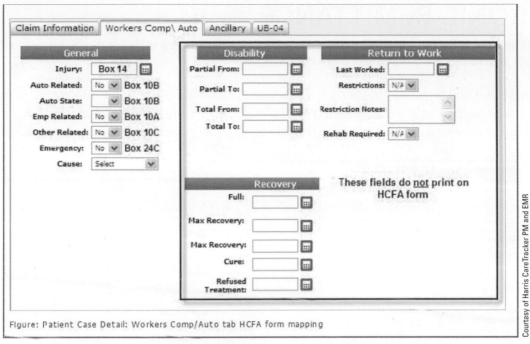

Figure: Patient Case Detail: Workers Comp/Auto tab HCFA form mapping

Figure 9-43   Workers Comp/Auto HCFA

TIP HCFA is an acronym for the Health Care Financing Administration. HCFA references the insurance claim form that a health care provider submits to an insurance company, the CMS-1500 Form.

FYI In a live practice, the steps to print paper claim batches are as follows:

1. Go to the *Home* module > *Dashboard* tab > *Billing* section > *Unprinted Paper Claim Batches* link.

2. Click *Go*. Harris CareTracker PM displays a list of paper claim batches that need to be printed. In your student version of Harris CareTracker, it will display "No Claims match your criteria."

3. (Optional) Click the plus sign [+] next to the word *Options* to display a set of filters (**Figure 9-44**). Use the filters to customize the list of paper claim batches displayed. (**Note:** The *Links Only* field applies to *Electronic Claim* batches only.)

4. If necessary, enter any notes regarding the printed paper claims in the *Notes* field.

5. Click *Save*.

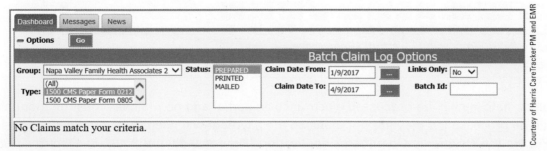

Figure 9-44   Batch Claim Log Options

ELECTRONIC REMITTANCE

Learning Objective 5: Perform activities related to electronic remittance including: posting payments and adjustments, and reconciling insurance payments.

Remittances received electronically in Harris CareTracker PM are identified in the *Electronic Remittances* application in the *Billing* section of the *Dashboard* (**Figure 9-45**). Harris CareTracker PM matches the transactions on the electronic remittance to a specific patient, date of service, CPT® code, and charge amount.

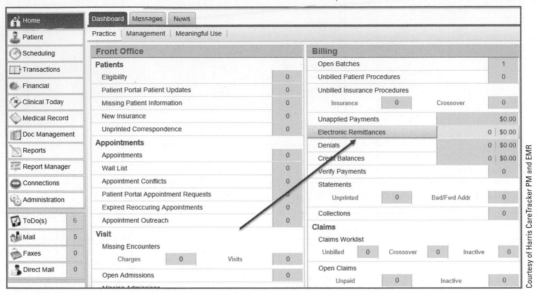

Figure 9-45   *Electronic Remittances Link*

 SPOTLIGHT There are three matching categories (**Figure 9-46**):

1. Complete (green)
2. Partial match (yellow)
3. No match (white)
4. Red indicates that someone manually unmatched the electronic remittance.

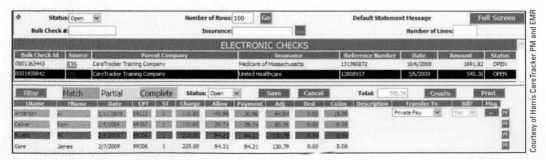

Figure 9-46   *Processing Electronic Remittance*

Only complete matches will be processed electronically; partial and no matches must be manually matched before they can be processed. If they are not matched the payment will need to be manually posted into Harris CareTracker PM via the *Payments Open Items* application (**Figures 9-47** and **9-48**). In *Electronic Remittances*, statement messages can be added for individual patients that will print on their statements generated from Harris CareTracker PM.

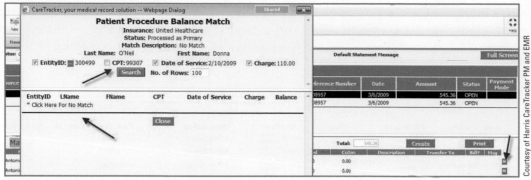

Figure 9-47   Patient Procedure Balance Match

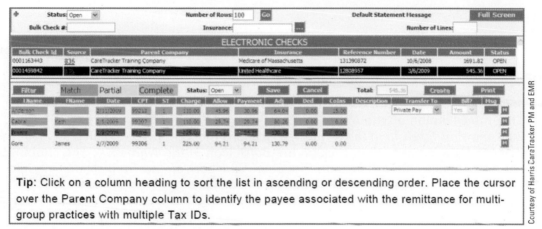

Tip: Click on a column heading to sort the list in ascending or descending order. Place the cursor over the Parent Company column to identify the payee associated with the remittance for multi-group practices with multiple Tax IDs.

Figure 9-48   Filter Patient Procedure Balance Match

Post Payments and Adjustments

Harris CareTracker PM provides a rich environment to record payments and ensures that these claims are being paid appropriately. *Transactions, Reports, Admin, Financial, Messages*, and *Scheduling* are the modules used in Harris CareTracker PM when entering and processing payments. Several applications within each module are made use of as well.

There is a normal flow of payment activity in Harris CareTracker PM that begins when a patient pays his or her copayment. Copayments are entered in Harris CareTracker PM when the patient checks in or checks out (depending on the office workflow). Next, a claim is sent to the insurance company after the patient visit. In Harris CareTracker PM, most claims are transmitted electronically; however, paper forms are sometimes mailed. When bills are transmitted electronically, the payment is received electronically or on a paper EOB/RA. Paper EOB/RAs received in the mail from primary or secondary insurers are entered in the *Transactions* module. If payments are not received, Harris CareTracker PM provides a work list of unpaid claims that need to be reviewed and followed up. Once a payment has been accepted in full, Harris CareTracker PM verifies the payment and the adjustment entered is based on contractual tables that can be loaded into the system for specific payers.

Open Items

Open Items is an application in the *Financial* module. There is an identical application accessed via the *Pmt Open Item* tab in the *Transactions* module, and this application can also be accessed as a window by clicking the *OI* button on the *Name Bar*. The *Open Items* application is used to view all dates of service and the associated procedures, financial transactions, and claims activity (**Figure 9-49**). In this application, you can enter many different types of financial transactions including patient payments, insurance payments, third-party payments, transfer balances, refunds, and apply unapplied money. You can also view the procedure details of each procedure, enter denial descriptions, attach statement messages to appear on patient statements, view a claim history, potentially rebill a claim, view electronic responses received from insurance companies, and view EOB/RAs attached to payments.

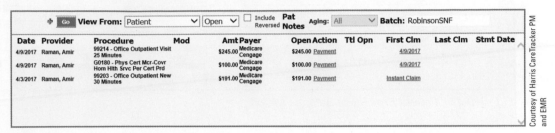

Figure 9-49   Open Items

 TIP You can access *Open Items* in the following ways:

- Left-click on an appointment in the *Book* application and select *Open Items.*
- Click the *OI* button on the *Name Bar.*
- Click the *Pmt Open Item* tab in the *Transactions* module. If you receive an error message that the batch in not open, click on the *Batch* icon in the *Name Bar.* The "RobinsonSNF" batch will display. Click *Edit,* then click *Save.* Click back on the *Transactions* module and the *Pmt Open Item* tab, and the *Open Item*(s) will display.

Processing Electronic Remittances

The total number and sum of remittances received electronically into Harris CareTracker PM displays on the *Dashboard* and a list of the received remittances that need to be posted into the system is accessed by clicking on the *Electronic Remittances* link. Electronic remittances should only be posted after the check (or electronic payment) is received from the insurance company.

Before posting payments via *Electronic Remittances*, select one patient from the remittance, pull the patient into context, click the *OI* button on the *Name Bar,* and verify that the date of service is still open in Harris CareTracker PM (**Figure 9-50**).

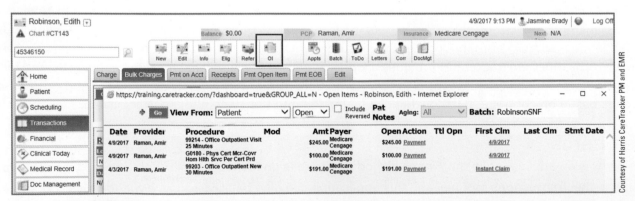

Figure 9-50   OI Electronic Remittance

You will process a simulated remittance in Activity 9-10.

FYI The *ClaimsManager* feature of Harris CareTracker PM is not active in your student version; however, the workflow to process electronic remittances in a live practice would be as follows:

> **ALERT!** *This FYI is informational only. Do not perform the steps outlined as it may conflict with your actual activity entries later. Only complete steps contained in Activity 9-10.*

1. Go to the *Home* module > *Dashboard* tab > *Billing* section > *Electronic Remittances* link. Harris CareTracker PM displays a list of electronic checks (**Figure 9-51**).

LName	FName	Date	CPT	ST	Charge	Allow	Payment	Adj	Ded	Coins	Description	Transfer To	Bill?	Msg
Cabral	*Antonio	1/10/2009	99306	1	225.00	94.21	94.21	130.79	0.00	0.00				
Cabral	*Antonio	2/10/2009	99307	1	110.00	29.74	29.74	80.26	0.00	0.00				
Laflamme	Carlos	2/10/2009	93000	1	70.00	74.78	24.78	45.22	0.00	0.00				
Laflamme	Jonathan	2/5/2009	99307	1	110.00	29.74	29.74	80.28	0.00	0.00				
O'Neil	*Donna	2/10/2009	99307	1	110.00	29.74	29.74	30.35	0.00	0.00				
Pitt	Brad	2/11/2009	99213	1	110.00	45.96	30.96	64.04	0.00	15.00				
Pitt	Brad	2/8/2009	99306	1	225.00	94.21	94.21	130.79	0.00	0.00				
Ramirez	Stephanie	2/7/2009	99306	1	225.00	94.21	94.21	130.79	0.00	0.00				

Figure 9-51   Electronic Remittance Screen   Courtesy of Harris CareTracker PM and EMR

2. Click the *plus sign* [+] to display the search fields (**Figure 9-52**). You would populate the desired search fields (**Figure 9-53**) as instructed in **Table 9-1**, Electronic Remittance Search.

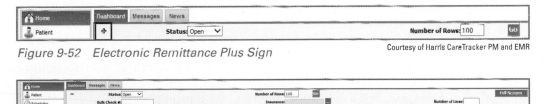

Figure 9-52   Electronic Remittance Plus Sign   Courtesy of Harris CareTracker PM and EMR

Figure 9-53   Electronic Remittance Search Fields   Courtesy of Harris CareTracker PM and EMR

Table 9-1   Electronic Remittance Search

SEARCH FIELD	DESCRIPTION
Status	Select the status of remittances you want to access.
Number of Rows	Enter the number of remittances you want to return in the search. Limiting the number of rows increases system response times.
Default Statement Message	Place your cursor over this field to view the default statement messages. Messages can be added for individual patients that will print on their statements generated from Harris CareTracker PM. (**Note:** You will not see the "Default Message" tab if you had not yet set this up in the *Administration* module.)
Bulk Check #	Enter the check ID number.
Reference #	Enter the system-generated reference number.
Number of Lines	Enter the number of check lines you want to work. Specifying a number of lines increases the response time by preventing the systems from loading all the lines from the electronic remittance. (**Note:** Limit the number of lines to 150 when processing large remittances.)
Date From/Date To	Enter the date range of the payments you want to access.

Courtesy of Harris CareTracker PM and EMR

(Continues)

(*Continued*)

3. Click *Go.* The application displays the remittances in the lower frame of the screen (**Figure 9-54**).

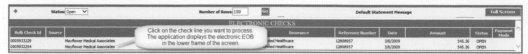
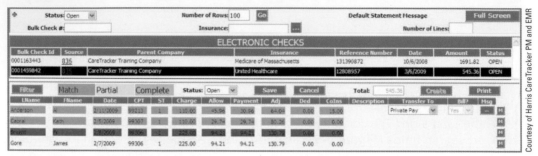

Figure 9-54   *Electronic Checks*

Courtesy of Harris CareTracker PM and EMR

4. Click the check line you want to process. The application displays the electronic EOB in the lower frame of the screen (**Figure 9-55**).

Figure 9-55   *Payment Window*

Courtesy of Harris CareTracker PM and EMR

 TIP Click on a column heading to sort the list in ascending or descending order. Place the cursor over the *Parent Company* column to identify the payee associated with the remittance for multigroup practices with multiple tax IDs.

5. Click *Save.* Harris CareTracker PM will automatically match as many unmatched transactions as possible, which is especially useful if you have received checks from secondary payers.

6. Manually match any remaining partial or unmatched transactions and then click *Save.*

7. You can transfer any balances to either a secondary payer or to private pay by selecting payer from the list in the *Transfer To* column. For balances transferred to private pay, Harris CareTracker PM automatically includes the default message set up in the *ERA Private Pay Message* application in the *Administration* module, *Practice* tab. **Note:** You will not see the "Default Message" tab if you had not yet set this up.

 SPOTLIGHT If the practice has not set up a default message, and you would like to select a different message, or add a new message:

- Click the ellipses (…) button in the *MSG* column. The application displays the *Statement Message* dialog box.

- In the *Msg Code* box, enter the message code or select a message from the *Stmt Msg* list.

- (Optional) Click *Msg* to view the entire message.

- Click *Save* to save the message and close the dialog box. The ellipses (…) button changes to a *MSG* button indicating that a message has been added.

8. Click *Create.* The application displays your current open batch information in a dialog box. **WARNING:** Do not click the *Create* button more than once.

9. Verify that the batch information is correct and then click *Confirm.* The application creates the financial transactions and displays a confirmation message in the lower frame of the screen.

10. Click on the highlighted check line. All of the payments created are highlighted in gray.

11. Click *Print*. The application displays a print options dialog box that displays the payments listed, the total of the check, and the reference number entered on the batch.

12. In the window, click the *Print* button to print out the document, and attach it to the EOB/RA. This document will replace your journal for payments processed via electronic remittances.

 TIP   If there are yellow or white lines on the remittance that were not manually matched, these payments are not posted; therefore, the payment amount on the EOB/RA will not match the total payments on this document.

---

13. From the *Status* list, change the status to *Close* and click the *Save* button which indicates that the remittance has been processed and removes it from open items. The status of manually posted remittances should be changed to "Inactive."

14. Click on the *Filter* button and de-select all options except "No Match" and "Partial Match." Click the *Accept* button, click the *Print* button, and then a list of all payments that were not posted will print. These partial or unmatched payments will need to be posted manually from the *Open Items* application in the *Financial* module.

15. Post your batch in Harris CareTracker PM.

16. Then work credit balances and denials.

 ## Activity 9-10
Save Charges; Process a Remittance

1. Before you begin this activity, pull Edith Robinson into context and refer back to Ms. Robinson's encounter from Activity 4-1. (**Hint:** refer to the *Scheduling* module, *History* tab to locate the appointment date.) Record the date of the encounter for this activity: _____

2. Create a new batch and name it "9-10PostRAs." Use today's date for the *Fiscal Period* and *Fiscal Year*.

3. Update the *Provider* and *Resource* to Edith Robinson's provider and PCP (Dr. Raman).

4. Click *Save and Close* on the newly created batch. If you receive a message that the "Service Date From is before today. Are you sure you want to save?", click *OK*.

5. Go to the *Home* module > *Dashboard* tab > *Visit* header > *Missing Encounters* > *Charges* link (**Figure 9-56**).

6. Set the fields as follows:
    • Change the beginning date to January 1, 20XX (current year) and change the ending date to today's date. (**Note:** By default, the ending date is yesterday and will not contain any entries made on the current date unless you change the ending date to today's date.) Be sure the dates include the date of the patient encounter from Activity 4-1.
    • Select *All providers*.
    • Select *All locations*.
    • Select *Visits Yes*.
    • Select *Charges No*.

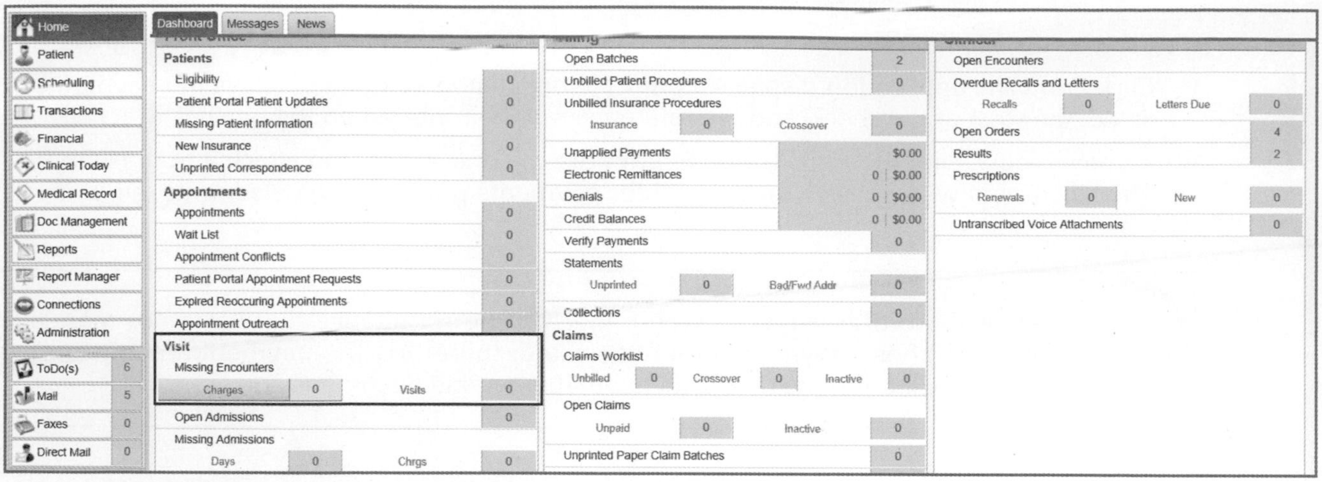

Figure 9-56 Missing Encounters/Charges Link

7. Then click *Go* (**Figure 9-57**). You will see the *Charges* that have not been saved (**Figure 9-58**). If multiple patients have appointments on the same date, you will notice that the *Visits* and *Charges* buttons only appear in the row for the first patient with an appointment on that date. This is because when you are working in *OI*, if more than one charge (e.g., multiple patient visits) appears on the same date, *Charges* are saved for all patients with appointments on that date (see **Figure 9-59**).

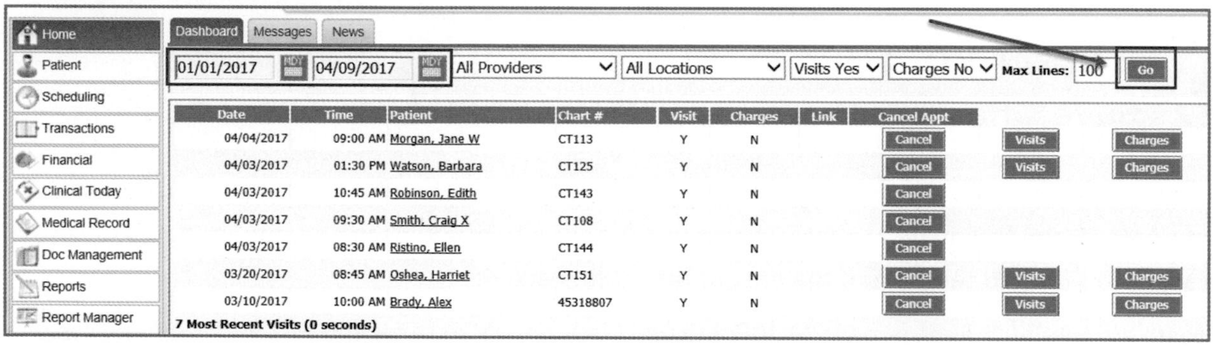

Figure 9-57 Visit YES/Charges NO

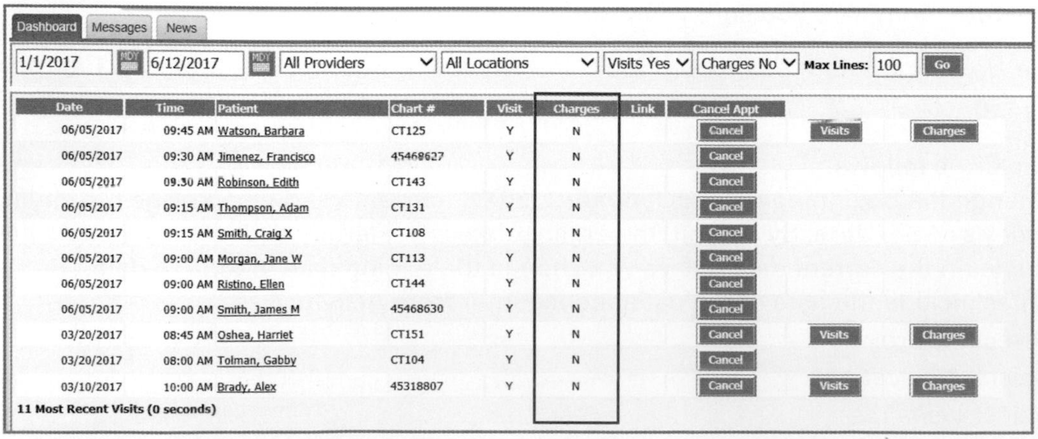

Figure 9-58 Charges Not Saved

8. In the *Date* column, locate the visit date (**Figure 9-59**) for patient Edith Robinson's appointment from Activity 4-1. Then click on the *Charges* button on the right side of your screen for the date of service corresponding to Edith's Activity 4-1 appointment. (Remember, the *Charges* button may not necessarily appear in Edith Robinson's row; it may appear in the row of a different patient who has the same date of service as her.)

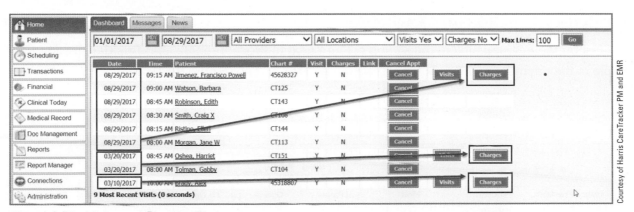

Figure 9-59   Visits and Charges Buttons

9. Now, click *Go* on the left side of your screen. The charges for all patient encounters on the Date of Service (DOS) display. **Note:** You may receive a pop-up message that says "Transaction Date must be within Period Start and End Dates: (of the date of your batch)." Click *OK* and the charges appear in the lower portion of your screen.

10. Since all the patients with charges display in the lower screen, you will need to scroll down to review the charges for patient Edith Robinson. We will assume here that the charges look okay.

11. Now, scroll down to the bottom of the lower screen, and click *Save* on the bottom left (**Figure 9-60**). (**Note:** If more than one charge [e.g., multiple patient visits] appear on the date, the *Charges* will be saved for all patients.)

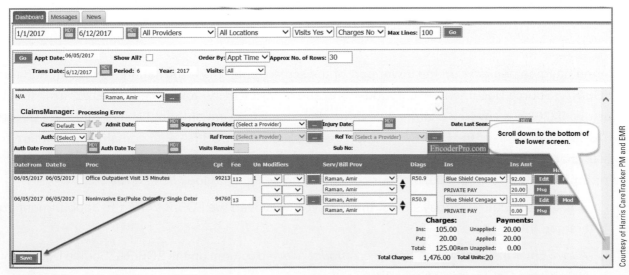

Figure 9-60   Save Visit—Jane Morgan

12. Wait until the "Transaction Saved" message appears before moving on. Then click *OK*. You will receive another pop-up stating "Bulk Charges Saved." Click *OK*.

13. With patient Edith Robinson in context, click on the *OI* button in the *Name Bar*. All captured charges for Ms. Robinson's Activity 4-1 appointment now display.

14. Click on *Instant Claim* in the *First Clm* column for Procedure 99203.

15. Place a checkmark next to the "99203" charge.

16. Click *Build Claim*. The *Open Items* dialog box will now display with a date in the *First Clm* column.

17. Click on the *Payment* link in the *Action* column next to Procedure 99203. Harris CareTracker PM displays the payment window in the lower frame of the screen (**Figure 9-61**).

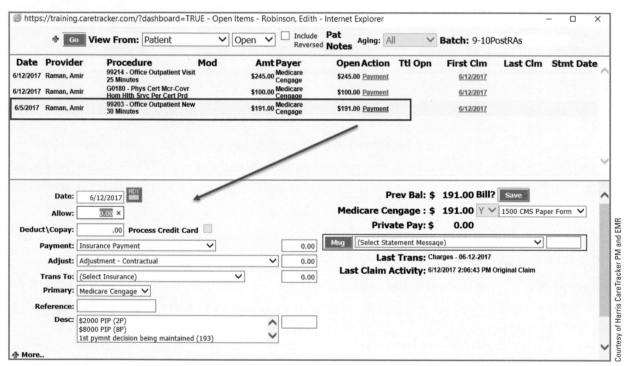

Figure 9-61   *Payment Window in OI*

18. In the payment window on the lower part of the screen, enter the information from Edith Robinson's EOB/RA (Source Document 9-1a, found at the end of this activity) for Procedure 99203 as instructed below. 92203 is a covered charge. A covered charge will have no amount listed in the "Not Covered (DENIAL)" column of the EOB/RA. You will also note that the EOB/RA also contains information for the SNF charge you entered in Activity 9-3 (Source Document 9-1b). **Important!!** Only enter the EOB/RA information for Procedure 99203. Your completed screen should look like **Figure 9-62**.

   a. *Date*: This should be today's date, the date you "received the EOB/RA" for the appointment you created in Activity 4-1.

   b. *Allow*: Enter the information from the *Amount Allowed* column on the EOB/RA (Source Document 9-1a). Now hit the [Tab] button on your keyboard.

c. *Deduct/Copay*: Enter the information from the *Deduct/Coins/Copay* column on the EOB/RA (Source Document 9-1a). Now hit the [Tab] button and this will populate the amount in the *Adjust* and *TransferTo* fields based on the information entered in the *Demographics* screen.

d. *Payment*: Confirm that *Insurance Payment* is selected.

e. *Adjust*: Confirm that *Adjustment—Contractual* is selected.

f. *TransTo*: Confirm that *Private Pay* is selected.

g. *Primary*: Confirm that *Medicare Cengage* is selected.

h. *Reference*: Leave blank.

i. *Desc*: Enter "45" in the blank box to the right of the *Desc* field and hit the [Tab] key.

j. *Msg*: Enter "CO" in the blank box to the right of the drop-down menu and hit the [Tab] key.

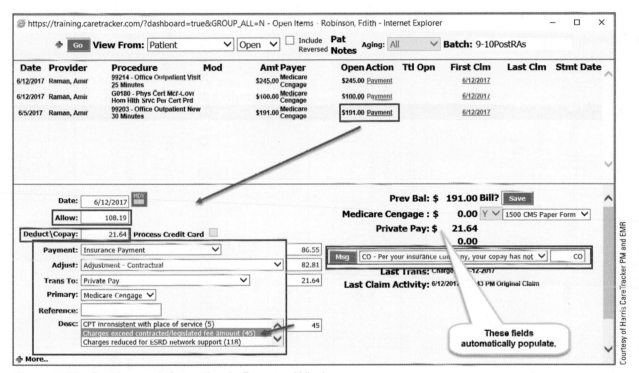

Figure 9-62   *Remittance Information in Payment Window*

🖫 **Print the Process Remittance (OI screen), label it "Activity 9-10a," and place it in your assignment folder.**

19. Once you have entered the EOB/RA information, click *Save*. Your transaction will be saved and the claim disappears.

20. (FYI) If you were working multiple charges, you would enter the additional charge information (following steps 18 and 19 for guidance) for each of the charges listed on the EOB/RA. (**Note:** Do <u>not</u> enter the additional payments at this point.)

21. Close out of the *Open Items* window by clicking the "X" in the upper-right corner of the window.

22. Run a *Journal* for batch "9-10PostRAs."

🖫 **Print the Journal, label it "Activity 9-10b," and place it in your assignment folder.**

Source Document 9-1A: Explanation of Benefits/Remittance Advice

MEDICARE CENGAGE

Medicare Cengage
P.O. Box 234434
San Francisco, CA 94137

AMIR RAMAN, D.O.
Napa Valley Family Health Associates (NVFHA)
101 Vine Street
Napa, CA 94558

Date: MM/DD/YYYY (use today's date)
Payment Number: 12808957
Payment Amount: $ 145.01

Account Number	Patient Name						Subscriber Number			Claim Number			
Dates of Service	Description of Service	Amount Charged	Not Covered (DENIAL)	Prov Adj Discount	Amount Allowed	Deduct/ Coins/ Copay	Paid to Provider	Adj Reason Code	Rmk Code	Patient Resp
CARE1357	Robinson, Edith									
(Appt. date used in Activity 4-1)	99203	$191.00		$82.81	$108.19	$21.64	$86.55	45*		$21.64

Source Document 9-1B: Explanation of Benefits/Remittance Advice

Account Number	Patient Name						Subscriber Number			Claim Number			
Dates of Service	Description of Service	Amount Charged	Not Covered (DENIAL)	Prov Adj Discount	Amount Allowed	Deduct/ Coins/ Copay	Paid to Provider	Adj Reason Code	Rmk Code	Patient Resp
CARE1357	Robinson, Edith									
(SNF date used in Activity 9-3)	99214	$245.00	$245.00		$0.00	$0.00	$0.00	96*		$245.00
(SNF date used in Activity 9-3)	G0180	$100.00		$26.93	$73.07	$14.61	$58.46			$14.61

Late charges, interest payments, and "take backs" are not processed from *Electronic Remittance* and must be applied manually via the *Payment Open Items* application. Post all primary before secondary checks (e.g., Medicare checks before Blue Shield checks in the case of a Medicare "primary" patient).

Insurance Payment Reconciliation and Follow-Up

Credit balances are created when either a patient or an insurance company pays more money for a specific procedure for a specific date of service than what was billed. Credit balances can be identified by the *Credit Balances* link under the *Billing* section of the *Dashboard* on the *Home* page for a specific batch or group. A credit balance should either be refunded to the patient or an insurance company or it can be applied to another date of service.

 TIP After you post payments via electronic remittances, it is best practice to work credit balances for the batch you were working on before posting the batch.

Matching Unmatched Transactions

Harris CareTracker PM matches the transactions on the electronic remittance to a specific patient, date of service, CPT® code, and charge amount. Only complete matches will be processed electronically; partial and no matches must be manually matched before they can be processed. If they are not matched, the payment must be posted manually into Harris CareTracker PM via the *Payments Open Items* application.

Print Insurance EOBs

From *Electronic Remittances,* Harris CareTracker PM can also print paper EOBs. Harris CareTracker PM has payer-specific EOBs that mimic payers' customized EOBs. Although not an active feature in your student version, in a live environment payer-specific EOBs can be printed for the payers listed below.

A generic EOB can be printed for all other payers. A generic EOB does not mimic a payer's customized EOB, but does include standard information such as patient name, allowed amount, paid amount, deductible/copayment, and adjustment. Generic EOBs are printed the same way as payer-specific EOBs.

In a live environment, payer-specific EOBs can be printed for the following payers:

- Medicare
- Aetna
- Blue Cross Blue Shield of Massachusetts
- Harvard Pilgrim
- Blue Shield of Texas
- Railroad Medicare
- Cigna, Unicare (GIC Indemnity)
- Tricare (North Region)

- United Healthcare
- Medicaid of Rhode Island
- Blue Cross Blue Shield of Rhode Island
- Medicaid of Massachusetts
- Tufts
- DME
- Connecticare
- GHI

FYI The workflow to print insurance EOBs in a live environment:

1. Access the *Home* module > *Dashboard* tab > *Billing* section > *Electronic Remittances* link.

2. Select the electronic remittance that you want to print. The application displays the EOB in the lower frame of the screen. (**Note:** Your screen will display "No Bulk Checks match your criteria" (**Figure 9-63**) because *ClaimsManager* is not active in your student version of Harris CareTracker PM.)

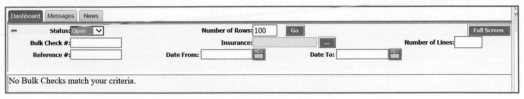

Figure 9-63   No Bulk Checks Match Your Criteria

3. Click *Print*. The application displays the *Print* window.

4. Click *Print EOB* to print the entire EOB. This will be a complete EOB without page breaks between patients. **Figure 9-64** is representative of a generic EOB, not one that would be electronically generated in Harris CareTracker.

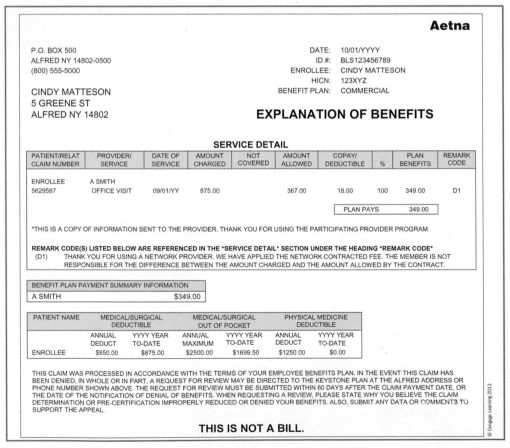

Figure 9-64   Generic EOB

5. To print an EOB for a patient or multiple patients, click on the corresponding patient's name in the *Associated Patient* box and then click *Add*.

TIP If a selection is made in error, click on the patient listed in the *Selected* box and then click the *Remove* button.

6. Click *Print EOB*. The application displays the *File Download* window.

7. Click *Open*. Adobe Acrobat opens the EOB in a window.

8. From the Adobe Acrobat menu, click *File > Print*.

Note: If printing multiple EOBs, each will print on a separate page by default.

Denials

Denials are claims that an insurance company has determined it will not pay, such as when a patient has not met his or her deductible. The *Denials* application identifies both the total number of denials and the total monetary value of the denials for a specific period, batch, or group. The application is updated overnight. In this application, you can work denials to adjust off balances. By working your denials separately from posting payments, you will improve the workflow and efficiency in your practice. Your student version of Harris CareTracker PM will not post *Denials* in your *Dashboard* because *ClaimsManager* is not active. If you were working in a live *Practice Management* system, best practice would be to work *Denials* after your batch has been posted. The *Dashboard* only shows *Denials* for the month. *Denials* are only tallied on the *Dashboard* if:

- The denial code or description was manually entered in the *Description* field in the *Open Items* application.

- Payments were posted electronically via *Electronic Remittances*. *Electronic Remittances* posted in Harris CareTracker PM will automatically post any denials. *Denials* remain in the *Denials* link on the *Dashboard* until they are paid or adjusted off.

Denial Details

Clicking on a denial in the work list displays the *Denial Details* tab (**Figure 9-65**). From the *Details* screen you can:

- Click the denial to display the *Procedure Line Item Details* in a new window

- Adjust procedure denials individually or in bulk

- Transfer one or more denial balances to private pay

- Launch the *Open Items* application for a denial

- View the *Claim Summary* for the denial

- Click the *Microsoft Excel®* icon at the bottom of the work list to export the denial details to a *Microsoft Excel®* file.

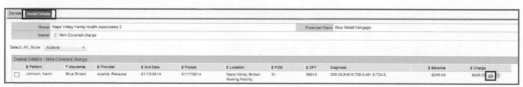

Figure 9-65   Denial Details Tab   Courtesy of Harris CareTracker PM and EMR

The *Denials* screen can be accessed by going to the *Home* module > *Dashboard* tab > *Billing* header > *Denials* link (**Figure 9-66**).

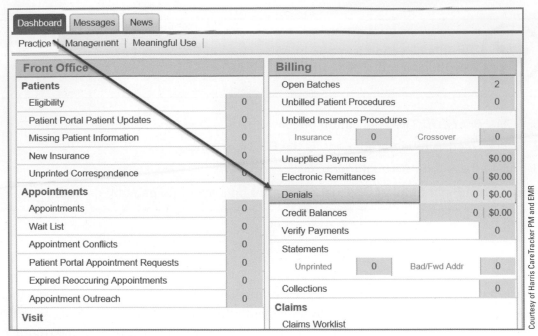

Figure 9-66 Denials Link

Using the same patient from Activity 9-10 (Edith Robinson), you will now post a denial and additional remittance to her account.

 ## Activity 9-11
Enter a Denial and Remittance 🚩

1. Before beginning this activity, click on *Batch* in the *Name Bar* and confirm you are still working in the "9-10PostRAs" batch.

2. With patient Edith Robinson in context, click on the *OI* button on the *Name Bar*.

3. You will see the charges for Ms. Robinson's *Open Items*. You are going to now work the SNF edited charges for Procedure codes 99214 and G0180.

TIP

1. **Important!!** Only if you do **not** see the edited SNF charges for Procedure codes 99214 and G0180, go to the *Home* module > *Dashboard* tab > *Visit* header > *Missing Encounters/Visit* link and you will see that the *Charge* has not been saved.

To save the *Charges*, set the fields as follows:

- Include the date of the patient encounter.
- Select *All providers*.
- Select *All locations*.
- Select *Visits Yes*.
- Select *Charges No*.
- Click *Go*.

2. In the *Date* column, locate the visit date (refer to Figure 9-59) for patient Edith Robinson's SNF charges from Activity 9-3. Then click on the *Charges* button on the right side of your screen for the date of service corresponding to Edith's Activity 9-3 charges. (Remember, the *Charges* button may not necessarily appear in Edith Robinson's row; it may appear in the row of a different patient who has the same date of service as her.)

3. Then click *Go* on the left side of your screen. The charges for all patient encounters on the Date of Service (DOS) display. **Note:** You may receive a pop-up message that says "Transaction Date must be within Period Start and End Dates: (of the date of your batch)." Click *OK* and the charges appear in the lower portion of your screen.

4. Scroll down to the bottom of the lower screen, and click *Save* on the bottom left. (**Note:** If more than one charge [e.g., multiple patient visits] appear on the date, the *Charges* will be saved for all patients.)

5. Wait until the "Transaction Saved" message appears before moving on. Then click *OK*. You will receive another pop-up stating "Bulk Charges Saved." Click *OK*.

6. With patient Edith Robinson in context, click on the *OI* ⬚ button on the *Name Bar*.

4. Click on *Payment* in the *Open Action* column for code 99214 and the *Open Items* dialog box will display in the lower portion of the screen. Procedure 99214 is not a covered charge. A charge that is not covered will have the dollar amount listed in the "Not Covered (DENIAL)" column of the EOB/RA.

5. Enter the "Not Covered (DENIAL)" information from Edith Robinson's EOB/RA (Source Document 9-1b, found on page 484) for Procedure 99214 as instructed below. Your completed screen should look like Figure 9-67.

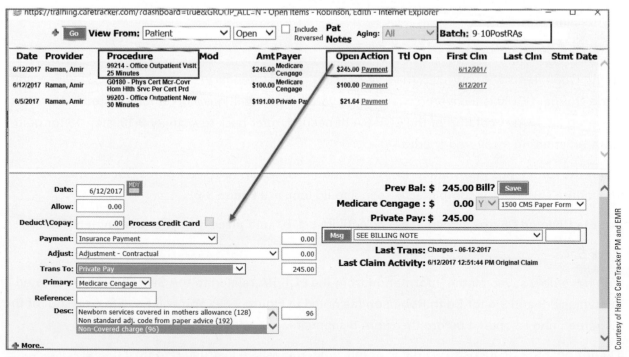

Figure 9-67 Open Action/Payment Screen $245 Charge

Note: Be sure to use the [Tab] key so that fields automatically populate.

    a. *Date*: Enter today's date (within the *Fiscal Period/Fiscal Year* set in your batch).

    b. *Allow*: Leave blank. (0.00)

    c. *Deduct/Copay*: Leave blank. (0.00)

    d. *Payment*: Using the drop-down, select "Insurance Payment." **Note:** You may need to change the field first to (Select Payment Type) and then back to "Insurance Payment." Be sure you use the [Tab] key so that amounts will populate in the proper fields.

    e. *Adjust*: Select "Adjustment – Contractual." Make sure this field is "0.00." If you need to enter "0.00," be sure you use the [Tab] key so that amounts will populate in the proper fields.

    f. *Transfer To*: Use the drop-down and select *Private Pay*. This will automatically populate the amount field to the right of *Trans To*, as well as the *Prev Bal* and *Private Pay* fields.

    g. *Primary*: Leave blank (or it can remain "Medicare Cengage").

    h. *Reference*: Leave blank.

    i. *Desc*: Type "96" in the blank box to the right of *Desc* and hit [Tab]. This will select "Non-Covered charge (96)."

    j. In the *Msg* field, use the drop-down list and select *SEE BILLING NOTE*.

    k. Your screen should reflect the same entries as noted in Source Document 9-1b (on page 484) for Procedure code 99214.

📇 **Print the Not Covered (DENIAL) Charge screen, label it "Activity 9-11a," and place it in your assignment folder.**

    l. Click *Save*. You will have to close out of the *OI* screen and re-open it before the claim disappears.

6. Click back on the *OI* button.

7. In the *Open Items* window, click the *Payment* link under the *Action* header for the G0180 Procedure code charge. G0180 is a covered charge. A covered charge will have *no* amount listed in the "Not Covered (DENIAL)" column of the EOB/RA (If needed, refer back to Activity 9-10, step 18 for guidance on entering a covered charge.)

8. Enter the remittance information from Edith Robinson's EOB/RA (see Source Document 9-1b) for Procedure G0180. Your completed screen should look like **Figure 9-68**.

📇 **Print the Covered Charge screen, label it "Activity 9-11b," and place it in your assignment folder.**

9. Click *Save*.

10. You have now saved all the information from the EOB/RA related to the SNF charge you created in Activities 9-3 and 9-4 for Edith Robinson (as noted in **Figure 9-69**). You will have to close out of the *OI* screen and re-open it before the claim disappears.

11. Do **not** post the "9-10PostRAs" batch at this time. You will be instructed to post it later.

Courtesy of Harris CareTracker PM and EMR

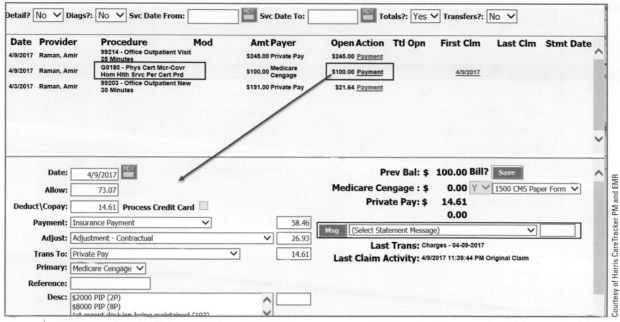

Figure 9-68 Open Action/Payment Screen $100 Charge

Courtesy of Harris CareTracker PM and EMR

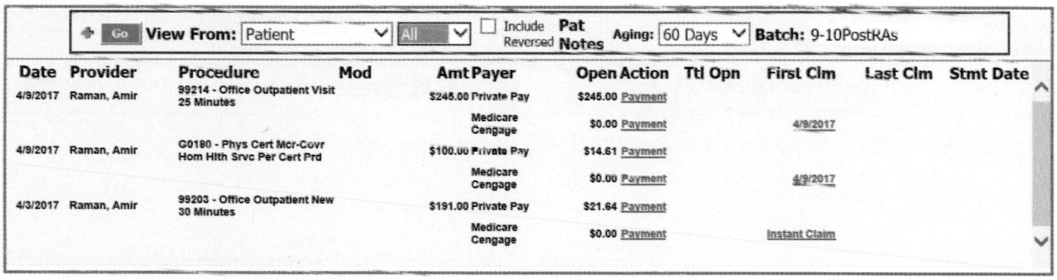

Figure 9-69 Denial and Remittance Information Saved—SNF Charge

Having entered the denial in Activity 9-11, the balance has now been transferred to private pay. **Note:** It is important to remember that it takes 24 hours for *Denials* to display in the *Dashboard* in a live environment. You can adjust your filters to set your display options. The *Dashboard* only shows *Denials* for the month.

Now that you have entered the EOB/RA and transferred the remaining balance to *Private Pay*, a typical workflow would be to adjust the denial balance. For instance, if after you transferred the balance to *Private Pay*, you determined that the CPT® code used should not have been billed; you would then adjust the denial balance to reflect the change.

Credit Balances

Working credit balances by batch should be done immediately after an electronic remittance has been posted in Harris CareTracker PM. Credit balances are created when either a patient or an insurance company pays more money for a specific procedure for a specific date of service than what was billed. Credit balances can be identified by the *Credit Balances* link under the *Billing* section of the *Dashboard* in the *Home* module for a specific batch or group (**Figure 9-70**). After you post payments via electronic remittances, it is best practice to work credit balances for the batch you were working in before posting the batch.

There are two ways to work credit balances: *by Batch* or *for Refunds* (**Figure 9-71**). Once you post the batch, this will create a charge on the patient's account. You can then post a payment to create the credit balance.

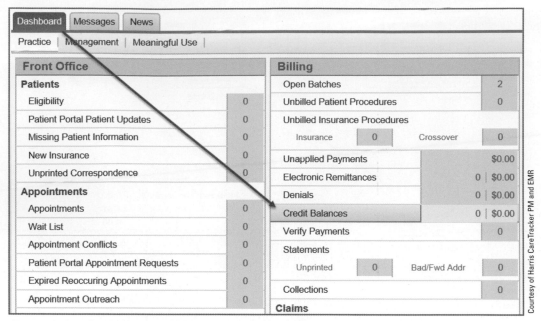

Figure 9-70   Credit Balances Link

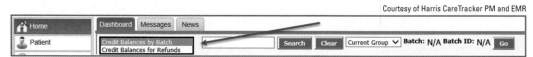

Figure 9-71   Work Credit Balances—By Batch or for Refunds

 TIP There is a big difference between a "Credit" and an "Unapplied Credit." A credit is an overpayment on an account, and an unapplied credit is only a patient payment (not insurance) that has not been attached to a DOS.

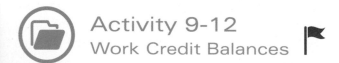

Activity 9-12
Work Credit Balances

In order to work a *Credit Balance*, you must first have a credit in the patient's account.

1. Pull patient Edith Robinson into context.

2. Create a new batch and name it "9-12CreditBalance" using the following parameters:

   a. *Fiscal Period*: The fiscal period of Ms. Robinson's SNF charge created in Activity 9-3.

   b. *Fiscal Year*: The fiscal year of Ms. Robinson's SNF charge created in Activity 9-3.

   c. *Provider*: Select Ms. Robinson's PCP (Dr. Raman).

   d. *Resource*: Select Dr. Raman as *Resource.*

   e. *Location*: Napa Valley Family Associates.

   f. Leave *Service Date From, Service Trans Date*, and *Payment Trans Date* blank.

3. Click *Save and Close* on the batch screen.

4. Click on the *OI* button on the *Name Bar*. Harris CareTracker PM displays the *Open Items* application.

5. To see a credit balance, you will need to post a payment to the patient's account first, following these instructions. The payment must be greater than the balance in the patient's account in *OI* in the *Open Action* column:

    a. Click on the *Payment* line in the *Open Action* column of her G0180 Procedure (which should be listed as "Private Pay" in the *Payer* column). The *payment* screen will display in the lower portion of the window.

    b. Using the *Payment* drop-down, select *Payment – Patient Cash (PATCSH)*.

    c. In the amount field next to the *Payment* drop-down, enter a payment in the amount of $50.00 more than the *OI* balance of her account. In this instance, her *OI* balance displays as $14.61, so you would add $50.00 to that amount for a total entry of $64.61. (**Note:** Do not enter the dollar sign.) You will see the *Private Pay* balance change to "$–50.00."

    d. In the *Msg* drop-down select (or leave as) "Select Statement Message." Your screen should look like **Figure 9-72**.

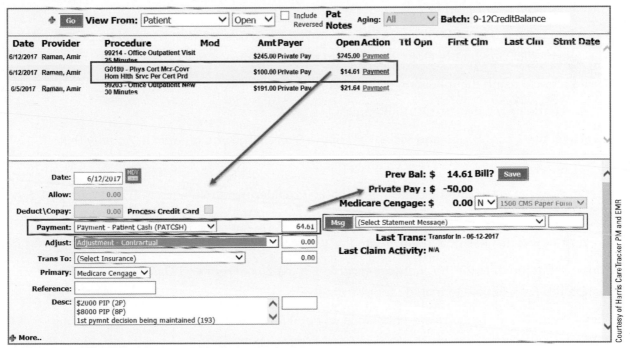

Figure 9-72   *OI Credit Balance Screen*

    e. Click *Save*.

    f. To close the *Open Items* screen, click "X."

    g. Run a *Journal* for the "9-12CreditBalance" batch.

    h. *Post* the "9-12CreditBalance" batch.

6. Go to the *Home* module > *Dashboard* tab > *Billing* header > *Credit Balances* link (see Figure 9-70).

7. Click on the *Search* button and Harris CareTracker PM displays a list of open batches in the *Search* dialog box.

    a. Because you have already posted your batch, it does not display in the *Search* box.

    b. Type in "9-12" and click the "Includes Closed Batches" and "All Groups" checkboxes (**Figure 9-73**), and then click *Search*.

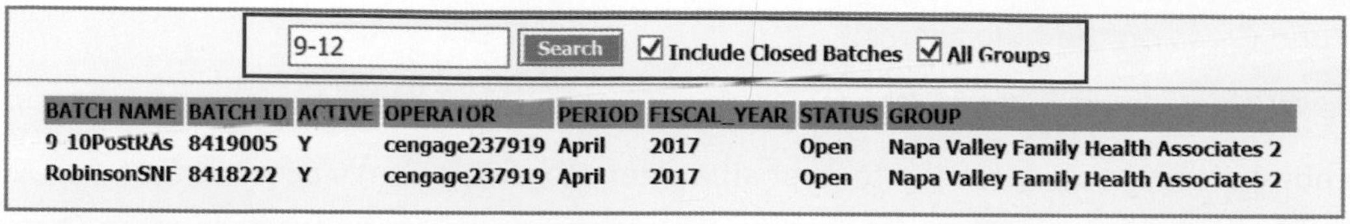

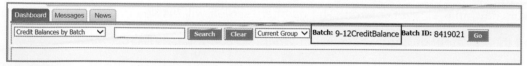

Figure 9-73   Credit Balance Search Criteria

Courtesy of Harris CareTracker PM and EMR

8. Click on the "9-12CreditBalance" batch and it is pulled into context (**Figure 9-74**).

Figure 9-74   Pull 9-12 Batch into Context

Courtesy of Harris CareTracker PM and EMR

9. Click *Go* and Harris CareTracker PM displays a list of credit balances including the patient's name, the financial class with the credit balance, the amount of the credit, and the patient's last transaction date.

10. Pull patient Edith Robinson into context on the *Name Bar* if you have not already done so.

11. In the drop-down menu found directly under the *Dashboard* tab, change "Credit Balances by Batch" to "Credit Balances for Refunds."

12. Since you posted the "CreditBalance" batch previously in this activity, you will be prompted to create a new batch. Click *Edit* on the *Operator Encounter Batch Control*. Click *Create Batch*.

13. Create a batch using the following parameters:

    a. Name the new batch "9-12CrBalRefunds."

    b. Select the *Fiscal Period* and *Fiscal Year* of the SNF charge you created in Activity 9-3.

    c. Click *Save*.

    d. Confirm the entries in the batch control box (Provider/Resource/Location) and then click *Save and Close*.

    e. Your new batch has now been created.

14. Confirm that the date for the charge is included in the *Date From* and *Date To* fields. **Hint**: Always change the *Date To* field to include today's date.

15. Click *Go* and Ms. Robinson's credit balance will pull in to the screen.

16. In the *Action* Column, use the drop-down and select *Refund-Patient (P)* (**Figure 9-75**).

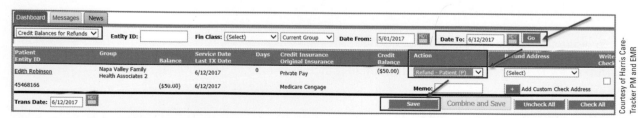

Figure 9-75   Select Patient for Credit Balances for Refunds

Courtesy of Harris Care-Tracker PM and EMR

🖨 **Print the Credit Balance for Refunds screen, label it "Activity 9-12," and place it in your assignment folder.**

17. Click *Save*.

18. The *Credit Balance Transfer* dialog box will display.

19. Click on *Write Transactions* (**Figure 9-76**).

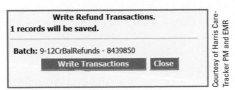

Figure 9-76   *Write Transactions*

20. The *Credit Balance Transfer* dialog box will confirm that the transaction has been saved (**Figure 9-77**).

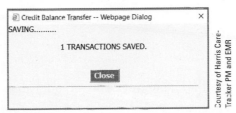

Figure 9-77   *Credit Balance Transfer Dialog Box*

21. Click *Close*, and the credit balance is removed from your screen.

In order to continue with billing and collections activities, you must build and generate claims, save the charges, and process the EOB/RAs for Jane Morgan, Ellen Ristino, Craig X. Smith, and Barbara Watson, as described in the following activity.

Activity 9-13
Save Charges, Process Remittance, and Transfer to Private Pay

In this activity, you will work with the following patients. Before you begin, refer back to the patient encounters and record the date of the encounters for this activity's patients:

9-13a: Jane Morgan (Source Document 9-2): _____

9-13b: Ellen Ristino (Source Document 9-3): _____

9-13c: Craig X. Smith (Source Document 9-4): _____

9-13d: Barbara Watson (Source Document 9-5): _____

1. Create a new batch and name it "9-13PostRAs" with the following parameters:

   a. Select the *Fiscal Period* and *Fiscal Year* for today's date.

   b. Click *Save*.

   c. Leave the *Provider/Resource/Location* as is.

   d. Click *Save and Close*.

TIP Since you have multiple batches open, it is best practice to confirm that you are work-ing in the correct batch. To confirm, click on the *Batch* icon. The batch you are working in will display. If the batch displaying is NOT the batch you are instructed to be working in, click *Edit*, and in the *Operator Encounter Batch Control* box, use the drop-down by each of the following batch fields: the *Encounter Batch Control*, *Payment Batch Control*, and *the Rever-sal Batch Control*, and change to the name of the batch you want to be working in. When finished, click *Save and Close*. You will now be working in the different batch you selected.

2. Check that charges have been saved for each of the patients listed above. To do this, go to the *Home* module > *Dashboard* tab > *Visit* header > *Missing Encounters* > *Charges* link and set the fields as follows:
    - Change the beginning date to January 1, 20XX (current year) and change the ending date to today's date. Be sure the dates include the date of the patient's encounter.
    - Select *All providers.*
    - Select *All locations.*
    - Select *Visits Yes.*
    - Select *Charges No.*

3. Then click *Go*. You will see *Charges*(s) that have **not** been saved. You may or may not see the charges for these four patients here. That is because charges for the four patients in this activity would have already been saved in Activity 9-10 if the patients had appointments on the same date as Edith Robinson. If an appointment was on a different date than Edith Robinson's, that appointment will appear here and the charges will need to be saved. If charges for any of these four patients are displaying, save the charges now. You can refer back to steps 8–12 of Activity 9-10 for assistance if needed. If no charges are displaying for any of these four patients, move forward to step 4.

4. Generate claims for all procedures listed for Ms. Morgan, Ms. Ristino, Mr. Smith, and Ms. Watson (refer to the steps noted below):
    - Pull patient into context.
    - *Click the OI* button *in the Name bar.*
    - Click on *Instant Claim* in the *First Clm* column (refer to **Figure 9-38**) for one of the procedures. Harris CareTracker PM displays the *Claims Summary* in the lower frame of the screen.
    - Place a check mark next to each claim and then click *Build Claim*. You will then note that the date you performed the activity is listed in the *First Clm* column.

5. For each patient noted above, process the EOB/RAs from Source Documents 9-2 through 9-5, provided at the end of this activity. Refresher steps are provided as a "Tip" below. **Hint**: Denials should be entered as they were in Activity 9-11, step 5. A denial is when the *Amount Charged* and the *Not Covered* is the same amount, and when the *Amount Allowed* is 0.00 on the EOB/RA.

 TIP *Refresher:* **Process an EOB/RA**
    1. If you are not already viewing the *Open Items* window, click on the *OI* button in the *Name Bar*.
    2. Click on the *Payment* link in the *Action* column next to the Procedure(s).
    3. Harris CareTracker PM displays the payment window in the lower frame of the screen (refer to **Figure 9-61**).
    4. In the payment window on the lower part of the screen, enter the information from the patient's EOB/RA (see the Source Documents provided at the end of this activity) for the

visit as follows. First determine if the charge is covered or not covered. To do this, look in the "Not Covered (DENIAL)" column of the EOB/RA. A covered charge will have no amount listed in the "Not Covered (DENIAL)" column. A not covered charge has an amount listed in the "Not Covered (DENIAL)" column. As described below, the process you follow for entering the charge will vary depending on if the charge is covered or not covered.

Covered Charges:
- *Date:* This should be today's date, the date you "received the EOB/RA" for the patient's visit.
- *Allow:* Enter the information from the *Amount Allowed* column on the EOB/RA. Now hit the [Tab] button on your keyboard.
- *Deduct/Copay:* Enter the information from the *Deduct/Coins/Copay* column on the EOB/RA. Now hit the [Tab] button and this will populate the amount in the *Adjust* and *Transfer To* fields based on the information entered in the *Demographics* screen.
- *Payment:* Confirm that *Insurance Payment* is selected.
- *Adjust:* Confirm that *Adjustment – Contractual* is selected.
- *Trans To:* Confirm that *Private Pay* is selected.
- *Primary:* Confirm that the patient's correct insurance is selected.
- *Reference:* Leave blank.
- *Desc:* Leave as is.
- *Msg:* Leave as is.

Not Covered Charges:
- *Date:* This should be today's date; the date you "received the EOB/RA" for the patient's visit.
- *Allow:* Enter the information from the *Amount Allowed* column on the EOB/RA. Now hit the [Tab] button on your keyboard.
- *Deduct/Copay:* Enter the information from the *Deduct/Coins/Copay* column on the EOB/RA. Now hit the [Tab] button and this will populate the amount in the *Adjust* and *Transfer To* fields based on the information entered in the *Demographics* screen.
- *Payment:* Confirm that *Insurance Payment"* is selected and $0.00 is the amount in the field.
- *Adjust:* Confirm that *Adjustment–Contractual* is selected. Delete the amount in the *Adjust* field, enter "0.00" and then hit the [Tab] button.
- *Trans To:* Confirm that *Private Pay* is selected. The *Trans To* field should then populate with *Private Pay* and the amount of the charge denied. (**Note:** If it does not populate, manually enter the amount to *Trans To Private Pay.* The *Private Pay* amount would be the same as noted in the "Patient Resp" column on the EOB/RA.)
- *Primary:* Confirm that the patient's correct insurance is selected.
- *Reference:* Leave blank.
- *Desc:* Leave as is.
- *Msg:* Leave as is.

5. Once you have entered the EOB/RA information, click *Save.* Your transaction will be saved and the claim disappears. (You have now saved all the entries from the EOB/RA related to the charge you created. You have to close out of the *OI* screen and re-open it before the claim disappears.)
6. If you were working multiple charges, you would repeat the steps to enter each of the charges listed on the EOB/RA. Refer to **Figure 9-62** for an example of what your completed screen should look like.
7. Close out of the *Open Items* window by clicking the "X" in the upper-right corner of the window.
8. Repeat the above steps for each patient.

6. Upon completion of *ALL* payment/denial entries, run a *Journal* (reference Activity 9-5 for assistance) and review for accuracy. Do **not** post the "9-13PostRAs" batch at this time.

🖳 Print the Journal after completing all the 9-13 activities, label it "Activity 9-13" and place in your assignment folder.

Source Document 9-2: Explanation of Benefits/Remittance Advice

BLUE SHIELD CENGAGE

Blue Shield Cengage
P.O. Box 32245
Los Angeles, CA 90002

Date: MM/DD/YYYY (use today's date)
Payment Number: 5564856
Payment Amount: $0.00

AMIR RAMAN, D.O.
Napa Valley Family Health Associates (NVFHA)
101 Vine Street
Napa, CA 94558

Account Number	Patient Name				Subscriber Number		Claim Number			
Dates of Service	Description of Service	Amount Charged	Not Covered (DENIAL)	Prov Adj Discount	Amount Allowed	Deduct/ Coins/ Copay	Paid to Provider	Adj Reason Code	Rmk Code	Patient Resp
BCBS97	**Morgan, Jane**									
(Appt. date used in Activity 4-1)	99213	$112.00		$36.00	$76.00	$76.00	$0.00			$56.00
(Appt. date used in Activity 4-1)	90746	$100.00		$23.00	$77.00	$77.00	$0.00			$77.00

Source Document 9-3:   Explanation of Benefits/Remittance Advice

ELUE SHIELD CENGAGE

Blue Shield Cengage
P.O. Box 32245
Los Angeles, CA 90002

Date: MM/DD/YYYY (use today's date)
Payment Number: 5564854
Payment Amount: $81.64

ANTHONY BROCKTON, M.D.
Napa Valley Family Health Associates (NVFHA)
101 Vine Street
Napa, CA 94558

Account Number	Patient Name				Subscriber Number			Claim Number			
Dates of Service	Description of Service	Amount Charged	Not Covered (DENIAL)	Prov Adj Discount	Amount Allowed	Deduct/ Coins/ Copay	Paid to Provider	Adj Reason Code	Rmk Code	Patient Resp
BCBS97	**Ristino, Ellen**									
(Appt. date used in Activity 4-1)	99213	$112.00		$36.00	$76.00	$15.20	$60.80			$15.20
(Appt. date used in Activity 4-1)	86308	$45.00			$16.55	$3.31	$13.24			$3.31
(Appt. date used in Activity 4-1)	3210F	$24.00			$9.50	$1.90	$7.60			$1.90
(Appt. date used in Activity 4-1)	36415	$15.00	$15.00		$0.00					$15.00
(Appt. date used in Activity 4-1)	94760	$13.00	$13.00		$0.00					$13.00

Source Document 9-4:   Explanation of Benefits/Remittance Advice

MEDICAID CENGAGE

Medicaid Cengage
P.O. Box 221352
Fresno, CA 93701

Date: MM/DD/YYYY (use today's date)
Payment Number: 5644425
Payment Amount: $46.00

AMIR RAMAN, D.O.
Napa Valley Family Health Associates (NVFHA)
101 Vine Street
Napa, CA 94558

Account Number	Patient Name					Subscriber Number			Claim Number			
Dates of Service	Description of Service	Amount Charged	Not Covered (DENIAL)	Prov Adj Discount		Amount Allowed	Deduct/ Coins/ Copay		Paid to Provider	Adj Reason Code	Rmk Code	Patient Resp
CAID8002	**Smith, Craig X.**											
(Appt. date used in Activity 4-1)	99213	$112.00		$79.00		$33.00	$0.00		$33.00			$0.00
(Appt. date used in Activity 4-1)	J7650	$25.00		$18.00		$7.00	$0.00		$7.00			$0.00
(Appt. date used in Activity 4-1)	71020	$13.50		$7.50		$6.00	$0.00		$6.00			$0.00

Source Document 9-5: Explanation of Benefits/Remittance Advice

BLUE SHIELD CENGAGE

Blue Shield Cengage
P.O. Box 32245
Los Angeles, CA 90002

Date: MM/DD/YYYY (use today's date)
Payment Number: 5564855
Payment Amount: $0.00

AMIR RAMAN, D.O.
Napa Valley Family Health Associates (NVFHA)
101 Vine Street
Napa, CA 94558

Account Number	Patient Name				Subscriber Number			Claim Number			
Dates of Service	Description of Service	Amount Charged	Not Covered (DENIAL)	Prov Adj Discount	Amount Allowed	Deduct/ Coins/ Copay	Paid to Provider	Adj Reason Code	Rmk Code	Patient Resp
BCBS97	**Watson, Barbara**									
(Appt. date used in Activity 4-2)	99213	$112.00		$36.00	$76.00	$76.00	$0.00			$56.00
(Appt. date used in Activity 4-2)	94760	$13.00		$11.00	$2.00	$2.00	$0.00			$2.00

Unapplied Payments

When a patient makes a payment before services are rendered (such as a copayment), or a payment is received that does not indicate a specific date of service, the payment is posted into Harris CareTracker PM as an *unapplied payment*. An unapplied payment is money that has been applied to a patient's account, but not to a specific date of service. The unapplied money can be applied automatically to the patient's charge through either the *Charges* or *Bulk Charges* application. If the unapplied money is not applied automatically, you will be able to apply the unapplied amount manually. The *Unapplied* application on the *Dashboard* lists each patient with an unapplied balance, the amount of unapplied money and the patient's last transaction date. As best practice, this list should be reviewed and reconciled daily.

Applying Unapplied Money

Not every Practice Management system has an *Apply/Unapplied* feature. Harris CareTracker PM does. A batch must be open to apply unapplied money and the patient must have a balance on his or her account. The total amount of unapplied money saved on the patient's account is displayed in the *Unapplied* field. When a monetary amount is entered in the field next to *Apply Unapplied*, Harris CareTracker PM deducts that amount from the *Unapplied* box. Refer to *Help* for additional information regarding applying unapplied money.

Billing Statements

Harris CareTracker PM generates and prints patient statements once a week; however, patients will only receive one statement every 30 days regardless of the number of services they have had. A statement will not be generated for a patient if the patient has an unapplied balance saved on his or her account equal to or greater than the current patient balance amount.

From the *Unprinted Statements* application, you can identify the batch of patients who should receive a statement, print billing statements, and identify patient statements that were undeliverable or forwarded to a new address.

Undeliverable and forwarding addresses are gathered through Express Bill, the company Harris CareTracker PM uses to distribute patient statements.

Verify Payments

The *Verify Payments* application compares the actual amount paid by an insurance company for a claim to the expected allowed amount, as defined on the *Allowed Schedule* linked to the physician billing contract, and is payer specific. If the payment made by the insurance company is different than the allowed amount, then *Verify Payments* indicates the discrepancy. You can then view the details of the over- or underpayment and use the work area to override, adjust, rebill, or transfer payment amounts as necessary to resolve the **variance (Figure 9-78)**.

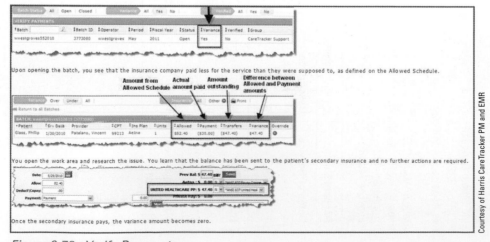

Figure 9-78   Verify Payments

For example, suppose you want to verify that the practice received the expected reimbursement for open payment batches. Using the *Verify Payments* application, you see that an open batch contains a payment item with a variance. Upon opening the batch, you see that the insurance company paid less for the service than it was supposed to as defined on the *Allowed Schedule.* You open the work area and research the issue. You learn that the balance has been sent to the patient's secondary insurance and no further actions are required. Once the secondary insurance pays, the variance amount becomes zero.

Viewing Payment Variances

The *Verify Payments* application displays a list of open batches containing one or more payment items with a variance. You can filter, sort, and search batches with payment variances, and filter and sort payment variances within a particular batch.

Table 9-2 describes the variance details that are displayed for the *Payment Item*.

Table 9-2　Payment Item Variance Details

DETAIL	DESCRIPTION
Patient	Name of the patient who received the service and incurred the charges.
Srv Date	Date on which the service was provided.
Provider	Physician responsible for providing the service.
CPT®	CPT® code identifying the service the patient received and for which the charge applies.
Ins Plan	Patient's primary insurance plan.
Units	Number of service units for which the charge applies.
Allowed	Negotiated amount of money the primary insurance is responsible for paying, as defined on the Allowed Schedule.
Payment	Amount of money received from the insurance company for the service to date.
Transfers	Amount of money outstanding. This is the total amount of money transferred to another party responsible for payment, such as a secondary insurance company, deductible or copay, and collections.
Variance	Difference between the Allowed and Payment amounts. This is the difference between the actual amount of money you received from the insurance company and the negotiated rate the insurance is responsible for paying. For example, Aetna's allowed amount for CPT® code 99213 is $82.40, but it paid only $35.00. Equation: Allowed − Payment = Variance Calculation: $82.30 − ($35.00) = $47.40 Therefore, the Variance is $47.40.
Override	If you want to allow the variance and verify the payment, then select a reason for overriding the variance. See the *Managing Payment Variances* section that follows for more information.

You also have the option to filter or sort the list. To filter the list, click the filter options at the top of the page.

- *Variance.* By default, only items that have been underpaid ("Under") are displayed. Click *Over* to display only items that have been over paid. Click *All* to display both under and over paid items and items with a variance that has been overridden.

- *Insurance.* By default, items for all insurance companies ("All") are displayed. To view only items for a particular company, click the company from the *Other* shortcut menu.

Managing Payment Variances

Managing payment variances involves first determining the cause and solution for the variance and then working the payment to resolve or override the variance. After resolving the variance, you can verify the payment batch.

Step 1 is to determine the cause and solution for a payment variance. Before you can work the payment to resolve the variance, you must first determine the cause of the variance and decide the appropriate way to resolve it. Determining the cause involves viewing the variance and looking at the item's payment history. When viewing the payment history for the item, you need to ask yourself questions about how to resolve the variance, such as:

- Does the payment need to be rebilled?

- Does the payment need to be adjusted?

- Will the payment be transferred to a secondary insurance?

- Is the patient responsible for the variance balance?

The way you will work the payment is determined by the answers to such questions, and is unique to the particular payment at hand.

Tables 9-3, 9-4, and **9-5** list scenarios, causes, and resolution details for payment variances. Each table contains variance details as they are displayed in the *Verify Payments* application. Underneath the variance details is a description of the variance scenario, how to determine the cause of the payment variance, and the steps you might take to resolve the variance.

Table 9-3   Scenario 1: Balance Transfer

INS PLAN	ALLOWED	PAYMENT	TRANSFERS	VARIANCE
Medicare	$62.50	($50.00)	($12.50)	$12.50

Payment variance scenario:

A claim in the amount of $62.50 is submitted to the patient's primary insurance, Medicare. Medicare's allowed payment for the service is $62.50, but it paid only $50.00, leaving an under-variance of $12.50. The *Transfer* amount of $12.50 indicates that the balance may be transferred to a co-insurance, private pay, or other party.

Step 1: Determine the cause of the payment variance.

View the open item payment history and determine where the unpaid $12.50 was sent. If a co-insurance is responsible for the payment, then the variance will be adjusted once the payment is made. If the patient is responsible for the payment, then you need to work the payment and send a bill to the patient.

Step 2: Work the payment.

If the patient is responsible for the remaining $12.50, then you must *Transfer* the balance to the patient and generate a bill.

Table 9-4　Scenario 2: Insurance Denial

INS PLAN	ALLOWED	PAYMENT	TRANSFERS	VARIANCE
Blue Cross	$0.00	($0.00)	($50.00)	$50.00

Payment variance scenario:

The lack of payment by the insurance company indicates that the insurance company may have denied payment, and the *Transfer* amount of $50.00 indicates that the amount may have been transferred to a co-insurance.

Step 1: Determine the cause of the payment variance.

View the open item payment history and determine why the insurance company did not pay its Allowed amount. You may need to take further steps to determine how to process the payment, such as contacting the insurance company to obtain more information about the payment status.

Step 2: Work the payment.

If the insurance company denied the claim, then you need to further process the payment. For example, you may need to bill the patient, override the variance, or resubmit the claim to the insurance company.

CRITICAL THINKING　"Solve the problem." Referring to Scenario 2: Insurance Denial (see Table 9-4), brainstorm about reasons the insurance company denied the claim. Come up with ideas to solve the problem for this claim and prevent denials of future claims. Further analyze and debate findings and discuss how you reached your conclusions.

Table 9-5　Scenario 3: Copay Transfer

INS PLAN	ALLOWED	PAYMENT	TRANSFERS	VARIANCE
Aetna	$50.00	($40.00)	($10.00)	$10.00

Payment variance scenario:

The under-variance of $10.00 implies that the primary insurance plus the patient copay equals 100% of the allowed amount.

Step 1: Determine the cause of the payment variance.

The $10.00 copay was transferred to private pay, and therefore, displays as a variance.

Step 2: Work the payment.

The remaining difference between the allowed amount and charge will be adjusted.

View or Edit Batch Deposits

Although typically practices do not use the steps to view or edit batch deposits, it is helpful to know that this feature is available. The total amount of money your group has deposited for the current month displays to the *Batch Deposits* link on the *Management* dashboard and allows you to view details of each deposit, add deposits, and edit deposits (**Figures 9-79** and **9-80**).

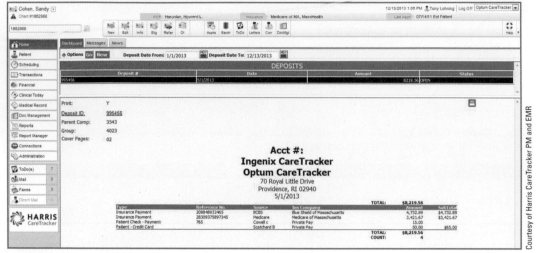

Figure 9-79   View or Edit Batch Deposits

Figure 9-80   Batch Deposits Link/Management Dashboard

CRITICAL THINKING There was a lot to cover in this chapter! Describe your understanding of the many different types of insurance plans and the effects on the practice when there is an issue regarding noncovered services.

If you are tasked with communicating the fees for services to patients, collecting copays, or billing/collections on overdue accounts, describe what communication skills you would use. How would you incorporate empathy toward the patient while performing your financial responsibilities? How would using an electronic health record help with your duties? Write out some scenarios and practice on a family member, classmate, or friend.

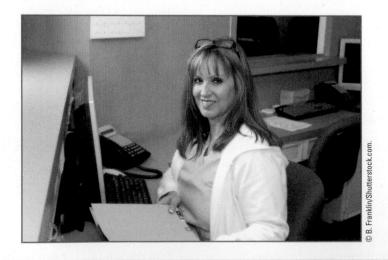

SUMMARY

The *Billing* function in Harris CareTracker PM and EMR provides a dynamic environment to ensure that the billing process goes smoothly and that the quality of the information sent to the insurance carriers is clean. The *Billing* function crosses many modules, applications, and functions.

The *batch* is the essential component required before entering and posting any financial transaction such as charges, payments, adjustments, and refunds. This helps identify transactions linked to the batch, the date of each transaction, and the operator who entered it into the system.

Prompt and accurate billing is vital to the revenue cycle and financial health of the medical practice. This chapter has provided instruction and activities that simulate workflows in a medical practice related to patient billing and entering payments and adjustments to accounts. Having completed this chapter, you should be proficient in the billing and revenue side of the practice and be able to demonstrate valuable knowledge and skills related to electronic health record billing functions. The application of skills related to the reconciliation of insurance payments, and the understanding of the *ClaimsManager* features leads to the advanced collection features and functions you will learn in Chapter 10.

CHECK YOUR KNOWLEDGE

Select the best response.

_____ 1. In *Batch Details*, the *Default Referral Provider* is set to "No." You should change the field to "Yes" if there is no referring provider in the patient's demographics or if there is no active referral/authorization for the patient. By changing the field to "Yes," who becomes the referring provider?

    a. None required   c. Designated practice

    b. Billing Provider   d. Resource

_____ 2. When manually entering a charge, how can you remove a diagnosis code in the *Diag* box?

    a. By left-clicking on the diagnosis code   c. By deleting the patient encounter

    b. By clicking on the *EncoderPro* button   d. By double-clicking on the diagnosis code

_____ 3. If a payment made by the insurance company is different than the allowed amount, then _____ indicates the discrepancy.

    a. *Allowed Schedule*   c. *Unmatched Remittance*

    b. *Verify Payments*   d. *Express Bill*

_____ 4. All transactions must be posted before running any *Month End* report in Harris CareTracker PM. Periods cannot be closed:

    a. When open batches are linked to   c. If you have not run a journal

        them   d. If there are multiple operators using the period

    b. When there are multiple periods open

_____ 5. Remittances received electronically in Harris CareTracker PM are identified in the *Electronic Remittances* application on the *Dashboard*. Harris CareTracker PM matches the transactions on the electronic remittance to a specific patient, date of service, CPT® code, and charge amount. Which is not one of the three matching categories?

    a. Complete (green)   c. Error (red)

    b. Partial match (yellow)   d. No match (white)

_____ 6. A(n) _____ is created when either a patient or an insurance company pays more money for a specific procedure for a specific date of service than what was billed.

      a. error

      b. credit balance

      c. debit balance

      d. Both b and c

_____ 7. Claims that an insurance company has determined they will not pay are known as:

      a. Undercoded

      b. Overcoded

      c. Copayments

      d. Denials

_____ 8. When a patient makes a payment before services are rendered (such as a copayment), the payment is posted into Harris CareTracker as a(n):

      a. Unapplied payment

      b. Credit balance

      c. Bulk charge

      d. Credit balance transfer

_____ 9. Denials are only tallied on the *Dashboard* if:

      a. The denial code or description was manually entered in the *Description* field in the *Open Items* application

      b. Payments were posted electronically via *Electronic Remittances*

      c. Both a and b

      d. None of the above

_____ 10. To reverse an unapplied payment (such as $30), in the *Amount* box, how would you enter it in Harris CareTracker?

      a. 30

      b. –30

      c. 60

      d. –60

CASE STUDIES

Case Study 9-1

1. Before beginning Case Study 9-1, create a new batch and name it "Ch9CS-Remit" with the following parameters:

    a. *Fiscal Period* and *Fiscal Year*: Select the current month and year for *Fiscal Period* and *Fiscal Year*. Click *Save*.

    b. Change *Provider* and *Resource* to Dr. Rebecca Ayerick.

    c. Location: Napa Valley Family Associates.

    d. Click *Save and Close*.

2. Pull patient Kevin Johnson into context.

3. Manually enter a charge for Kevin Johnson. Refer to Activity 9-3 and the following steps for help.

4. Select *Location* of "NVFA."

5. Select *POS*: Office

6. Search for and select ICD-10 code N41.0 in the *Dx Cd* field. (**Note:** This is a noncovered charge by Mr. Johnson's insurance.)

7. Using the following information, manually enter a charge for an "Online Service" for patient Kevin Johnson using today's date.

    a. Enter CPT code 99444 in the *Proc* field, and the *Fee* of $45.00.

8. Click *Save* and wait for the error message that the transaction has been saved.

9. Then click *OK*.

10. Upon completion, run a *Journal* (refer to Activity 9-5) and review. Do **not** post the "Ch9CS-Remit" batch at this time.

11. Enter a denial of the charge and transfer to private pay following instructions in Activity 9-11 and as noted on Mr. Johnson's EOB/RA (Source Document 9-6, located at the end of the Chapter 9 Case Studies). (**Hint**: First *Build the Claim* by clicking on *Instant Claim* in the *First Clm* column.)

12. Run the *Journal* again.

🖫 **Print the Journal after completing the 9-1 case study, label it "Case Study 9-1," and place in your assignment folder.**

13. Now *Post* the batch "Ch9CS-Remit."

Case Study 9-2

In order to complete Case Study 9-2, you must have completed the prior chapter Case Studies for patient Adam Thompson. Having captured the visit for Adam Thompson (in Case Study 7-3), you will now build the claim, and then enter the EOB/RA.

1. Create a new batch and name it "Ch9CS-RA" with the following parameters:

    a. *Fiscal Period* and *Fiscal Year*: Select the *Fiscal Period* and *Fiscal Year* of the encounters/visit(s) you created for Adam Thompson in Activity 4-1. Click *Save*.

    b. Change *Provider* and *Resource* to Dr. Anthony Brockton.

    c. Location: Napa Valley Family Associates.

    d. Click *Save* and *Close*.

2. Pull patient Adam Thompson into context.

3. Click on the *OI* button in the *Name Bar* and Mr. Thompson's charges will appear. **Hint**: If Mr. Thompson's charges aren't appearing in *OI*, you will need to first save the charges. To save the charges for Mr. Thompson's visit, refer back to Activity 9-13.

4. Click on *Instant Claim* in the *First Clm* column.

5. All of Mr. Thompson's charges appear in the lower screen.

6. Place a check mark next to each charge and then click *Build Claim*.

7. Now click on the *Payment* link in the *Open Action* column (repeat for each Procedure listed in the claim).

8. Referring to Source Document 9-7 located at the end of this case study, enter the EOB/RA amounts. Refer to Activities 9-9 and 9-10 for help.

9. Run a *Journal*.

🖫 **Print the screen after completing the 9-2 case study, label it "Case Study 9-2," and place in your assignment folder.**

10. Now *Post* the batch "Ch9CS-RA" (refer to Activity 9-6 for help).

Source Document 9-6: Explanation of Benefits/Remittance Advice

BLUE SHIELD CENGAGE

Blue Shield Cengage
P.O. Box 32245
Los Angeles, CA 90002

Date: MM/DD/YYYY (use today's date)
Payment Number: 2322144
Payment Amount: $0.00

REBECCA AYERICK, M.D.
Napa Valley Family Health Associates (NVFHA)
101 Vine Street
Napa, CA 94558

Account Number	Patient Name				Subscriber Number			Claim Number			
Dates of Service	Description of Service	Amount Charged	Not Covered (DENIAL)	Prov Adj Discount	Amount Allowed	Deduct/ Coins/ Copay	Paid to Provider	Adj Reason Code	Rmk Code	Patient Resp
9706416	**Johnson, Kevin**									
(Date of Case Study 9-1 manual charge)	99444	$45.00	$45.00	$0.00	$0.00	$45.00	$0.00			$45.00

Source Document 9-7:   Explanation of Benefits/Remittance Advice

Medicare Cengage
P.O. Box 234434
San Francisco, CA 94137

ANTHONY BROCKTON, M.D.
Napa Valley Family Health Associates (NVFHA)
101 Vine Street
Napa, CA 94558

MED CARE CENGAGE

Date: MM/DD/YYYY (use today's date)
Payment Number: 11235784
Payment Amount: $81.12

Account Number	Patient Name				Subscriber Number			Claim Number		
Dates of Service	Description of Service	Amount Charged	Not Covered (DENIAL)	Prov Adj Discount	Amount Allowed	Deduct/ Coins/ Copay	Paid to Provider	Adj Reason Code	Rmk Code	Patient Resp
CARE1357	Thompson, Adam									
(Appt. date from Activity 4-1)	94760	$13.00		$10.36	$2.64	$0.53	$2.11			$0.53
(Appt. date from Activity 4-1)	99213	$112.00		$53.11	$58.89	$11.78	$47.11			$11.78
(Appt. date from Activity 4-1)	71020	$13.50		$3.50	$10.00	$2.00	$8.00			$2.00
(Appt. date from Activity 4-1)	93000	$46.50		$16.50	$30.00	$6.00	$24.00			$6.00

BUILD YOUR PROFICIENCY

Proficiency Builder 9-1: Alternate Method to Access and Post Batches

1. Click on *Home* module > *Dashboard* tab > *Billing* header > *Open Batches* link (see **Figure 9-2**).

2. Print a copy of the *Open Batches* displaying on your screen.

💾 **Print the Open Batch screen after completing the BYP 9-1, label it "BYP 9-1," and place in your assignment folder.**

Proficiency Builder 9-2: Alternate Method to Apply Settings to Print Paper Claims

The alternative method to apply settings to print paper claims is to open an *Internet Explorer* browser window and launch the *Page Setup* from the menu bar; however, this method may require more adjustments than using the Harris CareTracker *Dashboard*. To apply a setting through Internet Explorer 11 complete the following steps. (**Note:** Harris CareTracker no longer supports Internet Explorer 7, 8, 9, or 10.)

1. Select the *File* drop-down menu and then click *Page Setup* (**Figure 9-81**).

2. In the *Page Setup* dialog box, remove any entries from the *Header* and *Footer* boxes. These boxes should be "-Empty-."

3. In the *Margins* section, set the Left, Right, Top, and Bottom margins to "0" (**Figure 9-82**). Click *OK*.

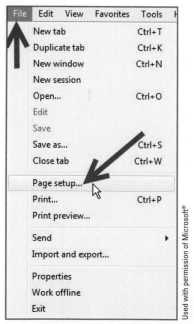

Figure 9-81   *Page Setup in Internet Explorer 11*

 TIP   To be able to print the 1500 Form, Mass Health Form, or UB92 Form from Harris Care-Tracker, you may have to adjust the *Offset Top* and *Offset Left* settings several times to get the form to line up properly.

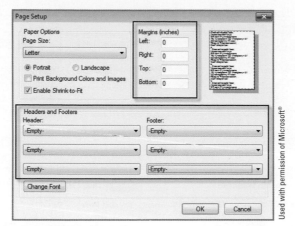

Figure 9-82   Page Setup in the Margins Setup

📧 **Print the Paper Settings screen after completing the BYP 9-2, label it "BYP 9-2," and place in your assignment folder.**

Proficiency Builder 9-3: Hospital Visits

Many times a provider will see patients in the hospital. When that occurs, you need to enter the charge for the provider's time (not the actual hospital-related charges) as noted below:

1. Create a new batch and name it "BYP-HospitalChg."

   a. Use today's date for *Fiscal Period* and *Fiscal Year*.

   b. Click *Save*.

   c. Change the *Provider* and *Resource* to Dr. Amir Raman.

   d. Click *Save and Close*.

2. Pull patient Eric Richard into context.

3. Click on the *Transactions* module. The *Charge* tab displays.

4. Enter the following information for the patient's hospital visit:

   a. Enter today's date for the *Trans Date*.

   b. *Location*: Use the drop-down and select "NVGH."

   c. *POS*: Use the drop-down and select "INPATIENT HOSPITAL."

   d. Enter the *Admit Date* of two days before today's date in MM/DD/YYYY format (see **Figure 9-83**).

   e. In the *Discharge Date* fields, enter today's date in MM/DD/YYYY format.

   f. Select Dr. Amir Raman as the *Ref Provider*.

   g. Complete the rest of the *Charge* with the following information:

   - Search Diagnosis for "DVT," and select ICD-10 code: I82.401

   - In the *Date* and *Date To* field enter yesterday's date.

   - In the *Proc* field, enter CPT code 99221.

   - In the *Fee* field, enter $145.00.

5. When finished, your screen should look like **Figure 9-83**.

(Continued)

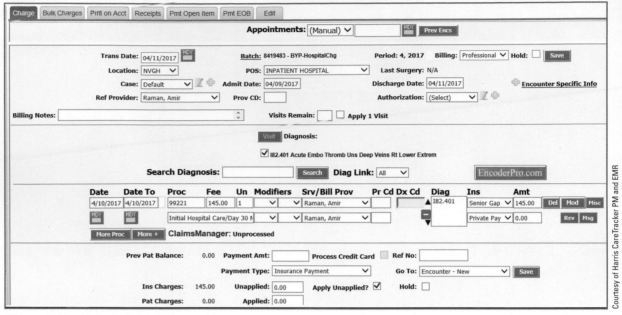

Figure 9-83   Hospital Visit Charge

▣ **Print the Hospital Charge screen after completing the BYP 9-3, label it "BYP 9-3A," and place in your assignment folder.**

6. Click *Save* and **wait** for the error message that the transaction has been saved.

7. Then click *OK*.

8. Do **not** post the batch at this time.

9. Now enter the information noted in the EOB/RA (refer to Source Document 9-8, located at the end of this Proficiency Builder). Refer to Activities 9-9, 9-10, and 9-11 for help. Make sure you are still working in the batch "BYP-HospitalChg."

▣ **Print the Hospital Charge screen after completing this Proficiency Builder, label it "BYP 9-3B," and place in your assignment folder.**

10. Click *Save* and then close out of the charge screen.

11. Run a *Journal* and then *Post* the "BYP-HospitalChg" batch.

Source Document 9-8:   Explanation of Benefits/Remittance Advice

PROPLAN

SENIOR GAP
P.O. Box 87956
Oakland, CA 94601

AMIR RAMAN, D.O.
Napa Valley Family Health Associates (NVFHA)
101 Vine Street
Napa, CA 94558

Date: MM/DD/YYYY (use today's date)
Payment Number: 2344570
Payment Amount: $82.53

Account Number	Patient Name							
					Subscriber Number	Claim Number		
Dates of Service	Description of Service	Amount Charged	Not Covered	Prov Adj Discount	Amount Allowed	Deduct/ Coins/ Copay	Paid to Provider	Adj Reason Code	Rmk Code	Patient Resp
9706416	Richard, Eric							
(Yesterday's date)	99221	$145.00		$52.47	$92.53	$10.00	$82.53			$10.00

ClaimsManager and Collections

10

Key Terms

accounts receivable
adjudicate
aging
American National
   Standards Institute
   (ANSI)
crossover

EncoderPro
inactive claim
National Drug Code
   (NDC)
private pay
unpaid claim

Learning Objectives

1. Use the features of ClaimsManager in Harris Care-Tracker PM and EMR.
2. Check status and work unpaid/inactive claims.
3. Generate patient statements.
4. Describe components of the patient collection process.
5. Review collection status and transfer private pay balances.
6. Perform collection actions.
7. Create collection letters.
8. Generate collection letters.

Real-World Connection

It cannot be overstated that all personnel, including office staff or collections agents, must act with the utmost professionalism during the collection process. Not only do numerous laws and regulations apply to the collection process, but also the sensitive nature of the relationship between provider and patient must be protected. Credit information of the patient is considered confidential and may not be released without the patient's expressed permission. Financial information regarding the patient is also confidential and must be protected according to the law. Both in-person and telephone discussions should be conducted in an area that is out of view and hearing of other patients.

Credit arrangements and interest charges must be disclosed in writing. Enforcing the credit policy can be uncomfortable for both patients and staff. You must overcome any inhibitions regarding discussion of fees and payments. The success of the practice relies heavily on the medical assistant's ability to politely yet firmly ask for payment from patients. The first step in the collection process is to advise patients of the office policy regarding payment when they call to schedule an appointment. It is important that you remain calm, compassionate, and empathetic to patients. If you encounter a difficult patient, follow these steps to diffuse and resolve the matter:

1. Let the patient vent.
2. Express empathy to the patient. The tone of your voice goes a long way. Use a genuinely warm and caring tone to enhance the meaning of empathetic phrases.
3. Begin problem-solving. Ask the patient questions to help clarify the situation and cause of the problem and double-check the facts.
4. Mutually agree on the solution. Be careful not to make a promise you cannot keep.
5. Follow up. You will score big points by following up with your patient to resolve the problem. This is sometimes referred to as service recovery.

You must demonstrate professionalism with every contact and treat each patient with the utmost respect. Your collection activities should be client-oriented and demonstrate the proper attitude and temperament with close attention given to protecting the goodwill established with your patient. Let me challenge you to role-play with your coworkers various collection scenarios that you might encounter. This will help with preparedness, conveying empathy, and noting the tone and inflection in your voice.

INTRODUCTION

This chapter continues many of the *Billing* and *ClaimsManager* features introduced in Chapter 9. The *ClaimsManager* and *Collections* applications in Harris CareTracker PM are where you begin the active process of reviewing and working claims, printing statements, and focusing collection efforts on patients with balances at least 30 days overdue.

Accounts receivable arises when a company provides goods or services on credit. For example, a medical practice may allow its patients to pay for services 30 days after they are provided and paid/adjusted by their insurance company. If patients do not pay as agreed, the practice could experience a cash flow problem. The term *aging* is often associated with a company's accounts receivable. **Aging** is the classification of accounts by the time elapsed after the date of billing or the due date. The aging of accounts receivable report will list each patient's outstanding balance and will then list the "age": current, 1–30 days past due, 31–60 days past due, 61–90 days past due, 91–120 days past due, and 120 + days past due. The aging of accounts receivable allows managers to quickly see which patients are behind in meeting the agreed-upon terms.

There are seven collection statuses in Harris CareTracker PM. Transferring private pay balances coincides with changing a patient's collection status. Harris CareTracker PM automatically moves patients into *Collections* when their overdue balance reaches the aging level assigned in the group settings and automatically removes patients from collections when their overdue balance is paid.

Understanding the concepts and performing collection action tasks demonstrate how an EHR can streamline workflows. As a medical assistant you will perform routine EHR clinical and/or administrative duties relating to the collection process per facility protocol. Duties include the transfer of balances, moving accounts to/from collection, creating custom form letters, adding the letters to *Quick Picks*, and generating and printing collection letters.

Billing and collection functions are vital to the medical practice and its revenue cycle and help maintain the provider database for the continuity of care of patients. When a patient misses or late cancels an appointment, revenue and care can be compromised.

> Before you begin the activities in this chapter, refresh your memory on working with Harris CareTracker by referring back to the Best Practices list on page xxiii of this textbook. This list is also posted to the student companion website. Following best practices will help you complete work quickly and accurately.

CLAIMSMANAGER

Learning Objective 1: Use the features of ClaimsManager in Harris CareTracker PM and EMR.

The *ClaimsManager* application in Harris CareTracker PM electronically screens a claim and the associated CPT®, ICD, and HCPCS codes and modifiers at the time the claim is created. A claim cannot be generated and sent to payers until charges for patient visits are saved in Harris CareTracker. In Chapter 9, you learned to use the *Charge* application of the *Transactions* module. The *Charge* application is typically used to:

- Enter visit information and create charges for patient visits that are not booked in Harris CareTracker PM, such as hospital visits

- Create charges for a scheduled appointment

- *Edit* unposted charges

When entering a charge, the basic visit information needs to be entered, including location, place of service, referring provider, servicing provider, billing provider, and a case or authorization, if applicable. Much of this information is pulled from the batch to which you are linking the charge and the patient's demographic.

The most important information that needs to be entered in the *Charge* application is the appropriate CPT® and ICD codes. Although there is no limit to the number of CPT® codes that can be entered for a charge, no more than four modifiers can be selected and no more than four ICD codes can be linked to each CPT® code.

Although *ClaimsManager* is not active in your student version, it is a very important tool for the medical practice. The instructions and screenshots included in this chapter provide useful information about the application. When the *Save* button is clicked during the claims process, the associated procedures (CPT®), diagnoses (ICD), and modifiers are sent to *ClaimsManager* instantly for screening. The screening can result in one of three statuses, including "Passed," "Failed," or "Warning" (**Figure 10-1**). If the screening results in a "Passed" status, the patient payment will be saved along with the charge and the two will be linked. If the *ClaimsManager* screening triggers an edit, the *ClaimsManager Edit* dialog box displays with detailed descriptions about the edits and provides action options to process the claim.

CLAIMSMANAGER SCREENING STATUS		
Color	**Status**	**Description**
	Not Processed	Not processed status indicates that the item has not been screened by the ClaimsManager.
	Passed	Passed status indicates that the item has passed the ClaimsManager screening.
	Warning	Warning status indicates that the item may fail or the ClaimsManager has suggested edits.
	Failed	Failed status indicates that the item does not meet the rules set by ClaimsManager and further edits are required.
	CMS Edits	This status indicates that the claim was flagged for CMS edits. Note: The CMS Edits status is deactivated by default. You must send a ToDo to CareTracker Support to request this feature.

Figure 10-1   ClaimsManager Screening Status

Harris CareTracker PM automatically splits out the private payment amount owed, such as the patient's copayment, for each procedure entered for the patient that requires a copayment. This only occurs if the amount of the patient's copayment is entered in the *Copay* field of the *Insurance* section in the *Demographics* application. The *Amt* field next to "Private Pay" displays the patient's copayment amount. If the patient's payment has not already been entered into Harris CareTracker PM, it can be entered now via the *Payments on Account* application fields that display in the bottom of the *Charge* screen. It is essential to enter the payment amount and the payment type.

EncoderPro

When all appropriate CPT® and ICD codes are entered, **EncoderPro**, Harris CareTracker's partner for online code verification, can be run to verify the procedures, diagnoses, and modifiers entered for a patient. Running *EncoderPro* (by clicking on the *EncoderPro.com* button [**Figure 10-2**]) helps ensure that correct coding information is entered and claims are processed and paid promptly.

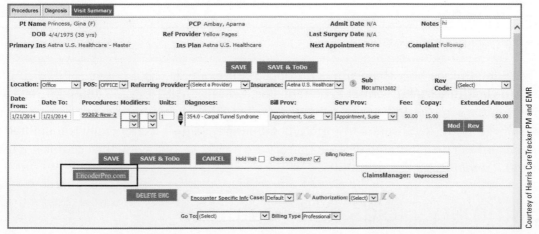

Figure 10-2   EncoderPro Button

SPOTLIGHT To launch *EncoderPro*:

1. Click the arrow ▼ next to the charge for which you want to view coding information. Harris CareTracker PM displays the *Actions* menu.
2. Click *EncoderPro* on the *Actions* menu. *EncoderPro* displays coding information for each of the codes included in the charge. This information can be used as a guide to correct the charge.
3. Review the coding information, and then close *EncoderPro*.

Claims Worklist Overview

Most claims are sent electronically in Harris CareTracker PM. Any claims identified with a problem that would prevent them from being paid will show up on a *Claims Worklist* to be resolved. The *Claims Worklist* identifies the following:

*   Newly prepared claims that will be transmitted during your next claim run
*   Claims that cannot be transmitted electronically due to a missing submitter number
*   Claims that cannot be transmitted from Harris CareTracker PM because of missing information
*   Claims that are not transmitted because of errors identified by *ClaimsManager*
*   Claims that will not be accepted by a payer because of missing information
*   Claims that you manually flagged as missing information or in review
*   Claims that a payer does not have on file and claims with a denial status

Any claims flagged in any of the *Claims Worklist* columns, except *New/Prepared*, need to be followed up on, which typically requires you to add and/or edit information and rebill the claim. Harris CareTracker PM performs an electronic claim status check and, based on its status, moves the claim to one of the *Claims Worklist* categories. You can also manually flag a claim to move it to a *Claims Worklist* category.

Claims Worklist Categories.

The *Claims Worklist* is grouped into four main categories: *New/Prepared*, *Claim Errors*, *Pending*, and *Other* (**Figure 10-3**). Claim categories are further subdivided as described in **Table 10-1**.

Financial Class	New/ Prepared	CLAIM ERRORS						PENDING		OTHER	
		Missing Submitter	Claim Edits	Payer Edits	Missing Info	Not Found	Set To Deny	In Review	Hold	Inactive	Crossovers
Commercial Insurance	1	0	0	0	0	0	0	0	0	1	0
Medicare Cengage	2	0	0	1	0	0	0	0	0	0	0
Total:	**3**	**0**	**0**	**1**	**0**	**0**	**0**	**0**	**0**	**1**	**0**

Figure 10-3 Claims Worklist Categories

The *form type* determines how the claim is produced, for example, on a paper 1500 form or in **American National Standards Institute (ANSI)** format to be sent electronically. ANSI (or CMS 1500) format can be changed to paper and Harris CareTracker PM ensures that the proper information is present on the claim form before releasing the claim to print. ANSI refers to form types that are claims electronically transmitted to a payer. If needed, a paper claim can be generated without Harris CareTracker PM verifying the accuracy of the information by clicking on the *Rebuild Paper Claim* button.

Claim Summary Fields and Features

Claim summary lines for each claim included in the *Claims Worklist* category you select for a particular financial class will display. Actions can be performed on multiple claims using this screen. **Table 10-2** details claim summary lines.

Table 10-1 Claims Worklist Categories

CATEGORY	COLUMN	DESCRIPTION
New	New/Prepared	Any claim listed in the *New/Prepared* column is a claim that will be transmitted during the next bill run. When a claim is edited and rebilled, it is added to this column. This column includes any claims that have been generated and that have been sent as well. Claims in the *New/Pending* column do not require follow-up.
Claim Errors	Missing Submitter	Claims will only appear in this column if there is a problem with the submitter numbers (as set up in the database). When a claim appears in this column, the enrollment specialist would be contacted to review/update. Claims in this column would either be rebilled when the enrollment is complete or dropped to paper.
	Claim Edits	Claims need to meet certain criteria to be transmitted from Harris CareTracker PM and EMR to a payer. When a claim does not meet these criteria (subscriber number, date of birth, and Harris CareTracker *ClaimsManager* database rules), the claim is placed in the *Claim Edits* column on the *Claims Worklist* screen. These claims have never been transmitted from Harris CareTracker PM. The required information needs to be added or edited to the claim and the claim needs to be rebilled in order for it to be removed from the *Claim Edits* column.
	Payer Edits	Claims in the *Payer Edits* column have been prepared by and transmitted from Harris CareTracker PM to a payer because they meet Harris CareTracker PM's claim criteria; however, the payer will not accept the claim because it is missing information the specific payer requires. These claims have not been reviewed by the payer because they cannot be accepted into its system electronically because the claims do not meet the payer's established claim criteria. These claims will appear on reports received back from insurance companies as rejected. Based on those reports, the status is automatically updated or you would be setting a claim with a status of *Payer Edit* manually. The required information needs to be added or edited to the claim and the claim needs to be rebilled in order for it to be removed from the *Payer Edits* column.
	Missing Info	When you manually flag a claim with having a status of *Missing Info*, the claim will appear in the *Missing Info* column. After reviewing a claim (an unpaid claim, and identifying information that the claim lacks), you can manually flag the claim as *Missing Info* and the claim will move to the *Missing Info* column. Claims remain in this column until the missing information is added or edited and the claim is rebilled. Claims are never automatically placed in this category. It must be a manual status change.
	Not Found	Claims are put into the *Not Found category* when you electronically check a claim's status and a claim is not on file with a payer. Harris CareTracker PM automatically flags the claim and moves it to this category. A claim will not be moved to the *Not Found Claims* category until seven days after the claim was originally transmitted, which allots time for transmission lag time and for the claim to be accepted into the payer's system. **Note:** When you electronically check a claim's status after the seven-day lag time and the payer does not have a claim accepted into its system, the claim will be moved to the *Not Found category*. When you call or check on claims with a payer not using the electronic claim status feature, you can manually flag a claim as *Not Found* and the claim will be moved to this category.
	Set to Deny	Claims are put into the *Claims Worklist* category of *Claim Status Denial* when you electronically check a claim's status and a payer flags a claim as set to deny. Harris CareTracker PM automatically flags the claim and moves it to this category. A claim will not be moved to the *Claim Status Denial* category until at least two weeks after the claim was originally transmitted, which allots time for transmission lag time, for the claim to be accepted into the payer's system, and for the payer to properly **adjudicate** the claim. Adjudication is the final determination of the issues involving settlement of an insurance claim, also known as a claim settlement. When you electronically check a claim's status after the two-week lag time, the payer has accepted into its system and has set the claim to deny, the claim will be moved to the *Claim Status Denial* category. The claim status window will show the details of each claim's denial. When you call or check on claims with a payer not using the electronic claim status feature, you can manually flag a claim as *Claim Status Denial*, and the claim will be moved to this category.
Pending	In Review	Claims are put into the *Claims Worklist* category of *In Review* when you electronically check a claim's status and the payer sends back a status of *In Review*. The claim is automatically moved to this category.
	Hold	A claim is only moved to the *Hold Claim category* if you manually flag the claim with a *Hold* status. For example, if there was an issue with a doctor's credentials, you would want to flag the claim with a *Hold* status to save it in the *Claims Worklist* screen until the issue was resolved and then you would rebill the claim. The status of claims saved in this category is not automatically checked by Harris CareTracker PM and EMR. However, you can do a manual recheck on the status of claims saved under this category if necessary.
Other	Inactive	A claim that has had no follow-up activity during the last 30 days is placed under this category.
	Crossover	Claims that are transferred from a patient's primary insurance to the supplementary insurance and are not paid within 30 days are placed under this category.

Courtesy of Harris CareTracker PM and EMR

Table 10-2   Claim Summary Lines

FIELD	DESCRIPTION
Back	Clicking on the *Back* button will bring you back to the *Unpaid/Inactive Claims* screen, where you can select an aged week of unpaid/*inactive claims* to work on for a particular financial class.
Select All	All claims included in the unpaid/inactive claims age for the financial class you chose to work on will be selected when the *Select All* button is clicked and a selected claim is indicated by a check mark in the *Select* column on the claim line. *Select All* is convenient to use if you need to perform an action on the selected batch of claims, such as electronically checking claim status, rebilling claims, or adding a note. When the *Select All* button is clicked, individual claims can be deselected by clicking on the check mark in the *Select* column.
Deselect All	Clicking on the *Deselect All* button will deselect any selected claim. A selected claim is indicated by a check mark in the *Select* column on a claim line. Deselecting a claim or all claims will remove the check mark.
Filing Limit	Claims approaching filing limit are highlighted red as a visual indication that these claims need to be handled in a timely manner. For most payers, a claim will turn red 25–30 days before its actual filing limit will be reached.
Inactive Limit	Claims that have not been worked in 30 days are considered inactive, and inactive claims are highlighted tan as a visual indication that these claims need to be worked.
Claim Summary Line	A claim summary line for each claim included in the unpaid/inactive claims age for the financial class you selected displays. The claim summary line shows the patient's name, Harris CareTracker PM and EMR patient ID number, the patient' date of birth, the insurance plan, the patient's subscriber number, the status of the claim, the claim's last activity date, the original claim date, the claim's age, the oldest service date, the provider, the original amount on the claim, the remaining open balance, the last transaction date, the description of the last transaction, the activity date, and the activity notes. More detailed claim summary information will display when an individual claim summary line is clicked.
Rebill	This *Rebill* button is used to rebill a batch of claims. Select the claims you need to rebill either by clicking on the *Select All* button or by clicking in the *Select* column for the appropriate claims and then click on the *Rebill* button. Rebilling claims changes their status to "New" and moves them to the *New/Pending* column on the *Claims Worklist* screen. Claims in the *New/Pending* column will be transmitted during your next bill run.
Claim Status	Every evening, Harris CareTracker PM and EMR automatically checks the status of every claim on which there is an outstanding balance. A claim is checked for the first time after it has been flagged as TRANS OPEN for seven days. If the claim status continues to remain "In process," the second automated check is performed three days after the first check. Because a third check is not performed by Harris CareTracker PM and EMR, it is best practice to call the payer and follow up on the claim or manually recheck the claim status. There are particular statuses returned from a payer when a claim's status is checked: *In Process, Finalized, Set to Pay, Set to Deny, Pending In Review,* and *Not Found.* Each claim will be updated accordingly when the automated batch claim status check is complete. When a status of *Set to Deny, Pending in Review,* or *Not Found* is returned during an automated batch claim status check, the claim will be updated and flagged in the *Claims Worklist* link under the *Billing* section of the *Dashboard.* Harris CareTracker PM does not check any claims moved to the "Hold" category automatically. However, you can perform a manual claim status check if necessary.
Notes	Enter an activity note in regard to the selected claims in the *Notes* field and click on the *Save* button. The note will be saved in the *Activity Notes* section of each selected claim and adding a note restarts the claims aging used to determine inactive claims.
Status	The *Status* field can be used to manually change the status of the selected claims. "Select" defaults in the *Status* field; however, the selected claims' statuses can be changed by selecting the appropriate status from the *Status* field drop-down list of "Payer Edits," "Not Found," "Claim Status Denial," "Missing Info," or "In Review." Manually changing the claim's status will move the selected claims to the corresponding column on the *Claims Worklist* screen.
Save	Clicking on the *Save* button will save an activity note that has been entered in the *Notes* field and/or a claim status that has been selected from the *Status* list.

CRITICAL THINKING Research claims filing limits for Medicare, Medicaid, Blue Cross/Blue Shield, and Aetna. Prepare a one-page paper on each insurer's claim filing limits. Contrast and compare and make best practice recommendations for the practice to process claims in a timely manner.

Claim Summary Screen

The *Claim Summary* screen (**Figure 10-4**) displays when an individual claim line is clicked. In this screen, actions can be performed on the selected claim only. The *Claim Summary* screen fields and descriptions are outlined in **Table 10-3**.

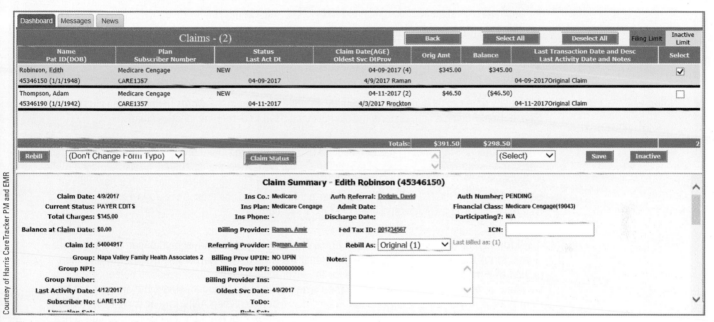

Figure 10-4   Claims Summary Screen

Courtesy of Harris CareTracker PM and EMR

Work the Claims Worklist

Having identified a problem (or problems) that would prevent a claim from being paid, you will work the *Claims Worklist* to resolve the issue(s).

Table 10-3   Claims Summary Screen

FIELD	DESCRIPTION
Claim Information	The top part of the *Claim Summary* screen displays all of the information that was included on the claim; the status, balance, last activity date, subscriber number, insurance company, insurance plan, billing and servicing provider, billing provider UPIN and NPI, referring provider, admission date (if applicable) and authorization number (if applicable), provider's tax ID, provider's enrollment status in insurance, and the effective date of enrollment. These fields cannot be edited; however, the billing provider and the referring provider's insurance number details can be viewed by clicking on the respective provider's name.
	Note: A provider's participating status can be one of the following:
	• *N/A*—This indicates that the insurance carrier does not require specific enrollment/credentialing to participate.
	• *No*—This indicates that the provider does not participate with the insurance listed on the claim.
	• *Yes*—This indicates that the provider is enrolled with the insurance and displays the date of effective date.

(continues)

Table 10-3   Claims Summary Screen *(continued)*

FIELD	DESCRIPTION
Rebill As	The *Rebill As* field is used to flag an electronically resubmitted claim (ANSI 837 format) with a code that indicates the claim is a resubmission. Flagging a resubmitted claim prevents the claim from being denied as a duplicate. Code definitions: • *Insurance Default (I)*: Rebills each claim with the default code that was set for the insurance on that claim. • *Claim Default (C)*: Rebills the claim with its current status. • *Original (1)*: First generation of claim. **Note:** This code is not used for rebilling. • *Corrected (6)*: Adjustment of a prior claim. • *Replacement (7)*: Replacement of a prior claim. • *Void (8)*: Void/Cancel of a prior claim.
Notes	An activity note can be added to the claim by entering the note in the *Notes* field and then clicking on the *Save* button. Adding a note restarts the claims aging used to determine inactive claims.
Rebill To ==>	When the needed information has been added to or edited to the claim or the patient's demographic, the *Rebill To* ==> button must be clicked to rebill the claim. When a claim is rebilled, it will be placed in the *New/Pending* column on the *Claims Worklist* screen and will be transmitted during your next bill run. Before clicking on the *Rebill To* ==> button, verify the form type selected in the *Form Type* field. A form type must be changed before clicking on *Rebill To* ==> button.
Form Type	ANSI form types are claims that are electronically transmitted to a payer, and paper form types are claims forms that are dropped to paper that must be printed from Harris CareTracker PM and then mailed to a payer. The default form type for the insurance plan the claim needs to be sent to is selected in the *Form Type* field. When a form type needs to be changed, select the appropriate form from the *Form Type* list and click on the *Rebill To* ==> button. When ANSI format is changed to paper, Harris CareTracker PM ensures that the proper information is present on the claim form before releasing the claim to print.
Rebuild Paper Claim	The *Rebuild Paper* claim button can be used to print paper claims without Harris CareTracker PM verifying the accuracy of the information. The form type selected in the *Form Type* field must be a paper form. When the *Rebuild Paper* claim button is clicked, the claim displays in a window. Right-click on top of it and select *Print* from the gray pop-up menu. The claim will be removed from *Claims Worklist* when the *Rebuild Paper* claim button is clicked.
View Paper	The claim will display in a window when the *View Paper* claim button is clicked. Clicking on the *View Paper* button does not remove the claim from the *Claims Worklist* link.
Edit	Clicking on the *Edit* button on the *Claim Summary* screen displays the *Encounter* window from which you can add and/or edit claim information including the location, place of service, *Additional Claim Info*, referring provider, modifiers, and diagnoses. Dates of service, procedure codes, fees, the insurance company, and the amount of the claim may not be edited from this pop-up. **Note:** When the billing provider, dates of service, procedure codes, fee, units, servicing provider, or insurance needs to be changed, the charge will need to be reversed from Harris CareTracker PM via the *Edit* application in the *Transactions* module. The charge will then need to be put back into the system.

FIELD	DESCRIPTION
Claim Status	Every evening, Harris CareTracker PM will automatically check the status of every claim submitted on which there is an outstanding balance. A claim is checked for the first time after seven days and it is flagged as "TRANS OPEN" in the *Claim Status* box. If the claim status continues to remain "In process," the second automated check is performed three days after the first check and if the claim is not finalized it will be flagged as "Not Found." Because a third check is not performed by Harris CareTracker PM, it is best practice to call the payer and follow up on the claim or manually recheck the claim status. There are particular statuses returned from a payer when a claim's status is checked: "In Process," "Finalized," "Set to Pay," "Set to Deny," "Pending In Review," and "Not Found." Each claim will be updated accordingly when the automated batch claim status check is complete. When a status of "Set to Deny," "Pending in Review," or "Not Found" is returned during an automated batch claim status check, the claim will be updated and flagged in the *Claims Worklist* link under the *Billing* section of the *Dashboard*. The *Claim Status* button on the *Claim Summary* screen enables manual recheck of claims' status without having to wait for the automated process. **Note:** Harris CareTracker PM does not automatically check any claims moved to the "Hold" category. However, you can perform a manual claim status check if necessary.
Status	The *Status* field can be used to manually change the status of the claim by selecting defaults in the *Status* field; however, the status can be changed by selecting the appropriate status from the *Status* list ("Payer Edits," "Not Found," "Claim Status Denial," "Missing Info," or "In Review"), and then clicking on the *Save* button. Manually changing the claim's status will move the claim to the corresponding column on the *Claims Worklist* screen.
Save	Clicking on the *Save* button will save an activity note that has been entered in the *Notes* field and/or a claim status that has been selected from the *Status* list.
Inactive	The *Inactive* button allows you to manually set an inactive date for one or more claims. When an inactive date is set, you can hover over the *Inactive* button to view the date. Additionally, Harris CareTracker PM adds an entry to the activity log below the *Claim Summary* each time an inactive date is set for a claim.
Status Column	The status column shows the claim's current status and all of the status steps the claim has gone through.
Activity Date	Activity date logs the date and time of all activity taken on the claim.
Activity Notes	Claim errors occur when a claim does not meet specific requirements set by Harris CareTracker PM and/ or payers. Errors display under the *Activity Notes* section of the *Claim Summary* screen as a mnemonic code along with the error description. Error descriptions direct you as to what pieces of claim information needs to be fixed before the claim can be successfully transmitted to a payer. Example: "BPINNO - Billing Provider/Insurance Number is missing for this particular Billing Provider/Insurance combination" instead of "BPINNO" only.
Key	By clicking on the *Key* link, a list of all the possible system note codes and their corresponding messages will display. This key can be used to decipher a code that you do not understand.
Link	The *Acknowledgement* and the *Report* electronically received into Harris CareTracker PM from a payer that included the claim will be accessible from the *Claim Summary* screen. The *Acknowledgement* report can be viewed by clicking on the *ANSI 837* link and the *Report* can be viewed by clicking on the *Report* link. The *Report* shows all the claims that were transmitted in the same claim batch as the current claim's summary you are viewing.
Operator	This logs the operator who performed each action that has been taken on a claim.
Claim Batch ID	This shows the claim batch identification number.

(continues)

Table 10-3 Claims Summary Screen *(continued)*

FIELD	DESCRIPTION
Procedures	Each procedure line included on the claim will display in the lower part of the *Claim Summary* screen. Under each procedure line will be a record of all the financial transactions linked to each procedure.
Payment	The *Payments* screen displays when the *Payment* link is clicked from a financial transaction where a payment, adjustment, or transfer for the respective procedure line can be entered.
Separate Claim	When multiple procedure codes appear on one claim, those procedures can be separated to different claims by clicking on the *Separate Claim* link.

Courtesy of Harris CareTracker PM and EMR

SPOTLIGHT In the medical setting, the **National Drug Code (NDC)** number identifies a listed drug product that is assigned a unique 10-digit, 3-segment number. This number, known as the NDC, identifies the labeler, product, and trade package size. The first segment, the labeler code, is assigned by the Food and Drug Administration (FDA). A labeler is any firm that manufactures (including repackers or relabelers) or distributes (under its own name) the drug. The second segment, the product code, identifies a specific strength, dosage form, and formulation for a particular firm. The third segment, the package code, identifies package sizes and types. Both the product and package codes are assigned by the firm. The NDC will be in one of the following configurations and is required to be reported: 4-4-2, 5-3-2, or 5-4-1. The NDC enhances safety by documenting drugs and establishes a method to recall.

Note: By clicking on the *Misc* button in the *Claim Summary* screen, you can enter an NDC code.

TIP When the billing provider, dates of service, procedure codes, fee, units, servicing provider, or insurance need to be changed, the charge must be reversed from Harris CareTracker PM via the *Edit* application in the *Transactions* module. The charge will then need to be put back into the system.

In the *Claim Summary*, select a claim frequency code from the *Rebill As* field to indicate why the claim is being resubmitted (if applicable). Each code is described in **Table 10-4**.

Table 10-4 Claims Frequency Codes

CODE	DESCRIPTION
Insurance Default (I)	Rebills each claim with the default code that was set for the insurance on that claim.
Claim Default (C)	Rebills the claim with its current status.
Original (1)	First generation of claim. **Note:** This code is not used for rebilling.
Corrected (6)	Adjustment of a prior claim.
Replacement (7)	Replacement of a prior claim.
Void (8)	Void/Cancellation of a prior claim.

Courtesy of Harris CareTracker PM and EMR

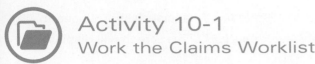

Activity 10-1
Work the Claims Worklist

1. Go to the *Home* module > *Dashboard* tab > *Billing* section > *Claims Worklist* link. There are three options: *Unbilled, Crossover,* and *Inactive* (**Figure 10-5**). Select *Unbilled.* This will take you to the *Claims Worklist* screen.

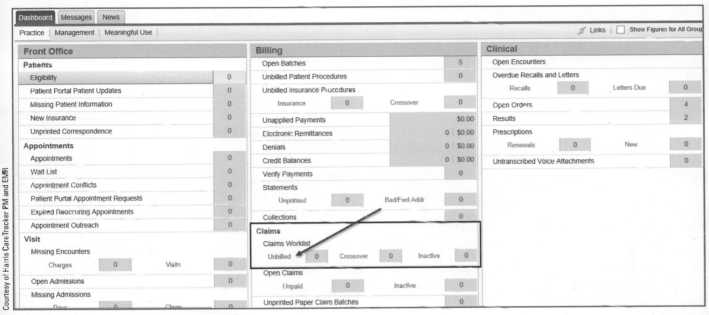

Figure 10-5   *Claims Worklist Dashboard*

2. The *Location* list defaults to "All Locations." You have the option to select a specific location if needed. Leave as is.

3. The *All Groups* list defaults to "N" for No. Select "Y" for Yes if you want to include claims for all groups. Select "Y."

4. Enter "180" in the *Crossover Days* field.

5. Select the *Incl. Crossovers?* checkbox to include crossover claims.

6. Leave the *Oldest Service Date From/To* as is. If you wanted to view claims from a specific time period, you would enter a date range here.

7. Click *Go.* The application displays a list of all claims broken down by financial class (**Figure 10-6**).

Financial Class	New/ Prepared	Missing Submitter	Claim Edits	Payer Edits	Missing Info	Not Found	Set To Deny	In Review	Hold	Inactive	Crossovers
Blue Shield Cengage	3	0	0	0	0	0	0	0	0	0	0
Commercial Insurance	3	0	0	0	0	0	0	0	0	1	0
Medicaid Cengage	1	0	0	0	0	0	0	0	0	0	0
Medicare Cengage	3	0	0	0	0	0	0	0	0	0	0
Total:	**10**	**0**	**0**	**0**	**0**	**0**	**0**	**0**	**0**	**1**	**0**

Figure 10-6   *Claims by Financial Class*

8. Click on a number in the *New/Prepared* column for the corresponding financial class you need to work (select the column for "Medicare Cengage"). The *New/Prepared Claims* screen will display (**Figure 10-7**).

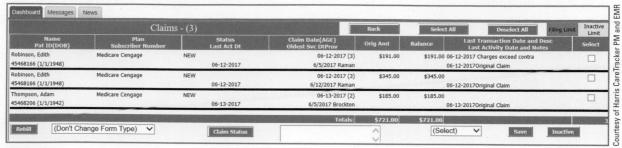

Figure 10-7   *New/Prepared Claims Screen*

 TIP   Click the column headings to re-sort the column data.

9. Select the checkbox in the *Select* column for each claim you want to work. Select the first claim for Edith Robinson and click the *Claim Status* button. (**Note:** You can select all of the claims by clicking *Select All.*) You will receive a pop-up (**Figure 10-8**) advising you of the claim's status (which displays "Processing. . . ."). **Do NOT** click the *Close* button in the pop-up as this will remove the claim from the *Unbilled Claims* screen. Rather, click on the "X" in the upper-right-hand corner to close out of the window.

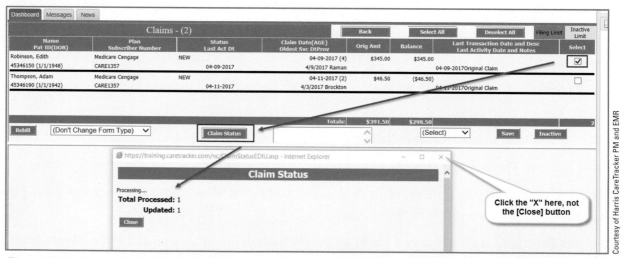

Figure 10-8   *Claim Status Pop-Up*

10. Click directly in the claim summary line containing Edith Robinson's first visit. The claim line now appears in yellow and the application displays the *Claim Summary* in the lower frame of the screen (see **Figure 10-4**). This allows you to review, edit, check claim status, or rebill an individual claim.

11. Scroll down and look under the *Activity Notes* column to determine the inaccurate or missing claim information that, triggered by *ClaimsManager*, prevented the claim from being transmitted from Harris CareTracker PM, that prevented the claim from being accepted by a payer, or that caused the claim to be denied by the payer (**Figure 10-9**).

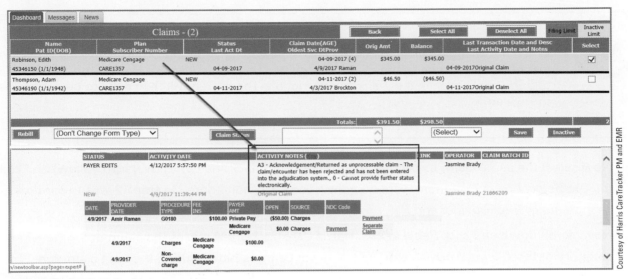

Figure 10-9   Activity Notes

12. Perform the desired action on the claim(s):

Confirm that *Billing Provider* and *Referring Provider* displays Dr. Raman. If not, scroll down and click *Edit* on the *Claim Summary* screen (**Figure 10-10**). The *Claim Transaction Summary* window displays the location, place of service, encounter specific claim information, referring provider, diagnosis code, and modifiers. Click *Save*. You may briefly receive the "error" message noted in **Figure 10-11**. Click *OK*. Your *Claim Summary* will now reflect the change to *Referring Provider*.

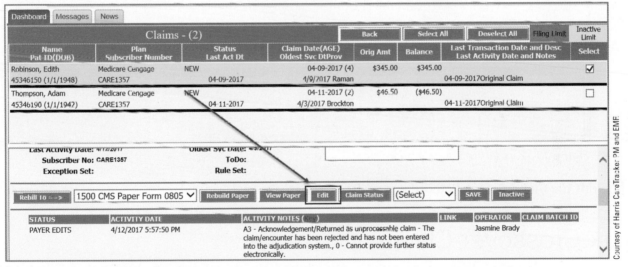

Figure 10-10   Edit Claim Summary

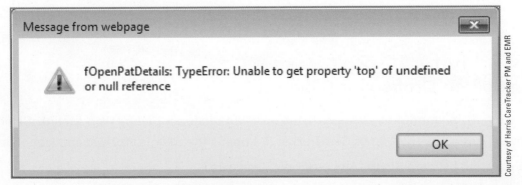

Figure 10-11   Update Claim Message

> **TIP**
> * When the billing provider, dates of service, procedure codes, fee, units, servicing provider, or insurance need to be changed, the charge must be reversed from Harris CareTracker PM via the *Edit* application in the *Transactions* module. The charge will then need to be put back into the system.
> * When rebilling claims, the form type is not typically changed.

13. Now select the same claim by clicking in the claim summary line (which will turn yellow) and checking the *Select* box even if there were no edits. (The only "edit" noted in step 12 was to confirm or change the *Billing Provider* and *Referring Provider* to Dr. Amir Raman).

14. Now, scroll down and click *Rebill To ==>*. Harris CareTracker PM places the claim in the *New/Pending* category of the *Claims Worklist*, and the claim will be transmitted during the next claim run.

15. Scroll down the screen and in the *Activity Notes* column, you will now see the activities completed (**Figure 10-12**).

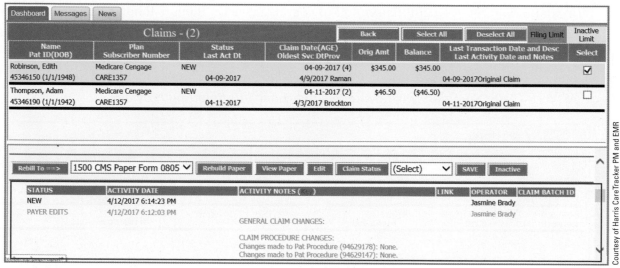

Figure 10-12   Claims Status Activity Note

🖷 **Print the Claim Status Activity screen, label it "Activity 10-1," and place it in your assignment folder.**

Work Crossover Claims

A **crossover** claim is a claim that is automatically forwarded from Medicare to a secondary insurer after Medicare has paid its portion of a service.

Activity 10-2
Search Crossover Claims

1. Go to the *Home* module > *Dashboard* tab > *Billing* section > *Claims Worklist* link. Select *Crossover* from the three options. Harris CareTracker PM opens the *Claims Worklist* application.

2. The *Location* list defaults to "All Locations." Leave as is.

3. The *All Groups* list defaults to "N" for No. Select "Y" for Yes to include claims for all groups.

4. Adjust the crossover days to 180.

5. Select the *Incl. Crossovers?* checkbox.

6. Leave the *Oldest Service Date From/To* as is. If you wanted to view claims from a specific time period, you would enter a date range here.

7. Click *Go*. Harris CareTracker PM displays a list of all claims organized by financial class (**Figure 10-13**).

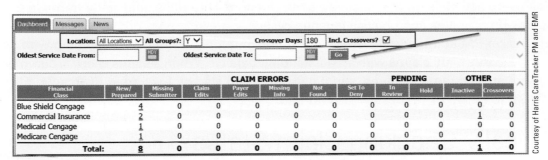

Figure 10-13   Crossover Claims

💾 **Print the Crossovers search screen, label it "Activity 10-2," and place it in your assignment folder.**

8. If there are crossover claims noted in the *Crossovers* column, click the number that corresponds to the financial class in which you want to work. Harris CareTracker PM displays a list of crossover claims (**Figure 10-14**). **Hint:** There are no *Crossover Claims* for you to work here.

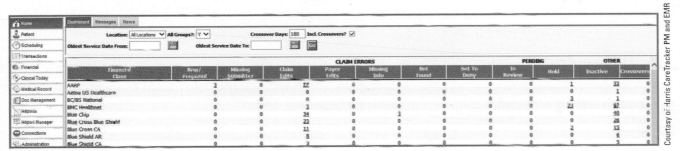

Figure 10-14   Crossover Claims Displayed

> **FYI** In a live environment, you would do the following:
>
> a. In the *Bill?* column, select the checkbox next to each claim you want to bill to secondary insurance. Alternatively, click *Check All* to bill all claims as crossover claims.
>
> b. Click *Set to Bill*. All crossover claims are saved as Secondary 1500 Forms under the *Unprinted Paper Claims* link for printing in the next bill run.

WORK UNPAID CLAIMS

Learning Objective 2: Check status and work unpaid/inactive claims.

Unpaid claims are claims that have been submitted to an insurance company but have not been paid. **Inactive claims** are claims that are not only unpaid, but also have not had any follow-up activity on them for the last 30 days. *Unpaid* and *Inactive* claims are aged by week, broken down by financial class, and can be worked from the *Unpaid/Inactive* links in the *Claims* section of the *Practice Dashboard*. Inactive claims are highlighted in tan and claims that are nearing their filing limit are highlighted in red as a visual alert that these claims need to be worked immediately. From this list, you can drill down into each *Unpaid/Inactive* claim that requires follow-up. When an inactive claim has been worked, it is removed from the inactive category; however, if there is no payment or additional activity on the claim for the next 30 days, it is recategorized as inactive.

The number of inactive claims should only be 5–10 percent of your unpaid claims. As best practice, you should focus your follow-up activities on the inactive claims category. This will significantly improve the efficiency of your claim follow-up activities and practice revenue cycle.

Harris CareTracker PM automatically checks the status of unpaid claims every evening with specific payers and will check the status of all claims with an outstanding balance. When a status check is complete, the claim's status is updated, attached to the claims, and if necessary will also be flagged in *Claims Worklist* if a status of "Not Found," "Set to Deny," or "In Review" is returned.

Electronically Checking Claim Status

Claim status is automatically checked every evening for every claim that has an outstanding balance. Typically, a manual claim status check is not necessary. However, if you need to manually check claim status, you do so individually or in a batch.

 SPOTLIGHT Harris CareTracker PM automatically performs a status check seven days after the claim is set to *Trans Open*. If the claim is not finalized, Harris CareTracker PM automatically performs another check three days later and then flags the claim as "Not Found."

Checking Individual Claim Status.

Claim status for individual claims can be checked from any application in Harris CareTracker PM where the *Claim Summary* screen displays. Possible statuses are noted in **Table 10-5**.

Table 10-5	Possible Claim Statuses
In Process	When a claim status check is complete and the payer returns that it is "In Process," Harris CareTracker PM sets the claim status to "In Process." When a claim is set to "In Process," its status will not be checked during a batch electronic claim status check for the next seven days. However, you can manually recheck the individual claim's status, overriding the seven-day period.
Finalized	When a claim status check is complete and the payer returns that it is "Finalized," Harris CareTracker PM sets the claim status to "Finalized." A "Finalized" claim will have the details of the finalization listed under the *Activity Notes* section of the *Claims Summary* screen. After a claim has been set to "Finalized," no additional electronic claim status checks can be performed.
Set to Pay	When a claim status check is done and the payer returns that it is "Set to Pay," Harris CareTracker PM will set the claim status to "Set to Pay." "Set to Pay" claims are going to be paid by the respective payer. These claims will remain in *Unpaid/Inactive* claims until they are paid or adjusted off in full. After a claim has been set to "Set to Pay," no additional electronic claim status checks can be performed.
Set to Deny	Any messages that constitute a claim status denial will set the claim's status to "Set to Deny." In addition to these claims being flagged in the *Unpaid/Inactive* link, they are flagged in the *Claims Worklist* link as well because they have been denied and will require follow-up. After a claim has been set to *Set to Deny*, no additional electronic claim status checks can be performed.

Pending in Review	There are *Claim Status* messages that will come back from the payer that the claim is "In Review." Any of these statuses will set the claim to *In Review. In Review* claims should be followed up on until they have been adjudicated by a payer.
Not Found	Any payer that has electronic claim status where the claim is not on file after seven days of the original claim date will be set to "Not Found" status.

Courtesy of Harris CareTracker PM and EMR

Activity 10-3
Individually Check Claim Status Electronically

1. Go to the *Home* module > *Dashboard* tab > *Billing* section > *Open Claims/Unpaid* link. Harris CareTracker PM displays the *Open Claims* application.

2. Select the desired filter options, as outlined (**Figure 10-15**):

   a. *Status*: NEW

   b. *Age By*: Oldest Service Date

   c. *Financial Class*: Leave as is

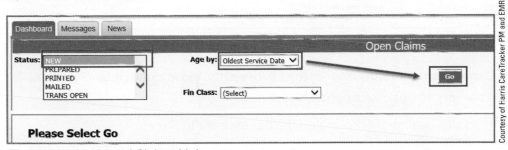

Figure 10-15   Unpaid Claims Link

3. Click *Go*. Harris CareTracker PM displays the *Unpaid/Inactive* claims, broken down by financial class and by week. The total inactive claims for a financial class displays in the *Inactive* column. Totals for all unpaid claims for a financial clas displays in the *Total* column, and for each week, the total number of unpaid claims displays in the *Totals* row (**Figure 10-16**).

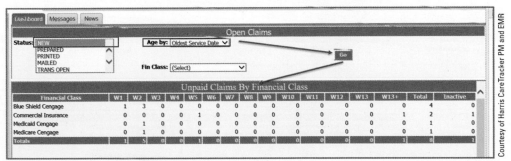

Figure 10-16   Open Claims

4. To work the "Blue Shield Cengage *Financial Class*" line, click on the corresponding number in the *Total* column. Harris CareTracker PM displays a claim line for all corresponding *Unpaid/Inactive* claims with the patient's name, ID number, date of birth, subscriber number, the insurance plan for which the claim was transmitted, the claim status, last activity date on the claim, claim date, claim age, oldest service date on the claim, the provider on the claim, the original amount, balance remaining, and the last activity notes saved for the claim.

5. Place a check mark in Ellen Ristino's *Select* column.

6. Then click directly on the patient's claim line. The line turns yellow and Harris CareTracker PM displays the *Claim Summary* in the lower frame of the screen.

7. You may need to scroll down the screen to be able to view the claim history (**Figure 10-17**). Click *Claim Status*.

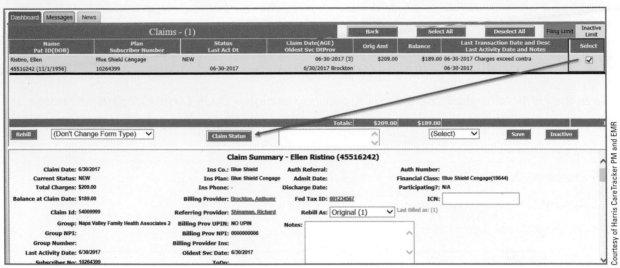

Figure 10-17   Claim History

8. When the *Claim Status* window has finished processing, close out of it by clicking only the "X" in the upper-right corner (do **not** click on the *Close* button).

9. Re-select the claim by directly clicking on the patient's claim line.

10. You must scroll down to locate the *Claim Status* button just above *Activity Notes* (**Figure 10-18**).

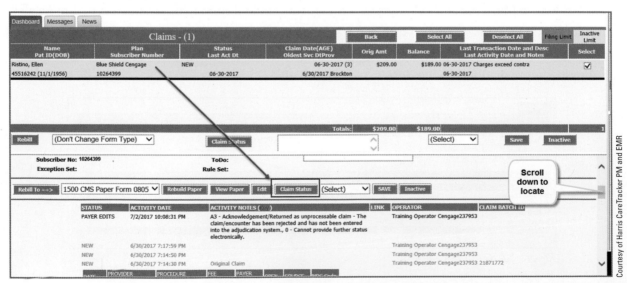

Figure 10-18   Select Claim Status Button

11. Click on the *Claims Status* button. Harris CareTracker PM displays the *Claim Status History* window (**Figure 10-19**), which includes all previous status checks that have occurred, including the date of the status check, the operator who performed the check, the claim status category, and the *Claim Status* code. (**Note**: If the message says no history, close the box and click it again.)

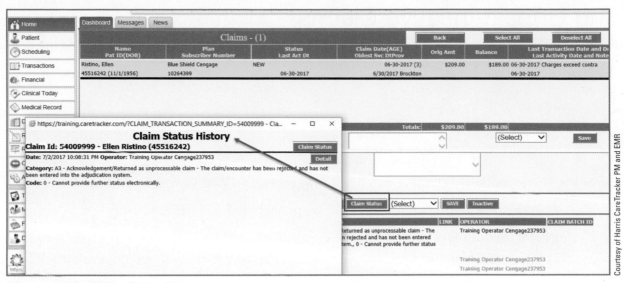

Figure 10-19   Claim Status History

12. Click on the *Claim Status* button on the top right corner of the *Claim Status History* window to perform another claim status check. When the claim status check is complete, the status of the current
claim is automatically updated. Click on the "X" in the upper-right corner of the *Claim Status* window
to close it (**do not** click on *Close*).

> **TIP** When a claim's status has been returned, except for "Set to Pay," the claim will be moved
> to the corresponding column on the *Claims Worklist* screen.

13. To view the details of the check, click on the *Detail* button in the *Claim Status History* box, and the
Claim Status Detail dialog box displays (**Figure 10-20**). (**Note:** The *Claim Status Detail* displayed will
not match your patient, provider, and insurance. That is because this is an educational environment.)

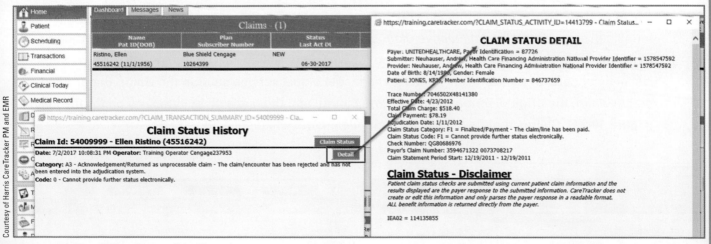

Figure 10-20   Claim Status Detail

📄 **Print the Claim Status Detail screen, label it "Activity 10-3," and place it in your assignment folder.**

14. Click "X" in the top right corner of the *Claim Status Detail* and the *Claim Status History* windows to
close out of them.

Working Unpaid/Inactive Claims

Now that you have checked the claim status, begin working the unpaid/inactive claims. The steps are similar to checking a claim status, but you are now working the claim.

Activity 10-4
Work *Unpaid/Inactive Claims*

1. Go to the *Home* module > *Dashboard* tab > *Billing* section > *Open Claims/Unpaid* link.

2. Harris CareTracker PM displays the *Open Claims* application. Enter the following:

   a. *Status* field: Do not make a selection; leave as is. (**FYI**) The *Status* field is where you select the status of the claims you want to view. To select multiple statuses, you would press the *[Ctrl]* key while clicking to select multiple statuses.

   b. In the *Age by* drop-down list, select the age of claims to view. Select "Oldest Service Date."

   c. (Optional) From the *Fin Class* drop-down list, select the financial class containing the claims you want to view. Leave as "(Select)."

   d. Click *Go*. Harris CareTracker PM displays the unpaid/inactive claims by financial class and by week.

TIP Unpaid claims by financial class:
- The *Inactive* column displays the total inactive claims for a financial class.
- The *Total* column displays the total unpaid claims for a financial class.
- The *Totals* row displays the total unpaid claims for each week.

---

3. Locate the claims you want to work. Select the number in the *Total* column for "Medicare Cengage," and click on the corresponding number. Harris CareTracker PM displays a claim line for each unpaid/inactive claim. (**Note:** You cannot click on a zero total.) (**Note:** When a number is clicked, a claim line for all corresponding *Unpaid/Inactive Claims* displays with the patient's name, ID number, date of birth, subscriber number, the insurance plan for which the claim was transmitted, the claim status, last activity date on the claim, claim date, claim age, oldest service date on the claim, the provider on the claim, the original amount, balance remaining, and the last activity notes saved for the claim (**Figure 10-21**). Claims that have reached their *Filing Limit* will display in red.)

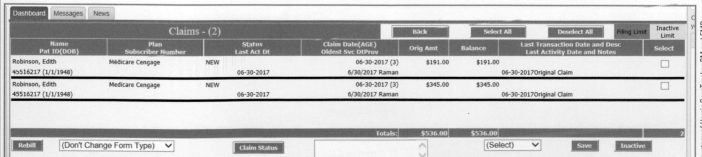

Figure 10-21 Unpaid/Inactive Claims

4. To work claims in a batch:

   a. To review or work an individual claim, click directly on the claim line (select Edith Robinson's first claim). The claim line will turn yellow. Harris CareTracker PM displays the *Claim Summary* in the lower frame of the screen.

   b. You will need to scroll down on both the upper and lower screens to view all the claims and the *Claim Summary* information for the claim selected.

   c. Scroll down and click *Edit* on the *Claim Summary* screen (**Figure 10-22**) to change the location, place of service, encounter-specific claim information, referring provider, diagnosis code, and modifiers. The *Claim Transaction Summary* window displays (**Figure 10-23**), where you can make changes. **Note:** Dates of service, procedure codes, fees, the insurance company, and the amount of the claim may not be edited from this window.

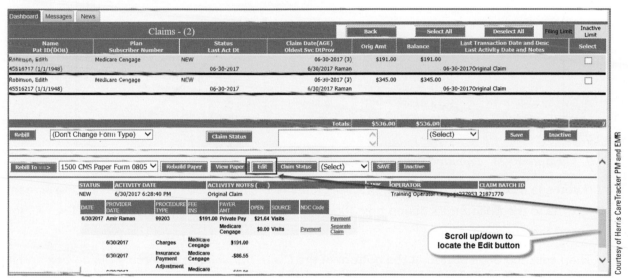

Figure 10-22   Edit Claim Summary

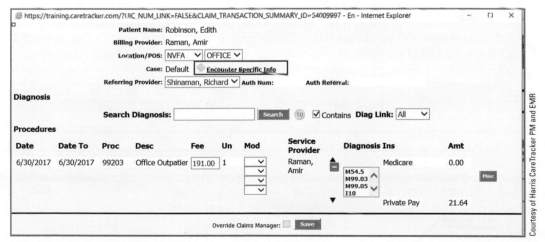

Figure 10-23   Encounters Window

   d. Click on the [+] icon next to *Encounter Specific Info* and a pop-up *Preferred Patient Case* dialog box will appear.

e. In the *Claim Information* tab, use the drop-down arrow and select "Dr. Raman" as both the *Supervising* and *Ordering Provider* (**Figure 10-24**).

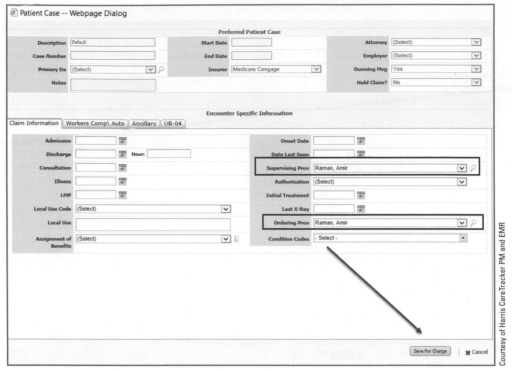

Figure 10-24   Preferred Patient Case Dialog Box

f. If you see a *Save For Charge* button, click on it and the dialog box disappears and the screen returns to the *Encounters* dialog box. If no *Save For Charge* button is displaying, click "X" to close out of the dialog box.

g. Then click the *Save* button at the bottom of the *Claim Transaction Summary* dialog box and it will close. **Hint**: If the box does not "close" automatically, click on the "X" to close the dialog box.

TIP If there is a number in *Rule Set*, click the number link next to *Rule Set* (**Figure 10-25**) to view descriptions of the rules for the insurance company. This can be helpful when determining the information that needs to be fixed. Click the *Key* link (in blue) next to the *Activity Notes* heading to view a key for deciphering each missing information code (**Figure 10-26**).

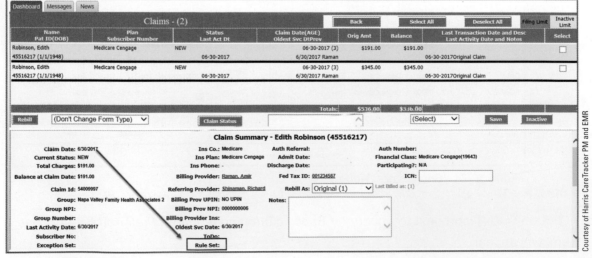

Figure 10-25   Rule Set

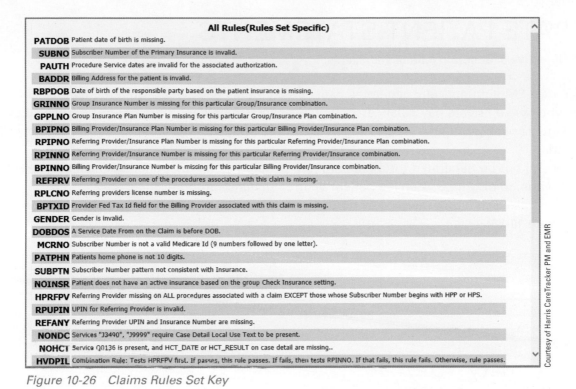

All Rules(Rules Set Specific)

PATDOB	Patient date of birth is missing.
SUBNO	Subscriber Number of the Primary Insurance is invalid.
PAUTH	Procedure Service dates are invalid for the associated authorization.
BADDR	Billing Address for the patient is invalid.
RBPDOB	Date of birth of the responsible party based on the patient insurance is missing.
GRINNO	Group Insurance Number is missing for this particular Group/Insurance combination.
GPPLNO	Group Insurance Plan Number is missing for this particular Group/Insurance Plan combination.
BPIPNO	Billing Provider/Insurance Plan Number is missing for this particular Billing Provider/Insurance Plan combination.
RPIPNO	Referring Provider/Insurance Plan Number is missing for this particular Referring Provider/Insurance Plan combination.
RPINNO	Referring Provider/Insurance Number is missing for this particular Referring Provider/Insurance combination.
BPINNO	Billing Provider/Insurance Number is missing for this particular Billing Provider/Insurance combination.
REFPRV	Referring Provider on one of the procedures associated with this claim is missing.
RPLCNO	Referring providers license number is missing.
BPTXID	Provider Fed Tax Id field for the Billing Provider associated with this claim is missing.
GENDER	Gender is invalid.
DOBDOS	A Service Date From on the Claim is before DOB.
MCRNO	Subscriber Number is not a valid Medicare Id (9 numbers followed by one letter).
PATPHN	Patients home phone is not 10 digits.
SUBPTN	Subscriber Number pattern not consistent with Insurance.
NOINSR	Patient does not have an active insurance based on the group Check Insurance setting.
HPRFPV	Referring Provider missing on ALL procedures associated with a claim EXCEPT those whose Subscriber Number begins with HPP or HPS.
RPUPIN	UPIN for Referring Provider is invalid.
REFANY	Referring Provider UPIN and Insurance Number are missing.
NONDC	Services "J3490", "J9999" require Case Detail Local Use Text to be present.
NOHCT	Service Q0136 is present, and HCT_DATE or HCT_RESULT on case detail are missing..
HVDPIL	Combination Rule: Tests HPRFPV first. If passes, this rule passes. If fails, then tests RPINNO. If that fails, this rule fails. Otherwise, rule passes.

Figure 10-26   Claims Rules Set Key

5. Scroll down and click *Rebill To ==>*. Harris CareTracker PM will place the claim in the *New/Pending* category of the *Claims Worklist* screen and will transmit the claim during the next bill run (**Figure 10-27**). When rebilling claims, the form type typically is not changed.

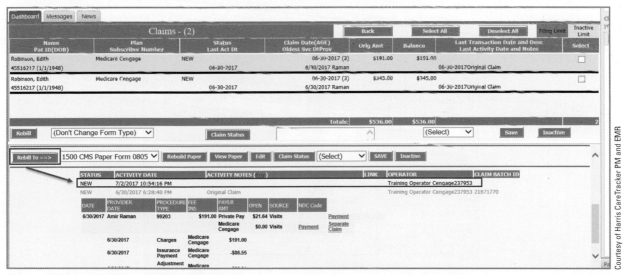

Figure 10-27   Last Transaction Update

📇 **Print the Unpaid/Inactive screen, label it "Activity 10-4," and place it in your assignment folder.**

GENERATE PATIENT STATEMENTS

Learning Objective 3: Generate patient statements.

Harris CareTracker PM automatically generates patient statements each week. Statements are sent to responsible parties who owe a private pay balance. Statements can also be sent for workers' compensation, nursing homes, and legal cases by setting up those organizations as an insurance company or an employer in Harris CareTracker PM.

A statement will not be generated for a patient if the patient has an unapplied balance saved on his or her account that is equal to or greater than the patient's current balance amount.

Patient statements will not be generated by Harris CareTracker PM until 5 p.m., regardless of when you submit the request (**Figure 10-28**).

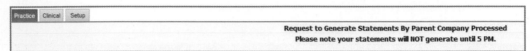

Request to Generate Statements By Parent Company Processed
Please note your statements will NOT generate until 5 PM.

Figure 10-28   Statements Generate at 5 p.m.

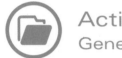

Activity 10-5
Generate Patient Statements

1. Before beginning this activity, post the following batches: "9-12CrBalRefunds," "9-10PostRAs," and "RobinsonSNF."

2. With patient Edith Robinson in context, go to the *Administration* module > *Practice* tab > *Daily Administration* section > *Financial* header > *Generate Statements* link (**Figure 10-29**). If a patient is in context, the application displays the option to generate statements for the parent company or the responsible party. You can generate statements for only the parent company when no patient is in context.

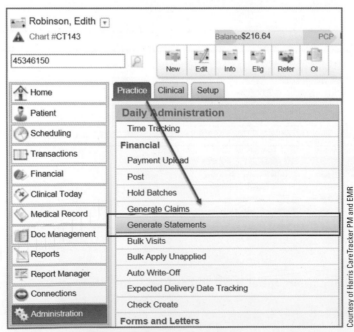

Figure 10-29   Generate Statements Link

3. In the *Generate Statements for Responsible Party* field, select the responsible party for whom you want to generate statements (select patient Edith Robinson) and then click *Go!* (**Figure 10-30**).

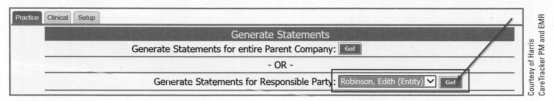

Figure 10-30   Generate Statements for Responsible Party—Edith Robinson

4. The application schedules the statements to be printed. Your screen will look like **Figure 10-31**.

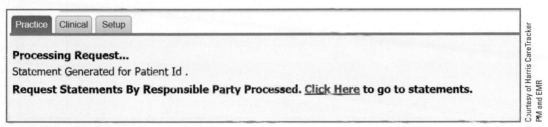

Figure 10-31   Statement Generated

SPOTLIGHT If no statements are displaying, recheck after 24 hours (or after 5 p.m. on the date the activity is performed). Continue with your activities, and repeat Activity 10-5 in 24 hours.

5. Click on the blue "Click Here" prompt (see **Figure 10-31**) to go to the statements. **Note:** You may need to click on *Generate* and *Click Here* (in blue) again for the statement(s) to appear. If you receive an error message, click out of the *Administration* module and repeat the activity steps. Your screen will now look like **Figure 10-32**. (**Note:** If no results are showing, change the *Date Range* to "All Dates.")

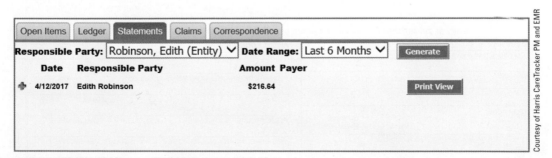

Figure 10-32   Statements Display

6. Click on the *Print View* button. The patient's statement will display in a new window (**Figure 10-33**).

7. Print the statement by right-clicking on the screen and selecting *Print* from the drop-down menu.

Napa Valley Family Associates

RESP PARTY ACCT #	101616-45346150	STMT DATE	4/12/2017
LAST PMT	$64.61	STMT TOTAL	$216.64

Statement - Page 1

DATE OF SERVICE	PATIENT	DESCRIPTION OF SERVICES	PROCEDURE CODE	SERVICING PROVIDER	AMOUNT	PATIENT AMT DUE
4/3/2017	Robinson, Edith (45346150)	Office Outpatient New 30 Minutes	99203	Raman, Amir	-$86.55	$21.64
		Per Your Insurance Company, Your Copay Has Not Been Paid In Full. The Balance Is Your Responsibility. Thank You.				
		Transaction 04/03/2017, Adjustment - Contractual			-$82.81	
		Transaction 04/03/2017, Charges			$191.00	
4/9/2017	Robinson, Edith (45346150)	Phys Cert Mcr-Covr Hom Hlth Srvc Per Cert Prd	G0180	Raman, Amir	$100.00	-$50.00
		Transaction 04/09/2017, Insurance Payment			-$58.46	
		Transaction 04/09/2017, Payment - Patient Cash			-$64.61	
		Transaction 04/09/2017, Adjustment - Contractual			-$26.93	
		Transaction 04/09/2017, Non-Covered charge				
4/9/2017	Robinson, Edith (45346150)	Office Outpatient Visit 25 Minutes	99214	Raman, Amir	$245.00	$245.00
		See Billing Note				
		Transaction 04/09/2017, Non-Covered charge				

MAKE CHECKS PAYABLE TO: Napa Valley Family Associates

PLEASE PAY THIS AMOUNT	$216.64

TO ENSURE PROPER CREDIT, PLEASE DETACH AND RETURN BOTTOM PORTION WITH YOUR PAYMENT

Napa Valley Family Associates
101 Vine Street
Napa, CA 94558

707- 555-1212 Ext:

RESP PARTY ACCT #	101616-45346150	STMT DATE	4/12/2017
AMT ENCLOSED $		STMT TOTAL	$216.64

PATIENT ID# 45346150

☐ CHECK BOX AND ENTER ADDRESS OR INSURANCE CORRECTIONS ON THE REVERSE SIDE

☐ IF PAYING BY CREDIT CARD, FILL OUT THE INFORMATION ON THE REVERSE SIDE

ADDRESSEE:

EDITH ROBINSON

3072 SACRAMENTO ST

SONOMA, CA 95476

REMIT TO:

NAPA VALLEY FAMILY ASSOCIATES

101 VINE STREET

NAPA, CA 94558

IF ANY OF THE INFORMATION HAS BEEN CHANGED SINCE YOUR LAST STATEMENT, PLEASE INDICATE...

ABOUT YOU:

YOUR NAME (Last, First, Middle Initial)

ADDRESS

CITY   STATE   ZIP

TELEPHONE   MARITAL STATUS
                   ☐ Single   ☐ Divorced
( )   ☐ Married   ☐ Widowed

EMPLOYER'S NAME   TELEPHONE
                          ( )

EMPLOYER'S ADDRESS   CITY   STATE   ZIP

IF PAYING BY CREDIT CARD, FILL OUT BELOW

☐ AMERICAN EXPRESS   ☐ MASTERCARD ☐ VISA

CARD NUMBER   CSV

CHARGE THIS AMOUNT   EXPIRATION DATE

SIGNATURE   CARDHOLDER NAME

ABOUT YOUR INSURANCE:

YOUR PRIMARY INSURANCE COMPANY'S NAME   EFFECTIVE DATE

PRIMARY INSURANCE COMPANY'S ADDRESS   PHONE

CITY   STATE   ZIP

POLICYHOLDER'S ID NUMBER   GROUP PLAN NUMBER

YOUR SECONDARY INSURANCE COMPANY'S NAME   EFFECTIVE DATE

SECONDARY INSURANCE COMPANY'S ADDRESS   PHONE

CITY   STATE   ZIP

POLICYHOLDER'S ID NUMBER   GROUP PLAN NUMBER

Courtesy of Harris CareTracker PM and EMR

Figure 10-33 Patient Statement

📑 **Print the patient statement, label it "Activity 10-5," and place it in your assignment folder.**

8. Close out of the Statement by clicking on the "X" in the upper-right-hand corner.

When statements have been generated, you can use several locations in Harris CareTracker PM to print them either by batch or individually, as outlined in **Table 10-6**.

Table 10-6 Print Statements, Bulk and Individual	
To Print Statements in Bulk	Go to the *Home* module > *Dashboard* tab > *Billing* section > *Statements/Unprinted Statements* link. Go to the *Reports* module > *Reports* tab > *Financial Reports* section > *All Statements* link.
To Print Individual Statements	Go to the *Financial* module > *Statements* tab. Go to the *Name Bar* > *Letters* button. (**Note:** This option is only applicable if your practice's statements are set up as a form letter.)

Courtesy of Harris CareTracker PM and EMR

Reprinting Statements

The *Statements* application in the *Financial* module (**Figure 10-34**) allows you to view and reprint statements that have been generated for the patient in context. A statement can be reprinted by clicking on the *Print View* button next to the appropriate statement line. When *Print View* is clicked, the patient's statement displays in a new window, and by right-clicking on top of it, the statement can be printed.

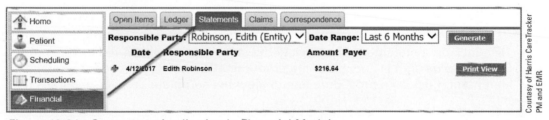

Figure 10-34   Statements Application in Financial Module

Activity 10-6
View and Reprint a Patient Statement Using the Financial Module

1. Pull patient Edith Robinson into context.

2. Click the *Financial* module. Click *Go.* The *Open Items* for the patient display (**Figure 10-35**). (**Note:** You can also access the open items by clicking the *OI* 📄 icon on the *Name Bar.*)

3. Click the *Statements* tab. Harris CareTracker PM opens the *Statements* application (see **Figure 10-36**).

    a. The *Responsible Party* list defaults to the responsible party set in the patient's demographic. Leave as is. (**Note:** You can select a different responsible party or "(All)" responsible parties, if applicable.)

    b. The *Date Range* list defaults to "Last 6 Months." Use the drop-down next to *Date Range* and select "All Dates."

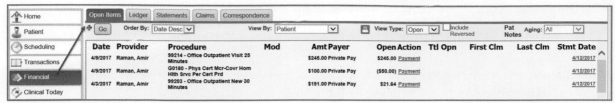

Figure 10-35   Financial Open Items

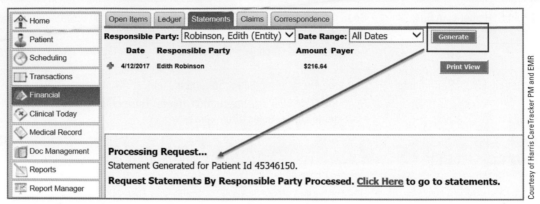

Figure 10-36   Financial Module/Statements Tab

4. Click *Generate*. Harris CareTracker PM generates a list of the patient's statements and displays a processing message in the lower frame of the screen.

5. Select the *Click Here* link in blue. The application displays the list of statements.

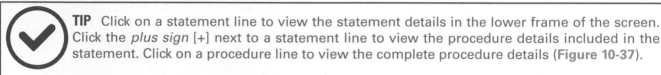

TIP Click on a statement line to view the statement details in the lower frame of the screen. Click the *plus sign* [+] next to a statement line to view the procedure details included in the statement. Click on a procedure line to view the complete procedure details (**Figure 10-37**).

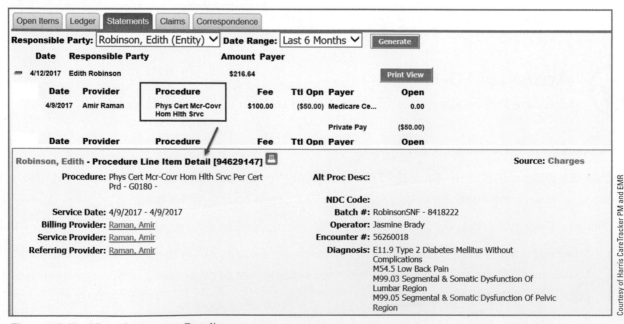

Figure 10-37   View Statement Details

6. Click *Print View* next to the statement you want to print. Select the most recent statement. The application displays the statement in a new window. **Note:** It may take a few moments to display.

7. Right-click on the statement and then select *Print* from the shortcut menu.

💾 **Print the statement, label it "Activity 10-6," and place it in your assignment folder.**

8. Close the statement window when the statement has printed.

PATIENT COLLECTIONS

Learning Objective 4: Describe components of the patient collection process.

The *Collections* application in Harris CareTracker PM allows you to focus collection efforts on patients with balances at least 30 days overdue. You can determine whether patients are identified by the collections system immediately or after their balance is 30, 60, 90, or 120 days overdue.

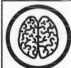 **CRITICAL THINKING** Identify the ways a medical practice can reduce the incidence of patient accounts going into collection status. How would a Practice Management/EMR program help facilitate this?

A patient balance will automatically appear in *Collections* when the balance ages past the days set in *Days Overdue* and one additional statement has generated. When "Immediate" is selected, the system will send a patient directly to the *Collections* module after his or her first statement is generated. The collections' setting applies to all groups in the company.

All new patients added to the *Collections* application will have a collection status of "New" and should be reviewed weekly to determine if they should be removed from *Collections* or if some type of collection action should be taken. However, when the patient balance reaches zero, Harris CareTracker PM automatically removes the patient from the *Collections* list. The *Collections Work List* is outlined in **Table 10-7**.

Table 10-7   Financial Classes (Collections Work List)

NAME	DESCRIPTION
Collections Pending	Balances are typically first transferred to an insurance plan that is linked to the *Collections Pending* financial class to indicate that these are the patient balances that you are actively working. The *Collections Pending* financial class is linked to the "Collect Pend Statement" and "Collect Pend No Statement" insurance plans.
Collections Actual	Once you have exhausted your own collection activity on an account and you would like to transfer the patient's balance, you can either transfer the balance to the insurance plan "Collections Actual" or the specific collection agency your office works with. These balances would then be found in the *A/R* link on your *Dashboard* under the financial class "Collections Actual." All balance transfers can be done in bulk from the *Collections System*. In addition to transferring the patient's balance, the patient's collection status should also be changed to the corresponding status. The *Collections Actual* financial class is linking to the *Collections Actual* insurance plan and any collection agency insurance plans.

Courtesy of Harris CareTracker PM and EMR

Financial Classes

While actively working on collecting **private pay** balances, you need to assign the private pay balances to a financial class. Private pay refers to patients without insurance or the balance due after insurance has adjusted the claim and paid any amount due under contract. In Harris CareTracker PM, the financial class is linked to the insurance plan. While working collection balances, many practices prefer to move the private pay balances out of the *Patient* financial class and into another financial class to differentiate these monies. If you would like to move the patient's balance to a different financial class for reporting purposes, you will have several options. There are two financial classes that private pay balances can be transferred to *Collections Pending* and *Collections Actual*, outlined in **Table 10-7**.

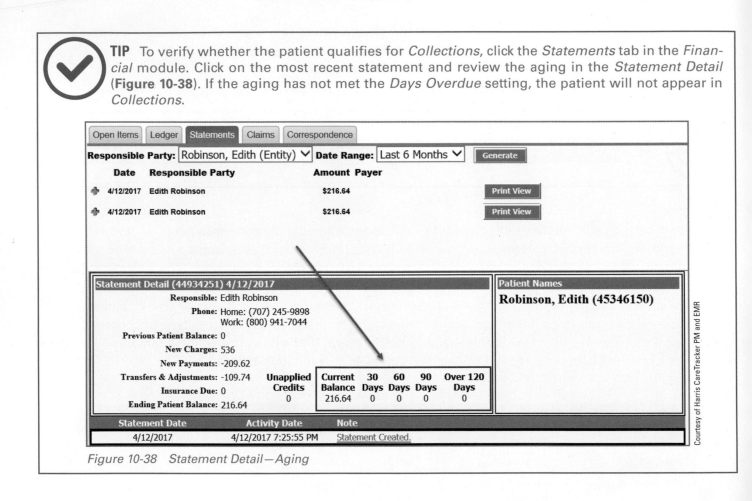

TIP   To verify whether the patient qualifies for *Collections*, click the *Statements* tab in the *Financial* module. Click on the most recent statement and review the aging in the *Statement Detail* (**Figure 10-38**). If the aging has not met the *Days Overdue* setting, the patient will not appear in *Collections*.

Figure 10-38   Statement Detail—Aging

In addition to managing the balance transfers, when you send a patient's balance to a collection agency, you should change his or her patient status to *Collections*. This can be done in the *Demographics* application by selecting "Collections" from the *Category* drop-down list (**Figure 10-39**). This status will always display next to the patient's name in Harris CareTracker PM (**Figure 10-40**) so all staff will know that this patient has been transferred to the collection agency. For the *Collections* notice to appear, you will have to take the patient out of context and then bring back into context before *Collections* status appears. **Table 10-8** describes the *Collections Reports* and *Last Activity Date* details.

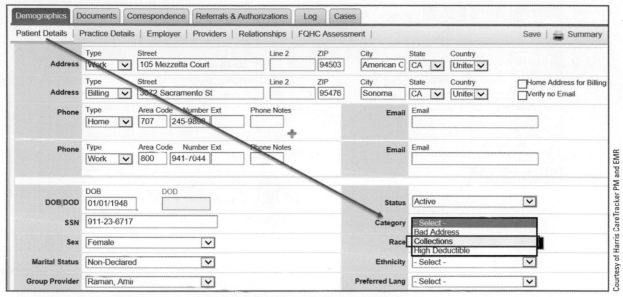

Figure 10-39   Patient Category–Collections in Demographics Screen

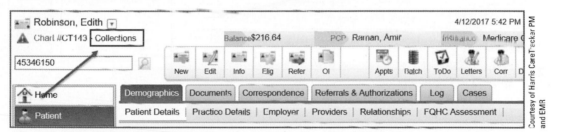

Figure 10-40   Collections Status Appears Next to Chart Number

Table 10-8   Collections

Collections Reports	There are *Collections* reports available in the *Reports* module > *Financial Reports* section > *Other Reports* link that can be used to identify balances to be transferred to your collections agency.
Last Activity Date	You can sort the collections list by last activity date by clicking the column heading. Harris CareTracker PM displays the last activity performed when the cursor is placed over the last activity date.

Courtesy of Harris CareTracker PM and EMR

COLLECTION STATUS

Learning Objective 5: Review collection status and transfer private pay balances.

The *Collections* application is accessed from the *Home* module > *Dashboard* tab > *Billing* section > *Collections* link (**Figure 10-41**). There are seven collection statuses in Harris CareTracker PM: New, Open Collections, Review, Collections Actual, Collections Pending, Collections Pending – NS, and Hold (**Figure 10-42**).

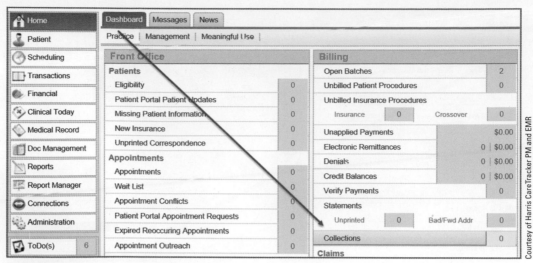

Figure 10-41   Collections Link

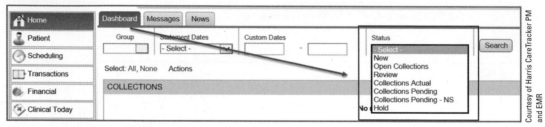

Figure 10-42   Seven Collection Statuses

New Status

After a patient has reached the set overdue period for your practice (i.e., immediate, 30, 60, 90, or 120 days over-due), they are automatically identified by the *Collections System* and assigned the status of "New." Patients and their balances with a status of "New" should be reviewed on a weekly basis to determine what action should be taken on the account and what collection status the patient should be assigned.

When a patient has been in the "New" status for more than six weeks, the system assumes that the item is not part of the collection process and is not included in the value displayed on the *Dashboard*. However, these collection items will continue to reside under the "New" status until the balance is paid off and removed from *Collections*.

If a patient in the "New" status is removed from *Collections* and he or she continues to have a patient bal-ance that is 30, 60, 90, or 120 days overdue, the patient will be flagged again for the *Collections System* when a statement is generated and will be placed in the "New" status.

Open Collection Status

When a collection letter is sent to a patient, change his or her status to "Open Collections." A patient in "Open Col-lections" will continue to receive statements until his or her balance is transferred to "Collections Pending-NS" or "Collections Actual."

Review Status

The "Review" status indicates that the physician or another office staff member should review the patient's account before any action is taken. Patients in the "Review" status should be reviewed on a weekly basis.

After "Review" patients have been reviewed, their status should be changed. Typically, the status would be changed to "Open" if an action is going to be taken (such as sending the patient a collection letter), or it should be changed to "Remove from Collections" if the patient needs to be removed from the *Collections System*.

Collections Actual Status

Any patient whose balance has been sent to a collection agency should be flagged with the "Collections Actual" status. These patients typically have been sent numerous collection letters but never made a payment or contacted the billing department/staff. When a patient is assigned the status of "Collections Actual," the patient's outstanding balance should be transferred to the "Collections Actual" insurance plan or to the actual collection agency your practice utilizes.

Collections Pending Status

The status "Collections Pending" identifies all patients with outstanding private pay balances transferred to the *Collect Pend Statement* insurance plan. Typically, patients are assigned to this status when you are still actively working on collecting owed money. Harris CareTracker PM continues to generate statements for patients in this status. When a patient is assigned the status of "Collections Pending," the patient's private pay outstanding balance should also be transferred to the *Collect Pend Statement* insurance plan.

 TIP You must have a batch open to transfer any balances from private pay to *Collect Pend Statement*.

Collections Pending – NS Status

The status "Collections Pending – NS" is assigned to all patients whose outstanding private pay balances have been transferred to the *Collect Pend No Statement* insurance plan. Typically, patients are assigned to this status in the *Collections System* and their balances transferred to this insurance plan to identify patients who are pending collections but from whom you are still actively working on collecting owed money. Harris CareTracker PM does not generate statements for patients in this status.

Hold Status

The "Hold" status is assigned to patients who you want identified by the *Collections System* but for whom you do not want to take action. For example, a patient may make a small payment after receiving his or her first collection letter. Instead of sending the patient a second collection letter alerting the patient of the remaining overdue balance, you can flag the patient as "Hold" to see if he or she makes additional payments. Patients who have been assigned a status of "Hold" should be reviewed weekly to determine if additional collection activity is required on their account or if they should be removed from the *Collections System*.

Transfer Private Pay Balances

Transferring private pay balances coincides with changing a patient's collection status. For example, if you want to transfer a balance from the financial class "Private Pay" to the financial class "Collections Pending," you must change the patient's status from "Open Collections" to "Collections Pending." Both a status change and a balance transfer can happen at one time from the *Collections* application.

After private balances have been transferred to either the *Collections Actual* plan or a collection agency, some practices choose to adjust off these outstanding balances using the code "Adjustment-Collections." Adjusting off outstanding private pay balances must be performed from the *Open Items* application. You can use the list of patients with a status of "Collections Actual" in the *Collections System* as a work list to pull each patient into context and then click on the *OI* icon on the *Name Bar* to complete the needed financial transaction.

Moving Patients to Collections

Harris CareTracker PM automatically moves patients into *Collections* when their overdue balance reaches the aging level assigned in the group settings and automatically removes patients from *Collections* when their overdue balance is paid. Operators can also move patients in and out of *Collections* manually. In *Open Items*, you can add a patient to *Collections* by clicking the *Add Responsible Party* link in the *Collections* work area or by transferring a balance to *Collections*.

Patients manually added to *Collections* are flagged with an asterisk (*) next to their name in the work area. Patients manually added to *Collections* must be removed from *Collections* manually as well. When manually adding a patient to *Collections*, Harris CareTracker PM pulls the patient into context and filters the *Collections* list to show the responsible party for that patient.

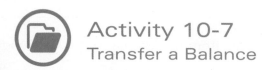

Activity 10-7
Transfer a Balance

1. Go to the *Home* module > *Dashboard* tab > *Billing* section > *Collections* link. Harris CareTracker PM displays a list of collection statuses and the number of patients in each status.

2. If there is no patient listed, click the *Add Responsible Party* link in the upper-right corner of the screen.

3. In the *Add Manual Collection* window, click the *Search* icon and enter the name of the patient you are searching for (select patient Edith Robinson). Click on the patient name in the *Results* window. The patient name now populates in the *Add Manual Collection* window.

4. Click *Save*.

5. Click the *Edit* icon next to the balance you want to transfer to a new financial class. Harris CareTracker PM displays the *Edit* window (**Figure 10-43**).

   a. *Insurance*: Leave blank (-Select-)

   b. *Overdue*: Leave blank (-Select-)

   c. *Letter*: Leave blank (-Select-)

   d. *Change Status*: Select "Open Collections"

6. Click *Save*.

7. In the *Updates Processed* window that appears, click *Close*. Harris CareTracker PM updates the patient's status in the *Collections* application, transfers the outstanding balance to the selected financial class, and adds the selected "Transfer To" financial class to the patient's *Demographics* record.

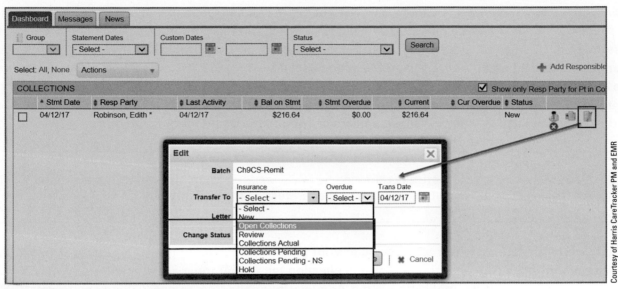

Figure 10-43   Edit Collections Dialog Box

TIP To transfer multiple balances to a new financial class, select the checkbox next to each balance you want to transfer and then click *Actions > Edit* (**Figure 10-44**).

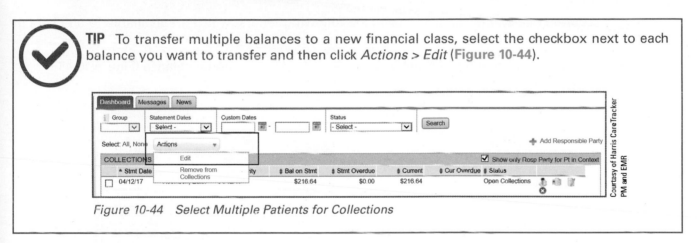

Figure 10-44   Select Multiple Patients for Collections

🖨 **Print the Balance Transfer screen, label it "Activity 10-7," and place it in your assignment folder.**

You can add the *Collections Pending Statement, Collections Pending No Statement, Collections Actual* financial classes, or your collection agency name to the *Insurance Plans* "quick pick" list in the *Quick Picks* application in the *Administration* module.

COLLECTION ACTIONS

Learning Objective 6: Perform collection actions.

There are four collection actions in Harris CareTracker PM: *Transfer, Remove from Collections, Group Collections,* and *Global Collection Letters.*

Transfer is used when a patient's private pay balance needs to be transferred to a different insurance plan/ financial class. Possible insurance plans you would be transferring to a private pay balance are:

- Collect Pend Statement
- Collect Pend No Statement
- Collections Actual
- Your practice's collection agency

Each insurance plan is linked to a financial class. There are two collection financial classes: *Collections Actual* and *Collections Pending*. After the private pay balance is transferred to the appropriate insurance plan, the money will automatically be moved to the appropriate financial class. A bulk transfer to one insurance plan can be done for multiple patients at one time from the *Collections* application.

The *Remove from Collections* action removes the patient from the *Collections System*. The patient will be put back into the *Collections System* if any portion of his or her private pay balance ages beyond the number of days set in the group's collections flag, when statements are generated again for the patient.

 TIP A patient is automatically removed from *Collections* when his or her private pay or collection balances are paid in full or adjusted off, regardless of the patient's collection status.

Group Collection Letters, which are specific to your practice, are built in the *Letter Editor* application in the *Administration* module. After creating a custom collection letter, you must add the letter to your *Form Letters Quick Picks* via the *Quick Picks* application in the *Administration* module. This will allow you to select the letter in the *Collections* module.

The *Global Collection Letters* application contains the following letters, which are available to all users in Harris CareTracker PM.

- "Collections 1": Explains that the account is overdue and lists the overdue balance (**Figure 10-45**).

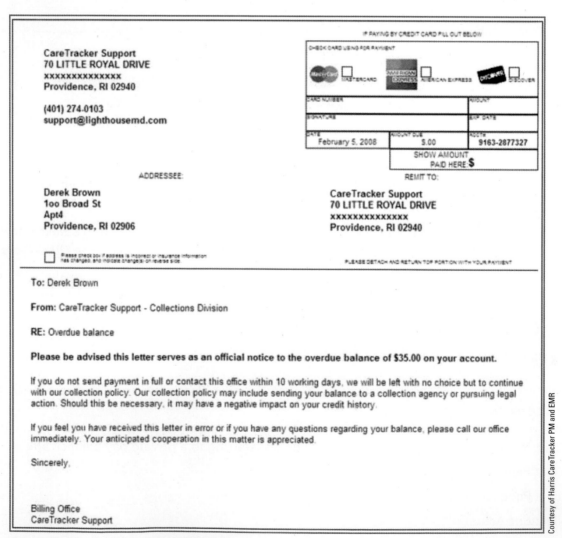

Figure 10-45   Collections 1 Letter

- "Past Due": Explains that the overdue balance or a portion of the balance is more than 60 days past due (**Figure 10-46**).

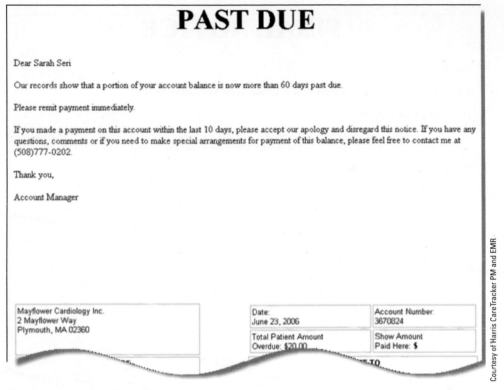

Figure 10-46   Past Due Letter

- "Delinquent": Explains that the overdue balance or a portion of the balance is more than 90 days past due (**Figure 10-47**).

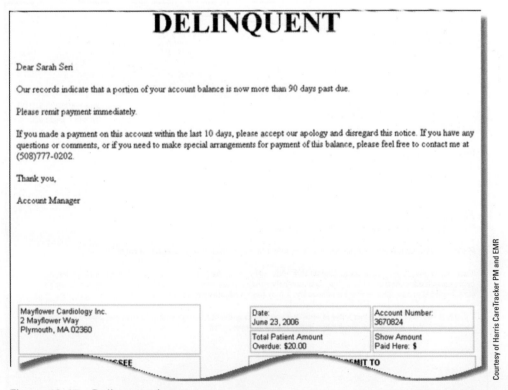

Figure 10-47   Delinquent Letter

- "Final Notice": Tells the patient that her overdue balance or a portion of her balance is more than 120 days past due. This is the final written notice the patient will receive, and, if payment is not received, the account will be sent to *Collections* (**Figure 10-48**).

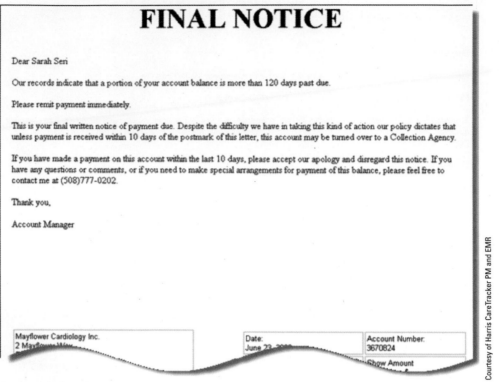

Figure 10-48 Final Notice Letter

- "75 Collection": States that if the overdue balance is not paid in full, the billing office will continue with its collection policy, which may include using a collection agency (**Figure 10-49**).

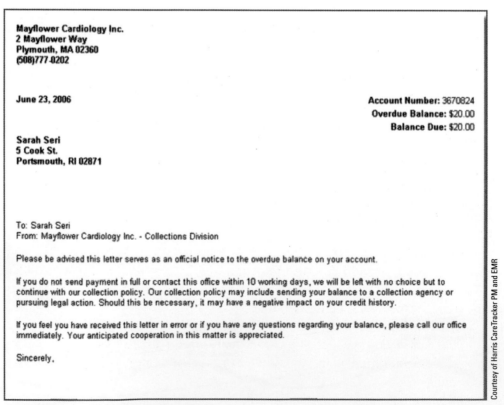

Figure 10-49 75 Collections Letter

- "Collection Payment Plan": Informs the patient that she can set up a weekly or monthly payment plan to pay off the overdue balance. On a "Collection Payment Plan" letter, the patient can also indicate if she has insurance that covered the services for which she has an overdue balance. When a patient indicates that he or she has insurance to cover the services, the patient must also complete the insurance section on the back of a statement (**Figure 10-50**).

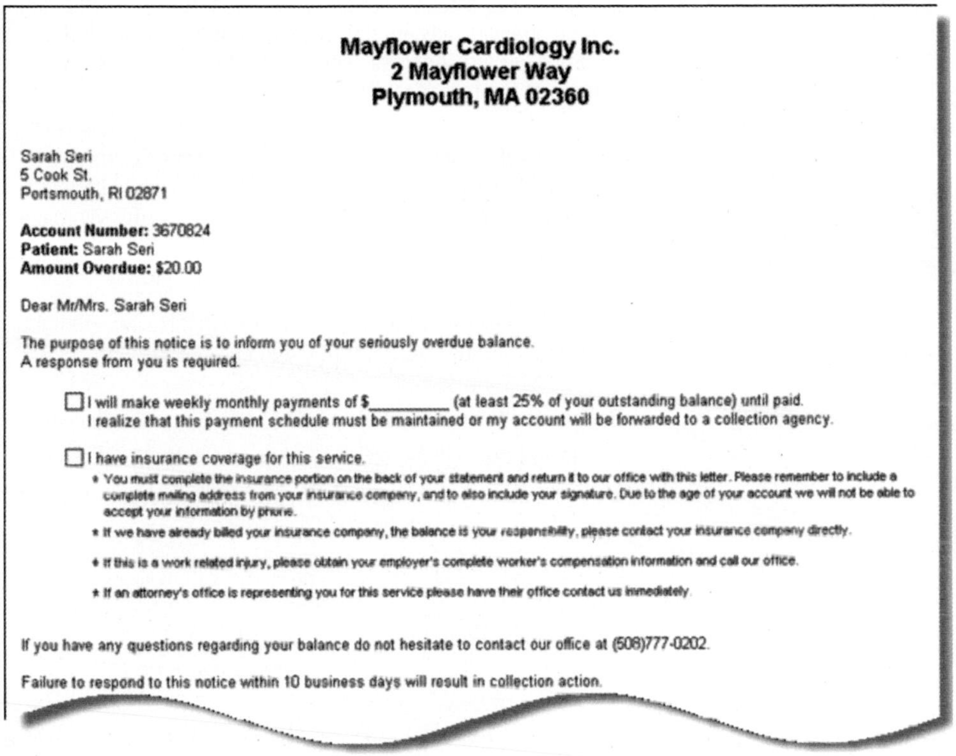

Mayflower Cardiology Inc.
2 Mayflower Way
Plymouth, MA 02360

Sarah Seri
5 Cook St.
Portsmouth, RI 02871

Account Number: 3670824
Patient: Sarah Seri
Amount Overdue: $20.00

Dear Mr/Mrs. Sarah Seri

The purpose of this notice is to inform you of your seriously overdue balance.
A response from you is required.

☐ I will make weekly monthly payments of $_____ (at least 25% of your outstanding balance) until paid.
I realize that this payment schedule must be maintained or my account will be forwarded to a collection agency.

☐ I have insurance coverage for this service.
* You must complete the insurance portion on the back of your statement and return it to our office with this letter. Please remember to include a complete mailing address from your insurance company, and to also include your signature. Due to the age of your account we will not be able to accept your information by phone.
* If we have already billed your insurance company, the balance is your responsibility, please contact your insurance company directly.
* If this is a work related injury, please obtain your employer's complete worker's compensation information and call our office.
* If an attorney's office is representing you for this service please have their office contact us immediately.

If you have any questions regarding your balance do not hesitate to contact our office at (508)777-0202.

Failure to respond to this notice within 10 business days will result in collection action.

Courtesy of Harris CareTracker PM and EMR

Figure 10-50   Collection Payment Plan Letter

You can also create custom collection letters in the *Letter Editor* application in the *Administration* module.

When you create a group-specific collection letter, the top portion of the letter by default includes patient information, such as name, address, and so on. The only portion of the letter you need to build in the *Letter Editor* is the text you want to appear in the letter. Refer to **Table 10-9** to view the *Letter Editor Tools* as you create your custom collection letter.

COLLECTION LETTERS

Learning Objective 7: Create collection letters.

Group-specific collection letters are built in the *Practice Letter Editor* in the *Administration* module. After creating a custom collection letter, you must add the letter to your *Form Letters Quick Picks* via the *Quick Picks* application in the *Administration* module. This will allow you to access the letter in the *Collections* module.

The *Letter Editor* is preset to double space when you hit the [Enter] key to enter a new line of text. For single spacing, hold the [Shift] key down as you press the [Enter] key.

Creating letters in the *Letter Editor* saves significant administrative time, especially for letters that are commonly used in the practice. In addition, using the *Letter Editor* feature locks the correspondence into the EHR for easy access and reference.

Refer to **Table 10-9** for the letter editor tools available in Harris CareTracker PM and EMR.

Table 10-9   Letter Editor Tools

TOOL	ICON	DESCRIPTION
Style	Normal	When you create a new letter, the text style defaults to "Normal" and the text displays as normal. There are also various Heading styles of different sizes that will present the selected text in a bigger, bolder format. A Heading format is typically how company names are displayed in headers of form letters. Other selections in the Style list are "Address" and "Formatted," and these will also change the formatting of the text accordingly.
Font & Font Size	Arial 1	Arial is the default font in *Letter Editor*. Tahoma, Courier New, Times New Roman, and Wingdings are the other available fonts for building a letter. These fonts appear in *Letter Editor* as they would in a Microsoft® Word document. Unlike in Microsoft® Word, the font sizes in *Letter Editor* only range from 1 to 7, with 1 being the smallest font and 7 being the largest. **Note:** You must have the small "IDAutomationHC39S" font installed on your computer to utilize the barcode font in the *Letter Editor*.
Bold, Italics, & Underline	**B** *I* <u>U</u>	**B:** Selected text will be **bolded** when this button is clicked. **I:** Selected text will be *italicized* when this button is clicked. **U:** Selected text will be <u>underlined</u> when this button is clicked.
Text Color		Allows you to change the color of the selected text.
Background Color		Allows you to highlight text with a background color.
Text Justification		Used to justify the text to the left, center, or right.
Numbering		Adds numbering to a list. Number 1 will be assigned to the first line, and when you hit [Enter], 2 will automatically be put on the second line, etc.
Bulleted		Adds bullets to a nonsequential list.
Indenting		Used to adjust the indentation of text in a paragraph. The left arrow decreases the indent. The right arrow increases the indent.
Edit Description/Status		Used to edit the description and status of a form letter already saved in Harris CareTracker PM and EMR. The status indicates whether a form letter is active or inactive. Before clicking on this icon, select the name of the letter you would like to edit or make inactive in the *Letters* field.
Selecting a Letter	Letters: (Select a Letter)	Form letters already created for your practice will be listed in the *Letters* list. To edit a letter, select the letter from the list, and then edit the letter accordingly. To create a new form letter, select "Create New Letter" from the *Letters* list and begin building your letter.
Search	Search:	Used to search all global form letters saved in Harris CareTracker PM and EMR. Enter the name of the letter you would like to search for and then click on the magnifying glass.

Table 10-9   Letter Editor Tools *(continued)*

TOOL	ICON	DESCRIPTION
New File		Creates a new form letter.
Save		Saves a new form letter or saves edits made to an existing form letter.
Cut		Selected text will be deleted from your form letter when this button is clicked.
Copy/Paste		Clicking on the first icon copies selected text. Then by clicking on the clipboard icon, you can paste the copied text into the current or another form letter. **Note:** You cannot copy fields from one letter type and paste them into another letter type. The letter types must be the same. For example, you cannot copy fields from an *Appointment* letter and paste them into a *Recall* letter.
Undo & Redo		Clicking on the Undo button will undo the last action performed while creating your form letter. Clicking on the Redo button will redo the last action you selected to undo while creating your form letter.
Select Field	{···}	Inserts a data field into the form letter. When your form letter is generated, the data fields pull in the respective data from Harris CareTracker PM and EMR. There are three types of data fields you can insert into a form letter: "Group," "Patient," or "Special." Within each of these categories are specific data fields that you can insert. To insert a field: 1. Place your cursor in the location where you want the data field to appear in the letter and then click the *Select Field* button. Harris CareTracker PM displays the *Select Field* dialog box. 2. Click the plus signs [+] to expand each category. 3. Click on the underlined link to insert the field in the letter. Harris CareTracker PM and EMR adds the data field to the letter in brackets. When a letter is generated for a patient, the patient-specific information will be pulled into the field from the patient's record.
Toggle HTML		Clicking on this button will allow you to toggle between the HTML code for the letter and the text format.
Numbers of Letters	Letters per page: 1 ⌄	When you create a form letter, Harris CareTracker PM and EMR defaults to generate and print one letter per 8½ × 11 inch page. However, you have the option of modifying the system so that more than one letter will be printed on one page.

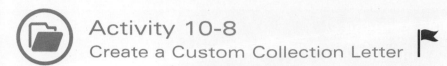

Activity 10-8
Create a Custom Collection Letter

1. Go to the *Administration* module > *Practice* tab > *Forms and Letters* section > *Practice Letter Editor* link (**Figure 10-51**).

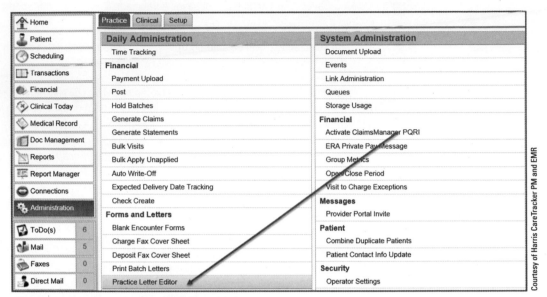

Figure 10-51   Practice Letter Editor Link

2. From the *Letters* drop-down list, select "Create New Letter" (**Figure 10-52**). The application displays the *New Letter* window (**Figure 10-53**).

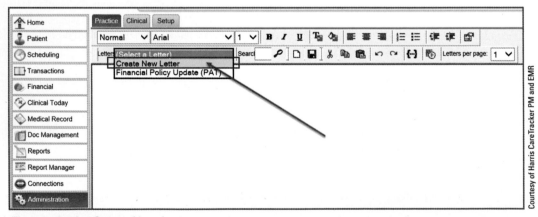

Figure 10-52   Create New Letter

3. Enter a descriptive name for the form letter in the *Letter Name* field. Enter "Missed Appointment Fee."

4. In the *Letter Type* field, select the radio button next to the type of form letter you are creating (select "Appointment").

5. Then click *Save* (see **Figure 10-53**). The application closes the *New Letter* window and pulls the new letter name and type into the *Letters* field (**Figure 10-54**). **Note:** It may take a few moments for the screen to refresh.

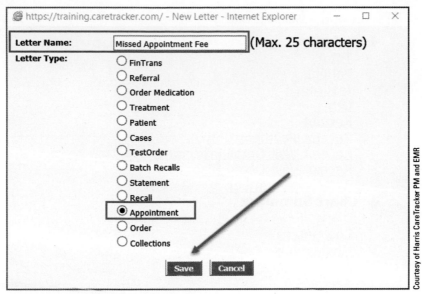

Figure 10-53   New Letter Window

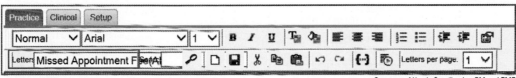

Figure 10-54   Letters Field

6. Enter the text to appear in the form letter and insert data fields where necessary using the *Select Field* {··}
   icon. Select data fields from the drop-down list in the *Select Field* list (Figure 10-55) to complete your letter. (For example, for the first line of the letter, select "Current Date – Long" from the *Special Fields* section in the *Select Field* list.) As a best practice, you should click *Save* ■ icon periodically while building
   your letter. Be sure to format the letter as you would like it to appear, following the instructions below:

   a. Click on the *Select Field* icon, scroll down to the *Special Fields* section, and select "Current Date
      – Long," then click [enter] to move the line. Recall that the *Letter Editor* is preset to double space
      when you hit the [Enter] key to enter a new line of text. For single spacing, hold the [Shift] key
      down as you press the [Enter] key.

   b. Click on the *Select Field* icon, scroll down, and in the *Patient Fields (General)* select "First Name."

   c. Staying on the same line, click on the *Select Field* icon, scroll down, and in the *Patient Fields
      (General)* select "Last Name."

   d. Staying on the same line, click on the *Select Field* icon, scroll down, and in the *Patient Fields
      (Billing Address)* select "Address 1."

   e. Staying on the same line, click on the *Select Field* icon, scroll down, and in the *Patient Fields
      (Billing Address)* select "City."

   f. Staying on the same line, click on the *Select Field* icon and scroll down, and in the *Patient Fields
      (Billing Address)* select "State Code."

   g. Staying on the same line, click on the *Select Field* icon, scroll down, and in the *Patient Fields
      (Billing Address)* select "Zip Code."

   h. Hit [Enter] to move to the next line.

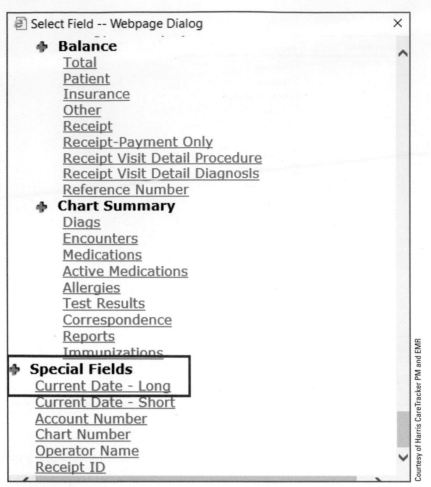

Figure 10-55   Select Field List

i.   Type "Dear", then a space.

j.   Then staying on the same line, click on the *Select Field* icon, scroll down, and in the *Patient Fields (General)* select "Title."

k.   Staying on the same line, click on the *Select Field* icon, scroll down, and in the *Patient Fields (General)* select "Last Name."

l.   Hit [Enter] to move to the next line.

m.   Type in the following message:

"You missed your last scheduled appointment with Dr. [click on the *Select Field* icon, scroll down, and in the *Primary Care Provider (PCP)* field select "Last Name"] on [click on the *Select Field* icon, scroll down, and in the *Appointment* field select "Date Only"]. We are concerned about your health and would like to reschedule the appointment at your earliest convenience. There is a $35 charge for appointments that are canceled with less than 8-business hours' notice. Please remit to our billing office.

Please call the office to schedule or select an appointment via the Patient Portal.

If you have any questions, please don't hesitate to call.

Sincerely,

Jasmine Brady, MA, Office Manager"

n. Your screen should look like **Figure 10-56**.

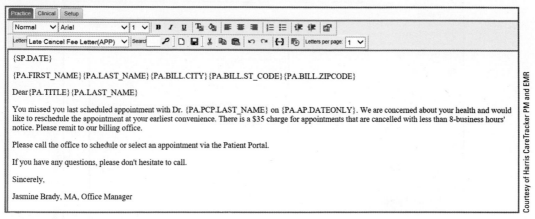

Figure 10-56   Late Cancel Fee Letter

7. Click the *Save File* icon when you are finished with your form letter.

Print the screen that displays the Custom Collection Letter, label it "Activity 10-8," and place it in your assignment folder.

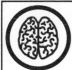

CRITICAL THINKING Using your experience as a medical assistant, create several custom letters, and cite their purpose. Submit the letters to your instructor for discussion. Add them to your *Quick Picks* (Activity 10-9) upon completion.

1. Custom Collection letter
2. Custom Missed Appointment letter
3. Custom Annual Physical Exam reminder letter

Adding a Form Letter to Quick Picks

After creating a new form letter, you must add it to your *Quick Picks* to make it available for use in Harris CareTracker PM and EMR.

Activity 10-9
Add a Form Letter to Quick Picks

1. Go to the *Administration* module > *Setup* tab > *Financial* section > *Quick Picks* link.

2. From the *Screen Type* drop-down list, select "Form Letters" (**Figure 10-57**).

3. In the *Search* field, enter part of the name of the new form letter you created in Activity 10-8 (enter "Missed") and then click the *Search* icon. The application displays a pop-up of all of the letters that match the search criteria (**Figure 10-58**).

4. Click on the form letter you want to add to your *Quick Pick* list (select "Missed Appointment Fee"). You will receive a pop-up *Success* box stating "Quick Pick information has been updated." Click *Close* on the *Success* box (**Figure 10-59**).

5. The application adds the letter to the *Quick Pick* list where it will be available to generate for patients.

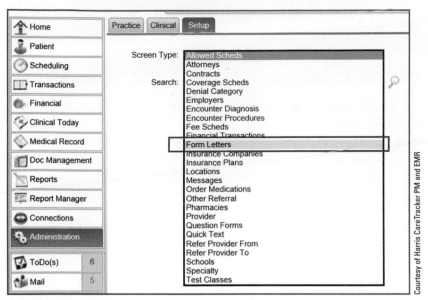

Figure 10-57   Screen Type—Form Letters

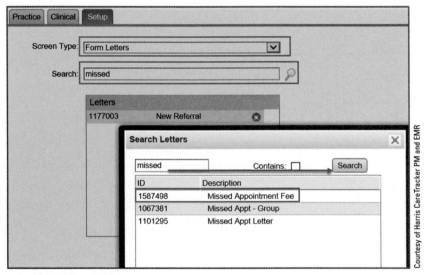

Figure 10-58   Search Letters Window

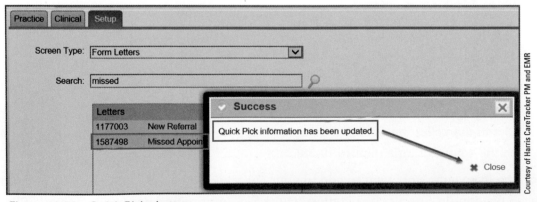

Figure 10-59   Quick Picks Letters

🖅 **Print the Quick Pick list screen with the Form Letter added, label it "Activity 10-0," and place it in your assignment folder.**

GENERATE COLLECTION LETTERS

Learning Objective 8: Generate collection letters.

To generate collection letters, use one of two options: Harris CareTracker PM and EMR's global collection letters, or build a custom collection letter specific to your practice. After collection letters have been generated, they must be printed from the *Print Batch Letters* application in the *Administration* module. Generated collection letters are saved in the patients' record in the *Correspondence* application of the *Financial* module.

  TIP You can click the column headings in the work area to sort the *Collections* list by statement date, responsible party, statement balance, overdue balance, current balance, and status.

 Activity 10-10
Generate Collection Letters

1. Go to the *Home* module > *Dashboard* tab > *Billing* section > *Collections* link. Harris CareTracker PM displays a list of collection statements (**Figure 10-60**).

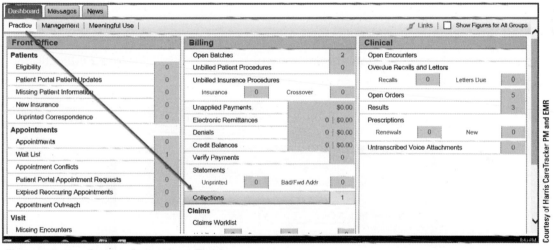

Figure 10-60   Search Collections Fields

2. (FYI) To search *Collections*, select an option from one or more of the following search fields and then click *Search* (**Figure 10-61**) to practice the options.
   - *Group*—*This field is only available when statements for the company are set up by group.*
   - *Statement Dates*—*This allows you to view a week's worth of statements.*
   - *Custom Dates*—*Enter a custom date range in the fields provided.*
   - *Status*—*Select the status of the collection statements you want to view.*

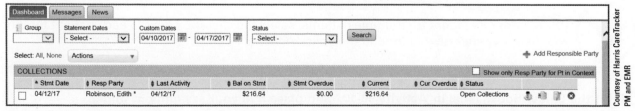

Figure 10-61   Search Collections Results

3. Use the filters at the top of the page to view statements by *Group, Status,* or date range. For this activity, in the drop-down list in the *Status* field, leave as (-Select-).

4. Double-click the name "Edith Robinson" in the line of the *Responsible Party* column to view the *State-ment Details* (**Figure 10-62**). It is helpful to review this information when determining a status change and/or deciding what action to take on a patient's balance. Close the *Statement Detail* dialog box.

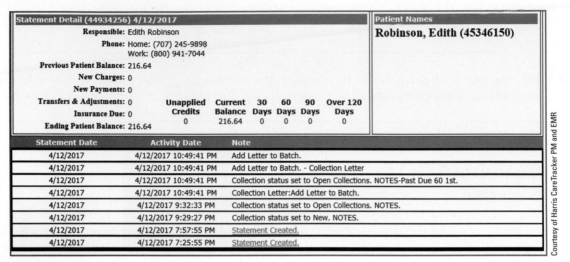

Figure 10-62   Statement Details

5. Close out of the *Statement Detail* dialog box.

6. Click the *Edit* icon next to the statement line for which you want to generate a collection letter (Edith Robinson). Harris CareTracker PM displays the *Edit* box.

7. From the *Letter* list, select the letter you want to generate. Select "Past Due 60 1st" (**Figure 10-63**)

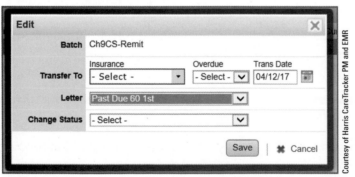

Figure 10-63   Generate Past Due 60 1st Letter

8. If needed, select a new status from the *Change Status* list. (Leave blank: "-Select-".)

 TIP To generate letters for multiple patients, select the checkbox next to each patient for whom you want to generate a letter and then click *Actions > Edit.*

🖳 **Print the Edit window, label it "Activity 10-10," and place it in your assignment folder.**

9. Click *Save*.

10. Then close out of the *Updates Processed* window. Generated collection letters can be printed from the *Print Batch Letters* application in the *Administration* module (**Figure 10-64**). You will receive an error message because you are not able to print batch letters in your student version of Harris CareTracker.

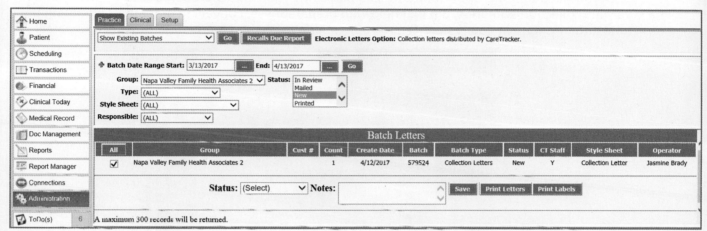

Figure 10-64   Print Batch Letters Application

Courtesy of Harris CareTracker PM and EMR

 TIP If you do not print the collection letters, Harris CareTracker PM and EMR will automatically print the letters to send out to the patient the next day.

 ## Activity 10-11
Run a Journal and Post All Remaining Batches

1. Go to the *Reports* module > *Todays Journals* link.

2. Click on *Add All >>*.

3. Scroll down and place a check mark in the *Includes Transfers* checkbox.

4. Click *Create Journal*.

🖫 **Print the Journal, label it "Activity 10-11a," and place it in your assignment folder.**

5. Go to the *Home* module > *Dashboard* tab > *Billing* section > *Open Batches* link. Harris CareTracker PM displays a list of open batches.

6. Place a checkmark in the *Batch Name* column by each unposted batch.

🖫 **Print the Batches to Post screen, label it "Activity 10-11b," and place it in your assignment folder.**

7. Click *Post Batches*.

CRITICAL THINKING Billing and collections activities require the utmost professionalism. Having completed your studies and activities in this chapter, do you feel more (or less) comfortable working collections? How would you apply professionalism skills to the situation where a patient desperately needs medical care and medication, but cannot afford either? How would you deal with an angry patient when you need to discuss finances? Can you think of ways to avoid difficult situations with patients and billing and collections? Consider also how the practice is affected by your ability to collect fees due.

If you have had the opportunity to role-play with your fellow students or a family member various collection scenarios, did that help with preparedness, conveying empathy, and noting the tone and inflection in your voice? Share your experiences with your instructor and classmates.

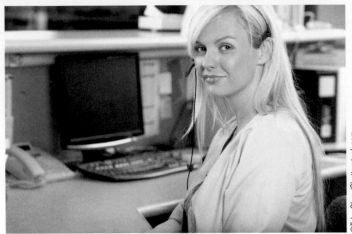

©Tyler Olson/Shutterstock.com

SUMMARY

The *ClaimsManager* application in Harris CareTracker PM and EMR is a feature that electronically screens a claim. A claim cannot be generated and sent to payers until charges for patient visits are saved in Harris Care-Tracker, which can be done in the *Charge* application of the *Transactions* module. *ClaimsManager* screens claims instantly, checking the CPT®, ICD, and HCPCS codes and modifiers. *EncoderPro* provides an online verification of codes. If *ClaimsManager* identifies an error or problem that would prevent the claim from being paid, it will display on the *Claims Worklist* to be resolved. Resolving any claim issue is a critical element of the billing and collection process. Although the *ClaimsManager* does not function in your student environment, it is important that you understand how it works.

Collections are the final step of the Harris CareTracker PM administrative and billing tasks. *Billing* and *Collections* are vital to the financial health of a medical practice. Harris CareTracker PM streamlines the billing and collection processes by providing global templates, the ability to create custom letters, and automatically generate statements. Patient information is pulled in to the collection letter template, eliminating the need to create and enter individual information and letters, improving accuracy and efficiency.

As with the entire text, the information learned and activities completed in this chapter will prepare you to successfully pass an EHR certification exam, a valued quality desired by medical practices. The comprehensive case studies in Chapter 11: Applied Learning Activities will provide you with more valuable "hands-on" experience with Harris CareTracker PM and EMR, allowing you to master the use of an integrated Practice Management and Electronic Medical Records program.

CHECK YOUR KNOWLEDGE

Select the best response.

_____ 1. The *Charge* application is where you enter the appropriate CPT® and ICD codes. What is the limit of CPT® codes? ICD codes? Modifiers?

    a. CPT® codes—4; ICD codes—4; Modifiers—4

    b. CPT® codes—no limit; ICD codes—4; Modifiers—4

    c. CPT® codes—4; ICD codes—no limit; Modifiers—4

    d. CPT® codes—no limit; ICD codes—no limit; Modifiers—4

_____ 2. Harris CareTracker PM automatically splits out the private payment amount owed, such as the patient's copayment, for each procedure entered for the patient that requires a copayment. This only occurs if the amount of the patient's copayment is entered where?

    a. In the *Billing* tab

    b. In the *ClaimsManager* field

    c. In the *Copay* field of the *Insurances* section in the *Demographics* application

    d. In the *Transactions* module

_____ 3. In which claims list category would you find claims that are transferred from a patient's primary insurance to the supplemental insurance and are not paid within 30 days?

    a. PENDING, In Review

    b. CLAIM ERRORS, Payer Edits

    c. OTHER, Set to Deny

    d. OTHER, Crossover

_____ 4. When the billing provider, dates of service, procedure codes, fee, units, servicing provider, or insurance need to be changed, the charge must be reversed from Harris CareTracker PM and EMR via the _____ application in the _____ module. The charge will then need to be put back into the system.

    a. *Edit; Transactions*

    b. *Edit; Patient*

    c. *Financial; Batch*

    d. *Batch; Edit*

_____ 5. A patient is automatically removed from *Collections* when the patient's private pay or collection balances are _____, regardless of his or her collection status.

    a. transferred

    b. paid in full

    c. adjusted off

    d. Both b and c

_____ 6. Of the four collection actions in Harris CareTracker PM, which is used when a patient's *Private Pay* balance needs to be assigned to a different insurance plan/financial class?

    a. Transfer

    b. Remove from *Collections*

    c. Group collections letter

    d. Global collections letter

_____ 7. Which *Global Collection* letter would be sent when an account balance is more than 60 days past due?

    a. Collection 1

    b. Past due

    c. Delinquent

    d. Final notice

_____ 8. After collection letters have been generated, they must be printed from the _____ application in the _____ module.

    a. *Batch Letters; Transactions*

    b. *Print; Patient*

    c. *Print; Transactions*

    d. *Print Batch Letter; Administration*

_____ 9. When a patient has reached the set overdue period for your company, the patient is automatically identified by the *Collections System* and assigned the status of:

      a. Collections actual   c. Collections pending

      b. New   d. Review

_____ 10. Patients manually added to *Collections* are flagged with [a(n)] _____ next to their name in the work area.

      a. asterisk (*)   c. exclamation point (!)

      b. plus sign [+] vs. (+)   d. brackets ([ ])

CASE STUDIES

Complete all case studies for the following patients

    a. Jane Morgan

    b. Adam Thompson (if you've completed Case Study 7-3 and 9-2)

    c. Ellen Ristino

    d. Barbara Watson

Case Study 10-1

Generate statements for all patients (a–d above). (Refer to Activity 10-5 for guidance.)

(**Note**: If statements are not displaying after you complete the steps or you receive an error message, click back on the *Administration* module, *Generate Statements* link, and repeat the steps.)

Print the Generated Statements, label them Case Study 10-1a through 10-1d, and place them in your assignment folder.

Case Study 10-2

Transfer any remaining balance to *Open Collections* for Jane Morgan, Adam Thompson, Ellen Ristino, and Barbara Watson. See Activity 10-7 for guidance. Note that you will need to click *Add Responsible Party* and add each of these four patients in order for them to appear in the *Add Manual Collection* window.

Once all balances have been transferred, print the screen showing all Transferred Balances, label it "Case Study 10-2" and place them in your assignment folder. Hint: If "**Show** only Resp Party for Pt in Context" is not checked, then you can take one screenshot that shows all of the patients.

Case Study 10-3

Generate collection letters (Past Due 60 1st) for all patients (a–d above). See Activity 10-10 for guidance. Once all patients (a–d above) have had the collections letter generated, click on the *Correspondence* icon after *Status* "Open Collections" of each patient. The *Patient Correspondence* dialog box displays. Print the *Correspondence Log* for each patient.

Print the Edit screens showing the Collection Letters generated for each patient, label them Case Study 10-3a through 10-3d, and place them in your assignment folder.

BUILD YOUR PROFICIENCY

Proficiency Builder 10-1: Remove a Balance from Collections:

There are times you will want to remove a balance from collections. For example, a patient has reached a payment agreement for the account balance. In order to understand the workflow for this task, for each of the following patients, remove a balance from *Collections* with the instructions noted below. (**Note**: You must have completed the Chapter 10 Case Studies to be able to perform this activity.)

    a. Edith Robinson

    b. Jane Morgan

    c. Adam Thompson

    d. Ellen Ristino

    e. Barbara Watson

1. Go to the *Home* module > *Dashboard* tab > *Billing* section > *Collections* link. Harris CareTracker PM displays a list of collection statuses and the number of patients in each status.

2. To remove an individual balance:

   Click the *Delete* icon next to the statement line you want to delete. Select the *Delete* icon for patient Edith Robinson (noted as "a" above). Harris CareTracker PM displays a confirmation dialog box. Click *OK*. Harris CareTracker PM removes the balance from the *Collections* application.

3. To remove multiple balances:

   a. Now select the checkbox next to each statement line you want to remove from *Collections* (refer to **Figure 10-65**). (Select the checkbox for patients Jane Morgan, Adam Thompson, Ellen Ristino, and Barbara Watson.)

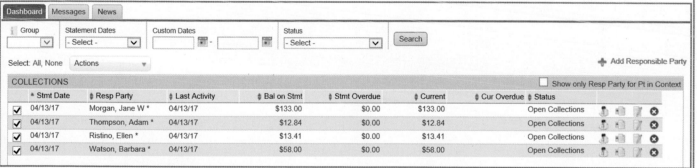

Figure 10-65   Remove From Collections   Courtesy of Harris CareTracker PM and EMR

   b. Click the *Actions* drop-down and select *Remove from Collections* at the top of the page. The application displays a confirmation dialog box.

   c. Click *OK*. Harris CareTracker PM removes the balance from the *Collections* application.

   🖫 **Print the screens showing the account has been removed from collections, label them "BYP 10-1a–e" and place them in your assignment folder.**

(continues)

BUILD YOUR PROFICIENCY *(continued)*

Proficiency Builder 10-2: Access Help and Review/Refresh Various Training Materials and Snipits

Having completed your chapter studies and prior to moving on to the Applied Learning Case Studies in Chapter 11, now is a good time to review any activities in *Help* that you might feel the need for a refresher or further clarification. To access the additional training materials, log in to Harris CareTracker, click on the *Help* icon, then click on the *Training* tab. In the *Training* tab, click on *Recorded Training* (or *Learn More* under *Recorded Training*) to display the training materi-. als. Choose from the wide variety of topics under the headers *Practice Management* or *EMR & Meaningful Use.* The sub-headings offer everything from *Patient* training, *Scheduling* training, *Front Office* training, *Reporting* training, *Billing & Claims* training, *Administrative* training, *EMR* training, and more. Recall that the training titles with (S) denote a recorded *Snipit*. Utilize these training materials to build your proficiency in Harris CareTracker PM and EMR.

🖫 **Print the screens showing the topics in Help you reviewed and write a summary of ways it improved your understanding and proficiency. Label them "BYP 10-2" and place them in your assignment folder.**

MODULE 5
Apply Your Skills

This module includes:

- Chapter 11: Applied Learning for the Paperless Medical Office

This chapter is the finale of the text and should be completed only after you have completed all of the other modules (Get Started, Administrative Skills, Clinical Skills, and Billing Skills).

This chapter follows a typical patient workflow in a medical clinic. You will apply the skills learned throughout this textbook by completing several case studies that test your comprehension of the material presented throughout the text without providing step-by-step instructions. You will build both competence and confidence from performing activities in this chapter.

Be sure you are working in a supported browser (Internet Explorer 11 or Safari for iPad) before you begin. Other browsers (such as Chrome and Firefox) are not supported. Review Best Practices.

Applied Learning for the Paperless Medical Office

Learning Objective

1. Perform EMR tasks related to registering and scheduling a patient, completing the visit, billing the appointment, and collecting payment

INTRODUCTION

This module is designed to apply the skills you have learned to several patient case studies without the step-by-step instruction given in the previous chapters. Completing these case studies will help you increase your proficiency in a real-world electronic health record.

If you need help completing these case studies, a guide has been posted to the student companion website. This guide references activities within the book that you can review for easy navigation.

> Before you begin the activities in this chapter, refresh your memory on working with Harris CareTracker by referring back to the Best Practices list on page xxiii of this textbook. This list is also posted to the student companion website. Following best practices will help you complete work quickly and accurately.

CASE STUDY 11-1: JULIA HERNANDEZ

Julia Hernandez calls the office this morning to schedule a new patient visit and would like to select Dr. Rebecca Ayerick as her primary care provider. (**Note:** Use the first date available that corresponds with Napa Valley Family Health Associates open office hours for Dr. Rebecca Ayerick.)

Step 1: Register a New Patient and Schedule an Appointment

Schedule a new patient CPE appointment for Julia Hernandez with Dr. Ayerick on the first available date. You will need to create a mini-registration to add the patient to the database before scheduling the appointment for her.

1. First search your database to see if Julia had ever been registered as a patient with the practice, using two patient identifiers: last name and date of birth. Upon confirming she is not already registered, create a new patient registration for Julia, starting with the following information (you will complete the full registration process when she arrives for her first appointment):

   - *Name:* Julia Hernandez
   - *Address:* 5224 Sunset Landing, Vacaville, CA 95688

- *Home Phone:* (707) 468-4457

- *Date of Birth:* 06/24/1992

- *Social Security Number:* 999-99-2137

- *Sex:* Female

2. Schedule an appointment for Julia with Dr. Ayerick, using the first available morning appointment slot. (**Note:** If you are entering data on a weekend, or a day when there is no availability in the schedule, select an appointment day on the first prior date available. This will ensure that you can complete activities by not working in a "future date." This applies to all of the case studies in Chapter 11.)

- *Appointment Type:* New Patient CPE

- *Chief Complaint:* New Patient

- *Location:* NVFA

While still on the phone with Julia, refer her to the Napa Valley Family Health Associates website to download the patient registration forms to complete and bring to her first appointment, along with photo ID and her insurance card(s). Advise Julia to arrive 15 minutes before her scheduled appointment to complete the registration process.

Step 2: Enter Payment, Check In Patient, and Complete Patient Registration

When you arrive at the office on the day of Julia's appointment, log in to Harris CareTracker and create a new batch titled "HernandezCS." When Julia arrives for her appointment, review her patient registration forms for completeness. You see from her insurance card that she has a $25.00 copay.

1. Accept and enter Julia's cash payment for her copay and print a receipt for her.

2. Check Julia in for her visit with Dr. Ayerick.

3. While Julia is waiting to see Dr. Ayerick, record her complete patient registration information (refer to Source Document 11-1 at the end of this case study).

📠 **Print the patient receipt and patient Demographics screen. Label them "Case Study 11-1a and 11-1b."**

Step 3: Patient Work-Up

To begin EMR activities, review your *Batch* to set up operator preference and update your *Login Application* to *Clinical*.

Background Information about Julia Hernandez

Julia Hernandez is a new patient here for a complete physical exam. Her company just started a new health and wellness program, which offers insurance premium discounts to employees who have one physical exam per year, as well as other preventive profiles and procedures. Julia does not have any current health concerns other than acid reflux. She is committed to a healthy lifestyle. Julia currently has an OB-GYN and is deferring a breast or genitourinary exam today.

1. *Transfer* Julia to Exam Room #1.

2. Referring to **Table 11-1**, enter Julia's medical information into her patient record.

Table 11-1   Medical Information for Julia Hernandez

Medication	Ortho Novum 1/35 (SIG: Take 1 tablet daily according to packet instructions.) Use the "begin date" of 5 years prior to today's date.
Allergies	Sulfa 10 (*Reaction*: Hives and Rash; *Start Date*: 06/15/2012; *Alert Status*: Popup Alert)
Immunizations	Skip this section. Julia does not have her immunization record with her and does not remember the dates of her immunizations. She states that her last tetanus shot was well over 10 years ago, so Dr. Ayerick will likely order a tetanus shot today. Julia signed a consent form for her medical records to be sent to Dr. Ayerick, but until her records arrive you will not be able to enter any information into this section.

3. Now enter the patient's medical history. Refer to **Tables 11-2** and **11-3** for Julia's history information. Recall that you will need to go through the *Clinical Today* module in order to enter information into the *History* section.

Table 11-2   Patient History for Julia Hernandez

SECTION	ITEM	ENTRY
General Medical History	*Fracture*	Spiral fracture of left tibia at age 14. Treatment: Leg cast for 10 weeks. No complications.
	GERD	Acid reflux problems at least 3–4 days/week. OTC meds give little relief.
		All other sections are negative.
Hospitalizations		None
Other Medical History		None
Tobacco Assessment	*Smoking Status*	Never smoker
Social History	*Alcohol Use*	Occasional
	Caffeine Use	2 servings per day
	Drug Use	"N"
	Sun Protection (SPF 30)	"Y"
	Tattoos	"Y"
	Sexually Active	"Y"
	Race	Hispanic
	Native Language	Spanish

(continues)

Table 11-2 *(continued)*

SECTION	ITEM	ENTRY
	Physical and Domestic Abuse	"N"
	Educational Level	Technical/vocational school
	Marital Status	Single
	Exercise Habits	strenuous >3×/wk
	Seatbelts	"Y"
	Body Piercings	"Y"
	Birth Control Method	Oral contraceptive
	Religion	Roman Catholic
	Occupation	Server
Depression Screening	*Little interest or pleasure in doing things*	At no time
	Feeling down, depressed, or hopeless	At no time
	Date of last depression screening	Leave blank
OB/GYN History	*LMP*	Enter a date that is 2 weeks ago from today's date
	Frequency of menstrual cycle	28 days
	History of abnormal Pap smears	"N"
	Sexually active	"Y"
	Ectopic pregnancy	"N"
	Birth Control	Oral contraceptive
		Leave remaining boxes in this section blank.
Pregnancy Summary	*Gravida*	0
		Leave all other boxes blank in this section.
Surgical/Procedural		Click on the box that states *No prior surgical history.*
Preventive Care	*Flu Vaccine*	First Monday in November of last year
	Pap Smear	First Monday in May of last year
		Leave all other boxes blank.
Self-Management Goal		1. Increase workout schedule to 7 days/week. 2. Get caught up on all preventive testing and procedures.

Table 11-3   General Family History for Julia Hernandez

DISEASE	COMMENT
Cardiovascular disease	Maternal grandmother died of a heart attack at age 65. (**Note:** In the *Finding Details* box, Grandmother is not an option. Free text the comment in the *Comments* section.)
COPD	Paternal grandfather died from complications of COPD at age 72. (**Note:** In the *Finding Details* box, Grandfather is not an option. Free text the comment in the *Comments* section.)
Hypertension	*Mother:* Controlled with medication
Osteoporosis	*Mother:* Controlled with medication
All other diseases should be marked "N."	

4. Next, take Julia's vital signs and record them in her chart. Refer to **Table 11-4** for Julia's vital sign information.

Table 11-4   Vital Signs for Julia Hernandez

Height	5" 4"	**Blood Pressure**	94/66	**Respiratory Rate**	12
Weight	115	**Pulse Rate**	66 bpm	**Pain Level**	0/10
LMP	14 days ago from today's date	**Temperature**	97.8°F	**Chief Complaint**	New Patient CPE. Patient here for a complete physical.

5. Because Julia is now ready to see Dr. Ayerick, create a *Progress Note* for her. Select a template of "IM OV Option 4 (v4) w/A&P." Refer to **Table 11-5** while completing the progress note.

Table 11-5   Progress Note for Julia Hernandez

TAB	ITEM	ENTRY
CC/HPI		Place a check mark next to *New Patient*.
		Free text in the *Other complaints* box: ICD-10 codes "Z00.00" and "K21.9."
ROS	*Gastrointestinal*	Click "N" on all the selections in this grouping.
	Other gastrointestinal symptoms	Free text: GERD
		Select "No symptoms" in all other sections.

(*continues*)

Table 11-5 *(continued)*

TAB	ITEM	ENTRY
PE		Click on "Y" for *patient deferred full body exam*.
	General	Select "awake," "well developed," and "well nourished."
	Head	Enter "Normocephalic" in the *Other head findings* box
	Eyes	Click "Y" for "PERRL" and "EOMI."
	Other eye findings	Fundi normal, vision grossly intact.
	Other ENT findings	External auditory canals and tympanic membranes clear. No nasal drainage, oral cavity and pharynx normal. No oral lesions or drainage. Teeth and gingiva in very good condition.
	Neck	Click "Y" beside "supple," click "N" beside "tenderness," "thyroid enlargement," and "carotid bruit."
	Lymphatics	Click "No" for "cervical adenopathy" and "tenderness."
	Chest	Click the box next to "Negative chest exam."
	Lungs	Click on "N" for "wheezing," "rhonchi," and "diminished breath sounds."
	Other lung findings box	Clear to auscultation
	Heart	Click on the "Y" beside "S1" and "S2." Click on the "N" beside "S3," "S4," and "irregular heart rhythm."
	Other heart findings box	No bruits, extremities are warm and well perfused, capillary refill is less than 2 seconds.
	Abdomen	Click on "Y" beside "soft"; click on "N" beside "rebound," "mass," "tenderness," "distention," and "muscle guarding."
	Other abdomen findings	Positive bowel sounds
	Musculoskeletal	Click on the "Y" beside "normal movement of all extremities"; click on the "N" beside "muscle tenderness," "joint tenderness," and "edema."
	Back	Negative back exam
	Neurologic	Click on the "Y" beside "cranial nerves II–XII intact"; click on the "N" beside "sensation," "motor," "gait and stance," and "reflexes."
	Other neurologic findings	Strength and sensation symmetric and intact throughout, reflexes good
	Mental Status Exam	Click on the "N" beside "affect," "attitude," and "mood."
	Skin	Click on the "Y" beside "warm," "dry," and "normal turgor."
Assess	*Today's Selected Diagnosis*	Free text in the *Assessment* box: Normal routine history and physical examination (Z00.00); GERD (K21.9)

TAB	ITEM	ENTRY
Plan	*Additional Plan Details*	Free text the following: 1. Basic metabolic panel in Blood; *Helicobacter pylori* Ag [Presence] in Stool by Immunoassay (*Fasting* 12 hours; *Routine*). 2. Rx for PriLOSEC oral capsules, delayed release, 20 mg, Sig 1 cap daily. # 30, 0 refills 3. Tetanus toxoid, adsorbed (VIS form) 4. Provide the patient with patient information sheets for "What is GERD?" and "MEDICATION: PRILOSEC." 5. Set up a referral for the patient to see Dr. David Wong, gastroenterologist in San Ramon. 6. Patient should follow up in one year for her next physical exam.

When you have completed **Step 3: Patient Work-Up**, print the patient's Chart Summary and label it **"Case Study 11-1c."**

Step 4: Review the *Plan* section of the *Progress Note* and complete the tasks noted in the *Plan*

Julia's visit is now over with Dr. Ayerick. It is your responsibility to complete orders as indicated in the *Plan* section of the progress note.

1. Enter the new lab order (selecting the first *Facility* in the drop-down list). (*Fasting* 12 hours; *Routine*).
   Hint: Be sure that each test is added and displays in the *Tests Summary* portion of the *Order*. You may need to click on *Add Test* more than once for the text to display in the *Tests Summary*. Enter the ICD-10 code that supports the lab order (K21.9).

Print the lab order and label it **"Case Study 11-1d."**

2. Create and reprint the new prescription related to the diagnosis for GERD (K21.9). (Use *Reprint Reason* "Pharmacy Did Not Receive E-Rx.")
   Label the prescription "Case Study 11-1e."

3. Add a new immunization: "tetanus toxoid, adsorbed." Refer to **Table 11-6** for additional immunization information.

Table 11-6   Immunization for Julia Hernandez

Manufacturer	Abbott Laboratories	**Dose Route**	IM
Lot Number	25698GBC	**Amount**	0.5 mL
Expiration Date	November 1 of next year	**Series**	1
Administration Date	Date of Julia Hernandez's appointment	**Site**	Left Deltoid
Administration Time	30 minutes following the start of the appointment	**VIS Date**	First Monday in October of Last year
Administered By	You	**Date VIS Given to Patient**	Date of appointment
Ordering Provider	Dr. Ayerick	**Adverse Reaction**	Patient tolerated well

4. Provide Julia with a copy of the *Patient Information* sheets ordered in the *Plan* section of the progress note.

💾 **Print the Patient Information sheets and label them "Case Study 11-1f-1 and 11-1f-2."**

5. Create an outgoing referral to the gastroenterologist noted in the *Plan* section of the progress note: Dr. David Wong in San Ramon.

💾 **Print the outgoing referral and label it "Case Study 11-1g."**

Step 5: Capture the Visit and Sign the Note

Having completed all the orders as indicated in the progress note, now capture the *Visit* and sign the progress note.

1. Capture the *Visit* by entering:

   a. *CPT® code(s):* 99203; 90471; and 90714.

   Source: Current Procedural Terminology © 2017 American Medical Association.

   b. *ICD-10 code(s):* Z00.00 and K21.9

2. Sign the progress note.

💾 **Print the signed progress note and label it "Case Study 11-1h."**

3. Before Julia leaves the office, add a *Recall* for her annual physical, scheduled one year from the date of this visit. Her recall appointment will be for an "Established Patient CPE."

Step 6: Other Clinical Documentation

(**Hint:** The detailed step instructions for this activity are in Proficiency Builder 8-1. Refer to Proficiency Builder 8-1 for guidance. If you have not completed Proficiency Builders while working through this text, skip this step.) The *Results* of Julia's lab order have been received.

1. Manually enter the lab order results for the "Basic metabolic panel in Blood" only. The results for the "*Helicobacter pylori* Ag [Presence] in Stool by Immunoassay" has not yet been received. Refer to **Table 11-7** to enter results. All results received on the lab report to date are normal and final. However, when saving the entries, do not mark as final at this point because additional results are due.

Prior to beginning this activity, make a note of the encounter date and collected time (if recorded) for which the lab order was created. You will need this information when you enter results manually. If the collected time is not recorded on the *Order*, refer back to the *Scheduling* module and *History* tab to identify the date and time of the patient's appointment. Date/Time: _____

 TIP Follow these general instructions when completing this lab order:

   a. In the *Value* field, enter the number listed in the Value column in Table 11-7.

   b. In the *Units* field, enter the units as shown in the Normal Range column in Table 11-7 (mg/dL).

   c. In the *Abnormal* field, indicate whether the results were "Normal" or "Abnormal." Compare the value listed in Table 11-7 to the normal range listed in Table 11-7 to determine if the result is normal or abnormal.

   d. In the *Reference Range* field, enter the range given in the Normal Range column of Table 11-7.

   e. In the *Status* list, select "Incomplete."

This activity requires in-depth review and careful data entry. Use the following table to make your entries:

Table 11-7   Results for Julia Hernandez Lab Order

TEST NAME	VALUE	NORMAL RANGE
Glucose	86	74–100 mg/dL
Creatinine	0.7	0.1–1.2 mg/dL
Calcium	9.2	8.7–9.7 mg/dL
Urea Nitrogen	16	6–22 mg/dL

Click on the *Print* icon in the upper-right-hand corner of the dialog box to print a copy of the lab results, label it "Case Study 11-1i," and place in your assignments folder.

2. Enter a *ToDo* to call the patient with the lab results.

Step 7: Process Remittance (EOB/RA) and Transfer to Private Pay

1. Save the charges.
2. Build all claims for the visit.
3. Refer to Julia's EOB/RA (Source Document 11-2 at the end of this case study) and process the remittance.
4. Run a journal to verify charges.

💾 **Print the journal and label it "Case Study 11-1j."**

Step 8: Work Claims and Generate Patient Statement

1. Work the *Claims Worklist*.
2. Post all open batches.
3. Generate a statement for Julia.

💾 **Print the statement and label it "Case Study 11-1k."**

Source Document 11-1

Patient Registration Form   NVFHA

Patient's Last Name	First (legal name)	First (Preferred name)	Middle Name
HERNANDEZ	JULIA		

Address (Number, Street, Apt #)	City	State	Zip Code
5224 Sunset Landing	Vacaville	CA	95688 - 5688

Mail will be sent to the address listed above, unless patient indicates a different address (leave blank if same as above)

Send mail to Address (Number, Street, Apt #)	City	State	Zip Code

Phone Options	Phone Number	Okay to leave detailed message	Call this number (circle one)
Home	(707) 468 - 4457	Yes _X_ No _____	(1st) 2nd 3rd choice
Cell	( ) -	Yes ____ No _____	1st 2nd 3rd choice
Work	(877) 883 - 7777	Yes ____ No __X__	1st (2nd) 3rd choice

Would you like to communicate by Email	Yes _X_ No __	Email Address	Jhernandez@email.com

Date of Birth	Sex	Social Security Number
06/24/1992	Female _X_ Male ___	000-00-2137

Marital Status (*circle one*)	What is your preferred language / secondary language
(Single) / Married / Divorced / Widow / Partner	Spanish/English

Race (*circle one*)

African American-Black / Asian / Bi-Multi-racial / Pacific Islander-Hawaiian / Caucasian–White / Native American Eskimo Aleut / Decline to state / Other

Ethnicity (*circle one*)

(Hispanic-Latino) / Non-Hispanic-Latino / Other

Religion	Roman Catholic	Organ Donor	Yes ____X____ No _____

Are you new to our practice	Who referred you to our practice	Who is your Primary Care Physician
Yes __X__ No _____	Rebecca Ayerick	Rebecca Ayerick

Additional Notes

Emergency Contact

Emergency Contact's Name	Relationship to patient	Phone
Cynthia Hernandez	SISTER	(707) 555 - 0454

On-Line Patient Portal Communication via Email

On-Line communication is used for non-urgent message/requests only. NVFHA uses secure technology to protect the privacy and confidentiality of your personal information. Only you, your physician, and authorized staff can read your message.

What is your preferred method of communication	Phone _X_ Letter _____ Patient Portal _____ Email _____

Insurance Information

Subscriber (Insurance Holder) Name	Date of Birth	Relationship to patient	Subscriber Phone Number
Self	/ /		( )

Health Plan Information	Primary Health Plan	Secondary Health Plan
Health Plan Name	Blue Shield Cengage	
Health Plan Address	PO Box 32245, Los Angeles, CA, 90002	
Group Number	BCBS 987	
Subscriber Number	BCBS 987	

Elig Date From	2/21/2011	Copay	$ 25.00

Patient Employer Information

Employer Name & Address (Number, Street, Apt #, City, State, Zip Code)	Employer Phone Number
River Rock Casino, 3250 Highway 128, Geyserville, CA, 95441	(877) 883 - 7777

Occupation	Server	Start Date	2/21/2011

Assignment of Benefits • Financial Agreement

I hereby give lifetime authorization for payment of insurance benefits to be made directly to **Napa Valley Family Health Assoc.,** and any assisting physicians, for services rendered. I understand that I am financially responsible for all charges whether or not they are covered by insurance. In the event of default, I agree to pay all costs of collection, and reasonable attorney's fees. I hereby authorize this healthcare provider to release all information necessary to secure the the payment of benefits.

I further agree that a photocopy of this agreement shall be as valid as the original.

Date: __XX/XX/20XX__   Your Signature: _Julia hernandez_

Method of Payment: ❑ Cash   ❑ Check   ❑ Credit Card

Source Document 11-2: Explanation of Benefits/Remittance Advice

BLUE SHIELD CENGAGE

Blue Shield Cengage
P.O. Box 32245
Los Angeles, CA 90002

Date: MM/DD/YYYY (use today's date)
Payment Number: 556774
Payment Amount: $176.80

REBECCA AYERICK, M.D.
Napa Valley Family Health Associates (NVFHA)
101 Vine Street
Napa, CA 94558

| Account Number | Patient Name | | | | | | | | |
Dates of Service	Description of Service	Amount Charged	Not Covered (DENIAL)	Prov Adj Discount	Amount Allowed	Deduct/ Coins/ Copay	Paid to Provider	Adj Reason Code	Rmk Code	Patient Resp
					Subscriber Number		Claim Number			
42507342	Hernandez, Julia									
(Appt. date used in Case Study 11-1)	99203	$191.00			$191.00	$38.20	$152.80			$38.20
(Appt. date used in Case Study 11-1)	90714	$15.00			$15.00	$3.00	$12.00			$3.00
(Appt. date used in Case Study 11-1)	90471	$15.00			$15.00	$3.00	$12.00			$3.00

CASE STUDY 11-2: DELORES SIMPSON

Delores Simpson is an established patient of the practice who calls the office this morning to schedule an appointment with Dr. Raman, her primary care provider. She tells you she has not been feeling well and complains of chest discomfort. She has taken her blood pressure at home several times this morning and says it is normal. Just to be on the safe side, you encourage the patient to call the EMS so that she can be evaluated. The patient refuses to call and insists on coming into the office. Due to her age and the severity of her complaint, you message Dr. Raman and he replies to have her come in to the office this morning. If there are no appointments open, double-book the first available appointment for her to be seen. Delores has not been in to see Dr. Raman since the office converted to electronic records, but she is registered in the database.

Step 1: Search the Database and Schedule an Appointment

1. Search the database for patient Delores Simpson. Update her demographics to include Dr. Raman as her PCP, update her insurance *Subscriber Number* to that of her *Group #*, and change her *Consent* and *NPP* to "Yes."

2. Schedule an appointment for Delores with Dr. Raman, using the first available morning slot, or by double-booking the 11:00 a.m. slot. (**Note**: If you are entering data on a weekend, or a day when there is no availability in the schedule, select an appointment day on the first prior date available. This will ensure that you can complete activities by not working in a "future date." This applies to all of the case studies in Chapter 11.)

    *   *Appointment Type:* Follow Up
    *   *Complaint:* Chest pain (resolved, normal BP readings)
    *   *Location:* NVFA

Step 2: Check In Patient

1. When Delores arrives for her appointment, view her *At-A-Glance* patient information to confirm that she is still insured with Medicare and has no copay.

2. Check Delores in for her visit with Dr. Raman.

Step 3: Patient Work-Up

To begin EMR activities, create a new *Batch* titled "SimpsonCS," and edit your operator preferences for clinical workflows with Dr. Raman as the provider.

When you have completed Step 3: Patient Work-Up, print the patient's Chart Summary and label it "Case Study 11-2a."

Background Information about Delores Simpson

Delores is a kind, older patient who rarely complains. This morning she has been experiencing some chest discomfort. Upon her arrival, you immediately escort Delores to the cardiac bay. This room has equipment that can be used during a cardiac event. Normally, you would update the patient's medical history information, but the provider tells you just to get the patient's medication and allergy information to expedite the process.

1. *Transfer* Delores to the cardiac bay. (**Hint**: You would have added the Cardiac Bay as a Room in Activity 5-7. If it is not displaying, add the room first.)

2. Referring to **Table 11-8**, enter Delores's medical information into her patient record.

Table 11-8 Medical Information for Delores Simpson	
Medications	Levothyroxine Sodium Oral Tablet, 100 mcg tab, 1 per day Lisinopril, 20 mg tab, 1 per day
Allergies	Codeine (*Reaction*: Hives and Rash; *Start Date*: 02/15/1999; *Alert Status*: Popup Alert)

3. Take Delores's vital signs and record them in her patient chart. Refer to **Table 11-9** for Delores's vital sign information.

Table 11-9 Vital Signs for Delores Simpson	
Height	5" 2"
Weight	143
Blood Pressure	122/68
Pulse Rate	68 bpm
Temperature	97.4°F
Respiratory Rate	14
Pulse Oximetry	96%
Pain Level	0/10

4. Because Delores is now ready to see Dr. Raman, create a *Progress Note* for her. Select progress note template "Cardio Option 3 (v4)." Refer to **Table 11-10** while completing the progress note. (**Note**: You will be acting as a scribe for the provider in this Case Study, meaning you will free text much of the medical record information in the *Progress Note*.)

Table 11-10   Progress Note for Delores Simpson

TAB	ITEM	ENTRY
CC/HPI	*Reason for Visit*	Click on the *REASON FOR VISIT* tab and check "Chest pain." In the *Other* box free text: "Chest pain (resolved)."
	HPI	Free text in the *HPI* box: Patient complains of early morning chest pain that lasted approximately 15 minutes and then subsided. No current chest pain. Patient described the pain as midsternal "tight, squeezing pressure radiating slightly to the left side of sternum." Pain rating at its worst around a "6." Patient denies any radiation of pain to other parts of the body, shortness of breath, or diaphoresis. There was no change in pain intensity upon movement. Patient took her blood pressure at least three times during the event but stated that each time her blood pressure was normal ("Around 110/68"). Patient denies any gastrointestinal or neurologic symptoms. Patient states that she has been under a great deal of stress lately because her daughter just moved to Boston. She feels that the pain may be related to stress. Patient does not recall any history of chest pain prior to this morning's event.
ROS		Select "N" for all categories in the *Cardiovascular ROS* sections, except select "Y" for chest pain. In the "other cardiovascular symptoms" box enter "Chest pain this morning, resolved."
		Do not mark any of the boxes in the *Review of Systems* section.
	Other Review of Systems box	Free-text the following entries: Denies fatigue, fever, weight changes, or pain (other than the chest discomfort she experienced this morning).
		HEENT: Denies headache, dizziness, or voice changes.
		CHEST: As stated in the HPI, patient denies any current chest pain or shortness of breath.
		CV: Refer to HPI.
		GI: Patient denies any nausea or vomiting, abdominal pain, or reflux. Has had some constipation lately but nothing out of the "ordinary."
		GU: Denies any frequency, dysuria, or changes in voiding habits.
		MUSC: Denies any muscular or joint pain or any joint swelling.
		NEURO: Denies vertigo, headache, ataxia, or syncope.
		PV: No changes in temperature or any swelling in extremities.
		PSYCH: As stated in the HPI, patient feels anxious over daughter moving to Boston. Feels like she will never see her daughter now that she is so far away.
PE		Select "N" for all applicable categories in the *Cardio PE* section. Click in the box beside *regular rate and rhythm*.
		Do not click on any of the responses in the *Physical Examination* box.
	Other Physical Findings box	Free-text the following: *General*: Patient appears alert and well.

TAB	ITEM	ENTRY
		HEENT: Head, normocephalic, no pharyngeal exudate or erythema, uvula midline.
		NECK: Supple, no palpable masses or nodules, thyroid normal in size, trachea midline.
		CHEST: Thorax without distortion. Respiration regular and unlabored, no cough. Lung fields normal. Negative rales or rhonchi. Breath sounds clear.
		HEART (CARDIOVASCULAR): EKG findings—12 lead with NSR without ST elevation or depression.
		ABDOMEN: Round and soft. No tenderness, rash, or palpable mass. Nail beds pink with less than 2-second capillary refill. Pedal pulse 2 + l.
		NEURO: Patient alert and oriented. No speech problems. Patient able to move all extremities and appears coherent. Other than being a little anxious regarding daughter's move, patient appears in good overall spirits.
EKG TESTS		Free text: EKG findings—12 lead with NSR without ST elevation or depression.
A&P	*Today's Selected Diagnosis*	Using the drop-down, scroll down and select "Chest pain, unspecified type (R07.9)"; search for and select "Anxiety (F41.9)." **Note**: You would need to click *Save* before the updates to all the fields display, including diagnosis updates.
	Assessment	In the *OTHER DIAGNOSES/CONDITIONS* of the A&P box, free-text the following: "R/O angina pectoris and MI. Chest discomfort may be related to the stress of her daughter's move."
	Other Plan Items box	1. 12-Lead EKG 2. Patient information sheet "Your Body's Response to Anxiety" 3. F/U in one week with Dr. Raman 4. Give patient a prescription for Xanax Oral Tablet MG (CIV) PRN (as needed), not to exceed 1 tablet in 24 hours, # 10, 0 refills; refill/reprint prescription for levothyroxine tabs, 100 mcg, Sig 1 tab daily, #30, 3 refills. 5. Order *Stat* lab test "Troponin I. cardiac [Mass/volume] in Serum or Plasma by Detection limit—0.01 ng/mL" for patient to have drawn at the lab tomorrow morning.

Step 4: Review the *Plan* section of the *Progress Note* and complete the tasks noted in the *Plan*

Delores's visit is now over with Dr. Raman. It is your responsibility to complete orders as indicated in the *A&P* section of the progress note.

1. Create and print the new prescription for Xanax.

Label the printed prescription "Case Study 11-2b."

2. In the *Procedures* tab within the progress note, type the following: "Performed 12-Lead EKG per Dr. Raman."

3. Provide Delores with a copy of the Patient Information sheet(s) ordered in the *Plan* section of the progress note.

Print the Patient Information sheet and label it "Case Study 11-2c."

Step 5: Capture the Visit and Sign the Note

Having completed all of the orders as indicated in the *Progress Note*, now capture the *Visit* and sign the progress note.

1. Capture the *Visit* by entering:

    a. *CPT® code(s):* 99213 and 93000

    Source: Current Procedural Terminology © 2017 American Medical Association.

    b. *ICD-10 code(s):* R07.9 and F41.9

2. Sign the progress note.

💾 **Print the signed progress note and label it "Case Study 11-2d."**

3. Before Delores leaves schedule her follow-up appointment noted in the *Plan* section of the progress note.

Step 6: Process Remittance (EOB/RA) and Transfer to Private Pay

1. Save the charges for the visit for Ms. Simpson. (**Hint**: Check your batch and make sure you are working in the batch "SimpsonCS." If not, edit the batch and using the drop-downs select the parameters as set in the original batch.)

2. Build all claims for Delores's visit.

3. Refer to Delores's EOB/RA (Source Document 11-3 at the end of this case study) and process the remittance.

4. Run a journal to verify charges.

💾 **Print the journal and label it "Case Study 11-2f."**

Step 7: Work Claims and Generate Patient Statement

1. Work the *Claims Worklist*.

2. Post all open batches.

3. Generate a statement for Delores.

💾 **Print the statement and label it "Case Study 11-2g."**

Source Document 11-3:   Explanation of Benefits/Remittance Advice

MEDICARE CENGAGE

Medicare Cengage
P.O. Box 234434
San Francisco, CA 94137

AMIR RAMAN, D.O.
Napa Valley Family Health Associates (NVFHA)
101 Vine Street
Napa, CA 94558

Date: MM/DD/YYYY (use today's date)
Payment Number: 1280977
Payment Amount: $126.80

Account Number	Patient Name				Subscriber Number		Claim Number			
Dates of Service	Description of Service	Amount Charged	Not Covered (DENIAL)	Prov Adj Discount	Amount Allowed	Deduct/ Coins/ Copay	Paid to Provider	Adj Reason Code	Rmk Code	Patient Resp
42399647	**Simpson, Delores**									
(Appt. date used in Case Study 11-2)	99213	$112.00			$112.00	$22.40	$89.60			$21.64

Account Number	Patient Name				Subscriber Number		Claim Number			
Dates of Service	Description of Service	Amount Charged	Not Covered (DENIAL)	Prov Adj Discount	Amount Allowed	Deduct/ Coins/ Copay	Paid to Provider	Adj Reason Code	Rmk Code	Patient Resp
CARE1357	**Simpson, Delores**									
(Appt. date used in Case Study 11-2)	93000	$45.50			$46.50	$9.30	$37.20			$9.30

CASE STUDY 11-3: ADAM ZOTTO

Adam Zotto is an established patient who calls the office this morning to schedule an appointment with Dr. Ayerick, his primary care provider. He says he wants to see Dr. Ayerick regarding his diabetes management. Adam has not been in to see Dr. Ayerick since the office converted to electronic records, but he is registered in the database. Search the database confirming his DOB, current address, phone number, and insurance, and then schedule the appointment for him.

Step 1: Search the Database and Schedule an Appointment

1. Search the database for patient Adam Zotto. Update his demographics to include Dr. Ayerick as his PCP; update his *Subscriber Number* to be the same as his *Group #*, and change his *Consent* and *NPP* to "Yes."

2. Schedule an appointment for Adam with Dr. Ayerick, using the first available appointment today. (**Note**: If you are entering data on a weekend, or a day when there is no availability in the schedule, select an appointment day on the first prior date available. This will ensure that you can complete activities by not working in a "future date." This applies to all of the case studies in Chapter 11.)

   - *Appointment Type:* Follow Up
   - *Complaint:* Follow-up; Diabetes management
   - *Location:* NVFA

Step 2: Enter Payment and Check In Patient

When Adam arrives for his appointment, view his *At-A-Glance* patient information and confirm that he is still insured with Senior Gap and has a $10.00 copay. Before accepting Adam's payment, create a new batch titled "ZottoCS."

1. Accept and enter Adam's cash payment for his copay and print a receipt for him.

   💾 **Label the printed receipt "Case Study 11-3a."**

2. Check Adam in for his visit with Dr. Ayerick.

Step 3: Patient Work-Up

To begin EMR activities, edit your *Batch* operator preferences for clinical workflows with Dr. Ayerick as the provider.

Background Information about Adam Zotto

Adam was diagnosed with type 2 diabetes mellitus approximately 20 years ago—around the same time he was diagnosed with hypertension. He has been very compliant over the years and remains on an oral hypoglycemic. He is here for a routine follow-up appointment exam. He recently discovered at a church health fair that his cholesterol is elevated and wants to discuss the findings with the doctor.

1. *Transfer* Adam to Exam Room #1.

2. Referring to **Table 11-11**, enter Adam's medical information into his patient record.

Table 11-11   Medical Information for Adam Zotto

Medications	MetFORMIN HCl Oral Tablet 1000 mg tablet by mouth twice a day. In the *Interaction Screening* dialog box, select the *Override Reason* "Benefit outweighs risk."
	Metoprolol Succinate Oral Tablet Extended Release: one 50 mg tablet by mouth daily. In the *Interaction Screening* dialog box, select the *Override Reason* "Benefit outweighs risk."
	Aspirin Oral Tablet Chewable 81 MG: Chew and swallow 1 tablet by mouth daily. In the *Interaction Screening* dialog box, select the *Override Reason* "Benefit outweighs risk."
	Lipitor: one 40 mg tablet by mouth at night. In the *Interaction Screening* dialog box, select the *Override Reason* "Benefit outweighs risk."
Allergies	None
Immunizations	Tetanus Toxoid Adsorbed; use the date of the first Monday in July of last year
	Influenza, seasonal injectable; use the date of the first Monday in October two years ago (**Note:** Enter the date of the injection in the VIS field. Continue with instructions of entering Immunization history as noted above.)

3. Now enter the patient's medical history. Refer to **Tables 11-12** and **11-13** for Adam's history information.

Table 11-12   Patient History for Adam Zotto

SECTION	ITEM	ENTRY
General Medical History	*DM Type 2*	Diagnosed in June of 2000. Controlled with diet and Metformin. Well controlled.
	Gastric Ulcer	April of 2013. Controlled with medication. Last EGD in April of 2015. Ulcer resolved. Medication discontinued.
	Hypertension	Diagnosed in March of 2000. Well controlled with metoprolol.
	Osteoarthritis	Diagnosed in May of 2009. Hands, hips, and knees affected.
		All other sections are negative.
Hospitalizations		Free text the following: Right TKA in August of 2014. No complications. Left TKA in July of 2016. No complications.
Other Medical History		None
Tobacco Assessment	*Smoking Status*	Former smoker
	# Pack Years	20

(continues)

Table 11-12 (*continued*)

SECTION	ITEM	ENTRY
Social History	*Alcohol Use*	Occasional
	Caffeine Use	3 servings per day
	Drug Use	"N"
	Sun Protection (SPF 20)	"Y"
	Tattoos	"Y"
	Sexually Active	"N"
	Race	Caucasian
	Physical Abuse	"N"
	Domestic Violence	"N"
	Educational Level	Grades 9-12
	Marital Status	Single
	Exercise Habits	Moderate >3×/wk
	Seatbelts	"Y"
	Body Piercings	"Y"
	Religion	Christian
	Occupation	Retired
Depression Screening	Select *Patient Refused.*	
	Date of last depression screening	Leave blank.
OB/GYN History		Skip
Pregnancy Summary		Skip
Surgical/Procedural	*Other Surgical History*	Right TKA in August of 2014. No complications. Left TKA in July of 2016. No complications.
Preventive Care	*A1c %*	10/12 of the previous year (6.5%)
	Blood Glucose	02/05 of last year (Fasting Value 110)

SECTION	ITEM	ENTRY
	Colonoscopy	02/12/2015 (Normal findings)
	Dilated Eye Exam	04/15 of last year
	PSA	04/22 of last year (based on old standards)
Preventive Care	*Td*	In comments box: "Check immunization table"
	Zoster Vaccine	09/02/2015
	Leave all other boxes blank.	
Self-Management Goal		1. Get caught up on all preventive testing and procedures. 2. Get a gym membership at the "Y."

Table 11-13   General Family History for Adam Zotto

DISEASE	COMMENT
Cardiovascular Disease	Father died of a heart attack at age 65.
CHF	Mother died at age 69 of congestive heart failure.
Diabetes	Mother, type 2; Age of onset, 42
Hypertension	Both mother and father
Kidney Disease	Mother
Osteoarthritis	Both mother and father
Leave all other sections blank.	

4. Next, take Adam's *Vital Signs* and record them in his chart. Refer to **Table 11-14** for Adam's *Vital Sign* information.

Table 11-14   Vital Signs for Adam Zotto

Height	5" 11"	**Pulse Rate**	78 bpm
Weight	205	**Temperature**	98.4°F
Blood Pressure	130/84	**Respiratory Rate**	16

5. Because Adam is now ready to see Dr. Ayerick, create a *Progress Note* for him. Select a template of "IM OV Option 4 (v4) w/A&P." Refer to **Table 11-15** while completing the progress note.

Table 11-15   Progress Note for Adam Zotto

SECTION	ITEM	ENTRY
CC/HPI	*Chief Complaint*	Established Patient; Follow-Up Visit; Diabetes Mellitus; Hypertension (stage 1 HTN)
ROS	*Constitutional*	No constitutional symptoms
	Eyes	No eye symptoms
	Cardiovascular	"Y" for "cold hands or feet" and "N" for all other symptoms in this category
	Genitourinary	No GU symptoms
	Neurological	"Y" for "tingling" (Both feet mainly when in a sitting position); "N" for all other symptoms in this category.
		Leave other sections blank.
PE	*General*	Select "awake," "alert," and "General appearance normal."
	Head/Other head findings	Normocephalic
	Eyes	"Y" for "PERRL" and "EOMI"
	Heart	"N" for "bradycardia," "tachycardia," "irregular heart rhythm," "murmurs," "rubs," and "gallop"; "Y" for "S1" and "S2" and "N" for "S3" and "S4"
	Genitourinary	Negative genitourinary exam
	Neurologic	"A" for "sensation" in feet with decreased sensation in monofilament testing
	Other neurologic findings	Some lower extremity numbness. Monofilament test shows two regions without sensation bilaterally. Bottoms of feet appear slightly calloused and dry. Skin is intact. Cranial nerves II–XII grossly intact. Cerebellar function intact demonstrated through RAM
	Skin	"Y" for "warm," "dry," and "normal turgor"
	Other skin findings	Feet slightly cooler than the rest of the body
Assess	*Today's Selected Diagnosis*	1. Diabetes mellitus type 2, uncomplicated (E11.9) 2. Diabetic peripheral neuropathy (E11.42) 3. Hypertension (I10)
Plan	*Additional Plan Details*	1. Hemoglobin A1c/Hemoglobin total in Blood by calculation (Routine/Fasting 12 hours) 2. Lipid panel with direct LDL in Serum or Plasma (Routine/Fasting 12 hours) 3. Rx: MetFORMIN HCl Oral Tablet: One 1000 mg tablet twice a day, 60 tabs, 3 refills 4. Rx: Metoprolol Succinate Oral Tablet Extended Release 24 Hour 50 MG: Take one 50 mg tablet daily, 30 tabs, 3 refills 5. Start Lipitor 40 mg one tablet at night for cardiovascular protection based on ACC/AHA 2013 guidelines; 30 tabs, 3 refills 6. Patient information sheet: "What is Peripheral Neuropathy?" **Note:** You may need to set the *Age* to "All" in your search. 7. 3-month follow-up appointment 8. Referral to podiatrist: Dr. Katrina Di Pasqua, DPM in Napa, CA

When you have completed Step 3: Patient Work-Up, print the patient's Chart Summary and label it "Case Study 11-3b."

Step 4: Review the *Plan* Section of the *Progress Note* and Complete the Tasks Noted in the *Plan*

Adam's visit is now over with Dr. Ayerick. It is your responsibility to complete orders as indicated in the *Plan* section of the progress note.

1. Enter the new lab orders.

Print the lab orders and label them "Case Study 11-3c."

2. Create and print the new prescriptions.
Label the printed prescriptions "Case Study 11-3d-1" and "Case Study 11-3d-2."

3. Provide Adam with a copy of the Patient Information sheet(s) ordered in the *Plan* section of the progress note.

Print the Patient Information Sheet and label it "Case Study 11-3e."

4. Create an outgoing referral to Dr. Katrina Di Pasqua, DPM. **Hint:** You must search her full last name, "Di Pasqua" in order to pull in to outgoing referral.

Print the referral and label it "Case Study 11-3f."

Step 5: Capture the Visit and Sign the Note

Having completed all the orders as indicated in the *Progress Note*, now capture the *Visit* and sign the progress note.

1. Capture the *Visit* by entering:

   a. *CPT® code(s):* 99213

Source: Current Procedural Terminology © 2017 American Medical Association.

   b. *ICD-10 code(s):* E11.9, E11.42, and I10

2. Sign the progress note.

Print the signed progress note and label it "Case Study 11-3g."

3. Before Adam leaves the office, add a *Recall* for his CPE one year from today's date.

Step 6: Other Clinical Documentation

The *Results* of Adam's lab order have been received. (**Hint:** The detailed step instructions for this activity are in Proficiency Builder 8-1. Refer to Proficiency Builder 8-1 for guidance. If you have not completed Proficiency Builders while working through this text, skip this step.)

1. Manually enter the lab order results. Refer to **Table 11-16** to enter results. All results are final.

Print a screenshot of the Manual Lab Results and label it "Case Study 11-3h."

2. Enter a *ToDo* to call the patient with the lab results.

Table 11-16 Lab Results for Adam Zotto

TEST NAME	RESULT	NORMAL VALUE
Hemoglobin A1c/Hemoglobin, total in Blood	6.8%	Less than 7%
Lipid Panel with Direct LDL in Serum or Plasma		
Cholesterol in LDL/Cholesterol in HDL [Mass Ratio]	Leave blank	Leave blank
Cholesterol in VLDL [Mass/volume] in Serum or Plasma	Leave blank	Leave blank
Cholesterol in LDL [Mass/volume] in Serum or Plasma	104 mg/dL	Less than 100 mg/dL
Cholesterol in HDL [Mass/volume] in Serum or Plasma	44 mg/dL	Greater than 40 mg/dL
Cholesterol in Serum or Plasma	232 mg/dL	Less than 200 mg/dL
Triglyceride in Serum or Plasma	160 mg/dL	Less than 150 mg/dL
Cholesterol Total/Cholesterol in HDL [Mass Ratio]	Leave blank	Leave blank

Step 7: Process Remittance (EOB/RA) and Transfer to Private Pay

1. Save the charges for the visit. **Hint**: Be sure you are still working in the "ZottoCS" batch.

2. Build all claims for Adam's visit.

3. Refer to Adam's EOB/RA (Source Document 11-4 at the end of this case study) and process the remittance.

4. Run a journal to verify charges.

💾 **Print the journal and label it "Case Study 11-3j."**

Step 8: Work Claims and Generate Patient Statement

1. Work the *Claims Worklist*.

2. Post all open batches.

3. Adam does not have an outstanding balance, so you do not need to generate a patient statement.

Source Document 11-4:   Explanation of Benefits/Remittance Advice

SENIOR GAP - CENGAGE

Senior Gap
P.O. Box 87956
Oakland, CA 94601

Date: MM/DD/YYYY (use today's date)
Payment Number: 4566751
Payment Amount: $102.00

REBECCA AYERICK, M.D.
Napa Valley Family Health Associates (NVFHA)
101 Vine Street
Napa, CA 94558

Account Number	Patient Name				Subscriber Number			Claim Number			
Dates of Service	**Description of Service**	**Amount Charged**	**Not Covered (DENIAL)**	**Prov Adj Discount**	**Amount Allowed**	**Deduct/ Coins/ Copay**	**Paid to Provider**	**Adj Reason Code**	**Rmk Code**	**Patient Resp**
42399658	Zotto, Adam									
(Appt. date used in Case Study 11-3)	99213	$112.00			$112.00	$10.00	$102.00			$10.00

Adj Reason Code (CP*) = patient's copay

CASE STUDY 11-4: BARBARA WATSON

Barbara is an established patient who was last seen in the office for a fever. She calls the office this morning to schedule a visit with Dr. Raman, her primary care provider. She is concerned about the flu that is going around and currently has cold symptoms.

Step 1: Search the Database and Schedule an Appointment

1. Search the database for patient Barbara Watson.

2. Schedule an appointment for Barbara with Dr. Raman, using the first available morning slot today. (**Note**: If you are entering data on a weekend, or a day when there is no availability in the schedule, select an appointment day on the first prior date available. This will ensure that you can complete activities by not working in a "future date." This applies to all of the Case Studies in Chapter 11.)

   - *Appointment Type:* Follow Up
   - *Complaint:* Follow-up; Fever and flu symptoms
   - *Location:* NVFA

Step 2: Enter Payment and Check In Patient

When Barbara arrives for her appointment, view her *At-A-Glance* patient information and confirm that she is still insured with Blue Cross Blue Shield and has $20.00 copay. Before accepting Barbara's payment, create a new batch titled "WatsonCS."

1. Accept and enter Barbara's cash payment for her copay and print a receipt for her.

🖬 **Print the receipt and label it "Case Study 11-4a."**

2. Check Barbara in for her visit with Dr. Raman.

Step 3: Patient Work-Up

To begin EMR activities, edit your *Batch* operator preferences for clinical workflows with Dr. Raman as the provider.

Background Information about Barbara Watson

Barbara is a fit older adult who recently retired. She has a history of osteoporosis but no other significant health problems. She likes to travel and is planning to fly out tomorrow morning to visit her friend in Texas. She is concerned that her symptoms will worsen because of the pressurized cabin on the plane. Barbara wants something that will help relieve her symptoms before tomorrow.

1. *Transfer* Barbara to Exam Room #1.

2. Review the patient's medical history with her. (Barbara tells you that there have been no changes since the last visit.) **Hint**: Be sure to access Barbara's appointment through *Clinical Today*.

3. Next, take Barbara's vital signs and record them in her chart. Refer to **Table 11-17** for Barbara's vital sign information.

Table 11-17 Vital Signs for Barbara Watson

Height	5" 10"	Temperature	98.8°F
Weight	131	Respiratory Rate	16
Blood Pressure	130/86	Pulse Oximetry	95%
Pulse Rate	78 bpm	Pain Level	6/10

4. Because Barbara is now ready to see Dr. Raman, create a *Progress Note* for her. Select a template of "IM OV Option 4 (v4) w/A&P." Refer to **Table 11-18** while completing the progress note.

Table 11-18 Progress Note for Barbara Watson

SECTION	ITEM	ENTRY
CC/HPI	*CC/Other Complaints*	Established patient Free text the following: Stuffy nose, sore throat, sinus headache, and frequent sneezing for the past week Intermittent dry cough.
	History of Present Illness box	Free text the following: Nasal congestion, rhinorrhea, and sinus congestion that began approximately one week ago. Reports frontal head pain (6/10) and facial pressure around cheekbones and eyes. Moderate amount of clear to green drainage from nose with intermittent congestion. Denies fever. Patient reports that she has a sore throat upon awakening in the mornings but it usually subsides by midday. No history of seasonal allergies.
ROS	*Constitutional*	"N" for "fever" and "Y" for "chills" and "headache"
	Eyes	"N" for "double vision," "blurred vision," and "photophobia"
	Other eye symptoms	Watery eyes
	ENT	"Y" for "nasal congestion," "nasal discharge," and "sore throat." "N" for "earache," "tinnitus," and "dysphagia"
	Other ENT symptoms	Intermittent bilateral ear pressure but no pain
	Neck	No neck symptoms
	Respiratory	"Y" for "cough" and "N" for all other symptoms
		Leave all other sections blank.
PE	*General*	Select "awake" and "alert."
	Other general findings	Denies significant changes in weight, fatigue, or appetite
	Head/Other head findings	Normocephalic with the exception of mild pressure reported upon palpation of forehead region

(continues)

Table 11-18 (*continued*)

SECTION	ITEM	ENTRY
	Eyes	"Y" for "PERRL" and "EOMI"
	Ears	"N" for all symptoms associated with the ear
	Nose	"Y" for "rhinorrhea," "coryza," and "sinus tenderness"
	Pharynx	"N" for "oropharyngeal hemorrhage" and "Y" for "oropharyngeal exudate" and "pharyngeal inflammation"
	Other ENT findings	Ears: Bilateral canals patent without erythema, exudate, or edema. Bilateral tympanic membranes intact, pearly gray with sharp cone of light. Nose: Bilateral nares congested with rhinorrhea, mild erythema of nasal mucosa. Throat: Posterior oropharynx has a moderate discharge (clear to white). No ulcerations. Uvula midline.
	Neck	"Y" for "supple" and "N" for all other symptoms in this category
	Lymphatics	Negative lymph node exam
	Chest	Negative lung exam
	Lungs/Other lung findings	Lungs clear upon auscultation
	Heart	"Y" for "S1" and "S2." "N" for all other symptoms
Assess	*Today's Selected Diagnosis*	1. Acute URI (J06.9) 2. Acute Sinusitis (J01.90) 3. Acute pharyngitis (R/O Strep) (J02.9)
Plan	*Additional Plan Details*	1. *Rapid Streptococcus Group Identification* (Kit) 2. Flonase Nasal Suspension 50 MCG/ACT. 2 sprays daily. Click on the *Dose* icon, and select "Inhale 2 sprays in each nostril daily"; Mucinex D 60-600 mg every 6 hours for 2 days; Tylenol 500 mg 1 tab by mouth every 4–6 hours as needed for pain; Cepacol lozenges as needed for sore throat. 3. Patient Information Sheet: Acute Sinusitis (**Hint:** You will need to select "All" in the *Age* category.) 4. Obtain an OTC decongestant to help with congestion.

When you have completed Step 3: Patient Work-Up, print the patient's Chart Summary and label it "Case Study 11-4b."

Step 4: Review the *Plan* Section of the *Progress Note* and Complete the Tasks Noted in the *Plan*

Barbara's visit is now over with Dr. Raman. It is your responsibility to complete the orders as indicated in the *Plan* section of the progress note.

1. Enter the results for the *Rapid Streptococcus Group Identification* test in the *Tests* tab of the patient's progress note. The result is negative.

2. Create and print the new prescription. **Hint**: For the Flonase prescription, select "Flonase Nasal Suspension 50 MCG/AC." Click on the *Dose* icon, and select "Inhale 2 sprays in each nostril daily." Select *Duration* of 30 days and no refills.

📧 **Print and label the printed prescription "Case Study 11-4c."**

3. Provide Barbara with a copy of the Patient Information sheet(s) ordered in the *Plan* section of the progress note.

📧 **Print the Patient Information sheet and label it "Case Study 11-4d."**

Step 5: Capture the Visit and Sign the Note

Having completed all the orders as indicated in the *Progress Note*, now capture the *Visit* and sign the progress note.

1. Capture the *Visit* by entering:
   CPT® code(s): 99213 and 87430
   Source: Current Procedural Terminology © 2017 American Medical Association.
   ICD-10 code(s): J06.9, J01.90, and J02.9

2. Sign the progress note.

📧 **Print the signed progress note and label it "Case Study 11-4e."**

Step 6: Process Remittance (EOB/RA) and Transfer to Private Pay

1. Save the charges for the visit.

2. Build all claims for Barbara's visit.

3. Refer to Barbara's EOB/RA (Source Document 11-5 at the end of this case study) and process the remittance.

4. Run a journal to verify charges.

📧 **Print the Journal and label it "Case Study 11-4f."**

Step 7: Work Claims and Generate Patient Statement

1. Work the *Claims Worklist*.

2. Post all open batches.

3. Generate a statement for Barbara.

📧 **Print the statement and label it "Case Study 11-4g."**

Source Document 11-5: Explanation of Benefits/Remittance Advice

BLUE SHIELD CENGAGE

Blue Shield Cengage
P.O. Box 32245
Los Angeles, CA 90002

Date: MM/DD/YYYY (use today's date)
Payment Number: 556776
Payment Amount: $93.60

AMIR RAMAN, D.O.
Napa Valley Family Health Associates (NVFHA)
101 Vine Street
Napa, CA 94558

Account Number	Patient Name				Subscriber Number			Claim Number			
Dates of Service	Description of Service	Amount Charged	Not Covered (DENIAL)	Prov Adj Discount	Amount Allowed	Deduct/ Coins/ Copay	Paid to Provider	Adj Reason Code	Rmk Code	Patient Resp
42399626	**Watson, Barbara**									
(Appt. date used in Case Study 11-4)	99213	$112.00			$112.00	$20.00	$69.60			$42.40
(Appt. date used in Case Study 11-4)	87430	$30.00			$30.00	$6.00	$24.00			$6.00

Adj Reason Code (CP*) = copay amount

CASE STUDY 11-5: CRAIG X. SMITH

Craig is an established patient who was last seen in the office for wheezing. He is returning today for a recheck from his prior visit.

Step 1: Search the Database and Schedule an Appointment

1. Search the database for patient Craig X. Smith.

2. Schedule an appointment for Craig with Dr. Raman, using the first available morning slot today. (**Note**: If you are entering data on a weekend, or a day when there is no availability in the schedule, select an appointment day on the first prior date available. This will ensure that you can complete activities by not working in a "future date." This applies to all of the case studies in this chapter.)

    *   *Appointment Type:* Follow Up
    *   *Chief Complaint:* Follow Up
    *   *Location:* NVFA

Step 2: Enter Payment and Check In Patient

1. When Craig arrives for his appointment, view his *At-A-Glance* patient information and confirm that he is still insured with Medicaid and has no copay.

2. Check Craig in for his visit with Dr. Raman.

Step 3: Patient Work-Up

To begin EMR activities, create a new *Batch* titled "CXSmithCS," and edit your operator preferences for clinical workflows with Dr. Raman as the provider.

Background Information about Craig X. Smith

Craig was seen two weeks ago for a fever and wheezing. His mother was unable to keep his follow-up appointment last week so she is following up today. Craig's symptoms have completely resolved. Fever has subsided and wheezing is gone.

1. *Transfer* Craig to Exam Room #1.

2. Now review the patient's medical history with his mother. Mom reports that there is no change since the last visit. (**Note**: This medical history was completed in Proficiency Builders 6-2a and 6-3a. If you did not complete that Proficiency Builder, you can skip this step without entering the medical history.) **Hint**: Be sure to access through *Clinical Today.*

3. Next, take Craig's vital signs and record them in his chart. Refer to **Table 11-19** for Craig's vital sign information.

4. Because Craig is now ready to see Dr. Raman, create a *Progress Note* for him. Select the template "Pediatric OV Option 4 (v1)." Refer to **Table 11-20** while completing the progress note.

📧 **When you have completed Step 3: Patient Work-Up, print the patient's Chart Summary and label it "Case Study 11-5a."**

Table 11-19   Vital Signs for Craig X. Smith

CATEGORY	ENTRY
Height	42 inches
Weight	49 lb 8 oz
Body Mass Index	Automatically populates after entering height and weight
LMP	N/A
Blood Pressure	94/60
Pulse Rate	96 bpm
Temperature	98.6°F
Respiratory Rate	20
Pulse Oximetry	98%
Pain Level	N/A
Head Circumference	N/A
Length	N/A

Table 11-20   Progress Note for Craig X. Smith

SECTION OF OV TAB	ENTRY
CC	Free text: Follow-up from last visit.
History of Present Illness	Free text: Patient's mother states that patient is doing much better. His symptoms have completely subsided and he is once again a happy and active boy.
Past Medical/Social/Family History	Free text: No changes since last visit.
Review of Systems	Free text the following: *General:* No acute distress at this time. *Ears, Nose, and Throat:* Symptoms have dissipated from previous exam. *Respiratory:* No wheezing or coughing at this time.
Physical Examination	Free text the following: *General:* Awake, well developed. *Ears, Nose, and Throat:* Normal oropharyngeal discharge, ears and nose clear. *Respiratory:* All lung fields clear, SaO_2 reading is 98% today. *Cardiovascular:* Normal rate and peripheral pulses are normal.

SECTION OF OV TAB	ENTRY
Tests	Leave blank.
Procedure Note	Leave blank.
Assessment	Free text: No active problems today.
Plan	Free text: Mother to call if symptoms return.

Step 4: Capture the Visit and Sign the Note

Having completed all the orders as indicated in the *Progress Note*, now capture the *Visit* and sign the progress note.

1. Capture the *Visit* by entering:

    a. *CPT® code(s):* 99392

    Source: Current Procedural Terminology © 2017 American Medical Association.

    b. *ICD-10 code(s):* R06.2 (**Note:** Although the symptoms have resolved, Craig is still being seen for a follow-up of this diagnosis.)

2. Sign the progress note.

📧 **Print the signed progress note and label it "Case Study 11-5b."**

Step 5: Process Remittance (EOB/RA) and Transfer to Private Pay

1. Save the charges for the visit.

2. Build all claims for Craigs's visit.

3. Refer to Craig's EOB/RA (Source Document 11-6) and process the remittance.

4. Run a journal to verify charges.

📧 **Print the journal and label it "Case Study 11-5d."**

Step 6: Work Claims and Generate Patient Statement

1. Work the *Claims Worklist*.

2. Post all open batches.

3. Craig does not have an outstanding balance, so you do not need to generate a patient statement.

Source Document 11-6:   Explanation of Benefits/Remittance Advice

MEDICAID CENGAGE

Medicaid Cengage
P.O. Box 221352
Fresno, CA 93701

AMIR RAMAN, D.C.
Napa Valley Family Health Associates (NVFHA)
101 Vine Street
Napa, CA 94558

Date: MM/DD/YYYY (use today's date)
Payment Number: 2321442
Payment Amount: $30.00

Account Number	Patient Name					Subscriber Number			Claim Number		
Dates of Service	Description of Service	Amount Charged	Not Covered (DENIAL)	Prov Adj Discount	Amount Allowed	Deduct/ Coins/ Copay	Paid to Provider	Adj Reason Code	Rmk Code	Patient Resp
42399649	**SMITH, CRAIG X.**									
(Appt. date used in Case Study 11-5)	99392	$195.00		$165.00	$30.00	$0.00	$30.00			$0.00

CASE STUDY 11-6: TRANSFER TO COLLECTIONS

Scenario: It has now been more than 60 days since you generated statements for Julia, Delores, and Barbara. Their final payments have not been received.

1. Manually transfer each of their accounts to *Collections.*

2. Generate a collection letter appropriate to the office policy for accounts older than 60 days.

🖬 **Print a screenshot of the Collections screen listing these outstanding accounts and label it "Case Study 11-6."**

CASE STUDY 11-7: OPERATOR AUDIT LOG

Having completed the activities in this textbook and the applied learning case studies, run an operator audit log to review the entries (refer to Activity 2-4).

🖬 **To print the log, click "Print Operator Audit Log", or right-click your mouse on the log and then select Print from the shortcut menu. Label the Operator Audit Log "Case Study 11-7."**

Resources

ABC News.com. (2009, July 16). *President Obama continues questionable "You Can Keep Your Health Care" promise*. Retrieved from http://abcnews.go.com/blogs/politics/2009/07/president-obama- continues-questionable-you-can-keep-your-health-care-promise/

American Academy of Family Physicians. (2003). The HIPAA privacy rules: three key forms. Retrieved from http://www.aafp.org/fpm/2003/0200/p29.html

American Association of Professional Coders (AAPC). https://www.aapc.com/

American Medical Association (AMA). https://www.ama-assn.org

Bureau of Labor Statistics, U.S. Department of Labor. (2014). *Occupational Outlook Handbook*. Medical Records and Health Information Technicians. Retrieved from http://www.bls.gov/ooh/healthcare/medical-records-and-health-information-technicians.htm

Centers for Medicare and Medicaid Services. (n.d.). Retrieved from http://www.cms.gov/Regulations-and-Guidance/HIPAA-Administrative-Simplification/Versions5010andD0/index.html

Centers for Medicare and Medicaid Services. (n.d.). Delivery system reform, medicare payment reform. Retrieved from https://www.cms.gov/Medicare/Quality-Initiatives-Patient-Assessment-Instruments/Value-Based-Programs/MACRA-MIPS-and-APMs/MACRA-MIPS-and-APMs.html

Centers for Medicare and Medicaid Services (CMS). (n.d.). Glossary. Retrieved from the CMS website http://www.medicare.gov/glossary/f.html

Centers for Medicare and Medicaid Services. (n.d.). *Meaningful use*. Retrieved from http://www.cms.gov/Regulations-and-Guidance/Legislation/EHRIncentivePrograms/Meaningful_Use.html

CertMedAssistants.com. (n.d.). Retrieved from http://www.certmedassistant.com/

Coding classification standards. (n.d.). Retrieved from www.ahima.org

Department of Health and Human Services (DHHS), *Centers for Medicare and Medicaid Services (CMS)*. (2003, June 6). Medicare hospital manual. Retrieved from http://www.cms.gov/Regulations-and-Guidance/Guidance/Transmittals/downloads/R804HO.pdf

Department of Health and Human Services (DHHS), Centers for Medicare and Medicaid (CMS). (n.d.). Remittance advice information: an overview. Fact sheet. Retrieved from https://www.cms.gov/Outreach-and-Education/Medicare-Learning-Network-MLN/MLNProducts/Downloads/Remit-Advice-Overview-Fact-Sheet-ICN908325.pdf

Duke Clinical Research Institute. (n.d.). Beers criteria medication list. Retrieved from https://www.dcri.org/beers-criteria-medication-list/

General information: Nurse practitioner practice. (2011, April 13). Retrieved from http://www.rn.ca.gov/pdfs/regulations/npr-b-23.pdf

Health Information and Management Systems Society. (2008, August). *Real time adjudication of healthcare claims* (HIMSS Financial Systems Financial Transactions Toolkit Task Force White Paper). Retrieved from http://himss.files.cms-plus.com/HIMSSorg/content/files/Line%2027%20-%20Real%20Time%20Adjudication%20of%20Healthcare%20Claims.pdf

Health Information Technology for Economic and Clinical Health (HITECH). (2013, November 27). HITECH Act Enforcement Interim Final Rule.

HealthIT.gov. (n.d.). *EHR incentives and certification*. Retrieved from https://www.healthit.gov/providers-professionals/ehr-incentive-payment-timeline

HealthIT.gov. (n.d.). Meaningful use definitions and objectives. Retrieved from https://www.healthit.gov/providers-professionals/meaningful-use-definition-objectives

HealthIT.gov. (n.d.). What does "interoperability" mean and why is it important. Retrieved from https://www.healthit.gov/providers-professionals/faqs/what-does-interoperability-mean-and-why-it-important

HealthIT.gov. (n.d.). What is meaningful use? Retrieved from http://www.healthit.gov/policy-researchers-implementers/meaningful-use

HealthIT.gov. (2013, January). Are there penalties for providers who don't switch to electronic health records (EHR)? Retrieved from https://www.healthit.gov/providers-professionals/faqs/are-there-penalties-providers-who-don%E2%80%99t-switch-electronic-health-record

Health Resources and Services Administration (of the HHS). (n.d.). Retrieved from http://www.hrsa.gov/index.html

Indian Health Service. (n.d.). Medicare and Medicaid incentives for EPs. Retrieved from https://www.ihs.gov/meaningfuluse/incentivesoverview/incentivesep/

Institute for Healthcare Improvement. (n.d.). The five rights of medication administration. Retrieved from http://www.ihi.org/resources/pages/improvementstories/fiverightsofmedicationadministration.aspx

Institute of Medicine of the National Academies. (2003, July 31). *Key capabilities of an electronic health record system.* Retrieved from http://www.iom.edu/Reports/2003/Key-Capabilities-of-an-Electronic-Health-Record-System.aspx

Internal Revenue Service. (2016, November). Questions and Answers about Reporting Social Security Numbers to Your Health Insurance Company. Retrieved from https://www.irs.gov/affordable-care-act/questions-and-answers-about-reporting-social-security-numbers-to-your-health-insurance-company.

Kaiser Family Foundation. (2016, September). Key facts about the uninsured population. Retrieved from http://kff.org/uninsured/fact-sheet/key-facts-about-the-uninsured-population/

Lowes, Robert. (2015, August). e-Prescribing controlled substances now legal nationwide. Retrieved from http://www.medscape.com/viewarticle/850268

"Meaningful Use." *Centers for Medicare and Medicaid Services.* (2014, February 8). Retrieved from http://www .cms.gov/Regulations-and-Guidance/Legislation/EHRIncentivePrograms/Meaningful_Use.html.

Medicare.gov. (n.d.). Your medicare coverage. Is my test, item, or service covered? Retrieved from https://www.medicare.gov/coverage/cervical-vaginal-cancer-screenings.html

Menachemi, N., & Collum, T. H. (2011). Benefits and drawbacks of electronic health record systems. *Risk Management and Healthcare Policy,* 4, 47–55. Retrieved from http://www .ncbi.nlm.nih.gov/pmc/articles/PMC3270933/

National Healthcareer Association. (n.d.). *Certified electronic health records specialist (CEHRS™).* Retrieved from http://www.nhanow.com/health-record.aspx

New Health Advisor. (2016). 10 rights of medication administration. http://www.newhealthadvisor.com/10-Rights-of-Medication-Administration.html

Rowley, R. (2011). *Ambulatory vs. hospital EHRs.* Retrieved from http://www.practicefusion.com/ehrbloggers/2011/07/ambulatory-vs-hospital-ehrs.html

SNOMED Overview: Clinical Terms and SNOMED Terminology Solutions. (2008, July 3). Retrieved from /files/HIMSSorg/content/files/snomed_101overview.pdf

The American Health Quality Association, Quality Update. (2003, August 22). Retrieved from www.ahqa.org

The Fiscal Times. (2016, May). Even with obamacare, 29 million people are uninsured; here's why. Retrieved from http://www.thefiscaltimes.com/2016/05/10/Even-Obamacare-29-Million-People-Are-Uninsured-Here-s-Why

U.S. Department of Commerce, U.S. Census Bureau, American National Standards Institute. (2013). Retrieved from http://www.census.gov/geo/www/ansi/ansi.html

U.S. Department of Health and Human Services. (n.d.). *HIPAA for Individuals.* Retrieved from http://www.hhs.gov/hipaa/for-individuals/index.html.

U.S. Department of Health and Human Services. (n.d.). *Summary of the HIPAA privacy rules.* Retrieved from http://www.hhs.gov/ocr/privacy/hipaa/understanding/summary/

U.S. Department of Health and Human Services. (2013, February 11). *Construction of LMS Parameters for the Centers for Disease Control and Prevention 2000 Growth Charts,* by Katherine M. Flegal, Ph.D., Office of the Director, National Center for Health Statistics; and Tim J. Cole, Ph.D., MRC Centre of Epidemiology for Child Health, Institute of Child Health, University College London, UK. National Health Statistics Report (No. 63). Retrieved from http://www.cdc.gov/nchs/data/nhsr/nhsr063.pdf

U.S. Department of Health and Human Services, National Institutes of Health. (n.d.). *What health information is protected by the privacy rule?* Retrieved from http://privacyruleandresearch.nih.gov/pr_07.asp

U.S. Drug Enforcement Administration. (n.d.). Retrieved from www.dea.gov

U.S. Food and Drug Administration. (2013, April 1). *CFR - Code of Federal Regulations Title 21.* Retrieved from http://www.accessdata.fda.gov/scripts/cdrh/cfdocs/cfCFR/CFRSearch.cfm?fr=155.3

Glossary

A

abstract. to abstract data means to condense a record. In the context of medical records, entering data from the patient's paper chart into an EHR is abstracting. For example, the patient's problem list, current medications, allergies, personal history, and family history are entered into the electronic chart as a baseline of medical history (Ch. 1).

accession. a unique identifier (usually a number) (Ch. 7).

accounts receivable (A/R). arise when a company provides goods or services on credit; money that is owed to your group broken out by financial class (e.g., Private Pay, Medicare, Blue Shield, Commercial, etc.) and also by age (e.g., current to 30 days old, 31–60 days old, etc.) (Ch. 2 and 10).

addendum. text that is added to a progress note after it is signed (Ch. 8).

adjudicate. final determination of the issues involving settlement of an insurance claim; also known as a claim; settlement (Ch. 7 and 10).

advance beneficiary notice (ABN). a written notice (the standard government form CMS-R-131) that a patient receives from physicians, providers, or suppliers before they furnish a service or item to the patient, notifying him or her that Medicare will probably deny payment for that specific/ service or item; the reason the physician, provider, or supplier expects Medicare to deny payment; and that the patient will be personally and fully responsible for payment if Medicare denies payment. ABNs alert beneficiaries that Medicare might not reimburse for certain services even though physicians have ordered them; ABNs ask for patients' consent regarding financial liability when Medicare denies coverage; ABNs notify patients with Medicare insurance that either a service or services rendered will be the patients' financial responsibility to the physician/ facility (lab) for payment (Ch. 7).

advance directive. legal documents, such as a living will, durable power of attorney, and health care proxy, that allow people to convey their decisions about end-of-life care ahead of time (Ch. 6).

aging. the classification of accounts by the time elapsed after the date of billing or the due date (Ch. 10).

American National Standards Institute (ANSI). form types that are claims electronically transmitted to a payer (Ch. 10).

American Recovery and Reinvestment Act (ARRA). also known as the "stimulus bill" signed into law by President Obama on February 17, 2009, which authorized the HHS to establish programs to improve health care quality through the promotion of HIT (Ch. 1 and 5).

anthropometric. refers to a measurement or description of the physical dimensions and properties of the body, especially on a comparative basis; typically used on upper and lower limbs, neck, and trunk (Ch. 6).

Ask at Order Entry (AOE). represents questions you must provide to the lab when sending an order electronically or submitting a printed order (Ch. 7).

attestation period. the date that begins the 90-day reporting period of meeting the core and menu measures for meaningful use (Ch. 5).

B

batch. establishes defaults and assigns a name to a batch (group) of financial transactions you will be entering into Harris CareTracker PM and EMR. A new batch must be created to enter financial transactions (Ch. 1, 2, 3, 4, and 9).

beers. the criteria for safe medication use in older adults— for people over 65 years of age (Ch. 7).

C

cache. a space in your computer's hard drive and random access memory (RAM) where your browser saves copies of recently visited web pages (Ch. 1).

carve-out. when charges are entered for the patient, Harris CareTracker PM and EMR will automatically calculate and "carve out" the copayment amount for private pay (the amount for which the patient is responsible) (Ch. 3).

Certification Commission for Health Information Technology (CCHIT®). An independent, not-for-profit group that certifies electronic health records (EHR) and networks for health information exchange (HIE) in the United States (Ch. 1).

chief complaint. in the patient's own words, the reasons for being seen for the visit (Ch. 4).

classification systems. organize related terms into categories for easy retrieval; used for billing and reimbursement, statistical reporting, and administrative functions (Ch. 1).

clearinghouse. a private or public company that processes health information and executes electronic transactions. It provides connectivity and often serves as a "middleman" between physicians and billing entities, payers, and other health care partners for transmission and translation of claims information (primarily electronic) into the specific format required by payers (American Medical Association) (Ch. 1, 2, and 9).

clinical templates. progress notes made within the EHR; allows documentation into EHR; must be interoperable (Ch. 1).

clinical vocabularies. a standardized system of medical terminology; set of common definitions for medical terms (Ch. 1).

compendium. a summary or abstract containing the essential information in a concise but brief form (Ch. 7).

Computer Physician Order Entry (CPOE). an application used by physicians and other health care providers to enter patient care information (Ch. 1).

context. a patient is "in context" when his or her information appears in the *Name* list and *ID* box. Pulling a patient into context populates the *Name Bar* with the patient's name and Harris CareTracker PM and EMR *ID* number, allowing you to perform patient-specific tasks. When a patient is in context, many transactions can take place in the patient's account, including editing the demographic record, rescheduling an appointment, and viewing any open balances (Ch. 3).

contraindication. a symptom or condition that makes a particular treatment or procedure inadvisable (Ch. 6 and 7).

copayment. a predetermined (flat) fee that an individual pays for health care services, in addition to what the insurance covers. For example, some HMOs require a $10 "copayment" for each office visit, regardless of the type or level of services provided during the visit. Copayments are not usually specified by percentages (Ch. 4).

covered entity. covered entities can include health plans, health care clearinghouses, and health care providers (Ch. 1).

credentials. access code; in an EHR, credentials are the login information required to access the software, which is the assigned username and password (Ch. 1)

crossover. a claim that is automatically forwarded from Medicare to Medicaid (or any other insurer) after Medicare has paid its portion of a service (Ch. 10).

crosswalk. (sometimes referred to as a "link") refers to a relationship between a medical procedure (CPT®/HCPCS code) and a diagnosis (ICD code). Not all HCPCS codes are linked via a crosswalk code set to CPT (R) codes. (Ch. 9).

Current Procedural Terminology (CPT®). a nationally recognizable five-digit numeric coding system maintained by the American Medical Association (AMA) that is used to represent a service provided by health care providers in an outpatient setting (Ch. 1).

D

demographics. basic patient identifying information; defining or descriptive information on the patient (e.g., name, address, phone number(s), gender, insurance information, DOB (age), ethnicity, etc.) and defined as relating to the dynamic balance of a population, especially with regard to density and capacity for expansion or decline (Ch. 3).

designated record sets (DRS). any item, collection, or grouping of information that includes protected health information and is maintained by a covered entity (Ch. 1).

dispensable (drug). capable of being dispensed, administered, or distributed (Ch. 7).

E

edit. modifying the content of the input by inserting, deleting, or moving characters, numbers, or data (Ch. 3).

electronic health record (EHR). refers to the interoperability of electronic medical records or the ability to share medical records with other health care facilities (Ch. 1).

electronic medical record (EMR). patient records in a digital format (Ch. 1).

electronic protected health information (ePHI). protected health information that is created, received, maintained, or transmitted in electronic form (Ch. 1).

eligibility. (checks) determining whether a person is entitled to receive insurance benefits for health care services (Ch. 3).

EncoderPro. Harris CareTracker's partner for online code verification. It can be run to verify all the procedures, diagnoses, and modifiers entered for a patient. Running *EncoderPro* helps to ensure that correct coding information is entered and that claims are processed and paid quickly (Ch. 1 and 10).

encounter. an interaction with a patient on a specific date and time. Encounter types include visits, phone calls, referrals, results of a test, and more (Ch. 5 and 6).

encryption. refers to the conversion of letter or numbers to code or symbols so that its contents cannot be viewed or understood (Ch. 3).

explanation of benefits (EOB). detail of the amount of claim to the insurance company (or Medicare), any discounts for contracted rates, the percentage paid by the insurance or Medicare, denial reasons (codes), and balance due from the patient; sometimes accompanied by a benefits check (Ch. 9).

explosion codes. In Harris CareTracker PM and EMR, explosion codes can be built to include multiple CPT codes, which eliminates the need to enter each procedure individually. Creating one explosion code for this procedure reduces the amount of time it takes to enter the charge into the system. Valid modifiers for each procedure code can also be linked to them. Explosion codes are practice-specific and you can determine the descriptive name of the code set along with the CPT codes it will include (Ch. 9).

F

family history. displays part of a patient's medical history in which questions are asked in an attempt to find out whether the patient has hereditary tendencies toward particular diseases. Family history is to be present in all members' charts, including children (Ch. 6).

fee schedule. determines the amount charged for each CPT® code entered into Harris CareTracker PM and EMR (Ch. 2).

flowsheet template. a profile with selected items. Data in a patient medical record can be pulled into a flow sheet, eliminating the need for double entry. It accommodates multidisciplinary documentation requirements and is linked to progress notes, vital signs, and the results applications (Ch. 6).

formulary. defined by the Centers for Medicare and Medicaid Services as a list of prescription drugs covered by a prescription drug plan or another insurance plan offering prescription drug benefits (also called a drug list) (Ch. 7).

G

group number. typically identifies the employer (insurance) related (Ch. 3).

growth chart. provides a graphical method to compare a child's achieved growth with that of children of the same age and sex from a suitable reference population (Ch. 6).

guarantor. also known as the patient's responsible party (Ch. 3).

H

Health Information Technology for Economic and Clinical Health (HITECH) Act. created as part of the ARRA (Stimulus Bill), that was signed into law on February 17, 2009 to promote the adoption and meaningful use of health information technology (Ch.5).

Health Insurance Portability and Accountability Act (HIPAA). passed in 1996, providing new directives for protecting patient information and providing security measures as well as specific instruction for electronically transmitting patient data where required (Ch. 1).

Health Level 7 (HL7). one of the world's leading developers of health care standards for exchanging information between medical applications, to devise a common industry standard for EHR functionality that will guide the efforts of software developers; a messaging standard used to transfer data between applications (Ch. 1).

Healthcare Common Procedure Coding System (HCPCS). (called level II) managed by CMS and classifies medical equipment, injectable drugs, transportation services, and other services not classified in CPT® (Ch. 9).

history of present illness (HPI). the patient's account of related symptoms for today's visit. The HPI is generated with the use of problem-focused templates, voice dictation, or handwriting and voice recognition (Ch. 4).

hybrid conversion. using a combination of paper and electronic data (Ch. 1).

I

inactive claims. claims that are not only unpaid, but also have not had any follow-up activity on them for the last 30 days (Ch. 10).

International Classification of Diseases (ICD). the internationally recognizable three- to five-digit code set representing medical conditions or signs and symptoms (standardized categorization of diseases); diagnosis codes used in a health care setting; standards developed by the World Health Organization (WHO) (Ch. 1).

interoperable. refers to the architecture or stands that make it possible for diverse EHR systems to work compatibly in a true information network (Ch.5).

iteration. the act of repeating (Ch. 6).

K

Knowledge Base. a repository of constantly updated product troubleshooting tips and procedures (Ch. 2).

L

Logical Observation Identifiers Names and Codes (LOINC®). a universal code system for identifying laboratory and clinical observations. LOINC® enables the exchange and aggregation of electronic health data from many independent systems and includes standardized terms for all kinds of observations and measurements (Ch. 1).

lot. a collection of primary containers or units of the same size, type, and style manufactured or packed under similar conditions and handled as a single unit of trade (Ch. 5).

M

meaningful use. the set of standards defined by the Centers for Medicare and Medicaid Services (CMS) incentive programs that governs the use of electronic health records and allows eligible providers and hospitals to earn incentive payments by meeting specific criteria; a term used by the CMS to ensure that electronic medical records are being used in a meaningful way or to their fullest potential. Medicare and Medicaid payments are affected by meaningful use; using certified electronic health record technology to: improve quality, safety, efficiency, and reduce health disparities; Engage patients and family; improve care coordination, and population and public health; Maintain privacy and security of patient health information (Ch. 1 and 5).

member number. a number that is typically assigned to individual family members on the insurance policy (Ch. 3).

minimum necessary. must provide only PHI in the minimum necessary amount to accomplish the purpose for which use or disclosure is sought (Ch. 1).

mnemonics. assisting memory (Ch. 9).

modifier. a two-character code added to a CPT® or HCPCS code that is used to help in the reimbursement process. For example, a modifier is used to explain that a procedure not normally covered when billed on the same day as another is actually a separate and significant process, or that it is a rural health procedure that gets higher reimbursement. Up to four modifiers can be attached to each CPT®, although in most cases, only one or two are used (Ch. 1 and 9).

multi-resource appointment. an appointment that requires two or more resources. For example, if a patient is to be seen by a provider, but also needs an ultrasound at the same visit, the *Advanced* application allows you to book one appointment for both resources (Ch. 4).

N

National Drug Code (NDC). a code that identifies all medications recognized by the Food and Drug Administration (FDA) by vendor (manufacturer), product, and package size; number identifies a listed drug product that is assigned a unique 10-digit, 3-segment number (Ch. 1 and 10).

nomenclature. a system of terms used in a particular science (Ch. 1).

nonparticipating payer. a payer who chooses not to enter into a participating agreement to provide electronic eligibility checks for free (Ch. 3).

nonverbal communication. includes body language, gestures, eye contact, and expressions to communicate a message (Ch. 4).

notice of privacy practices (NPP). a document that describes medical practices policies and procedures regarding the use and disclosure of PHI (Ch. 1 and 3).

O

open encounter. documentation of a patient visit that took place that was never completed (Ch. 6).

open order. test or X-ray that the provider has ordered for a patient but the practice has not received the results of that test or X-ray (Ch. 2 and 6).

order. consists of a list of tests to perform on one or more patient specimens, for example, blood or urine (Ch. 7).

order set. a grouping of treatment options for a specific diagnosis or condition; predefined groupings of standard orders for a condition, disease, or procedure (Ch. 1).

override. used to either restrict an operator's access to certain applications and functionality, or it can be used to grant an operator additional privileges that may not be included in the operator's role (Ch. 2).

P

patient history. part of the medical record where you enter the patient's personal medical history, past medical history, and family medical history (Ch. 6).

practice management. referring to the "front office" of a medical practice, including functions such as the patient's record, financial, demographic, and nonmedical information (Ch. 3).

primary. first in order (Ch. 3).

private pay. refers to patients without insurance, or the balance due after insurance has adjusted the claim and paid any amount due under contract (Ch. 10).

progress note. the heart of the patient record, written by the clinician or provider, that describes the details of a patient's encounter and is sometimes referred to as a chart note. It serves as a chronological listing of the patient's overall health status. Data pertaining to the findings from the visit are entered into a progress note (Ch. 6 and 8).

protected health information (PHI). individually identifiable health information, held or maintained by a covered entity or its business associates acting for the covered entity that is transmitted or maintained in any form or medium (including the individually identifiable health information of non-U.S. citizens). This includes identifiable demographic and other information relating to the past, present, or future physical or mental health or condition of an individual, or the provision or payment of health care to an individual that is created or received by a health care provider, health plan, employer, or health care clearinghouse. For purposes of the Privacy Rule, genetic information is considered to be health information (HHS/NIH) (Ch. 1 and 3).

providers. people or organizations that furnish, bill, or are paid for health care in the normal course of business (Ch. 1).

R

Real Time Adjudication (RTA). refers to the immediate and complete adjudication of a health care claim upon receipt by the payer from a provider (Ch. 7).

recall. reminders to patients that an appointment needs to be booked. Rather than scheduling a future appointment, a recall (reminder) date is set for the appointment (Ch. 2 and 4).

receipt. receipts in Harris CareTracker PM and EMR identify a patient's previous balance, the activity of charges and payments for that date of service, and the new patient balance (Ch. 4).

remittance advice (RA). notice of payment that explains and itemizes the payment and any adjustment(s) made to a payer during the adjudication of claims (Ch. 9).

resource. can be people, places, or things. Providers are always considered a resource, but an exam room or a piece of equipment can also be considered a resource. Something that requires a schedule is considered a resource because it has specific availability with days and times it can provide certain services. If the resource does not need a set schedule then it is not considered a "resource" in Harris CareTracker PM and EMR (Ch. 2 and 4).

responsible party. the individual who is responsible for any private pay balances; the remaining amount, if any, after insurance has paid its portion; also referred to as guarantor (Ch. 3).

revenue codes. practice-specific codes that give you an alternative way of reporting financial data in Harris CareTracker PM and EMR. Revenue codes can either be linked to specific CPT® codes on your fee schedule (e.g., "New Patient Office Visits"), or can be selected during the visit or charge entry to represent a specific servicing provider, billing provider, and location combination (e.g., "Evening Clinic") (Ch. 2).

roles. determine which Harris CareTracker PM and EMR modules and applications an operator can access (Ch. 2).

routed (drug). refers to the way that a drug is introduced into the body, such as oral, enteral, mucosal, parenteral, or percutaneous (Ch. 7).

Rx Norm. a standardized nomenclature for clinical drugs and drug delivery devices produced by the National Library of Medicine (NLM). The Rx Norm code supports interoperability between EHR systems (Ch. 7).

S

scope of practice. there is no single definition of a medical assistant and his or her scope of practice. All medical assistants must work under the direction of a physician or licensed health care professional. The employer is ultimately responsible and accountable for actions of the medical assistant. A medical assistant is not allowed to independently assess or triage patients, make medical evaluations, independently refill prescriptions, or give out drug samples without the approval of the physician (Ch. 1).

scrub. to verify technical and coding accuracy before claims are filed by identifying potential problems that will cause claim rejection or reduction in payment. The claim scrubber provides a comprehensive set of coding and technical edits. Each individual edit may be enabled or disabled completely for a specific claim type or for an individual payer (Ch. 1 and 9).

secondary. second in order (Ch. 3).

sensitive information. information regarding the patient's STD and HIV history as well as alcohol and drug history (Ch. 6).

sequelae. an after-effect of disease, condition, or injury; a secondary result (Ch. 1).

SIG. an abbreviation for *signa* in Latin (meaning "label" or "sign"). SIG codes are specific dosage instructions that are given when prescribing medications (Ch. 6 and 7).

stat. refers to "immediately" or "without delay" (Ch. 7).

subscriber. an individual who is a member of a benefits plan. For example, in the case of family coverage, one adult is ordinarily the subscriber. A spouse and children would ordinarily be dependents (Ch. 3).

subscriber number. refers to the insurance policy number (Ch. 3).

Surescripts®. the largest network of its kind and provides electronic connectivity between pharmacies (Ch. 6).

sustainability. the responsible use of resources (Ch. 1).

Systematized Nomenclature of Medicine, Clinical Terms (SNOMED-CT®). a comprehensive clinical terminology covering diseases, clinical findings, and procedures that allows for a consistent way of indexing, storing, retrieving, and aggregating clinical data across specialties and sites of care (Ch. 1).

T

"Tall Man" lettering. medication names that have mixed case lettering in the description name, for example, NEXium. This is to comply with the patient safety initiative endorsed by the Food and Drug Administration (FDA) and Institute for Safe Medication Practices (ISMP), which helps reduce errors between medication names that either look or sound alike (Ch. 7).

task classes. determine what types of appointments can be seen at what times; are the building blocks for a resource's schedule (Ch. 2).

TeleVox®. an automated appointment reminder and confirmation system that can be used to notify patients of upcoming appointments (Ch. 4).

tertiary. third in order (Ch. 3).

titer. (having labs drawn) determines how much antibody is present in the patient's blood to fight a specific antigen (disease-causing agent) (Ch. 8).

ToDo. Harris CareTracker's internal messaging system (Ch. 6).

total conversion. when all paper records are converted to electronic records at once (Ch. 1).

transfer. the status of a patient when he or she has been taken to an exam room (Ch. 6).

treatment, payment, and operations (TPO). conditions under which protected health information can be released without consent from the patient (Ch. 1).

U

Unified Medical Language System (UMLS®). another clinical standard, which is a set of files and software that brings together many health and biomedical vocabularies and standards to enable interoperability between computer systems; that is, a thesaurus database of medical terminology (Ch. 1).

unknown status. results when the patient's primary insurance is a non-participating (non-par) payer (Ch. 3).

unpaid claims. claims that have been submitted to an insurance company but have not been paid (Ch. 10).

unsigned note. a progress note that was never signed (Ch. 6).

V

variance. difference between the allowed and payment amounts; the difference between the actual amount of money you received from the insurance company and the negotiated rate the insurance is responsible for paying (Ch. 9).

verbal communication. the use of language or the actual words spoken (Ch. 4).

W

workflow. how tasks are performed throughout the office (usually in a specific order); for example, the patient is checked in, insurance cards are scanned, the patient is taken to the exam room, vital signs are taken/recorded, and so on (Ch. 1 and 3).

Index